Pediatric
Sonography

Pediatric Sonography

Editor

Marilyn J. Siegel, M.D.

Professor of Radiology
Associate Professor of Pediatrics
Department of Radiology
The Edward Mallinckrodt Institute of Radiology
Washington University Medical Center
St. Louis, Missouri

Raven Press ☙ New York

Raven Press, 1185 Avenue of the Americas, New York, New York 10036

Made in the United States of America

Library of Congress Cataloging-in-Publication Data

Pediatric sonography / editor, Marilyn J. Siegel.
    p.   cm.
   Includes bibliographical references.
   Includes index.
   ISBN 0-88167-680-2
   1. Children—Diseases—Diagnosis.   2. Diagnosis, Ultrasonic.
I. Siegel, Marilyn J.
   [DNLM: 1. Ultrasonic Diagnosis—in infancy & childhood.
2. Ultrasonic Diagnosis—methods.   WS 141 P3682]
RJ51.U45P43   1991
618.92′007543—dc20
DNLM/DLC
for Library of Congress   90-8840
                                         CIP

The material contained in this volume was submitted as previously unpublished material, except in the instances in which some of the illustrative material was derived.

Great care has been taken to maintain the accuracy of the information contained in the volume. However, neither Raven Press nor the editor can be held responsible for errors or for any consequences arising from the use of the information contained herein.

9 8 7 6 5 4 3 2 1

To my husband, Barry,
who taught me the art of writing
and to my parents,
for their love and encouragement.

Preface

In the early 1940s, the initial use of sonography in medical diagnosis was to image the brain. Since that time, major technical advancements have improved image quality, with the result that sonography has become accepted as an important imaging technique for nearly every part of the body. In fact, it is the screening procedure of choice in evaluating intracranial and abdominal diseases, and it is recognized as a useful tool in guiding aspiration and biopsy.

The information provided by sonography has redirected the imaging evaluation of some disease processes in children. Most notably, sonography has replaced excretory urography for diagnosing or excluding suspected renal and adrenal masses and hydronephrosis. Hepatic scintigraphy for diagnosing masses and staging malignancies also has been replaced as has oral cholecystography.

This volume provides a comprehensive text on the applications of sonography in the head and extracranial regions of the body. It is intended primarily for use by radiologists in training and in clinical practice. Ultrasound technologists and pediatricians can also benefit from the information on the relative indications and value of sonography in various parts of the body.

The initial chapter presents an overview of the various technologies available for sonography and serves as a reference for those not entirely familiar with the subject. In the succeeding chapters, sonographic techniques, basic anatomy, and findings in a variety of pathologic conditions are described and illustrated for each region of the body. Both technical and interpretative errors that can occur with sonography are stressed. The final chapter describes the role of sonography in interventional procedures. To keep sonography in proper perspective, discussions of the relative values of sonography and other imaging studies for a variety of clinical problems are included within individual chapters.

The experience in this book and the suggested uses of sonography reflect the experience of the diagnostic radiology staff at the Mallinckrodt Institute. Each member has established an interest and expertise in a specific area. We recognize that our recommendations for the optimal use of sonography may need to be varied depending on personal expertise and available equipment and that alternative approaches to evaluating some clinical problems are possible. We are also aware that sonography is a rapidly changing field, and, as instrumentation continues to improve and new techniques develop, the clinical applications of sonography will continue to evolve.

Marilyn J. Siegel, M.D.

Acknowledgments

I wish to thank my colleagues at the Edward Mallinckrodt Institute of Radiology who kindly contributed chapters in their areas of expertise. Special thanks are extended to Janet Hurt and Deborah Reiter for their tireless cooperation in performing the studies illustrated in this book. I would also like to acknowledge Deborah Larson and Jane Woods for typing the manuscripts and verifying the references, and Thomas Murry, Sue Alexander, and Vicki Friedman for preparing the illustrative material.

Finally, a note of gratitude to Mary Rogers and Kathy Cianci of Raven Press for their encouragement and advice throughout this entire project.

Contents

Contributors

Thomas E. Herman, M.D.
Assistant Professor of Radiology

Marshall E. Hicks, M.D.
Assistant Professor of Radiology

William H. McAlister, M.D.
Professor of Radiology and Pediatrics

William D. Middleton, M.D.
Associate Professor of Radiology

Gary D. Shackelford, M.D.
Professor of Radiology and Pediatrics

Marilyn J. Siegel, M.D.
*Professor of Radiology and
Associate Professor of Pediatrics*

*The Edward Mallinckrodt Institute of Radiology
Washington University School of Medicine
510 South Kingshighway Boulevard
St. Louis, Missouri 63110*

1

Physical Principles and Instrumentation

William D. Middleton

Ultrasonography has been an attractive means of displaying normal and abnormal anatomy for many years. In radiology, it has been used most extensively in imaging abdominal and pelvic abnormalities in adults and in evaluating maternal and fetal disorders in pregnancy. However, in the early and mid-1980s it became increasingly evident that ultrasonography could be used just as effectively in the pediatric patient.

There are many reasons why sonography is an appealing imaging technique for the pediatric age group, perhaps the most compelling of which is its lack of ionizing radiation. One important goal of the pediatric radiologist is to obtain diagnostic information with as little radiation exposure to the child as possible. Sonography often can provide the information necessary to determine clinical management without having to resort to radiographic methods, and therefore is often the method of choice for evaluating specific clinical problems.

A second appealing aspect of sonography is the real-time nature of the examination. This makes it possible to evaluate rapidly moving structures such as the heart. It also makes it possible to obtain diagnostic examinations in patients who cannot suspend respiration, do not cooperate, or cry—all common problems in the pediatric patient.

The third major advantage of sonography is its multiplanar imaging capability. With modern real-time equipment, sonography provides unparalleled flexibility in the choice of imaging planes and ease of altering the imaging plane. This is often extremely helpful in determining the origin of pathologic masses and in analyzing spatial relationships among various structures.

Another advantage of sonography in the pediatric age group relates to patient size. For a given sonographic unit and a given type of transducer, the higher the transmitted frequency the better the image resolution, but the poorer the penetration. These conflicting characteristics of transducer frequency force a

compromise in adults, where lower frequencies must be used to obtain adequate depth of penetration at the expense of image resolution. In small children and infants, however, the required penetration depth is significantly less than in adults so that higher frequency, higher resolution transducers can be used routinely. In addition, the lack of significant body wall and intraabdominal fat in most small children is a great advantage since fat generally causes a degraded ultrasound image.

The examination's portability is another characteristic that separates sonography from other cross-sectional examinations (computerized tomography [CT] and magnetic resonance imaging [MRI]). This is obviously important in evaluating patients who cannot be transported to the radiology department.

Finally, the relatively lesser expense of sonography makes it a more appropriate initial imaging examination than CT or MRI for many clinical problems. In addition, the issue of cost makes ultrasonography attractive in situations where multiple follow-up examinations are necessary or when screening large patient populations is desired.

All of these factors have made ultrasonography an extremely valuable tool for investigating pediatric disorders. Therefore, any radiologist dealing with pediatric patients must have a basic understanding of sonographic examination instrumentation.

ACOUSTICS

The term ultrasound refers to sound above the audible range (i.e., greater than 20 KHz) (1,2). Diagnostic sonography generally operates at frequencies of 1 to 20 MHz. The ultrasonic pulses used for diagnostic sonography are generated by ceramic crystal elements housed within the ultrasound transducer. These ceramic crystals deform when electric voltage is applied across them. Short voltage pulses will cause the crystal to vibrate and create a pulse of sound that can be transmitted into the body. The frequency of this ultrasonic pulse is equal to the resonant frequency of the crystal element, which in turn is dependent on the thickness of the crystal. When this ultrasonic pulse returns to the transducer, it distorts the crystal element and generates an electric pulse which can then be used to generate image information. Because the crystal element converts electric energy to sound energy and vice versa, it is referred to as a piezoelectric crystal (i.e., ''pressure electric'').

After the ultrasonic pulse is generated and transmitted into the body, it can be reflected, refracted, scattered, and absorbed. Reflection occurs whenever the ultrasonic pulse encounters an interface between tissues that have different acoustic impedances. Acoustic impedance is equal to the tissue density times the speed of sound propagation in the tissue. The amount of sound that is reflected at an interface depends on the difference in acoustic impedance between the tissues and the angle of insonation of the sound beam. The greater the acoustic impedance mismatch, the more sound will be reflected.

Refraction refers to a change in sound direction as it passes from one tissue into another. Refraction occurs when sound encounters an oblique interface between two tissues that transmit sound at different speeds. Because the sound frequency remains constant, the sound wavelength must change to accommodate the difference between the speed of sound in the two tissues. It is this change in wavelength that causes the pulse to be redirected as it passes through the interface.

When the ultrasonic pulse encounters an acoustic interface that is not smooth, the sound is redirected in many different directions. This is referred to as scattering. Scattering also occurs to some degree within a single tissue due to the heterogeneity of biological tissues.

Absorption refers to the loss of sound energy due to conversion to thermal energy. Absorption is less in fluids than in soft tissues and is less in soft tissues than in bone.

The combined effects of reflection, scattering, and absorption result in decreasing intensity of the ultrasonic pulse as it passes through tissues. This decrease in intensity is referred to as sound beam attenuation. Because of attenuation, an acoustic interface in the deeper tissues will produce a weaker reflection than will an identical interface in the superficial tissues. To compensate for this, echoes returning from the deeper portions of the image are electronically amplified. This is referred to as distance gain compensation (DGC) or time gain compensation (TGC), and is displayed graphically as a curve which indicates the amount of echo amplification for various depths in the image. The TGC curve can be seen displayed to the right of the image on Figures 1 through 4.

ULTRASOUND IMAGING TECHNIQUES

The concept of using sound waves to analyze internal structures in the human body has been exploited for many years. Original devices transmitted sound into the body and displayed the reflections arising from tissue interfaces in graphic form, with time on the horizontal axis and echo amplitude on the vertical axis. This was referred to as the A (amplitude) mode. Another means of showing the information is to display the echo as a dot, with higher amplitude echoes appearing as brighter dots. This is referred to as the B (brightness) mode. In both A and B-mode sonography, the distance of the reflector from the transducer can be worked out based on the time taken for sound to travel to the reflector and back along with the knowledge that the speed of sound in soft tissues is normally assumed to be 1,540 meters per sec.

Early two-dimensional units attached B-mode transducers to an articulated arm that was capable of determining the exact location and orientation of the transducer in space. This provided the ability to locate the origin of the returning echoes in two dimensions. Then, by sweeping the transducer across the patient's body, a series of B-mode lines of information could be added together to generate a two-dimensional image. The field of view was variable depending on the organ of interest. However, one of the major advantages of static B-mode imaging was its capability to produce images showing large organs, such as the liver or the gravid uterus in one cross-sectional image. The major disadvantage of static B-mode imaging was its lack of real-time capabilities. Because of this limitation, static, articulated arm, B-mode devices have now been almost completely replaced by real-time units.

Modern real-time units use a variety of transducer designs to generate gray-scale ultrasound images. Perhaps the simplest design is the mechanical sector transducer (Fig. 1). Such transducers use a single, large crystal element to generate the ultrasound pulses and to listen to the returning echoes. Beam steering is accomplished by mechanical motion of the crystal element itself (either oscillating or rotating) or by reflection of the sound pulse off an oscillating acoustic mirror. Beam focusing is performed by using differently shaped crystal elements or by attaching an acoustic lens to the transducer. Unfortunately, for a given mechanical sector transducer, the level of focus is not variable. To vary the focal distance, one must switch to a different transducer.

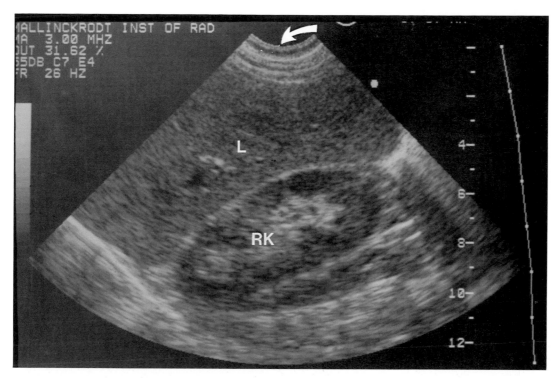

FIG. 1. Longitudinal view of the right kidney (*RK*) and liver (*L*) obtained with 3 MHz mechanical sector transducer. The superficial portion of the image is concave and curvilinear (*arrow*) because the single element transducer steers the beam by mechanically rotating the transducer element. Because the focal zone is fixed, no focal zone indicator is seen adjacent to the scale on the right aspect of the image.

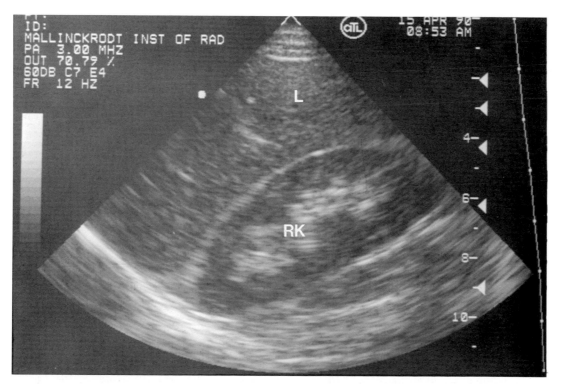

FIG. 2. Longitudinal view of the right kidney (*RK*) and liver (*L*) obtained with a 3 MHz electronic phased array transducer. The superficial aspect of the image comes to a point because the beam is steered electronically, not mechanically. The multiple focal zone indicators to the right of the image reflect the ability of phased array transducers to focus at variable and multiple depths.

The electronic phased array sector transducer is the other major transducer design (Fig. 2). These transducers use an array of multiple small crystal elements that are stacked adjacent to each other. Each line of sight in the sonographic image is produced by the composite sound pulse generated by all of these multiple crystal elements. This composite pulse can be steered and focused by electronically altering the activation sequence of the individual crystal elements. Because the focusing is created electronically, the focal zone can be controlled electronically. Therefore a single transducer can be focused at different depths, de-pending on the location of the structure of interest. This represents a significant practical advantage over mechanical sector transducers. Another unique capability of phased array sector transducers is the ability to focus at multiple levels simultaneously. Although this is accomplished at the expense of a decreased frame rate, it can still be a very useful feature in many situations.

Multi-element electronic phased arrays can also be arranged in a linear format to produce a rectangular-shaped image (Fig. 3). The sound beam in these linear arrays is always oriented perpendicular to the trans-

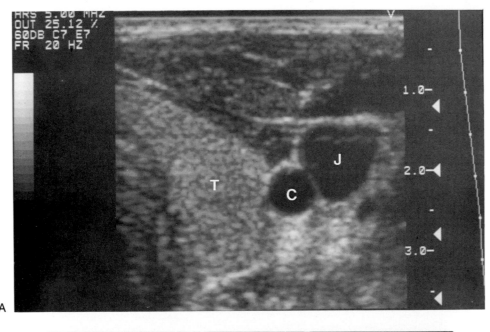

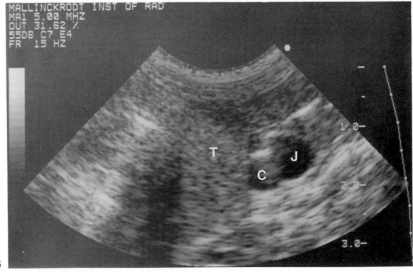

FIG. 3. Transverse scan of the thyroid (*T*), common carotid (*C*), and jugular vein (*J*) obtained with a 5 MHz linear array transducer **(A)** and a 5 MHz mechanical sector transducer **(B)**. As with the phased array sector transducer shown in Fig. 2, the linear array transducer can focus at variable levels. It also provides excellent resolution in the superficial field of view. The mechanical sector transducer provides much poorer resolution overall, particularly in the superficial field of view.

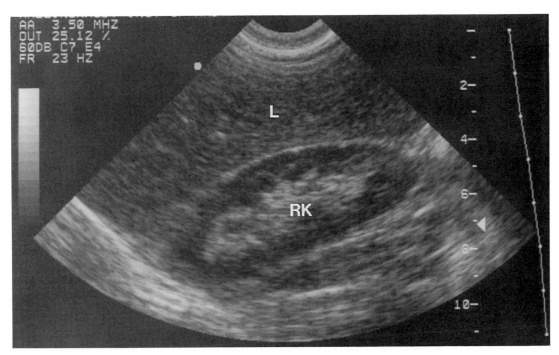

FIG. 4. Longitudinal view of the right kidney (*RK*) and liver (*L*) obtained with a 3.5 MHz annular array. Because the beam is steered mechanically, the format of the annular array is similar to that of a mechanical sector transducer, with the superficial field of view being concave and curvilinear. However, electronic focusing allows the focal zone to be varied, therefore a focal zone indicator must be shown to the right of the image.

ducer face. It is steered by activating a limited number of adjacent elements and sequentially shifting the active elements down the length of the transducer. Focusing is accomplished in a manner similar to phased array sector transducers. The major advantage of linear phased array transducers is their high resolution in the superficial field of view adjacent to the transducer. The major disadvantage is their size, which sometimes limits their use in situations where acoustic access to the organ of interest is limited, such as in intercostal scanning. This limitation can be decreased somewhat by arranging the crystal elements of the linear array in a convex orientation. This decreases the size of the transducer while maintaining the superb near-field resolution of conventional linear arrays.

The final group of transducers in current widespread use are the annular phased array transducers (Fig. 4). These transducers are composed of multiple, ring-shaped, concentrically located annular crystal elements. With such a design, the beam can be electronically focused both in the plane of the image and perpendicular to the plane of the image. Theoretically, this allows for detection of smaller structures such as cysts and stones. Steering of the annular array is accomplished mechanically as with mechanical sector transducers.

As mentioned earlier, lower frequency transducers must be utilized in larger patients in order to obtain the sound penetration necessary to image deep body structures. Recently, transducers have been designed to be placed within various body lumens in order to position the transducer in closer proximity to the organ of interest. The two most common intraluminal probes are the transrectal and transvaginal transducers (Fig. 5). These are currently in widespread use in adult patients to image the prostate and female pelvic organs. Because the transducer itself is positioned immediately adjacent to the organ of interest, higher frequencies can be used and thus higher resolution images can be obtained. In addition, the ability to image the organs without having to transmit the sound beam through the abdominal wall fat avoids the image-degrading properties of body wall fat. The overall result is images of much higher quality compared with standard transabdominal images.

Even more recently, small transducers have been added to flexible endoscopes in order to evaluate both upper and lower gastrointestinal pathology. In the upper gastrointestinal tract these transducers can aid in evaluating esophageal and periesophageal abnormalities, as well as gastric wall lesions and perigastric organs. In the lower gastrointestinal tract, these en-

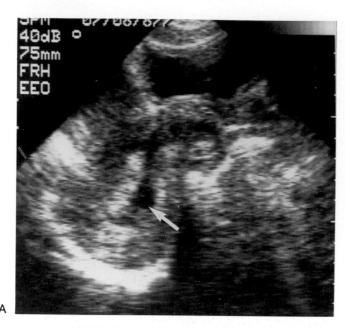

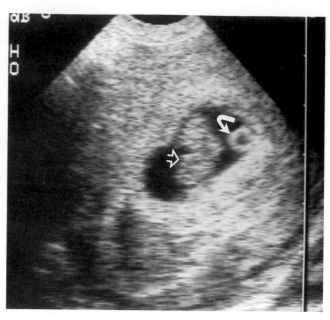

FIG. 5. Early intrauterine pregnancy demonstrated with a 3.5 MHz mechanical sector transducer from a transabdominal approach **(A)** and a 7.5 MHz mechanical sector transvaginal approach **(B)**. **A:** A nonspecific intrauterine fluid collection is seen on the transabdominal scan (*arrow*). **B:** The improved resolution on the transvaginal scan demonstrates a definite intrauterine pregnancy with a fetal pole (*open arrow*) and a yolk sac (*curved arrow*).

doscopic probes have been used to evaluate colonic carcinoma and other mucosal and submucosal lesions.

The most recent addition to the intraluminal sonographic armamentarium is the intraarterial probe. Investigations are currently underway to determine its ability to evaluate a variety of arterial wall abnormalities. Other applications will undoubtedly be determined in the future.

DOPPLER SONOGRAPHY

The previous discussion focuses on the various transducer designs used to produce real-time, two-dimensional images. All of these designs rely ultimately on analysis of the amplitude of the returning echo to generate gray-scale information. However, analysis of the frequency of the returning echo can also yield important information. The Doppler principle as it relates to ultrasound imaging states that sound reflecting off a moving target will undergo a change in frequency. The difference between the transmitted and received frequency is called the Doppler frequency shift. The magnitude of the Doppler frequency shift is determined by the equation:

$$Fd = 2 \times Ft \times (V/c) \times \cos \theta,$$

where Fd = Doppler frequency shift, Ft = transmitted frequency, V = speed of moving target (blood flow velocity), c = speed of sound in soft tissue, and θ =

angle between direction of blood flow and sound beam (3,4).

A number of transducer designs have evolved to take advantage of the Doppler principle. The earliest and simplest was the continuous wave Doppler probe, which consisted of one crystal that continuously transmitted sound and a second crystal that continuously received the returning echoes. Continuous wave Doppler was, and continues to be, an extremely sensitive method of detecting blood flow. However, it cannot determine the exact source of the returning Doppler signal since motion at any depth along the sound beam will produce a signal.

Pulsed Doppler, as its name implies, transmits a short pulse of sound and then listens for the returning echo. Because the speed of sound is constant, the delay in time between transmission and reception is proportional to distance. By varying the delay between transmission and reception, it is possible to select defined points along the Doppler beam from which the signal arises. With this capability, one can then use standard gray-scale ultrasonography as a road map to visualize the vessels of interest, and to position the Doppler sample volume at various points within the vessel. This combination of gray-scale sonography with pulsed Doppler has been labeled duplex Doppler (Fig. 6).

Duplex Doppler has been and continues to be a very powerful tool for evaluating blood flow. Its major dis-

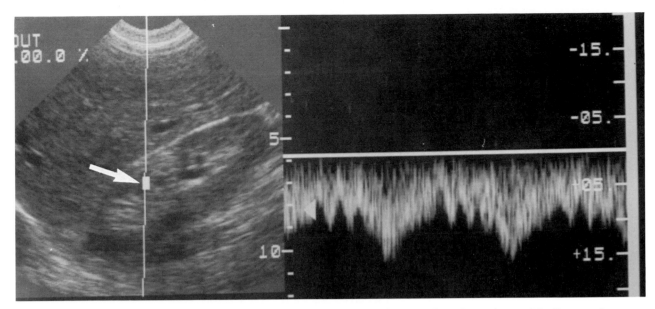

FIG. 6. Duplex Doppler scan of the right kidney showing the sample volume (*arrow*) in the renal sinus and a corresponding renal venous waveform to the right of the image.

advantage is its inability to perform Doppler interrogation of more than one point within a vessel at a time. Therefore evaluation of an entire vessel can be quite time consuming, and requires meticulous technique and a great deal of persistence. In addition, analysis of vessels in small organs (such as the testis) can be extremely difficult since the vessels are too small to be resolved with gray-scale imaging.

Color Doppler ultrasonography represents a major advance over duplex Doppler because it is sensitive to Doppler signals throughout the field of view. It can provide a real-time image of tissue morphology in gray scale while simultaneously displaying blood flow in color, thereby eliminating the major disadvantages of duplex Doppler. Color Doppler ultrasonography operates by analyzing the returning echoes for amplitude, frequency, and phase information. Moving targets produce a phase shift and will be assigned a color based on the direction of phase shift (direction of blood flow

toward or away from the transducer). The shade of color will depend on the mean Doppler frequency shift arising from the pixel. High-frequency shifts are assigned a lighter color while lower frequency shifts are assigned a darker color. Stationary objects produce no phase shift and, therefore, are assigned a gray-scale value based on echo amplitude as in conventional gray-scale imaging.

REFERENCES

1. Curry TS, Dowdey JE, Murry RC. *Christensen's introduction to the physics of diagnostic radiology*, 3rd ed. Philadelphia: Lea & Febiger, 1984;351–400.
2. Kremkau FW. *Diagnostic ultrasound: physical principles and exercise*, 1st ed. New York: Grune & Stratton, 1980.
3. Taylor KJW, Holland S. Doppler US. Part I: basic principles, instrumentation, and pitfalls. *Radiology* 1990;174:297–307.
4. Burns PN. The physical principles of Doppler and spectral analysis. *J Clin Ultrasound* 1987;15:567–590.

2

Brain

Marilyn J. Siegel

Attempts at sonographic imaging of the neonatal head began in the 1950s when investigators reported their experience with A-mode scanning for detecting midline shift and localizing brain tumors. This early work was followed by attempts at B-mode scanning and later by waterbath head scanning, both of which were not much more successful because of the poor resolution and crude quality of the scans related to the use of the compound sector scanning technique and low-frequency transducers. Significant improvements in image quality and resolution were seen in the 1980s with the advent of high-resolution, real-time imaging, coupled with the use of the anterior fontanelle as an acoustic window. With those advances, sonography became the primary imaging study in the evaluation of the neonatal brain (99,106).

Sonography has proven to be extremely valuable in identifying normal and abnormal intracranial anatomy. Because of its portability and ease of performance, particularly in unstable premature infants, it has replaced computerized tomography (CT) as the initial examination of choice in the identification of hydrocephalus, periventricular, intraventricular, and intracerebral hemorrhages, and congenital anomalies.

This chapter will review the indications for sonography in evaluating the neonatal head and compare its accuracy with that of computerized tomography. A discussion of scanning techniques and normal sonographic anatomy also will be presented.

TECHNIQUE

A 5-MHz transducer is generally adequate for the evaluation of most neonatal brains. Occasionally a lower frequency transducer is needed to ensure adequate penetration, especially in larger infants or older infants with closing fontanelles. Higher frequency transducers, such as 7.5- or 10-MHz transducers, are helpful in evaluating superficial structures, such as the extracerebral spaces or cortex.

The anterior fontanelle is available as an acoustic window through the first year of life. Closure begins at about 9 months and is usually complete at about 15 months of age. The real-time examination begins with the transducer positioned on the anterior fontanelle to produce images in the coronal plane. Then the transducer is rotated 90° on the fontanelle to obtain images in a sagittal plane (109,122) (Fig. 1). Standardized sections (see below) are obtained and photographed with a hard copy camera. Occasionally transcranial scanning through a coronal suture or the squamosal portion of the temporal bone is useful in identifying extracerebral fluid collections not visualized with the transfontanelle approach, and in assessing the vascular structures of the circle of Willis (85). Scanning through the posterior fontanelle may be helpful to delineate abnormalities of the posterior fossa associated with spinal dysraphism, such as Arnold-Chiari or Dandy-Walker malformations.

CROSS-SECTIONAL SONOGRAPHIC ANATOMY

Coronal Sections

The ventricular system and some cerebrospinal fluid (CSF) spaces serve as the reference standard for identifying intracranial anatomy and selecting scan planes. Coronal scans usually are obtained through five levels of the ventricles: (a) frontal horns anterior to the foramen of Monro; (b) foramen of Monro; (c) posterior aspect of the third ventricle through the thalami; (d) quadrigeminal cistern, and (e) trigones of the lateral ventricles (79,106,122). A sixth routine image is obtained through the periventricular white matter posterior to the trigones of the lateral ventricles.

The most coronal scan is anterior to the third ventricle through the frontal horns, which appear as an-

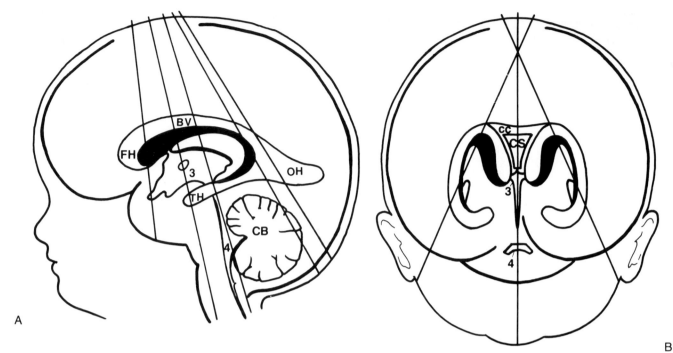

A

B

FIG. 1. Schematic representations of standard scanning planes. **A:** Coronal and **B:** sagittal planes. *FH,* frontal horns; *BV,* body of ventricle; *OH,* occipital horn; *TH,* temporal horn; *CB,* cerebellum; *3,* third ventricle; *4,* fourth ventricle; *CC,* corpus callosum; *CS,* cavum septi pellucidi. (Modified from ref. 109).

echoic, paramedian fluid-filled spaces with a crescentic configuration (Fig. 2). The hypoechoic corpus callosum forms the roof of the frontal horns; the anechoic cavum septi pellucidi forms the medial wall; and the echogenic head of the caudate nucleus forms the lateral wall. Superior to the corpus callosum is the hy-

perechoic pericallosal sulcus that separates the corpus callosum from the hypoechoic cingulate gyrus. Immediately lateral and inferior to the caudate nucleus are the putamen and globus pallidus. Pulsations from the anterior and middle cerebral arteries may be observed in the interhemispheric and sylvian fissures, re-

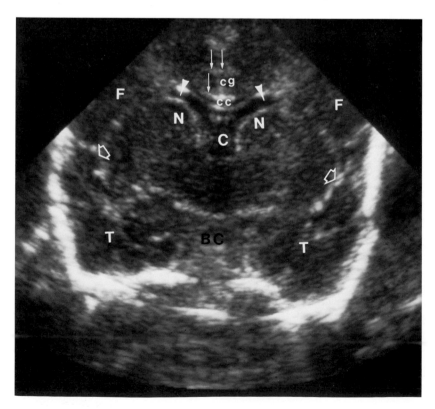

FIG. 2. Coronal scan through the frontal horn. At this level, the frontal horns appear as crescentic fluid-filled spaces (*arrowheads*) separated by the cavum septi pellucidi (*C*). The heads of the caudate nuclei (*N*) lie adjacent to the lateral walls of the ventricles. The hypoechoic corpus callosum (*CC*) forms the roof of the cavum and the lateral ventricles. Paralleling the corpus callosum is the hypoechoic cingulate gyrus (*cg*) surrounded by the echogenic callosal sulcus (single *white arrow*) and cingulate sulcus (two *small white arrows*). Also note the echogenic sylvian fissure (*open arrows*) between the frontal (*F*) and temporal (*T*) lobes. *BC,* basilar cistern.

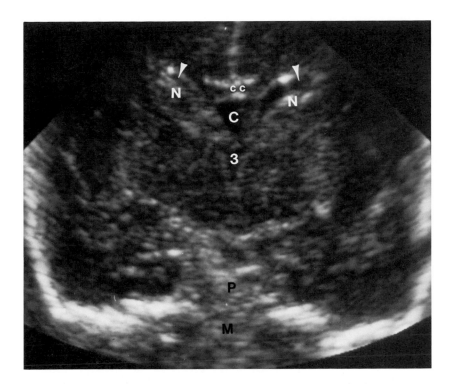

FIG. 3. Coronal scan through foramen of Monro. The lateral (*arrowheads*) and third (*3*) ventricles are identified as fluid-filled structures, with the bodies of the caudate nuclei (*N*) lying adjacent to the lateral ventricles. Between the lateral ventricles and superior to the third ventricle is the triangular cavum septi pellucidi (*C*). The corpus callosum (*CC*) is again noted superior to the cavum and lateral ventricles. *P,* pons; *M,* medulla oblongata.

spectively (144). The relatively hypoechoic frontal and temporal lobes also are imaged at this level.

The next most posterior scan is through the foramen of Monro (Fig. 3). At this level, the lateral and third ventricles communicate through the foramen of Monro. The third ventricle usually is not visualized when normal in size because its transverse diameter is so small. When dilated, however, it can be visualized as an anechoic structure beneath the bodies of the lateral ventricles. The anechoic cavum septi pellucidi is again seen between the lateral ventricles. The lateral recesses of the lateral ventricles are bordered by the echogenic body of the caudate nucleus. Pulsations from the pericallosal artery in the interhemispheric fissure and middle cerebral artery in the sylvian fissure may be noted. The echogenic brainstem, containing pons and medulla, also is easily visualized in this plane.

On a scan at the level of the posterior aspect of the third ventricle, the bodies of the lateral ventricles are bordered by the body of the caudate nucleus laterally and thalami inferiorly (Fig. 4). The thalami are separated from each other by the third ventricle, although

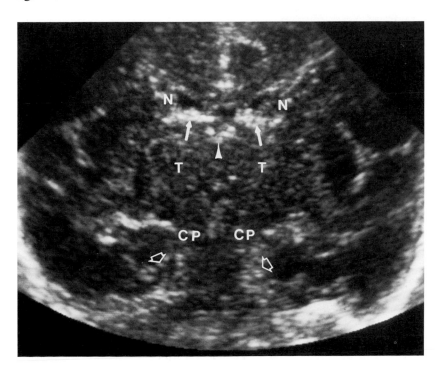

FIG. 4. Coronal scan through posterior aspect of third ventricle. At this level, the bodies of the lateral ventricles are imaged with the bodies of the caudate nuclei (*N*) lying at the lateral aspects of the ventricles and the thalami (*T*) lying inferiorly. The three central echogenic areas represent the choroid plexus in the floor of the lateral ventricle (*arrows*) and in the roof of the third ventricle (*arrowhead*). The hypoechoic cerebral peduncles (*CP*) and the echogenic tentorium (*open arrow*) are also seen.

the latter usually is not imaged in the absence of hydrocephalus. In this section, the body of the corpus callosum forms the roof of the bodies of the lateral ventricles. The choroid plexus lies in the groove between the thalamus and lateral ventricle and in the roof of the third ventricle. Inferior to the thalami are the hypoechoic cerebral peduncles. These are separated from the hypoechoic cerebellar hemispheres by the highly echogenic tentorium. A portion of the anechoic cisterna magna may be seen inferior to the vermis.

On a slightly more posterior scan, the highly echogenic quadrigeminal cistern is visualized lying superior to the echogenic cerebellar tentorium (Fig. 5). The cause of the hyperechogenicity of this fluid-filled space is unknown, but it has been postulated that it may be secondary to the presence of arachnoid septations or due to pulsations of large vessels within the cistern (47). The bodies of the lateral ventricles, bordered by the caudate nucleus and thalamus, are seen superiorly and the temporal horns are seen inferiorly. The echogenic midline structure in the posterior fossa is the cerebellar vermis. Posterior and inferior to the vermis is the cisterna magna. On this section, pulsations can be detected in the middle cerebral and pericallosal arteries.

The most posterior coronal scan is through the trigones of the ventricles, which often appear asymmetrical in size (Fig. 6A). At this level, the lateral ventricles diverge laterally and are separated superiorly by the echogenic splenium of the corpus callosum. Within the trigones is the highly echogenic glomus of the choroid plexus. Lateral to both trigones are normal areas of increased periventricular echogenicity (48). The degree of echogenicity of the normal periventricular halo is less than that of the choroid plexus. Inferior to the ventricles and superior to the cerebellum is the echogenic V-shaped tentorium.

Scans obtained posterior and cephalad to the trigones are particularly useful if there is a suspicion of parenchymal abnormality (Fig. 6B). At this level there are no vessels or ventricles; instead, the superficial sulci and gyri and interhemispheric fissures are seen. The number of gyri and sulci that can be seen increase directly as a function of age. The white matter cephalad to the trigones of the lateral ventricles is visible as echogenic areas on either side of the midline.

Sagittal Sections

Midline sagittal images are obtained by turning the transducer 90° on the fontanelle from the coronal plane. Planes are obtained through: (a) the midline, (b) caudothalamic groove, and (c) body of the lateral ventricle. On midline images, the cavum septi pellucidi appears as a fluid-filled structure lying between the anterior horns of the lateral ventricles (Fig. 7). The cavum vergae is visualized more posteriorly, lying between the bodies of the lateral ventricles. These structures vary from slit-like spaces to large, cystic structures. Superior to the cavi septi pellucidi and vergae is the thin, crescentic, hypoechoic corpus callosum surrounded by the echogenic sulcus of the corpus callosum (i.e., pericallosal sulcus) (3) which contains the

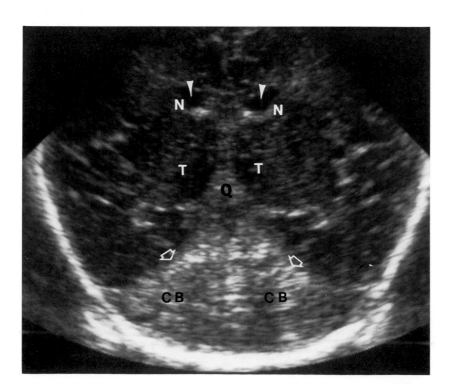

FIG. 5. Coronal scan through quadrigeminal cistern. The quadrigeminal cistern (*Q*) appears as an echogenic, star-shaped structure inferior to the bodies of the lateral ventricles (*arrowheads*). The thalami (*T*), bodies of the caudate nucleus (*N*), cerebellum (*CB*) and tentorium (*open arrows*) also are imaged on this section.

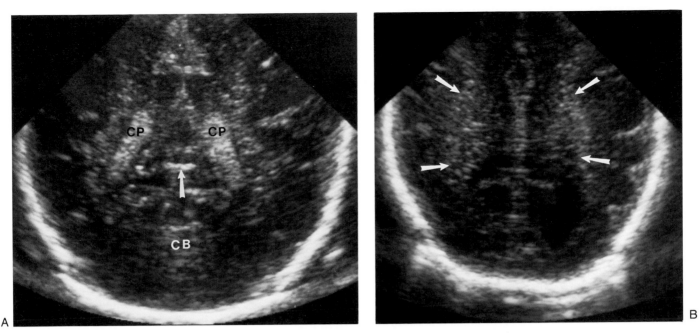

FIG. 6. A: Coronal scan through trigones of lateral ventricles. At this level, the lateral ventricles containing the echogenic choroid plexus (*CP*) diverge laterally. The splenium of the corpus callosum is seen as a horizontally oriented echogenic line (*arrow*) between the ventricles. Note also the top of the echogenic cerebellum (*CB*). **B:** Coronal scan posterior to occipital horns shows normally echogenic white matter (*arrows*) on either side of the midline. Also seen are echogenic cortical sulci extending medially from the lateral margins of the brain.

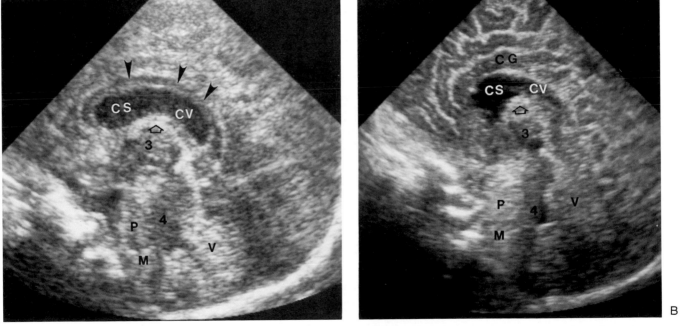

FIG. 7. Normal midline sagittal plane. **A:** Immature brain and **B:** mature brain. The cavum septi pellucidi (*CS*) and vergae (*CV*) are easily identified as a comma-shaped, fluid-filled structure. Superior to the cavi is the hypoechoic corpus callosum (*arrowheads*) and cingulate gyrus (*CG*). Below the cavi is the third ventricle (*3*) with the echogenic choroid plexus (*open arrow*) forming its roof. The pons and medulla are seen as moderately echogenic structures anterior to the fourth ventricle (*4*). The echogenic cerebellar vermis (*V*) is posterior to the fourth ventricle. The number of convolutions increases with gestational age. Thus, gyri and sulci are more easily seen in the term infant than in the preterm infant. The sulci extend to the cingulate gyrus, never to the ventricles. *P*, pons; *M*, medulla.

pericallosal arteries. Cephalad and superior to the sulcus of the corpus callosum is the cingulate gyrus appearing as a broad, curvilinear hypoechoic band. The cingulate sulcus, appearing as a thin, hyperechoic line, separates the cingulate gyrus from the more superficial gyri. The sulci between the superficial gyri on the medial surface of the brain appear as short, thin, hyperechoic lines coursing at an angle to the cingulate gyrus and terminating at the cingulate sulcus. They never extend to the third ventricle. Within the cerebral sulci are branches of the anterior cerebral artery. Pulsations from these vessels can be noted on real-time examinations.

The normal-sized third ventricle also can be visualized on the midline sagittal plane. The massa intermedia is a soft tissue structure within the third ventricle and usually is visualized only in the presence of hydrocephalus. Posterior to the third ventricle is an echogenic band representing the quadrigeminal plate cistern. Immediately inferior to the cistern is the very echogenic cerebellar vermis, which is indented anteriorly by the triangular-shaped fourth ventricle. The brainstem, lying anterior to the ventricle and posterior to the clivus, is of medium echogenicity in contrast to the higher level echoes of the surrounding clivus and vermis.

Slight lateral and oblique angulation of the transducer produces a parasagittal image of the frontal horns

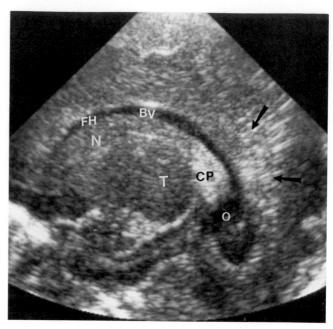

FIG. 9. Parasagittal scan through body of lateral ventricles. At this level, the frontal horn (*FH*), body (*BV*), and occipital horn (*O*) of the lateral ventricle can be defined. The highly echogenic choroid plexus (*CP*) is noted within the trigone of the lateral ventricle. Below the lateral ventricle is the caudate nucleus (*N*) and thalamus (*T*). Superoposterior to the trigone of the lateral ventricle is the normal periventricular halo (*arrows*). Although this area is echogenic, it is less so than the adjacent choroid plexus.

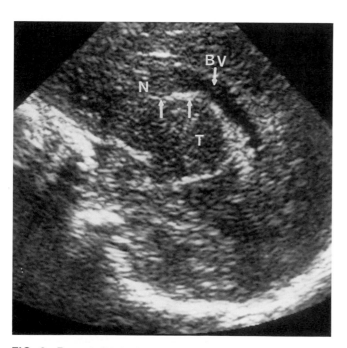

FIG. 8. Parasagittal plane through head of the caudate nucleus. At this level the body (*BV*) of the lateral ventricle is seen. The head of the caudate nucleus (*N*) anteriorly and thalamus (*T*) posteriorly lie inferior to the lateral ventricle. Between these structures is the caudothalamic groove containing the anterior extent of the choroid plexus (*arrows*).

and bodies of the lateral ventricles (Fig. 8). The anatomic landmark on this image is the caudothalamic groove, a thin, echogenic band lying between the caudate nucleus anteriorly and thalamus posteriorly. The caudate nucleus normally is slightly more echogenic than the thalamus. In premature infants, the germinal matrix is located immediately anterosuperiorly to the caudothalamic groove.

Further lateral angulation of the transducer produces a section through the bodies and through occipital and temporal horns of the lateral ventricles (Fig. 9). The highly echogenic glomus of the choroid plexus in the trigone of the lateral ventricle is noted on this image. The choroid plexus extends anteriorly from the glomus into the body of the lateral ventricle to the foramen of Monro, at which point it courses inferiorly into the third ventricle. Normally the choroid plexus has a smooth contour. The amount of CSF present in the lateral ventricles may vary widely, ranging from a tiny anechoic rim above the choroid plexus to a larger volume, C-shaped collection filling the entire lateral ventricle. The frontal, parietal, occipital, and temporal lobes surround the lateral ventricles. Posterior to the occipital horns, the normal area of increased echogenicity (periventricular halo or blush) can be observed.

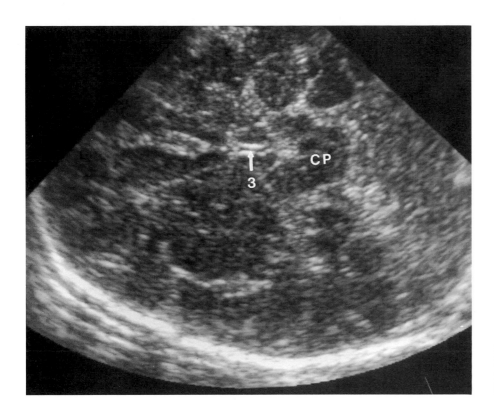

FIG. 10. Axial scan through the brainstem. The cerebral (*CP*) peduncles and third ventricle (*3*) are identified.

Generally, images are not obtained further lateral to the ventricles since there are no major vascular or ventricular structures to serve as landmarks. Instead, a variable number of cerebral convolutions can be seen, which increases with gestational age. This section, however, can be useful to confirm an abnormality noted on coronal images.

Axial Scans

For axial scans, the transducer is placed in front of the ear and superior to the zygomatic process, over the squamosal portion of the temporal bone (Fig. 10). With this approach, images of the brainstem, cerebral peduncles, middle cerebral and posterior cerebral arteries, and the anterior communicating artery of the circle of Willis are obtained.

Normal Variants

Lateral Ventricles

Asymmetry of the lateral ventricles, particularly the occipital horns, is a normal finding in up to 40% of premature infants and in slightly under 20% of term infants (66,145). In most cases, the left ventricle is larger than the right and the occipital horns are larger than the frontal horns.

Ventricular size also changes with maturity. With increasing fetal age, the size of the lateral ventricle decreases relative to the size of the cerebral cortex. Thus, on sonography, the ventricles of the premature infant appear relatively larger than those of the term infant (106). In the term infant the lateral ventricles, especially the frontal horns, may appear compressed or slitlike (145). The slitlike appearance has been reported in about 60% of normal subjects (126). This variation needs to be recognized when assessing the neonatal brain for the presence of cerebral edema. Slitlike ventricles occur in infants with cerebral edema secondary to hypoxia or ischemia, but they usually are associated with other findings, such as increased parenchymal echogenicity, poor definition of sulci and gyri, and decreased vascular pulsations (7,126).

Cavi Septi Pellucidi and Vergae

Two structures that are frequently visualized on sonograms of normal infants are the cavum septi pellucidi and vergae (31). The cavum septi pellucidi lies between the anterior horns of the lateral ventricles, while the cavum vergae is interposed between the bodies. These anechoic, fluid-filled spaces communicate with each other but not with the ventricular or subarachnoid spaces (121). Occasionally linear echoes are identified in the cavum septi pellucidi and are believed to represent septal veins (40). The cavi septi pellucidi and vergae are normally found in the fetus; however, during the sixth month of gestation, the cavum vergae begins to close from posterior to anterior. Just before term, the cavum septi pellucidi begins to close. Closure is complete in most infants by approximately 2 months of postnatal life (121).

The cavum veli interpositi is a fluid-filled space situated posterior-inferior to the cavum vergae. It is virtually always found in neonates who also have both a prominent cavum septi pellucidi and cavum vergae. The cavum veli interpositi usually projects behind the quadrigeminal cistern. On sonography, this space often is separated from the cavum vergae by a septation.

Germinal Matrix

The germinal matrix is a highly vascular structure found in premature infants, but not seen in term infants. It is situated inferolateral to the ependyma lining the floor of the lateral ventricle, and superior to the head and body of the caudate nucleus. It is also present in the roof of the third and fourth ventricles. Involuation begins about the third month of gestation in the area of the body of the caudate nucleus; by 6 months gestation the germinal matrix persists mainly over the head of the caudate. At term it is no longer identifiable as a discrete structure. The clinical significance of the germinal matrix is discussed below.

Choroid Plexus

The choroid plexus of the lateral ventricle courses posteriorly from the tip of the temporal horn to the trigone and then continues anteriorly along the floor of the lateral ventricle to the foramen of Monro. It then extends through the foramen, joins the choroid from the opposite side, and courses posteriorly in the roof of the third ventricle to the suprapineal recess (32). The choroid plexus within the body of the lateral ventricle and the temporal horn is normally thin with a smooth outline. It becomes bulbous in the region of the trigone where it forms the glomus. Focal thickening in areas other than the glomus should arouse suspicion of hemorrhage. The choroid plexus never extends into the frontal or occipital horns. There is also choroid plexus in the roof of the fourth ventricle, but it is not normally sonographically visible.

Periventricular Halo

A periventricular echogenic halo exists around the posterior part of the lateral ventricles in almost all nor-

mal neonates (48). Ninety-seven percent of newborns with a mean gestational age of 32 weeks demonstrate a normal periventricular halo or blush (28). The halo is also present in full-term infants, although not as prominently. The normal periventricular echogenicity has a homogeneous appearance, an intensity less than that of the normal choroid plexus, and is separated from the normal choroid by an anechoic rim of CSF. The etiology of the echogenic halo is unclear. It has been postulated that it is related to the white matter fibers and vascular plexus that course radially from the cortex to the subependymal layer of the ventricle (28). Alternatively, the echogenicity may be a scanning artifact since the echogenic area cannot be reproduced in all scan planes. Differential diagnostic considerations include cerebral hemorrhage and periventricular leukomalacia. Either of the latter should be suspected if the periventricular halo is abnormally dense, globular, coarse, or heterogeneous (28).

Cisterna Magna

The cisterna magna is an arachnoid-lined structure lying inferior to the vermis and communicating with the fourth ventricle. The midsagittal height of the cisterna magna varies from 3- to 8-mm, with a mean of 4.5 mm $\pm$ 1.29 mm (41). Dimensions are smaller with Arnold-Chiari malformation and are larger than normal in Dandy-Walker syndrome.

DUPLEX AND COLOR DOPPLER IMAGING

Duplex Doppler sonography is a noninvasive method of evaluating cerebral blood flow and velocity. Vessels can be sampled either with an anterior fontanelle or transtemporal approach (Fig. 11) (50,67).

The anterior cerebral (ACA), pericallosal, basilar, and internal carotid arteries are best evaluated via the anterior fontanelle, while the middle (MCA) and posterior (PCA) cerebral arteries are best evaluated by the transtemporal approach at the level of the circle of Willis. The ACA is insonated at approximately 0°, the MCA at 10° to 30°, and the PCA at 45° to 65° (67). Use of the anterior fontanelle for evaluating velocity flow of the MCA and PCA should be avoided, since this approach produces a high angle of Doppler insonation and results in underestimation of velocity (50,67).

Absolute systolic and diastolic velocities progressively increase with gestational age (67,116). As expected, the resistive index (RI) (peak systolic minus end diastolic divided by peak systolic velocity) decreases with increasing gestational age. The decrease is mainly due to a greater increase in end diastolic flow

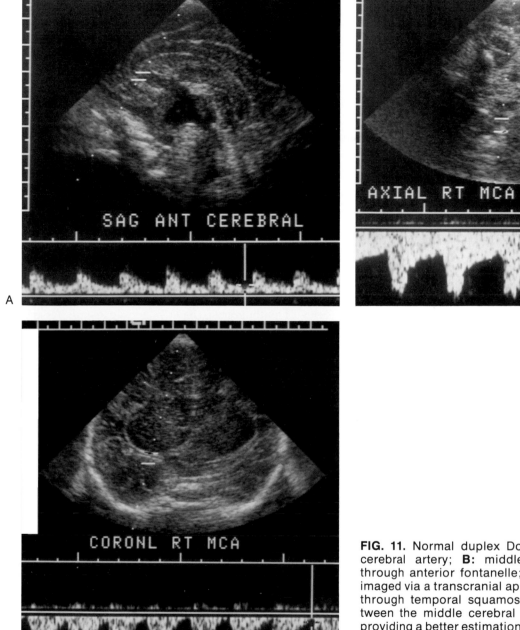

FIG. 11. Normal duplex Doppler images. **A:** Anterior cerebral artery; **B:** middle cerebral artery imaged through anterior fontanelle; **C:** middle cerebral artery imaged via a transcranial approach. Note that scanning through temporal squamosa optimizes the angle between the middle cerebral artery and Doppler beam, providing a better estimation of true blood-flow velocity. Also note that antegrade flow is present in the cerebral arteries throughout diastole.

velocity when compared with systolic flow velocity, reflecting decreasing cerebrovascular resistance. Maximum spectral velocity and resistive indexes for the major intracranial vessels have been established (101). In full-term infants, average RI is 75 ± 10 (S.D.) (116). Antegrade flow is always present during systole and diastole.

An elevated RI may indicate either an intra- or extracranial abnormality affecting cerebral blood flow. Intracranial abnormalities that can elevate RIs include hemorrhage, brain edema, subdural effus-

ions, periventricular leukomalacia, and hydrocephalus (12,65,116). The increased RI is due to increased cerebral resistance. Extracranial abnormalities increasing RIs include patent ductus arteriosus, cardiac failure, hypoxic-ischemic encephalopathy, and hypotension (83). These conditions increase the RI because of decreased cerebral perfusion rather than increased cerebral impedance. Although elevated RIs are nonspecific, they can be used to follow patients with increased intracranial pressures and to assess the effectiveness of ventricular tapping or shunting (116).

More recently, color Doppler imaging (CDI) has proven effective in the evaluation of intracranial vessels (Fig. 12, see Colorplate 1) (86–88,147). Similar to duplex Doppler sonography, the anterior fontanelle approach is the most useful for demonstrating the anterior cerebral, pericallosal, internal carotid, basilar, and vertebral arteries. The axial approach through the squamosal portion of the temporal bone provides better quality images of the middle and posterior cerebral arteries of the circle of Willis and the anterior and posterior communicating arteries, because of a more optimal Doppler angle. Sagittal views can confirm findings on coronal and transtemporal views.

Color Doppler imaging can assist in more precise placement of the cursor for quantitative duplex Doppler interrogation. It also can be useful in diagnosing vascular abnormalities, such as the vein of Galen malformation. Recently CDI has been used to evaluate flow in neonates before and after extracorporeal membrane oxygenation (ECMO) (86,147). In ECMO, the right common carotid artery and jugular vein are cannulated. Deoxygenated blood from the right atrium is shunted to an external membrane for oxygenation and then returned to the aorta via the carotid artery. Perfusion of the right cerebral hemisphere is by collateral flow from the basilar artery and contralateral common carotid artery via the circle of Willis. This collateral flow appears as flow reversal within the proximal segment of the anterior cerebral artery (86,147). In this situation, CDI can be useful to assess the adequacy of collateral pathways and to document flow to both cerebral hemispheres.

INTRACRANIAL HEMORRHAGE

There are four major, clinically important types of intracranial hemorrhage: (a) periventricular-intraventricular (PVH-IVH), (b) subarachnoid, (c) subdural, and (d) intracerebellar. Of these types of hemorrhage, PVH-IVH is the most common and serious lesion (97,103,141,142).

Periventricular-Intraventricular Hemorrhage

PVH-IVH is almost exclusively a lesion of the premature infant, with an incidence of approximately 40% in infants weighing less than 1,500 gm or under 32 weeks of gestation (76,97). The most common site of origin of PVH-IVH is the germinal matrix at the junction of the head of the caudate nucleus and choroid plexus in the floor of the lateral ventricle. This tissue gives rise to spongioblasts and neuroblasts which dur-

ing development migrate peripherally to form basal ganglia and cerebral cortex (53,97). The germinal matrix is a highly vascular structure which is present in premature but not in term infants. The vessels are composed of a single layer of fragile endothelial cells which are prone to injury.

Bleeding into the germinal matrix may be limited to this structure and of little clinical significance. However, it may at times rupture through the ependyma resulting in intraventricular hemorrhage which may lead to posthemorrhagic hydrocephalus. Germinal matrix hemorrhage also may extend into the cerebral parenchyma, eventually resulting in areas of encephalomalacia (45,113).

Pathogenesis

The exact cause of germinal matrix hemorrhage in the premature infant is uncertain and numerous theories of pathogenesis have been suggested. As mentioned previously, the germinal matrix is a very vascular structure with thin-walled, friable vessels. These vessels are supported by a delicate, gelatinous matrix which lacks connective tissue support and is easily injured (139,142). The vascular supply to the germinal matrix also is particularly sensitive to fluctuations in arterial blood pressures. The major factor in elevating blood pressure appears to be ischemia. Ischemia increases cerebral blood flow leading to hypercapnia, preferential flow of blood to the brain, arterial hypertension, and distention of fragile arterioles and capillaries (139,142). Elevations in venous pressure also predispose the vessels in the germinal matrix to rupture. Elevated venous pressure usually is the result of myocardial failure due to perinatal asphyxia or elevated intrathoracic pressure, particularly secondary to pneumothorax.

Currently it appears most likely that several factors are responsible for germinal matrix hemorrhage. In most cases, hypoxia or ischemia leads to hyperperfusion or venous distention, followed by increased vascular pressure and then rupture of vessels in the germinal matrix.

Grading Intracranial Hemorrhage

Several grading systems have been used to describe intracranial hemorrhage (97,120). These vary depending on the presence or absence of inclusion of intraparenchymal hemorrhage. The most popular classification includes intraparenchymal hemorrhage (IPH) as the most severe form of PVH-IVH (97,120). In this classification, hemorrhage is graded as follows: grade

1, confined to the subendymal matrix; grade 2, intraventricular hemorrhage without ventricular dilatation; grade 3, intraventricular hemorrhage with ventricular dilatation; and grade 4, intraventricular hemorrhage with intraparenchymal hemorrhage.

Other authors have excluded intraparenchymal hemorrhage from the grading system based on the belief that intraparenchymal hemorrhage is not an extension of PVH-IVH, but instead is caused by primary cerebral infarction (84,114). In this system, hemorrhage is classified as follows: grade 1, subependymal hemorrhage with minimal or no intraventricular hemorrhage and normal ventricular size; grade 2, intraventricular hemorrhage without complete filling of the ventricular lumen by blood and with or without mild ventricular dilatation; and grade 3, hemorrhage filling and distending at least one lateral ventricle.

The debate on the precise cause of intraparenchymal hemorrhage is ongoing in view of emerging data on hemorrhage and ischemia (140,142). Recent reviews have suggested that hemorrhagic and ischemic insults frequently coexist (42,46,84,119). For the purpose of discussion, intracranial hemorrhage will be discussed separately from hypoxia/ischemia. It should be noted, however, that distinguishing between them is often difficult on the basis of sonography alone.

Grade 1 Hemorrhage

Germinal matrix hemorrhage, also referred to as subependymal hemorrhage (SEH), appears echogenic, presumably due to the formation of fibrin mesh within the organized clot. On coronal scans, the echogenic focus is observed inferolateral to the floor of the frontal horn or ventricular body, typically near the head of the caudate nucleus. On parasagittal sections, SEH appears as a bulge anterior to the termination of the caudothalamic groove (20,77) (Fig. 13). The lesion may be unilateral or bilateral, and may be isolated or found in association with more extensive hemorrhage. Occasionally SEH may be large enough to compress or obliterate the frontal horns or bodies of the lateral ventricles. Caution must be taken not to confuse SEH with normal specular reflections from the ventricular floor and roof or with normal choroid plexus, which also are intensely echogenic (124). Normal choroid plexus, however, tapers anteriorly in the caudothalamic groove and does not extend anterior to the foramen of Monro (20,32).

Many subependymal hemorrhages disappear entirely over a period of days or weeks. Some leave a thin, echogenic linear density behind, whereas others undergo central liquefaction, resulting in formation of

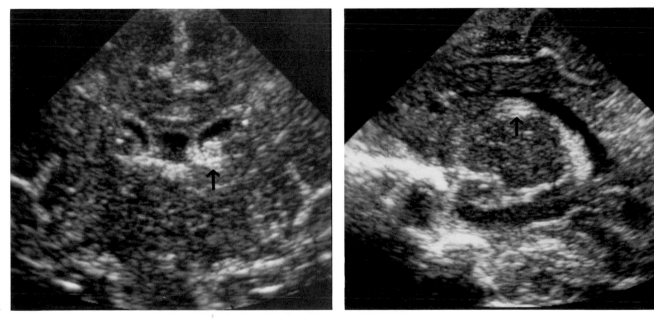

FIG. 13. Acute subependymal hemorrhage. **A:** Coronal and **B:** right parasagittal sonograms show a focus of increased echogenicity (*arrow*) at the level of the head of the caudate nucleus. The hemorrhage is just anterosuperior to the termination of the choroid plexus in the caudothalamic groove.

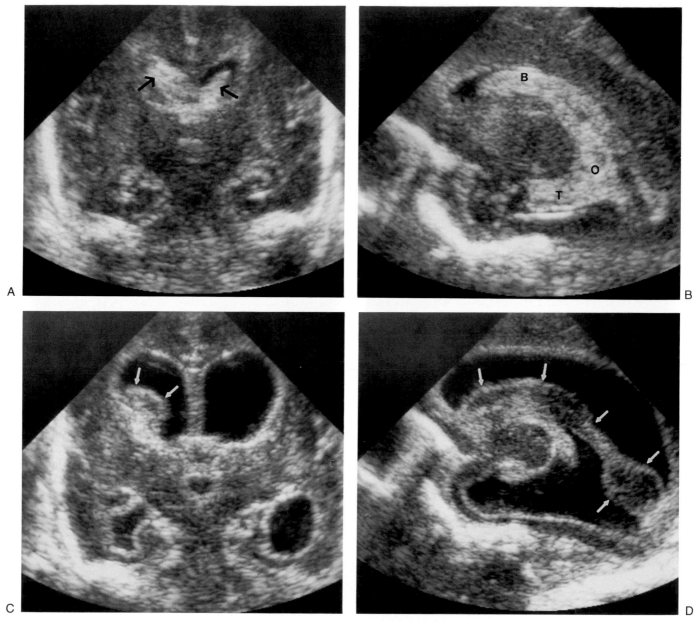

FIG. 17. Evolution of grade 3 hemorrhage. **A:** Coronal scan demonstrates dilated, blood-filled lateral ventricles (*arrows*). **B:** Parasagittal scan through right lateral ventricle shows blood filling dilated body (*B*), and temporal (*T*) and occipital (*O*) horns of the lateral ventricle. The intraventricular hemorrhage is inseparable from the subependymal hemorrhage where it originated. **C:** Coronal and **D:** sagittal scans 2 weeks later demonstrate retraction of the intraventricular clot (*arrows*). Note that the hematoma has decreased in echogenicity and is surrounded by a well-defined rim. Note also that the lateral ventricles have become larger.

Grade 3 IVH usually becomes smaller and disappears over 5 to 6 weeks. As they are being resorbed, most hematomas decrease in echogenicity, fragment, and retract. With retraction, a cleavage plane develops between the clot and ventricular wall or choroid plexus, creating the appearance of a "ventricle within a ventricle" (Fig. 17). Resorption continues until there is complete clearing of blood from the ventricles. Occasionally, residual septations or bands may be observed. With grade 3 hemorrhage, there usually is residual mild or moderate hydrocephalus, which may be asymmetric (19). At times, there is development of pronounced ventriculomegaly, requiring diversionary shunt placement.

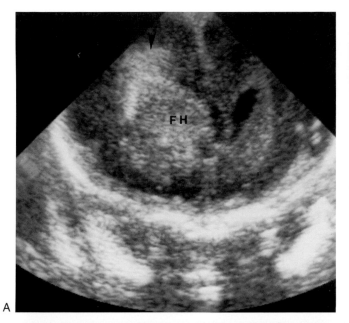

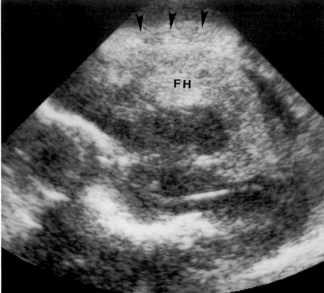

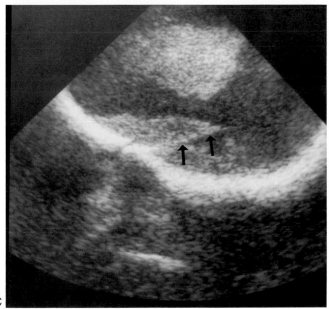

FIG. 18. Grade 4 hemorrhage. **A:** Coronal and **B:** right parasagittal images demonstrate clot in the frontal horn (*FH*) of the right lateral ventricle as well as extension of hematoma in a frontoparietal distribution (*arrowheads*). There is shift of the midline to the left. **C:** Right parasagittal image adjacent to the lateral ventricle shows the extent of parenchymal hemorrhage. Arrows point to sylvian fissure which is widened secondary to blood.

Grade 4 Hemorrhage

Intraparenchymal hemorrhage appears as an intensely echogenic focus adjacent to the lateral ventricle (Fig. 18). Initially the bleed has irregular but well-circumscribed margins with homogeneous internal echogenicity. Intraparenchymal hemorrhage is most common in the frontal and parietal lobes on the same side as PVH-IVH. Rarely, the thalamus may be involved by extension of SEH. Occasionally, IPH is so massive that it extends almost to the periphery of the brain or into the occipital lobe. With larger hemorrhages, mass effect with shift of the midline structures to the unaffected contralateral side is observed. Extensive coexisting IVH is a frequent finding.

Pitfalls in diagnosis of IPH do exist. Increased periventricular echogenicity is not specific for IPH but also can be seen with nonhemorrhagic ischemic lesions. The nonhemorrhagic lesions are usually smaller than IPH. In addition, they are often bilateral and lack mass effect. Another problem in diagnosis can be the differentiation between a hematoma limited to the ventricle and a hematoma adjacent to the ventricle. Intraparenchymal hemorrhage usually has irregular, ragged borders, whereas IVH tends to have sharp, well-defined margins.

Intraparenchymal hemorrhage may regress and gradually disappear over several weeks. However, large lesions tend to undergo liquefaction 1 to 2 weeks after the hemorrhage, and appear hypoechoic with a

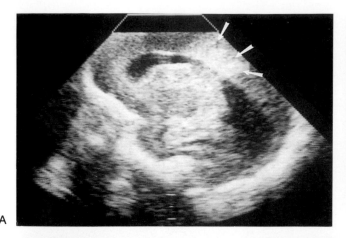

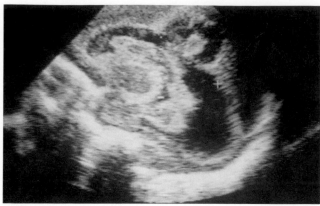

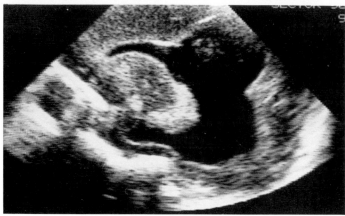

FIG. 19. Evolution of intraparenchymal hemorrhage. **A:** Parasagittal image at 9 days of age demonstrates intraventricular hemorrhage and echogenic clot (*arrows*) within the parietal region. **B:** Two weeks later the resolving hematoma has retracted and fragmented, becoming partially hypoechoic. **C:** At 2 months, the hematoma has resolved, leaving an area of encephalomalacia. (From Shackelford and Volpe, ref. 119, with permission.)

well-defined echogenic rim. By 2 to 4 weeks, retraction of the clot from the surrounding brain parenchyma can be observed. Finally, by 2 to 3 months retraction, fragmentation, and phagocytosis of the hematoma are complete, with development of an area of encephalomalacia (8,35,44,45) (Fig. 19). Communication of the encephalomalacic areas with the adjacent ventricle may be observed.

Timing of PVH-IVH

Periventricular-intraventricular hemorrhage typically occurs in the first 3 days of life, with 36% occurring on day 1, 32% on day 2, and 18% on day 3 (110). By the sixth day, approximately 90% of intracranial hemorrhage has occurred. Rarely, hemorrhage occurs between the first and eighth postpartum weeks (57). Optimal scanning for detection of PVH-IVH is 4 to 7 days after birth, with a follow-up scan at 14 days.

Anatomic Sequelae

Posthemorrhagic hydrocephalus, i.e., progressive ventricular dilatation, occurs in approximately 75% of surviving infants with IVH by 3 weeks of age (142). Spontaneous resolution or arrest of ventricular dilatation occurs in approximately 75% of patients. The resolution commences within 4 weeks of development

of ventricular dilatation (1,59). In 25% of patients, ventricular dilatation will continue to progress (142). This sequelae is more likely to occur in patients with severe intraventricular and intraparenchymal hemorrhage (35). Placement of a ventriculoperitoneal shunt that diverts CSF from the lateral ventricles to the peritoneal cavity will be required in <10% of patients (75,142).

On sonography, the trigones and occipital horns dilate before the frontal horns. These may be the only areas to enlarge in infants with small ventricular hemorrhages, whereas the entire ventricle may enlarge in infants with large hemorrhages (Fig. 20). Posthemorrhagic ventricular dilatation may be asymmetric and affect the lateral ventricles more than the third or fourth ventricles. Significant enlargement of the fourth ventricle is very unusual and suggests ventriculitis superimposed on hemorrhage or combined obstruction of the aqueduct of Sylvius and the foramina of Luschka and Magendie, resulting in a trapped or isolated fourth ventricle.

Prognosis

The outcome of PVH-IVH relates to the hemorrhage severity (120). With grades 1,2,3, and 4 hemorrhage, mortality rates are 15%, 20%, 40%, and 60%, respectively, and the incidence of ventricular dilatation is 5%, 25%, 55%, and 80%, respectively. The incidence of

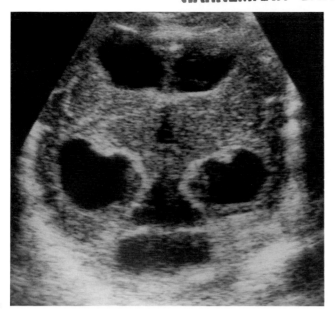 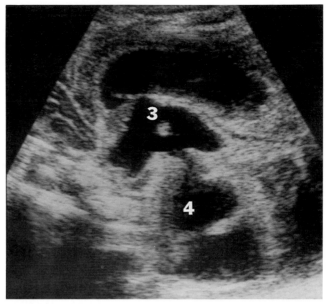

A

B

FIG. 20. Posthemorrhagic hydrocephalus in an infant with a grade 3 hemorrhage. **A:** Coronal and **B:** midline sagittal images demonstrate dilated lateral, third (*3*) and fourth (*4*) ventricles. These findings are consistent with extraventricular obstruction, presumably from obliterative arachnoiditis in the posterior fossa.

long-term neurological sequelae, particularly spastic diplegia or quadriparesis and intellectual retardation, in infants with grades 1,2,3, and 4 hemorrhage is 15%, 30%, 40%, and 90%, respectively (142).

Subarachnoid Hemorrhage

Primary subarachnoid hemorrhage is more frequent in the premature than in the term infant and is generally common but almost always clinically benign (141). It is occasionally related to neonatal asphyxia or trauma, although often the pathogenesis is unclear. Sonography is relatively insensitive in detecting subarachnoid hemorrhage because the brain periphery is normally echogenic, making differentiation between blood and normal tissue difficult. Sometimes, however, a large subarachnoid hemorrhage may be apparent on coronal scans as hyperechoic widening of the sylvian fissures (see Fig. 18), although caution must be taken to distinguish between a sylvian fissure distended with blood and the normally prominent fissures seen in premature infants. In general, identification of subarachnoid hemorrhage in premature infants is very difficult.

Subdural Hemorrhage

Subdural hemorrhage is more frequent in the full-term infant than in the premature infant, and is relatively uncommon but usually clinically serious (141). It is related primarily to trauma and is the result of falx laceration, tearing of bridging veins in the supra- or infratentorial regions, tentorial laceration, or occipital

osteodiastasis. With falx laceration, the subdural hematoma collects over the inferior aspect of the interhemispheric fissure, while rupture of bridging veins results in hemorrhage over the cerebral convexity. Interhemispheric subdural collections can be seen on sonography, appearing as fluid between the two hemispheres. Large convexity hematomas also can be visualized as fluid collections adjacent to the surface of the frontoparietal lobes (Fig. 21). Small convexity hematomas may be more difficult to identify by sonography because of the difficulty in angling the trans-

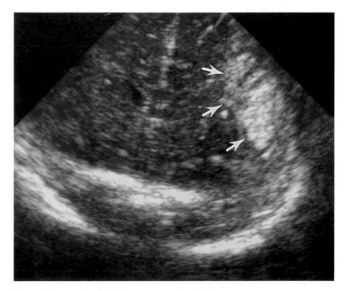

FIG. 21. Acute supratentorial subdural hematoma. Coronal sonogram demonstrates echogenic fluid (*arrows*) depressing the surface of the brain medially.

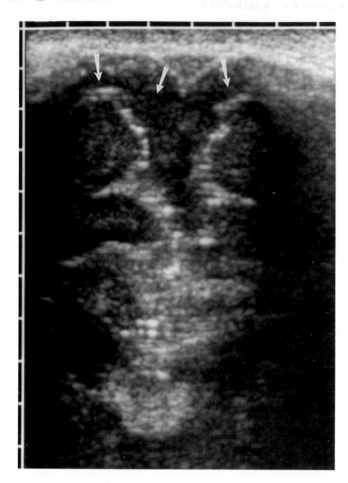

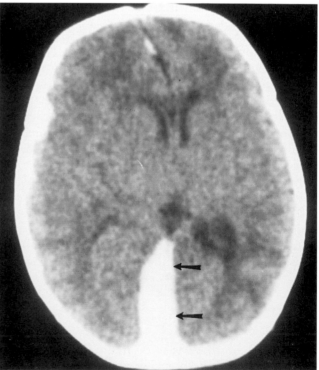

FIG. 22. Subacute subdural hematoma in an 8-month-old boy. Coronal scan with a high-resolution linear array transducer shows a large sonolucent fluid collection (*arrows*) over the cerebral hemispheres. The patient had head trauma 2 weeks previously.

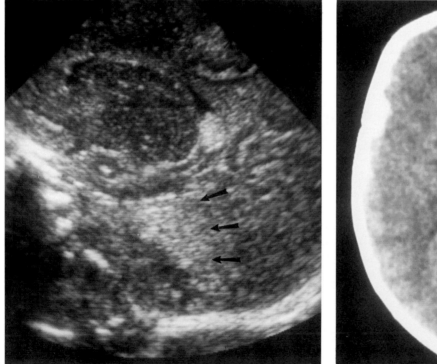

A

B

FIG. 23. Infratentorial subdural hematoma. **A:** Left parasagittal sonogram shows increased echogenicity along the tentorium or falx (*arrows*). **B:** CT scan demonstrates interhemispheric subdural hematoma (*arrows*).

ducer to image the curved surface of the brain. When hemorrhage is acute, the subdural space appears echogenic (37). As the hematoma evolves, it becomes hypoechoic (Fig. 22). Associated findings include flattened gyri and distorted, compressed ventricles.

Tentorial laceration and occipital osteodiastasis result in infratentorial subdural hematomas. Acute posterior fossa subdural hematomas appear as echogenic fluid collections beneath the tentorium and over the cerebellar hemisphere (47) (Fig. 23). Large hematomas may compress the cerebellum and brainstem, obstructing the prepontine cisterns, fourth ventricle, and aqueduct. An interhemispheric subdural hematoma also may be present when the falx is lacerated. Scanning in the axial plane is sometimes helpful in assessing the presence and extent of inferiorly located collections (85).

Intracerebellar Hemorrhage

Intracerebellar hemorrhage is more frequent in the premature than in the full-term infant, being found at autopsy in 15% to 25% of infants under 32 weeks gestation (52,82). In general it is an uncommon, but usually serious lesion (141). Possible causes include rupture of the germinal matrix of the fourth ventricle secondary to ischemia, traumatic breech deliveries, and direct occipital compression by compressive straps for face mask ventilation (96). On sonography, the cerebellum is asymmetrically echogenic with altered parenchymal echotexture (98,105) (Fig. 24).

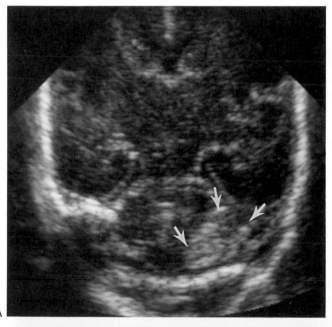

A

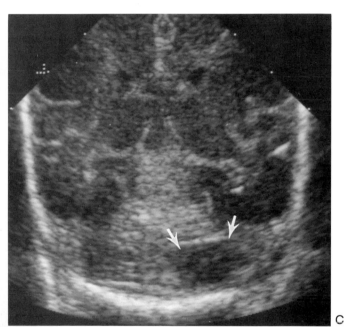

C

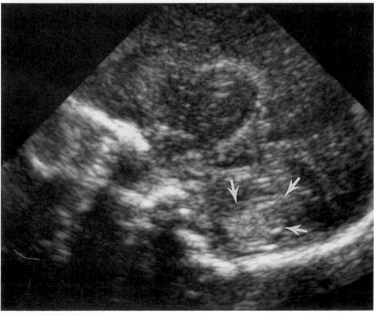

B

FIG. 24. Intracerebellar hemorrhage. **A:** Coronal and **B:** left parasagittal images show a well-defined area of increased echogenicity (*arrows*) within the cerebellum. **C:** On a follow-up scan 10 days later, the hemorrhage (*arrows*) has become relatively sonolucent.

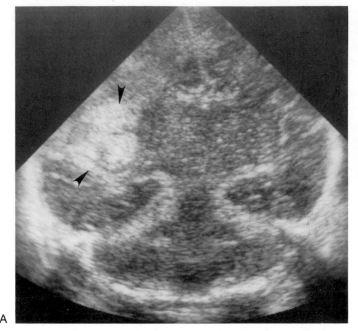

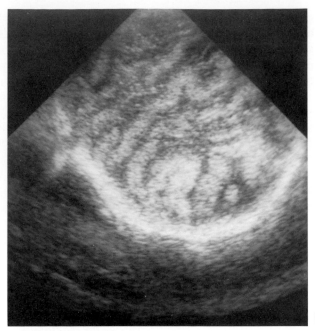

FIG. 25. Gyral hemorrhage. **A:** Coronal and **B:** right parasagittal scans show abnormally echogenic cerebral gyri (*arrowheads*). CT scans confirmed gyral hemorrhage.

Intracerebral Hemorrhage

Isolated intracerebral hemorrhage without PVH-IVH occurs primarily in term infants in association with trauma. Less commonly, it is secondary to coagulation defects or bleeding diatheses. Rarely, it is the result of hemorrhagic infarction due to venous or arterial thrombosis. Intraparenchymal hemorrhage almost always is supratentorial and frequently associ-

ated with extraaxial hemorrhage. The appearance is that of an abnormal area of increased echogenicity in the cerebral cortex or basal ganglia (25) (Figs. 25,26).

HYPOXIC-ISCHEMIC ENCEPHALOPATHY

The major types of neuropathologic lesions in children with hypoxic-ischemic encephalopathy include: (a) periventricular leukomalacia, (b) focal and diffuse

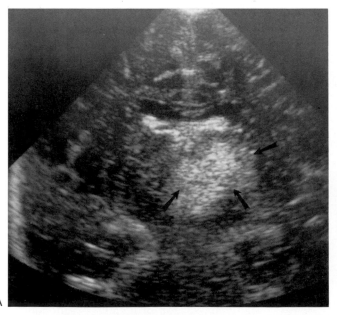

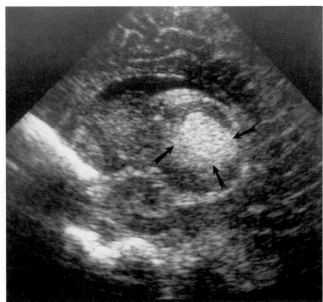

FIG. 26. Thalamic hemorrhage in a 1-month-old infant. **A:** Coronal and **B:** left parasagittal scans show increased echogenicity of the region of the left thalamus (*arrows*). The left ventricle is mildly compressed posteriorly.

ischemic brain injury, (c) hemorrhagic necrosis of basal ganglia and thalamus, (d) selective neuronal injury, and (e) parasagittal cerebral injury. Sonography is useful in evaluating the first three varieties of injury, but is not valuable in defining either selective neuronal necrosis or parasagittal neuronal necrosis because the lesions are too peripherally situated or too localized to be visualized (126,140).

Periventricular Leukomalacia

Periventricular leukomalacia is an infarction of deep white matter adjacent to the external angles of the lateral ventricles. This area represents a watershed region between the end branches of major vascular distributions. With microangiographic techniques, it has been shown that the site of infarction is the border zone between the penetrating ventriculopetal and deep ventriculofugal arteries, 3 to 10 mm from the ventricular wall (132,133). Pathologically, the lesions may be hemorrhagic or nonhemorrhagic. The incidence of periventricular leukomalacia has been observed to be between 7% and 26% on autopsy studies (2,18,28,140). The frequency is higher in infants weighing <1500 g at birth and in those surviving longer than one week on assisted ventilation.

Periventricular leukomalacia (PVL) is especially common in premature infants with a history of severe cerebral hypoxia or ischemia or cardiorespiratory difficulties in the neonatal period. Pathologically, the earliest finding is coagulation necrosis, followed by a proliferation of astrocytes and macrophages. Phagocytosis of the necrotic tissue begins within 5 to 7 days, leading to cavitation after about 2 weeks. If there is concomitant destruction of the ependyma, these cavities may communicate with the ventricles. Focal or diffuse hemorrhage within the affected white matter has been found in 25% of cases (2). Associated subependymal, intraventricular, and subarachnoid hemorrhage also have been reported in between 28% and 59% of cases (115,123). Clinically, affected neonates have nonspecific signs including seizures, apnea, abnormal muscle tone, and leg weakness. The major long-term sequelae of PVL are spastic diplegia or quadriplegia; visual, auditory, and speech disturbances; and convulsive disorders.

The earliest sonographic finding of PVL, occurring in the first 2 weeks of life, is a broad band of increased echogenicity (18,23,27,42,46,61,76,111,115) located lateral to the frontal horns and trigones of the lateral ventricles (Fig. 27). Approximately 36% of premature infants with intraventricular hemorrhage on sonography exhibit periventricular echodensities (84). Approximately one-half of these echodense lesions are large, coarse, and unilateral, and one-half are small, linear, and mainly bilateral (28,84). Large lesions are often hemorrhagic infarcts associated with major PVH-IVH; smaller lesions are more likely nonhemorrhagic and associated with minor degrees of PVH-IVH. The distinction between hemorrhagic and nonhemorrhagic forms of PVL is difficult by sonography, since the degree of echogenicity is similar in both lesions (115).

The increased periventricular echogenicity occurring with periventricular leukomalacia must be differentiated from the periventricular echogenic halo seen in normal neonates. In general, the echogenicity with

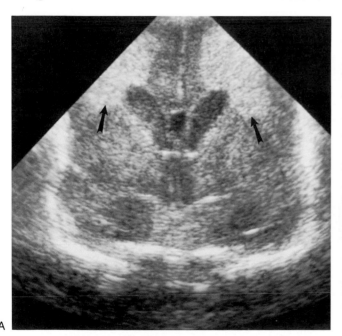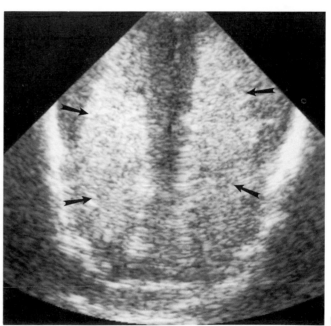

A   B

FIG. 27. Periventricular leukomalacia. **A, B:** Two coronal images show marked symmetric echogenicity (*arrows*) around the lateral ventricles.

periventricular leukomalacia is more intense, hetero-geneous, and discretely defined than that seen with the normal periventricular halo. In some instances, defin-itive diagnosis may require weekly follow-up sono-grams and demonstration of periventricular cysts.

The smaller, bilateral periventricular echodensities usually disappear within 2 to 3 weeks; however, in about 15% of patients cyst formation occurs. On the other hand, the larger unilateral lesions are almost al-ways followed by cyst formation. Cyst development occurs between 2 and 3 weeks after the initial ap-pearance of the increased periventricular echogenicity (115) (Fig. 28). With this development, the diagnosis of PVL becomes certain (18,23). The cysts are thick-

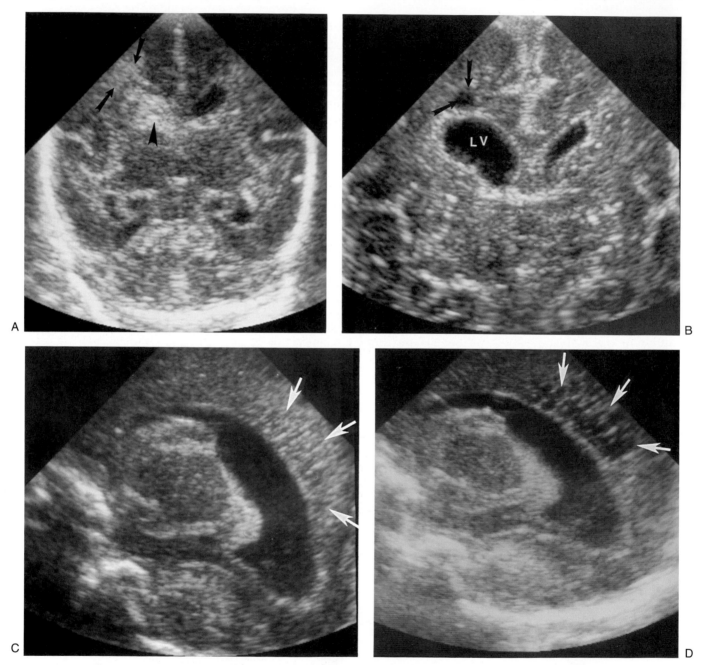

FIG. 28. Evolving periventricular leukomalacia. **A:** Coronal scan demonstrates an area of in-creased echogenicity (*arrows*) radiating from the right frontal horn. Also noted is clot in the right lateral ventricle (*arrowhead*). **B:** Follow-up scan 2 weeks later shows a small cystic lesion adjacent to the lateral angle of the right ventricle (*LV*) which has undergone progressive dilatation. **C:** Sagittal sonogram in another patient demonstrates periventricular echogenicity (*arrows*) pos-terior to the left lateral ventricle. Although the periventricular echoes appeared normal, they were noted to be brighter than those on the right. **D:** Follow-up scan reveals small cystic areas (*arrows*). In certain patients, differentiation between normal and abnormal periventricular echogenicity may be impossible on initial studies; serial scans eventually provide a diagnosis when cysts become evident or fail to develop.

walled, multiple, and usually do not communicate with the ventricular system. They may be limited to the anterior or posterior areas of the ventricles, or in more severe cases, they can extend around the entire border of the lateral ventricle. In some cases the septae separating the cysts from each other and from the lateral ventricles degenerate, producing the appearance of ventricular outpouchings (42,46). Findings on long-term follow-up of PVL include generalized cerebral atrophy manifested by widening of the interhemispheric fissure and cerebral sulci, and varying degrees of ventriculomegaly (46).

Prognosis for infants with large and small periventricular echodense lesions differs markedly. Infants

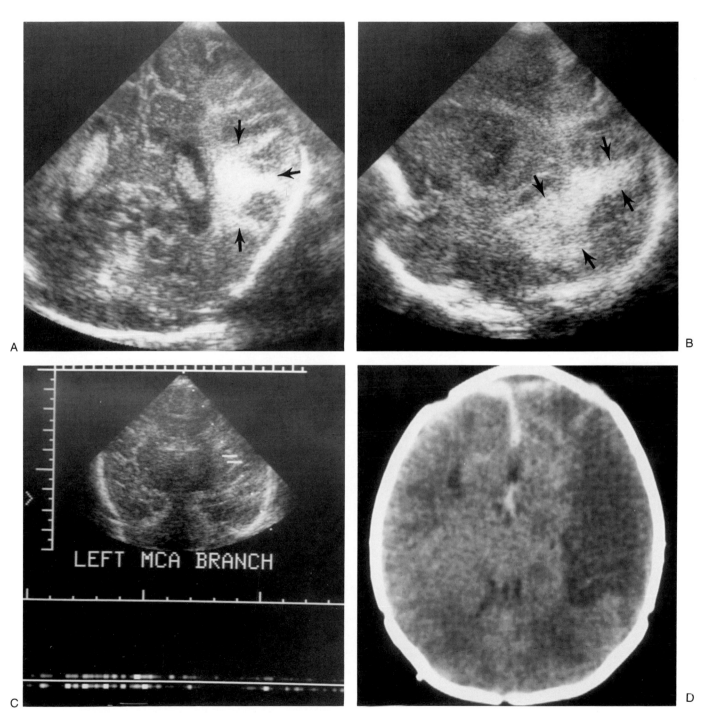

FIG. 29. Focal infarct. **A:** Coronal image shows an irregular area of increased echogenicity in the distribution of the left middle cerebral artery. **B:** Parasagittal image lateral to the left lateral ventricle confirms the area of increased echogenicity (*arrows*). **C:** Duplex Doppler image reveals no perfusion of the left middle cerebral artery within the sylvian fissure. **D:** CT scan shows a homogeneous, low density, wedge-shaped lesion consistent with infarct. Mass effect with midline shift is present.

with small, linear echodensities have no or mild neurological deficits; infants with large, dense echoes have moderate to severe neurologic deficits (84).

Focal and Diffuse Ischemic Injury

Focal or multifocal ischemic brain injury affects term more often than premature infants. The ischemic lesions are localized in the watershed area of the cerebral cortex and subcortical white matter, between the three major cerebral arteries (140). Factors predisposing to focal or multifocal infarction include prolonged hypoxia, congenital heart disease, polycythemia, trauma, meningitis, emboli, and most recently extracorporeal membrane oxygenation (ECMO) (7,11, 58,134). Pathologically, the earliest findings are

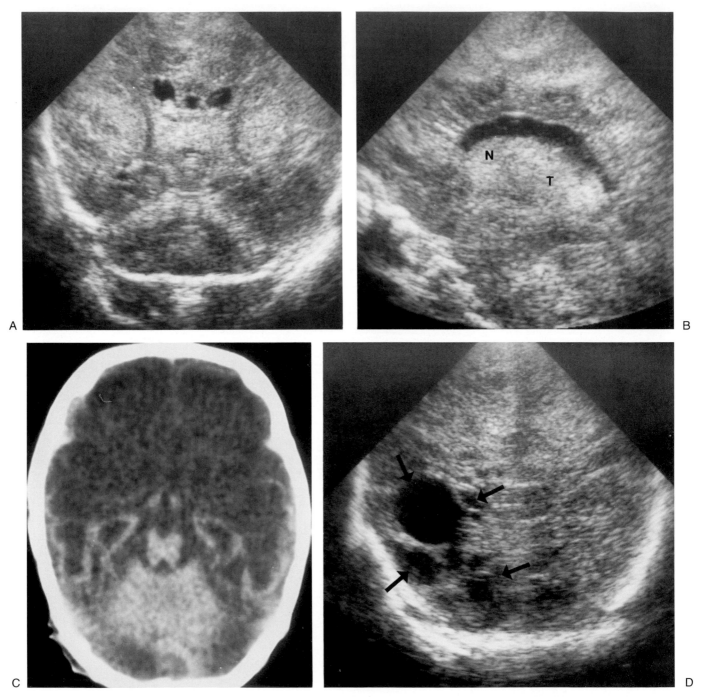

FIG. 30. Diffuse hypoxic-ischemic injury in a full-term infant. **A:** Coronal and **B:** sagittal images show generalized increased parenchymal echogenicity with obliteration of the normal sulcal interfaces. Increased echogenicity of the thalamus (*T*) and caudate nucleus (*N*) also is noted. **C:** CT scan demonstrates low attenuation throughout gray and white matter with relative sparing of the cerebellum. **D:** Follow-up coronal sonogram 4 weeks later reveals areas of encephalomalacia in the temporal area (*arrows*).

cerebral edema and cellular disruption. The edematous areas may resolve completely, produce variable degrees of cortical atrophy, or proceed to infarction with extensive areas of brain necrosis and cavitation (58). Focal ischemic injury commonly occurs in the distribution of one of the major cerebral vessels, with the middle cerebral artery being affected most often (140).

Both focal and diffuse ischemic injury cause highly echogenic areas within the cerebral cortex, poor definition of gyral-sulcal interfaces, and absent vascular pulsations (7,58,60,126,127) (Figs. 29,30). When injury is diffuse, the ventricles are small due to edema, although this finding is not specific for ischemic brain damage, but also can occur in normal full-term infants (126). Once infarction has occurred, atrophy, mild ventricular enlargement, parenchymal calcifications, and cystic encephalomalacia may be observed (127,129).

Neurologic outcome varies with the presence or absence of cerebral echogenicity. Ninety percent of patients with hypoxic-ischemic encephalopathy and abnormal parenchyma on sonography die or have neurologic sequelae. In contrast, only 10% of patients with normal parenchyma have neurologic deficits (126).

Basal Ganglia and Thalamic Injury

Ischemic injury to the basal ganglia and thalami is a relatively infrequent lesion observed in both premature and term infants (140). Causes of infarction include perinatal asphyxia and thrombosis due to meningitis. Basal ganglia and thalamic injuries are visualized especially well when concomitant hemorrhagic necrosis is present (73) (Fig. 31). Sonographic

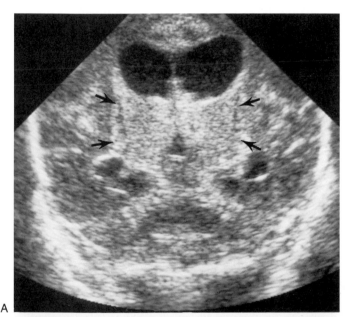

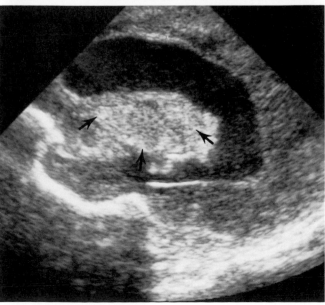

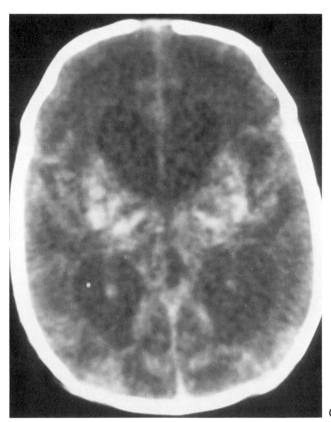

FIG. 31. Ischemic injury of the basal ganglia. **A:** Coronal and **B:** left parasagittal scans of a 1-week-old infant with severe perinatal asphyxia reveals bilateral increased echogenicity in the region of the basal ganglia and thalami (*arrows*). Note also ventricular dilatation. **C:** CT demonstrates diffuse decreased attenuation of white and gray matter and increased attenuation of basal ganglia. At autopsy, there were multiple areas of hemorrhagic necrosis involving caudate, putamen, and thalamus. Cortical edema also was noted.

findings include increased echogenicity of the basal ganglia and decreased vascular pulsations.

CONGENITAL MALFORMATIONS

Cerebral malformations may be the result of errors in cytogenesis (development of molecules into cells), histogenesis (development of cells into tissues), and organogenesis (development of tissues into organs) (139). Alterations of brain development due to errors in cytogenesis are not identifiable by sonography, whereas alterations in histogenesis and organogenesis produce gross anatomic changes readily recognizable by sonography (6). Defects of histogenesis give rise to the vein of Galen malformation, Sturge-Weber syndrome, neurofibromatosis, and tuberous sclerosis. Errors of organogenesis produce a wide variety of abnormalities. Most of these are related to alterations of neural tube closure and include dysrhaphic disorders, Dandy-Walker syndrome, and agenesis of the corpus callosum. Rarer errors of organogenesis include disorders of diverticulation, cellular migration, size and myelination, and destructive lesions (38).

Disorders of Histogenesis

Vein of Galen Malformation

The vein of Galen malformation is an arteriovenous malformation resulting from failure of embryonic arteriovenous shunts to be replaced by capillaries. The end result is shunting of blood flow directly from arteries into the deep venous system. This lesion is typically found in the area of the quadrigeminal plate cistern and may compress the cerebral aqueduct, producing secondary obstructive hydrocephalus. Affected neonates often present with high output cardiac failure due to the large arteriovenous shunt. Older infants may present with an enlarging head due to obstructive hydrocephalus or seizures, whereas older children or adults present with hemorrhage (26).

On coronal sonography, the dilated vein appears as an anechoic mass in the midline, posterior to the third ventricle. On sagittal views, the dilated vein of Galen can be followed posteriorly into the straight sinus and torcular Herophili (26,70,95,107) (Fig. 32). There may be associated parenchymal atrophy secondary to shunting of blood away from the cerebral cortex or hydrocephalus. Pulsations within the mass or surrounding dilated feeding arteries can be noted with real-time sonography. Doppler imaging confirms the

markedly increased flow in the vein of Galen and allows differentiation of this dilated vessel from a cyst, but it cannot readily determine the flow pattern. Color Doppler sonography can be helpful in characterizing flow patterns and in assessing the effect of embolization therapy (137).

Tuberous Sclerosis

Tuberous sclerosis is a heredofamilial condition transmitted as an autosomal dominant trait with variable penetrance. It is characterized by hamartomas in a variety of organs and systems, including brain, skin, skeleton, and kidneys. A clinical diagnosis can be made with certainty if the triad of adenoma sebaceum, mental retardation, and seizures is present. Brain tubers composed of astrocytes, spindle cells, and glial tissue are present in all patients with tuberous sclerosis. Most are located beneath the ependyma of the lateral ventricles, but they also may be found in cortical gray matter or cerebellum. On sonography, subependymal tubers appear as echogenic nodules in the walls of the lateral ventricles (Fig. 33). Ventricular dilatation, secondary to obstruction of the foramen of Monro, may be present.

Disorders of Closure of the Neural Tube

Dysrhaphic Disorders

Dysrhaphic disorders include anencephaly, encephalocele, and meningocele or myelomeningocele. Anencephaly is the result of failure of brain development except at the base of the skull. An encephalocele is herniation of meninges through a defect in the skull. Most are located in the midline, with 70% occurring in the occipital region (33). Occipital encephaloceles frequently contain ventricles, occipital lobes, and cerebellum as well as meninges. Anencephaly and encephalocele are usually diagnosed by direct observation of the newborn, and imaging studies are rarely needed. If additional studies are required, CT is currently the method of choice to demonstrate the bony defect as well as the contents of the encephalocele.

Chiari II Malformation

The Arnold-Chiari malformation is a spectrum of anomalies associated with spinal dysrhaphism and a meningocele or myelomeningocele (90–93). Pathologically, there is caudal displacement of the cerebellum and fourth ventricle, with varying degrees of cerebellar dysplasia. Three types of Chiari malformations

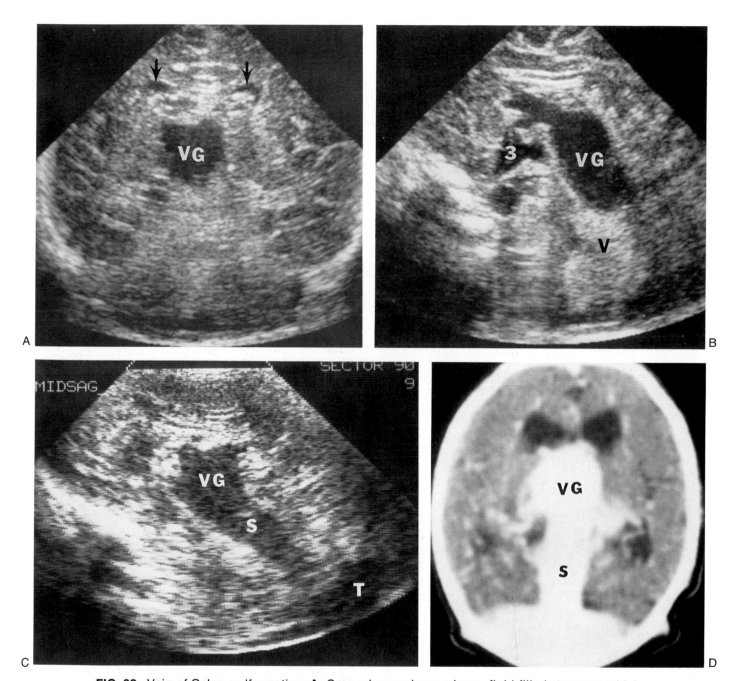

FIG. 32. Vein of Galen malformation. **A:** Coronal scan shows a large, fluid-filled structure which is the vein of Galen (*VG*) beneath the lateral ventricles (*arrows*). **B:** Midline sagittal scan shows the dilated vein of Galen (*VG*) located superior to the vermis (*V*). *3,* third ventricle. **C:** On a midline sagittal scan from another patient, the dilated vein of Galen (*VG*) can be followed posteriorly into the straight sinus (*S*) and torcular Herophili (*T*). **D:** CT scan confirms the aneurysmal vein of Galen (*VG*), straight sinus (*S*), and torcular Herophili, and shows the arterial feeders.

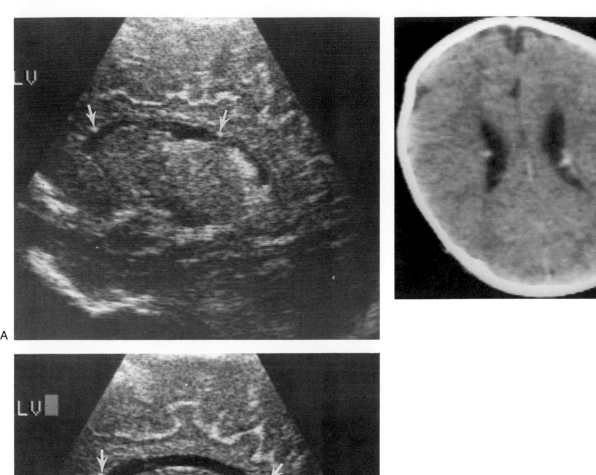

FIG. 33. Tuberous sclerosis in a 2½-year-old boy with seizures. **A,B:** Parasagittal scans through bodies of right and left lateral ventricles (respectively) show nonshadowing, highly echogenic foci (*arrows*) situated in the subependymal regions along the frontal horns and bodies. Also noted is minimal prominence of the frontal horns. **C:** CT demonstrates calcified subependymal nodules.

have been described. Type I deformity is characterized by downward displacement of the tonsils and inferior cerebellum but without displacement of the medulla and fourth ventricle. This type usually is recognized in adulthood and is rare in children. Type II malformation consists of downward displacement of the inferior cerebellum and tonsils, as well as caudad displacement of the pons, medulla, and fourth ventricle into the upper spine. A myelomeningocele invariably is associated with this type of Chiari malformation. Type III deformity is rare and consists of displacement

of the medulla, fourth ventricle, and all of the cerebellum into a high cervical or occipital encephalomeningocele. Type II malformation is the most common and usually is diagnosed in infancy, presenting as a meningocele, or more commonly, a myelomeningocele.

Sonographic findings include caudal displacement of the cerebellum, a poorly visualized fourth ventricle, and an obliterated cisterna magna (47). An enlarged massa intermedia often partially or totally fills an enlarged third ventricle. The lateral ventricles may be enlarged, with the occipital horns larger than the frontal horns, although ventricular dilatation may not be present until repair of the meningocele. Typically, there is anterior and inferior pointing of the frontal horns, referred to as a "bat-wing" appearance (9) (Fig. 34).

Dandy-Walker Complex

The Dandy-Walker complex consists of the Dandy-Walker malformation and the Dandy-Walker variant. The former is characterized by a markedly enlarged posterior fossa secondary to cystic dilatation of the

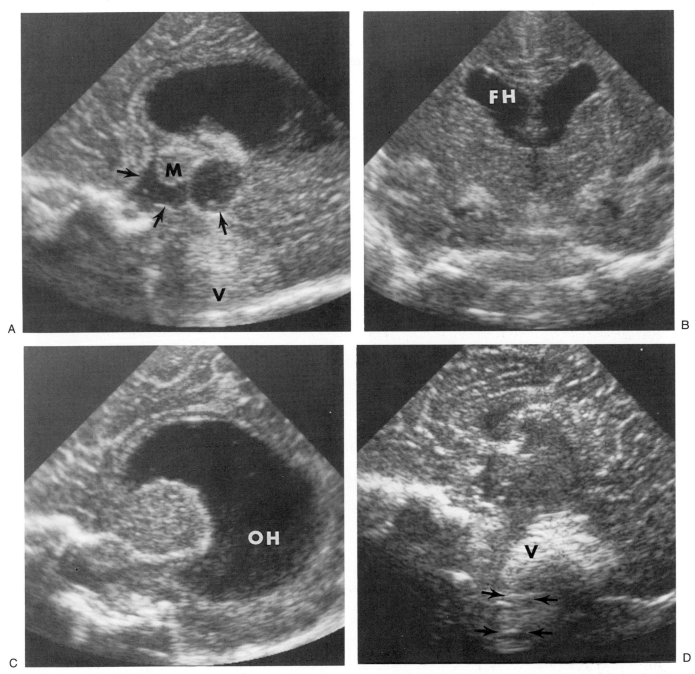

FIG. 34. Chiari II malformation. **A:** Midline sagittal scan shows the low-lying vermis (*V*) in the posterior fossa. The fourth ventricle and cisterna magna are obliterated. Also noted is a prominent massa intermedia (*M*) within the enlarged third ventricle (*arrows*). **B:** Anterior coronal and **C:** left parasagittal scans show inferior and anterior pointing (batwing appearance) of the frontal horns (*FH*). The lateral ventricle is enlarged, with the occipital horn (*OH*) more dilated than the frontal horn. **D:** Midline sagittal scan in another patient shows the cerebellar vermis (*V*) to extend through the foramen magnum into the upper cervical spine (*arrows*).

fourth ventricle and cerebellar vermian dysgenesis or agenesis. Dandy-Walker variant is characterized by a mildly enlarged posterior fossa, a posterior fossa cyst in continuity with the fourth ventricle by a narrow channel and a dysgenetic cerebellar vermis. It has been postulated that Dandy-Walker malformation is the result of an insult to the developing fourth ventricle and cerebellum and that Dandy-Walker variant results from a more limited insult to the cerebellar hemispheres (14).

Patients with both anomalies may present with developmental delay or an enlarged head circumference. The degree of developmental delay is directly related to the severity of associated supratentorial anomalies, which include hydrocephalus, agenesis of the corpus callosum, gray matter heterotopias, polymicrogyria,

and occipital encephaloceles. Hydrocephalus may be present at birth, but more frequently develops later and is present in about 75% of patients by 3 months of age. The most common systemic anomalies are cardiac anomalies and polydactyly.

The features of the Dandy-Walker complex are best seen on the midline sagittal image. These include: (a) a large, fluid-filled posterior fossa cyst that is actually a ballooned fourth ventricle; (b) partial or complete absence of the vermis; (c) hypoplasia of the cerebellar hemispheres; and (d) superior elevation of the tentorium (135). Coronal sonograms confirm the presence of the posterior fossa cyst and high position of the tentorium (Fig. 35). Occasionally, a posterior fossa arachnoid cyst or an enlarged cisterna magna may be confused for the Dandy-Walker syndrome, but the latter

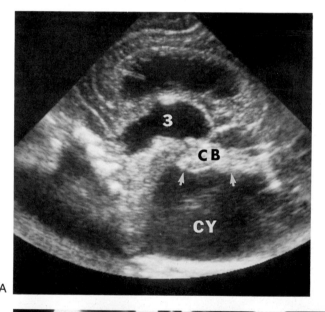

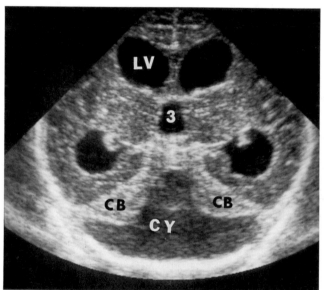

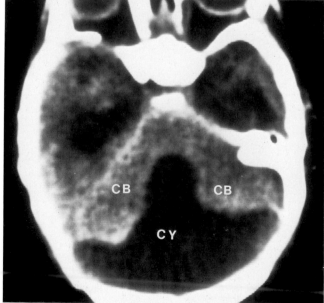

FIG. 35. Dandy-Walker syndrome. **A:** Midline sagittal scan demonstrates a large posterior fossa cyst (*CY*) which actually represents a huge fourth ventricle. The tentorium (*arrowheads*) and hypoplastic cerebellum (*CB*) are elevated by the cyst. **B:** Coronal scan shows the large cyst (*CY*) nearly filling the posterior fossa and the small cerebellar hemispheres. Also noted are dilated lateral (*LV*) and third (*3*) ventricles. The vermis is absent. **C:** CT shows enlarged posterior fossa filled with a large cyst (*CY*) that is actually the fourth ventricle and hypoplastic cerebellar hemispheres (*CB*).

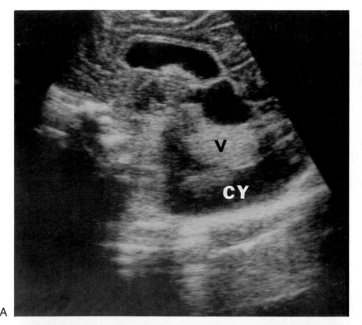

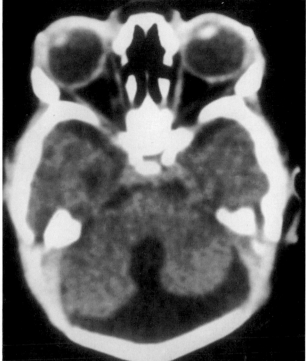

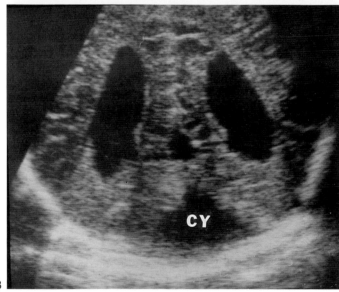

FIG. 36. Dandy-Walker variant. **A:** Midline sagittal scan demonstrates a posterior fossa cyst (*CY*) and minimally hypoplastic vermis (*V*). On this scan alone, distinguishing between Dandy-Walker malformation and a large cisterna magna may be difficult. **B:** Coronal sonogram shows the small posterior fossa cyst (*CY*), minimally hypoplastic cerebellum, and dilated ventricles. **C:** CT scan shows continuity of the cyst with the fourth ventricle, as well as the presence of a hypoplastic vermis.

two conditions have an intact cerebellar vermis and fourth ventricle.

In Dandy-Walker variant, the cerebellar hemispheres may almost appose each other, so that on a midline sagittal image they create the appearance of an intact vermis. Coronal images or CT scans through the posterior fossa will show the narrow channel between the anterior part of the fourth ventricle and the posterior fossa cyst and the absence of intervening vermis (38) (Fig. 36).

Agenesis of the Corpus Callosum

The corpus callosum is a midline interhemispheric commissure that allows the two cerebral hemispheres to share learning and memory. In callosal agenesis, the interhemispheric, commissural fibers fail to cross the midline and intersect, leaving thick bundles of fibers (Probst bundles) coursing along the superior medial aspect of each ventricle. Callosal agenesis may be complete or partial and isolated or associated with other malformations such as midline intracerebral lipoma, interhemispheric cysts, Dandy-Walker malformation, Chiari II malformation, polymicrogyria, gray matter heterotopias, and porencephaly (16). Patients with isolated callosal agenesis are usually asymptomatic. When present, symptoms are usually due to the associated anomalies and include seizures and mental retardation.

Complete absence of the corpus callosum is caused by either an *in utero* vascular or inflammatory lesion occurring before the twelfth week of gestation. Sonographic findings include absence of the corpus callosum with marked separation of the frontal horns. The frontal horns are sharply angulated laterally and indented medially by the thickened Probst bundles. The occipital horns are relatively larger than the frontal horns. Other findings include elongation and a variable degree of dorsal displacement of the third ventricle between the lateral ventricles, and distortion of the sulcal pattern. Instead of the sulci paralleling the corpus callosum and cingulate sulcus, the medial cerebral gyri and sulci have a radial pattern extending to the roof of the elevated third ventricle, through the area usually occupied by the corpus callosum (3,5,38,39) (Fig. 37).

Midline interhemispheric cysts occur in about 30% of patients with complete callosal agenesis and usually represent marked dilatation of the third ventricle (Fig. 38). Less frequently, these are arachnoid cysts or communicating porencephalic cysts. Sonographic findings include a large midline cyst widening the interhemispheric fissure and displacing the cerebral hemispheres laterally. Communication of the cyst with the lateral ventricles may be present, especially when the cyst is a markedly enlarged third ventricle (3). Associated in-

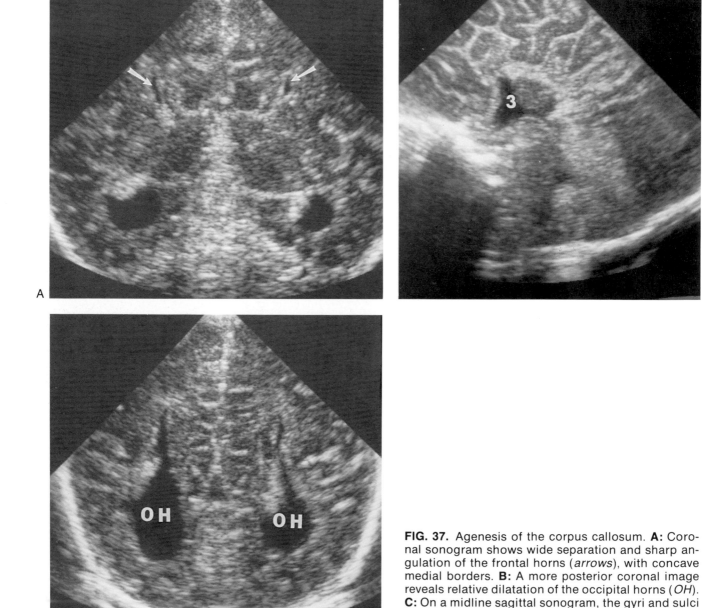

FIG. 37. Agenesis of the corpus callosum. **A:** Coronal sonogram shows wide separation and sharp angulation of the frontal horns (*arrows*), with concave medial borders. **B:** A more posterior coronal image reveals relative dilatation of the occipital horns (*OH*). **C:** On a midline sagittal sonogram, the gyri and sulci radiate toward the roof of the elevated third (*3*) ventricle, creating a "sunburst" pattern.

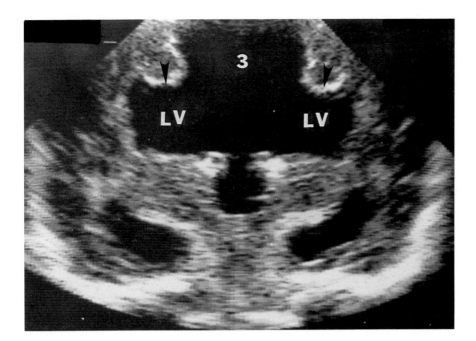

traparenchymal lipomas also can be demonstrated with sonography, appearing as highly echogenic lesions (Fig. 39).

Partial absence is the result of destruction of a previously well-formed corpus callosum and usually involves the posterior portion of the corpus callosum. Rarely, a partial anterior callosal defect is present. The third ventricle herniates cephalad, but only in the region where the corpus callosum is absent.

Disorders of Diverticulation

Holoprosencephaly

Holoprosencephaly is a deformity of the forebrain characterized by failure of separation of the prosencephalon into the telencephalon (cerebral hemispheres) and diencephalon (thalamus, hypothalamus) (34). This error usually occurs between the fourth to

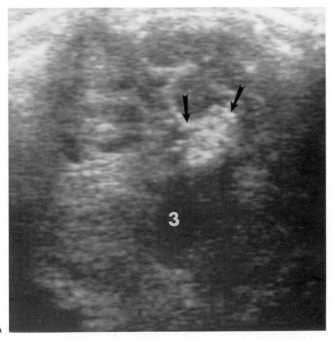

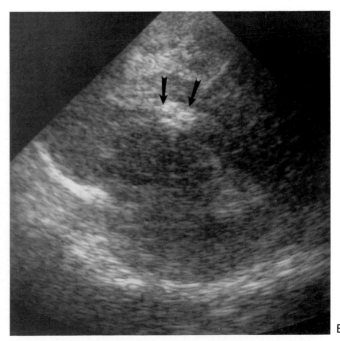

FIG. 39. Agenesis of corpus callosum with lipoma. **A:** Coronal and **B:** left parasagittal sonograms demonstrate an area of increased echogenicity (*arrows*) superior and to the left of the elevated third ventricle (*3*).

eighth weeks of intrauterine development and is believed to be the result of lack of induction of the forebrain due to an abnormality of the rostral end of the notochord. The end result is variable degrees of fusion of the paired olfactory tracts, optic tracts, and cerebral hemispheres. The severity of the anomaly varies directly with the degree of fusion of the cerebral hemispheres.

Three subtypes of holoprosencephaly have been recognized: alobar, semilobar, and lobar. Alobar holoprosencephaly is the most severe form of this condition. Clinically, patients have associated midline

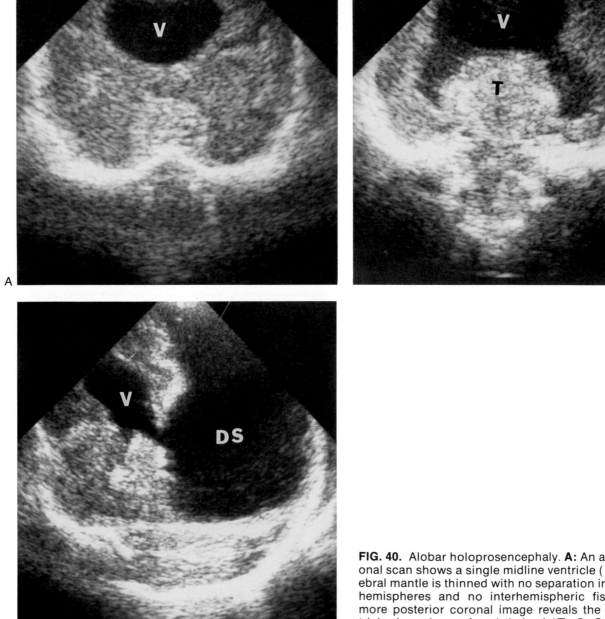

FIG. 40. Alobar holoprosencephaly. **A:** An anterior coronal scan shows a single midline ventricle (*V*). The cerebral mantle is thinned with no separation into cerebral hemispheres and no interhemispheric fissure. **B:** A more posterior coronal image reveals the single ventricle draped over fused thalami (*T*). **C:** On a midline sagittal sonogram, the midline ventricle (*V*) communicates posteriorly with a large dorsal sac (*DS*).

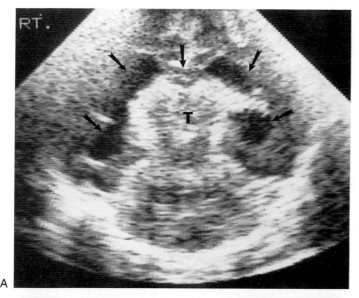

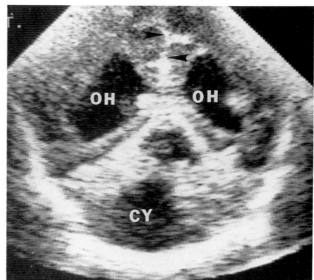

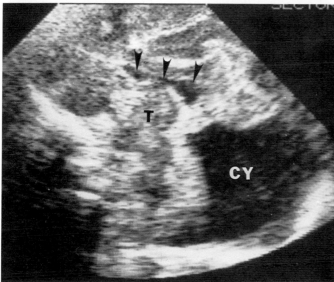

FIG. 41. Semilobar holoprosencephaly. **A:** Anterior coronal scan demonstrates a single ventricle (*arrows*) draped over fused thalami (*T*). **B:** A more posterior coronal sonogram demonstrates separate occipital horns (*OH*), a partially developed interhemispheric fissure (*arrowheads*), and a large posterior fossa cyst (*CY*). **C:** Midline sagittal sonogram shows the single ventricle (*arrowsheads*) superior to the fused thalami (*T*). The third ventricle is incorporated into the single ventricle. The large posterior fossa cyst (*CY*) is due to the Dandy-Walker malformation. (From Funk and Siegel, ref. 38, with permission.)

defects such as cyclopia, hypotelorism, cleft palate and cleft face, micrognathia, and absence of the nasal septum. On sonography there is a single midline ventricle, often associated with a dorsal sac; fused echogenic thalami; and an undifferentiated mantle of parenchyma superior to the monoventricle. There is no differentiation of frontal, temporal, or occipital horn. The third ventricle, falx, and interhemispheric fissures are absent. The cerebellum and brainstem, however, are relatively normal (Fig. 40).

Lobar and semilobar holoprosencephaly are characterized by variable separation of the cerebral hemispheres. Milder facial anomalies are present, including cleft lip and palate and hypotelorism. Semilobar

holoprosencephaly has a single ventricular body with fused thalami. Separate occipital horns are present and there is partial development of the interhemispheric fissure, usually posteriorly. The third ventricle is small or absent (Fig. 41). The fourth ventricle, brainstem, and cerebellum usually are normal.

Lobar holoprosencephaly is the mildest form of this anomaly. On sonography, there is absence of the septum pellucidum, resulting in fused frontal horns having a square shape, flat roof, and angular corners. The occipital horns are separated, but the bodies of the lateral ventricles are closely apposed. The anterior interhemispheric fissure is present but shallow. The posterior interhemispheric fissure, thalami, and posterior horns of the lateral ventricles usually are normal (Fig. 42).

Septo-optic dysplasia is believed to be in the spectrum of holoprosencephaly (34). It is characterized by agenesis of the septum pellucidum but, in addition, there is hypoplasia of the optic nerves. Affected patients often have hypopituitarism, nystagmus, and diminished visual acuity. On sonography, the septum pellucidum is absent, the frontal horns are box-like, and the anterior recess of the third ventricle is enlarged. The interhemispheric fissures are normal. Isolated absence of the septum pellucidum is a rare anomaly that needs to be differentiated from lobar holoprosencephaly and septo-optic dysplasia. In patients with isolated absence of the septum pellucidum, the frontal horns have minimally flattened roofs and are less squared than those of lobar holoprosencephaly or septo-optic dysplasia. The sonographic examina-

tion, as well as the clinical examination, is otherwise normal.

Disorders of Sulcation and Migration

Between the third and sixth months of brain development, neuroblasts in the subependymal matrix migrate radially to the cerebral cortex. Concurrent with this migration, a tangential migration of neuroblasts occurs within the cortex. Errors in migration result in lissencephaly, schizencephaly, heterotopia, and polymicrogyria.

Lissencephaly is the result of failure of neuronal migration producing a four-layered cortex, in contrast to the normal six-layered cortex. Consequently, there is failure of development of the cerebral sulci and gyri, which usually develop with the last two layers of cor-

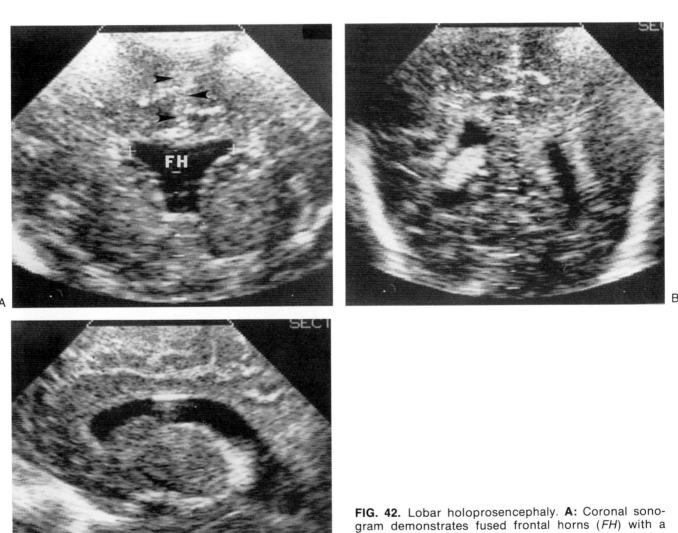

FIG. 42. Lobar holoprosencephaly. **A:** Coronal sonogram demonstrates fused frontal horns (*FH*) with a squared, flat roof, absent septum pellucidum, and a slightly shallow anterior interhemispheric fissure (*arrowheads*). **B:** Posterior coronal and **C:** parasagittal scans through the left lateral ventricle show normal bodies and occipital horns of the lateral ventricles.

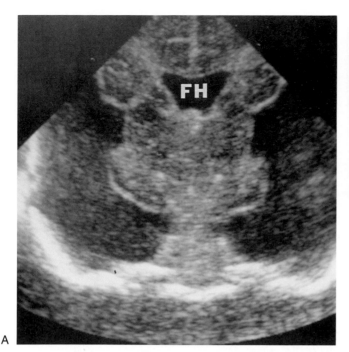

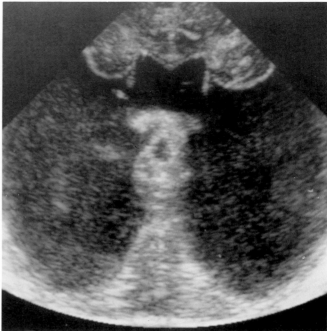

A

B

FIG. 43. Open lip schizencephaly. **A:** Anterior and **B:** posterior coronal scans show large symmetric clefts extending from the periphery of the brain into the ventricular system. The septum pellucidum is absent, creating a squared appearance of the frontal horns (*FH*).

tex. On sonography, the sylvian fissures and subarachnoid space are widened and the cortical surface of the brain is smooth without sulcal or gyral formation (4). The ventricles usually are mildly to moderately enlarged, with the occipital horns dilating more than the frontal horns (89). Although sonography can suggest the diagnosis, it is more easily recognizable on CT.

Schizencephaly is characterized by irregular full-thickness clefts extending from the lateral ventricles to the cortical surface of the brain. Presumed theories of pathogenesis include failure of germinal matrix formation or failure of migration of primitive neuroblasts within the matrix. Pathologically, these clefts are lined by cortical gray matter, frequently in the form of polymicrogyria. The clefts may be unilateral or bilateral and the lips of the clefts may be fused or open. Clefts with closed lips are very narrow with apposed walls obliterating the CSF space. Open lip clefts are large, widely separated, and distended with CSF; large portions of the hemispheres are absent. Clinically, symptoms are related to the amount of destroyed brain tissue and include microcephaly, retardation, seizures, and developmental delay.

On sonography, open lip clefts appear as large, fluid-filled spaces within the hemispheres communicating with the lateral ventricles. The edges of the clefts are echogenic because of the presence of cortical tissue. The ventricles are often enlarged with squaring of the frontal horns due to associated partial absence of the septum pellucidum (Fig. 43). Clefts with fused lips usually are difficult to diagnose by sonography.

Heterotopic gray matter represents localized abnormalities in neuronal migration. On sonography it has the same echogenicity as normal gray matter and usually is difficult to recognize. Polymicrogyria is characterized by abnormal thickening of the cortex due to the presence of many small gyri with fused surfaces. Histologically, there is a four-layer cortex. The diagnosis usually cannot be made by sonography, but instead requires tissue sampling.

Destructive Brain Lesions

Hydranencephaly

Hydranencephaly is a condition characterized by absent brain mantle and subadjacent white matter, with replacement of the cerebral hemispheres by a thin-walled, membranous sac containing CSF. The outer layer of the sac is composed of leptomeningeal connective tissue and the inner layer is composed of remnants of cortex and white matter. The pathogenesis of hydranencephaly remains unclear. Some cases may be due to intrauterine infection while others may represent *in utero* occlusion of the carotid arteries. Pathologically, the thalami, inferior parts of the frontal

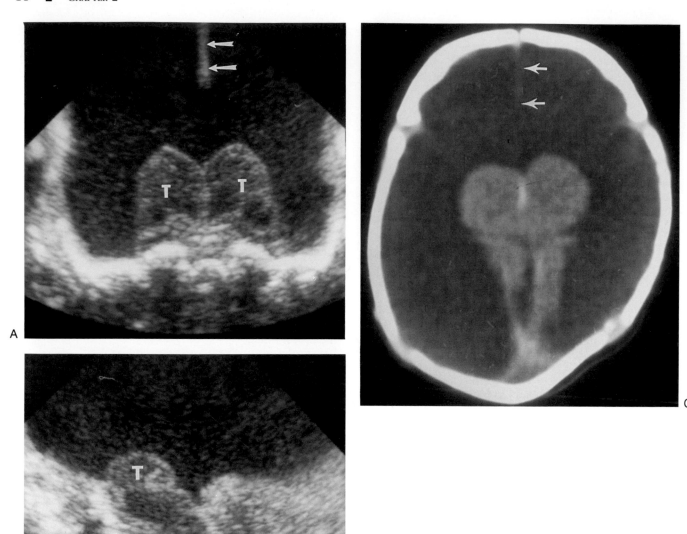

FIG. 44. Hydranencephaly. **A:** Coronal and **B:** midline sagittal images show replacement of the cerebrum by a large, fluid-filled sac. The thalami (*T*), cerebellar vermis (*V*), and falx cerebri (*arrows*) are preserved. Increased echogenicity in the occipital area on the sagittal image represents through-transmission, related to the fluid content of the cerebral hemispheres. **C:** CT scan shows complete absence of the cerebral hemispheres with the exception of the thalami and some occipital cortex. The falx cerebri (*arrows*) is present.

lobes, and inferomedial aspects of the temporal lobes are present. The cerebellum also is normal, although the brainstem is atrophic.

The sonographic features of hydranencephaly are: (a) complete absence of the cerebral hemispheres, (b) a large, fluid-filled supratentorial cavity, (c) normal thalami and cerebellar hemispheres, and (d) an intact falx cerebri (Fig. 44). The major diagnostic problem is differentiation of hydranencephaly from severe hydrocephalus. In severe hydrocephalus, there is a thin rim of brain parenchyma surrounding the ventricles, whereas there is no peripheral tissue in hydranencephaly. This distinction is important because children with hydrocephalus may respond well to CSF shunting if it is performed early, and they can have normal intelligence. In contrast, CSF diversion will not improve intellectual development in children with hydranencephaly. Although sonography occasionally can be used to identify the thin rim of white matter and cortex that is present in severe hydrocephalus, CT or magnetic resonance imaging (MRI) are superior in imaging the periphery of the brain.

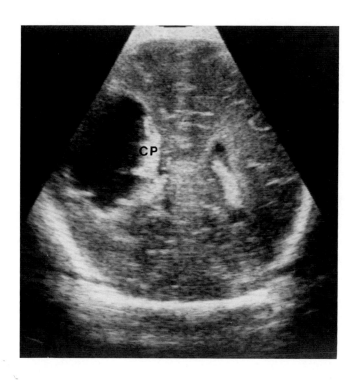

FIG. 45. Porencephaly. Coronal scan shows a smooth-walled, fluid-filled cavity adjacent to and including the right frontal horn. *CP,* choroid plexus.

Porencephaly

The term "porencephaly" has been used to describe both congenital and acquired focal cavities within the brain parenchyma. Here it will be used to refer to brain destruction during the first half of gestation, which is the time before the brain is able to make a glial response. Typically, the porencephalic cyst appears as a unilocular, smooth-walled, fluid-filled cavity. Porencephalic cysts also have been called encephaloclastic porencephalies. They need to be differentiated from agenetic porencephalies (i.e., the schizencephalies) which are the result of an early developmental error, and from encephalomalacia which occurs either late in gestation or postpartum, after the brain is able to make a glial scar. Pathologically, porencephalic cysts have a white matter lining without surrounding glial reaction, whereas encephalomalacic cavities contain glial septations and an irregular glial wall. The capability of the fetal brain to produce glial reaction occurs sometime during the late second or third trimester. On sonography, porencephaly appears as a fairly smooth-walled anechoic cavity (Fig. 45). Differentiation between porencephaly and a single area of encephalomalacia is difficult unless septations are present. The latter features would favor encephalomalacia. Schizencephaly can be recognized by the presence of unilateral or bilateral clefts that extend the full thickness of the cerebrum from the ependymal to the pial surfaces. There is no evidence of any glial scar along the clefts (15).

INTRACRANIAL INFECTION

Viral and Parasitic Infections

A large number of viral and protozoan infections involve the central nervous system. In the neonate, the most common causative organisms of meningoencephalitis are cytomegalovirus, *Toxoplasma gondii,* rubella virus, and herpes simplex virus. Herpes simplex virus type 2, which affects the maternal genital tract, causes most of the perinatally acquired infection (143). Herpes simplex infection is acquired at the time of birth, usually during passage through an infected birth canal. Cytomegalovirus, toxoplasmosis, and rubella virus generally are transmitted via the transplacental route. Pathologically, the various viruses produce a necrotizing inflammatory process.

Sonography is useful in identifying the parenchymal and ventricular abnormalities associated with pre- and perinatal infections. The spectrum of sonographic findings of viral and protozoan infections include dystrophic calcifications, ventricular dilatation, cystic degeneration, and echogenic vasculature in the basal ganglia (36,136). Calcifications appear as brightly echogenic foci with or without distal acoustic shadowing. Their distribution varies with the causative organism and severity of infection (51). Calcifications are common in cytomegalic inclusion disease. In mild cases, the calcifications are scattered in the periventricular

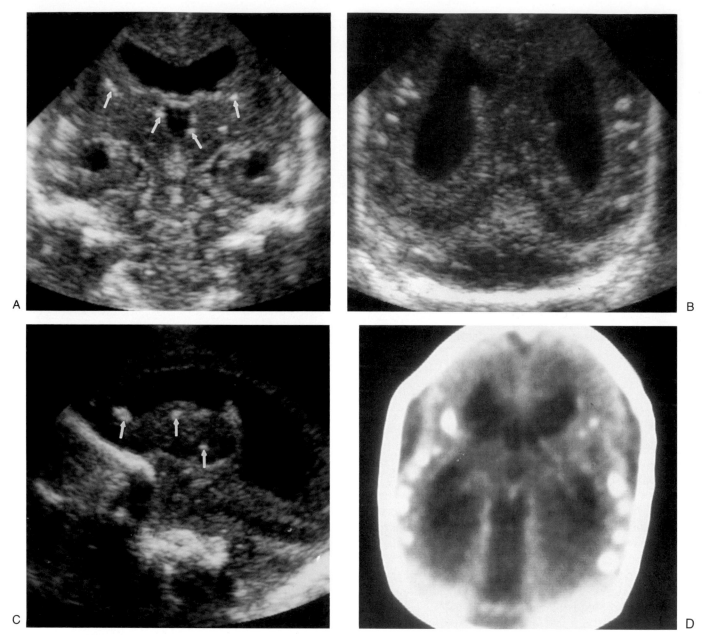

FIG. 46. Cytomegalovirus infection. **A,B:** Two coronal and **C:** left parasagittal scans show scattered foci (*arrows*) of increased echogenicity, representing subependymal and parenchymal calcifications. Also noted is ventricular dilatation. **D:** *CT* confirms extensive cortical calcifications, ventricular enlargement, and enlarged sylvian fissure.

regions of dilated lateral ventricles. In severe cases there is extensive cortical calcification (Fig. 46). Calcifications also are common in toxoplasmosis; they usually involve the periventricular region, basal ganglia, and cortex. As with cytomegalovirus infection, there is a spectrum from mild disease with a few periventricular calcifications, to severe involvement with diffuse cortical calcification. In herpes simplex type 2 infection, the calcifications tend to be massive, involving both gray and white matter; occasionally they have a gyriform appearance (Fig. 47). In congenital

rubella, calcifications are small and may involve either the periventricular region or cortex.

Ventricular dilatation also can be seen and is thought to be secondary to either obstruction of CSF flow by inflammatory exudate (22) or secondary to diffuse brain atrophy. Hydrocephalus and atrophy can coexist with either being dominant. Cystic degeneration associated with intrauterine infections may be periventricular or parenchymal, and focal or diffuse (118,129) (Fig. 48). Recently, brightly echogenic basal ganglia and thalamic vessels have been described in congenital

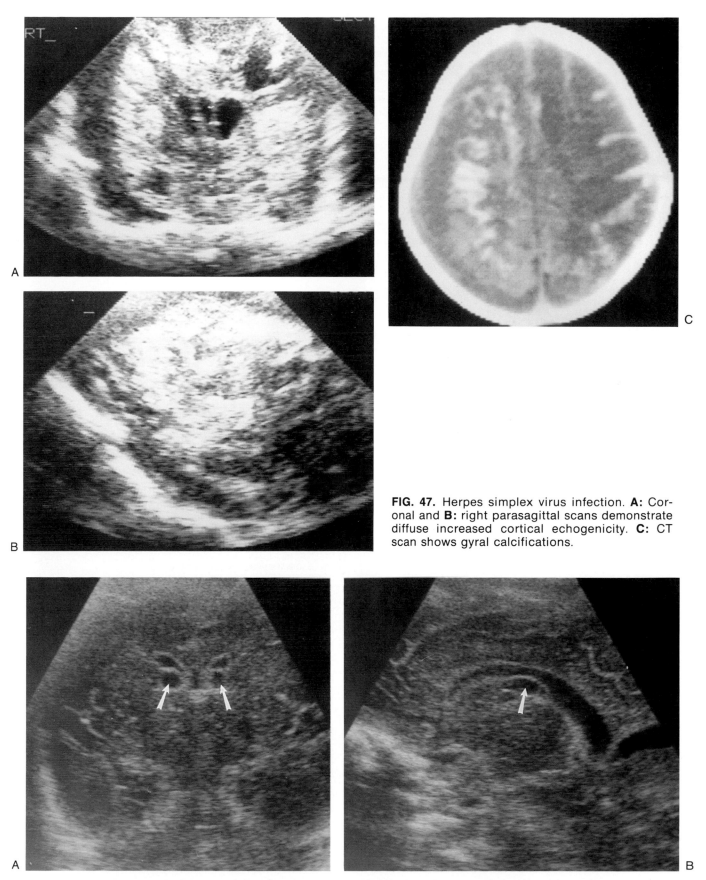

FIG. 47. Herpes simplex virus infection. **A:** Coronal and **B:** right parasagittal scans demonstrate diffuse increased cortical echogenicity. **C:** CT scan shows gyral calcifications.

FIG. 48. Postinfectious subependymal cysts. **A:** Coronal and **B:** left parasagittal scans demonstrate well-defined cystic lesions (*arrows*) superior to the caudothalamic groove.

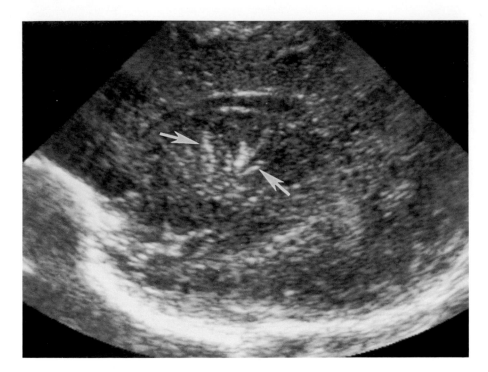

FIG. 49. Echogenic vasculature of the basal ganglia. Parasagittal sonogram reveals several linear, echogenic structures (*arrows*) within the basal ganglia, representing vessels. Cultures were positive for cytomegalovirus.

infections. Mineralization of arterial walls or hypercellular arterial walls are the most likely reasons for the echogenicity of these vessels (136) (Fig. 49).

Bacterial and Fungal Infection

Bacterial infection of the brain in neonates may be acquired perinatally by spread of bacteria from the cervix to the amniotic fluid or postnatally by hematogenous spread (36). The organisms most commonly responsible for intracranial infection in the newborn infant are group B streptococci and *Escherichia coli.* After the neonatal period, the most common inciting organisms are *Haemophilus influenzae, Streptococcus pneumoniae,* and *Neisseria meningitidis.* Pathologically, the acute changes of bacterial meningitis or meningoencephalitis are arachnoiditis, ventriculitis, vasculitis, cerebral edema, and infarction (17). The disease may progress into a widespread cerebritis, evolve into a localized abscess, or resolve completely. Late complications include multicystic encephalomalacia, atrophy, and hydrocephalus. Subdural effusions may be present early or late in the course of disease. Fungal infections are rare and have a propensity to affect premature infants or those on long-term antibiotic therapy. The most common causative organism is *Candida albicans. Candida* invades blood vessels and causes hemorrhagic infarcts as well as abscesses.

Sonography has been shown to be useful in evaluating the complications of meningoencephalitis. Sonographic findings of acute bacterial infection include echogenic sulci, abnormally increased parenchymal echogenicity, abscess, extraaxial fluid collections, ventriculitis, and ventricular enlargement (10,21,29, 54,108). The most common finding of bacterial meningitis is echogenic sulci, occurring in about 40% of patients (54). The increased sulcal echogenicity is believed to be due to accumulation of inflammatory exudate in fissures and sulci around the pial and subarachnoid vessels. In some instances, the sulci are widened as well as echogenic.

Abnormal parenchymal echogenicity may be focal or diffuse, and probably reflects cerebritis, brain edema, or infarction due to vasculitis (Fig. 50). When the increased echogenicity is focal, particularly when limited to a gyral distribution, the likelihood of infarct increases (10). In general, abnormal parenchymal echogenicity appears to be related to significant neurologic sequelae, unlike increased sulcal echogenicity which is not associated with significant neurologic deficit (54).

Brain abscess occurs as a complication of cerebritis, particularly cerebritis caused by virulent gram-negative organisms, such as *Proteus mirabilis* or *Citrobacter diversus.* The abscesses are usually located in the cerebral hemispheres, with the frontal lobe most often affected. On sonography, the abscess appears as a well-defined hypoechoic area surrounded by an echogenic rim (30). The evolution from cerebritis (increased parenchymal echogenicity) to abscess formation is 7 to 14 days. Compression of the ipsilateral

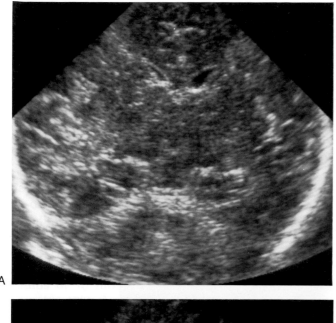

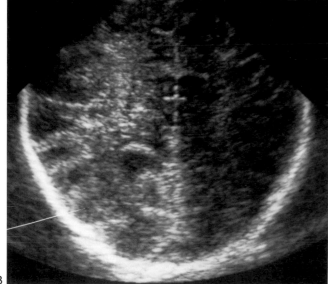

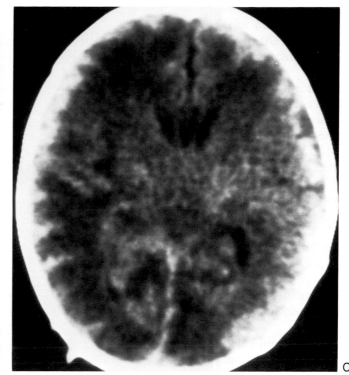

FIG. 50. Bacterial meningitis. **A,B:** Two coronal sonograms show increased echogenicity throughout the right hemisphere. **C:** CT demonstrates decreased attenuation of gray and white matter, greater on the right than the left, representing cortical infarction. Follow-up CT scan one month later showed changes of cystic encephalomalacia.

ventricle and displacement of midline structures are associated findings.

Subdural or subarachnoid fluid effusions are often seen as transient findings in patients with bacterial meningitis, especially *Haemophilus influenzae*. In most instances, these are not clinically significant and do not require aspiration or drainage unless there is a significant shift of intracranial structures or protracted fever and seizure activity suggesting empyema (54). Extraaxial fluid collections are generally hypoechoic relative to brain and are located over the frontal temporal regions of the brain (Fig. 51). Subdural fluid collections along the convexity displace the brain away from the cranial vault, while fluid collections in the interhemispheric fissure appear as widening of the fissure. Subdural empyema cannot be differentiated from a sterile fluid collection by sonography. Computerized tomography is required to demonstrate the enhancing subdural membrane.

Ventriculitis has been reported in 65% to 90% of cases of neonatal meningitis and contributes significantly to morbidity and mortality (62). It is believed to be the result of hematogenous spread of infection to the choroid plexus where bacteria produce a choroid plexitis, ependymitis, and inflammatory exudate in the ventricular fluid. Later, glial septa may develop and

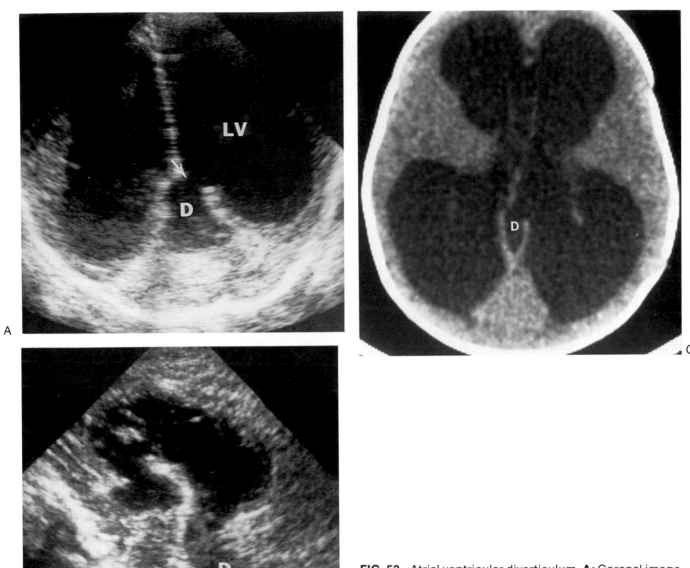

FIG. 53. Atrial ventricular diverticulum. **A:** Coronal image shows dilated lateral ventricles and a diverticulum (*D*) in communication (*arrow*) with the left lateral ventricle (*LV*). **B:** Midsagittal sonogram through the left lateral ventricle clearly shows the communication between the diverticulum (*D*) and the dilated ventricle. *CB*, cerebellum. **C:** CT confirms dilated lateral ventricles and the left ventricular diverticulum (*D*).

(71) (Fig. 53). These diverticula can be mistaken for arachnoid cysts, but demonstration of continuity of the trigone of the lateral ventricle with the diverticulum establishes the diagnosis. Other sites of herniation include the suprapineal and anterior recesses of the third ventricle. In some cases, ventricular herniation occurs at the site of a needle puncture of a dilated ventricle. The anatomic basis of ventricular diverticula is believed to be a focal dehiscence of the lateral wall through which pia and CSF protrude.

The primary sonographic criterion for determining the site of intraventricular hydrocephalus is the point of transition from a dilated to nondilated ventricle. The

site of obstruction varies with etiology. If the foramen of Monro is obstructed, there is lateral ventricular enlargement which may be asymmetric. Aqueductal stenosis is associated with dilatation of third and lateral ventricles; the fourth ventricle is normal or small (Fig. 54). It usually results from hemorrhage in premature neonates, although it may be inherited as an X-linked dominant trait. Obstruction of the foramina of Magendie and Luschka produces cystic dilatation of the fourth ventricle and variable degrees of dilatation of the third and lateral ventricles. Extraventricular obstructive hydrocephalus and dysfunctional or nonobstructive hydrocephalus are characterized by dilated

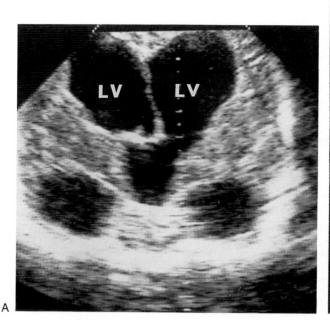 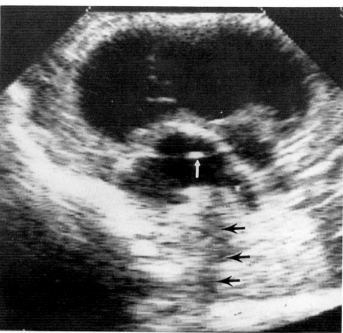

FIG. 54. Hydrocephalus secondary to aqueductal stenosis. **A:** Coronal and **B:** midline sagittal images show dilated lateral (*LV*) and third ventricles with a normal sized fourth ventricle (*black arrows*). Also note the massa intermedia (*white arrow*) within the third ventricle. (Fig. 54B from Siegel, et al., ref. 125, with permission.)

lateral and third ventricles and varying degrees of fourth ventricular dilatation (Fig. 55). In as many as 25% to 35% of cases of extraventricular obstructive hydrocephalus, there is little or no dilatation of the fourth ventricle (94).

Two common causes of hydrocephalus are PVH-IVH and meningitis. Acute hydrocephalus due to hemorrhage is most often the result of blood clot obstructing the ventricular system or arachnoid villi. In the

acute phase of meningitis, hydrocephalus may be caused by clumping of cellular debris in the ventricles or it may result from inflammation of the arachnoid granulations. Chronic hydrocephalus after hemorrhage or meningitis is the result of fibrosis of the subarachnoid space with subsequent adhesive arachnoiditis (59,63,64).

Following placement of shunt catheters, sonography can be utilized to document the position of the shunt,

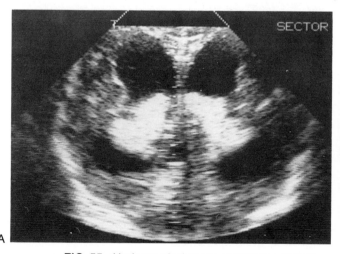 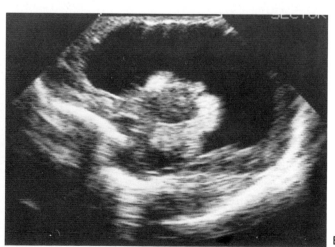

FIG. 55. Hydrocephalus secondary to villous hypertrophy of the choroid plexus. A CT scan several months earlier had shown ventriculomegaly. **A:** Posterior coronal and **B:** parasagittal scans following ventriculoperitoneal shunting demonstrate ventricular dilatation and enlarged choroid plexus. Hydrocephalus was due to excessive CSF production. (From Shackelford, ref. 117, with permission.)

monitor ventricular size, and detect intracranial complications, including recurrent obstruction, trapped fourth ventricle, intraventricular hemorrhage, and subdural hematomas. On sonography, intracranial shunts are highly echogenic and easily recognizable (117). Less common complications of ventriculo-peritoneal shunting include ascites, pseudocyst formation, and bowel perforation or obstruction.

INTRACRANIAL CYSTS AND NEOPLASMS

Intracranial Cysts

Intracranial cystic lesions may be congenital, inflammatory, neoplastic, traumatic, or vascular in etiology. Arachnoid cyst is the most common cause of

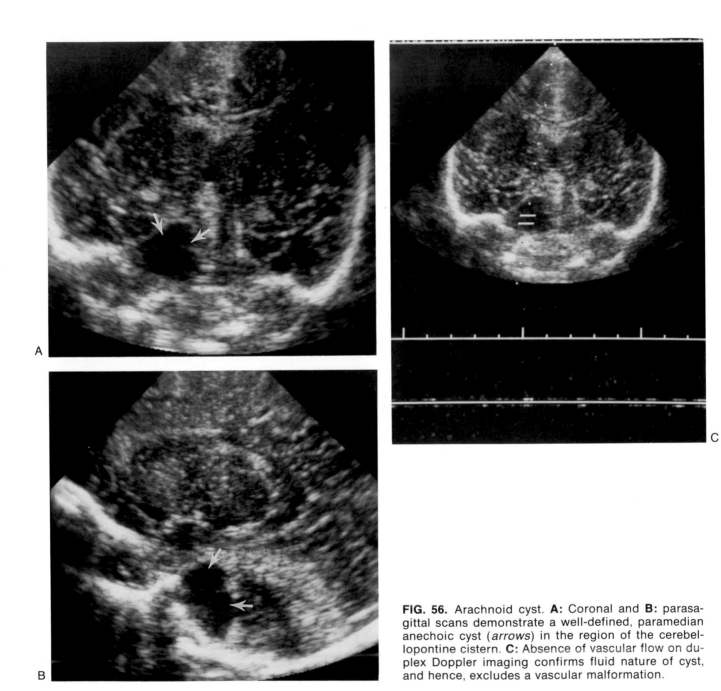

FIG. 56. Arachnoid cyst. **A:** Coronal and **B:** parasagittal scans demonstrate a well-defined, paramedian anechoic cyst (*arrows*) in the region of the cerebellopontine cistern. **C:** Absence of vascular flow on duplex Doppler imaging confirms fluid nature of cyst, and hence, excludes a vascular malformation.

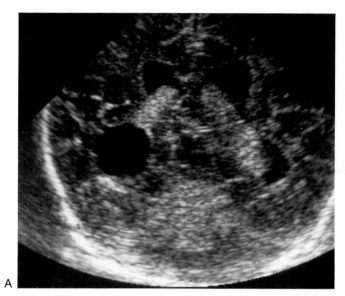 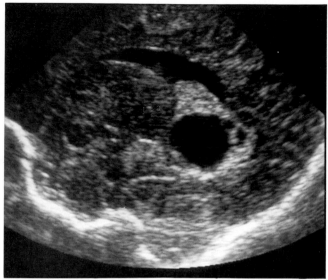

FIG. 57. Choroid plexus cyst in a patient with trisomy 13. **A:** Coronal and **B:** right parasagittal images demonstrate a large anechoic mass, representing a cyst of the choroid plexus.

an intracranial cyst and accounts for 1% of all space-occupying intracranial masses in childhood. It may be primary due to abnormal splitting of the arachnoid, or acquired due to entrapment of CSF by arachnoid adhesions. The cyst is located between the brain and dura, is lined by arachnoid, contains CSF, and has no communication with the ventricle. The most common locations for arachnoid cysts are the sylvian fissure, and the suprasellar, quadrigeminal plate, cerebellopontine, and infratentorial midline cisterns. Rarely, they are found in the interhemispheric fissure and cerebral convexity. On sonography, an arachnoid cyst appears as a fluid-filled lesion with an indiscernible wall that displaces adjacent structures (24) (Fig. 56).

Congenital intracranial cysts also may occur in association with other congenital malformations. Agenesis of the corpus callosum and alobar holoprosencephaly are the two malformations most frequently associated with large midline dorsal cysts (see earlier discussion). Intracranial cysts can also be seen in association with Dandy-Walker malformation and variant (80). As discussed previously, the intracranial cyst in the Dandy-Walker complex is a large, dilated fourth ventricle. Congenital syndromes associated with cysts include Zellweger (cerebro-hepato-renal) syndrome and trisomy 13 (78) (Fig. 57).

Care must be taken not to confuse intracranial cystic masses with normal cystic areas, including the cisterna

magna and cavum septi pellucidi and vergae. These normal structures are associated with normal ventricles and lack mass effect. Midline cystic masses also may be noted after shunting of patients with Chiari II malformation. The precise origin of these cysts is uncertain, but they are typically found near the quadrigeminal cistern.

Acquired cystic lesions include areas of encephalomalacia and subependymal and periventricular cysts (72). Subependymal and periventricular cysts and encephalomalacic cavities are the result of brain necrosis secondary to hemorrhage, infarction, or infection and occur after the brain has developed the capacity for glial response to injury. Encephalomalacia may be localized and may mimic porencephaly or schizencephaly (see earlier discussion), or it may be multifocal. On sonography, localized encephalomalacia appears as a fluid-filled lesion, frequently containing septations.

Multiple cystic encephalomalacia results from a diffuse insult to the brain. Pathologic examination reveals bilateral, supratentorial cavities of variable size separated by glial septations. Typically, the cavities are found in the cortex and peripheral white matter. The periventricular white matter, inferior temporal lobes, and cerebellum are usually spared. Sonographic findings are those of multiple, bilateral cysts of diverse size and shape separated by echogenic septae; ventricu-

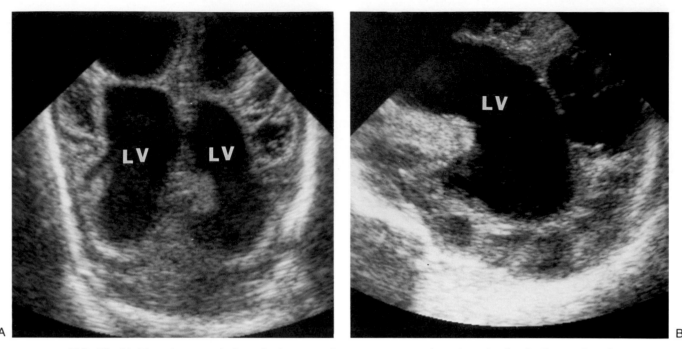

FIG. 58. Multicystic encephalomalacia secondary to severe perinatal asphyxia. **A:** Coronal and **B:** parasagittal images 2 weeks after a hypoxic episode shows dilated ventricles (*LV*) and multiple cystic lesions within the brain parenchyma.

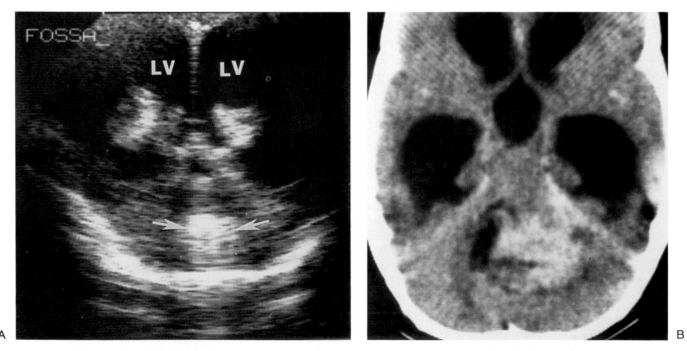

FIG. 59. Cerebellar astrocytoma. **A:** Coronal sonogram shows a poorly defined echogenic mass (*arrows*) in the posterior fossa. Moderate dilatation of the lateral ventricles (*LV*) is also present. **B:** CT scan demonstrates an enhancing mass with calcification in the cerebellum, proven at operation to be an astrocytoma.

lomegaly; and well-defined, thickened ventricular walls (Fig. 58).

Neoplasms

Approximately 10% of all intracranial tumors are detected in the first 2 years of life, and of these, only 35% are seen in the first year of life. Identification of a tumor in the newborn is even rarer. The most frequent tumors in young infants are astrocytomas, primitive neuroectodermal tumors, choroid plexus papillomas, teratomas, and ependymomas (24,69).

Intracranial neoplasms discovered in the neonatal period are generally quite large and echogenic relative to surrounding cerebral cortex (55,102,112) (Fig. 59). Areas of cystic degeneration and necrosis appear as anechoic components and have been noted in teratomas and ependymomas. Occasionally calcifications are present, appearing as areas of increased echogenicity with acoustic shadowing. Obstructive hydrocephalus and displacement of midline structures are associated findings (131).

Although sonography is not very specific for intracranial tumors, it can identify the presence of a lesion. However, CT scans or MRI are required to show the precise site and extent of the tumor. Intraoperatively, sonography can be used to localize the tumor for biopsy and complete excision, reducing the extent of brain exploration and decreasing damage to normal brain.

COMPARATIVE IMAGING

Computerized tomography and sonography are equally effective in identifying hydrocephalus (125). However, CT occasionally is superior to sonography in determining the level of ventricular obstruction, particularly in distinguishing between intra- and extraventricular hydrocephalus. It also is better in characterizing lesions, particularly masses, associated with obstruction. Therefore, a CT scan is recommended if sonography fails or cannot determine the level and cause of ventricular obstruction or if sonography demonstrates a parenchymal mass that needs to be characterized further.

Computerized tomography is generally better than sonography in showing calcifications and is recommended in any infant suspected of having intracranial infection if the sonogram is normal (51). Sonography, however, is superior to CT for demonstrating intraventricular septations or debris following infection that cause hydrocephalus via compartmentalization of the ventricles. This information is important in assisting drainage tube placement (138).

Sonography and CT are equally reliable in detecting SEH, moderate to large intraventricular hemorrhage or subdural collections, and large focal parenchymal lesions (43,68,125). Computerized tomography is somewhat better than sonography in demonstrating blood within normal sized ventricles, choroid plexus hemorrhages, and small extraaxial hematomas or fluid collections (81). These lesions often are not clinically significant; therefore, the inability of sonography to detect these abnormalities is probably not a significant limitation. The one exception is infants who are suspected to be abused; in this circumstance, the diagnosis of subarachnoid hemorrhage and other small blood collections is important for management. Hence, most authors believe that sonography should be the initial screening procedure in infants with suspected intracranial bleeding (125). Computerized tomography is recommended only if there is a clinical suspicion of serious traumatic injury or child abuse and the sonogram is normal (56).

Sonography is superior to CT in detecting the non-hemorrhagic form of periventricular white matter disease or leukomalacia because of the normal decreased attenuation of the neonate brain on CT scans. The latter makes it difficult to define the exact border between abnormal and normal parenchyma. Sonography also appears somewhat superior to CT in depicting small periventricular cysts, probably related to density averaging on CT (115). Sonography, therefore, is the procedure of choice for screening infants with suspected hypoxic-ischemic encephalopathy. Computerized tomography or MRI probably should be reserved for further investigation after sonography in those patients with hypoxia and progressive neurologic deterioration. It is particularly useful in the study of selective neuronal and parasagittal cerebral injuries.

Magnetic resonance imaging is more sensitive than sonography and CT in the diagnosis of congenital malformations (13,15). It is particularly sensitive in detecting neuronal migration anomalies such as agyria, polygyria, polymicrogyria, schizencephaly, and gray matter heterotopias, because of its exceptional ability to differentiate between gray and white matter (13,128). Magnetic resonance imaging is also known to be superior to sonography and CT in demonstrating complex anomalies around the craniovertebral junction, such as Arnold-Chiari malformation (146). At the present time, sonography remains the screening procedure of choice for detecting intracranial anomalies in children with enlarged head circumference or myelomeningoceles. Magnetic resonance imaging is the examination of choice to follow sonography if more information is required about the extent of abnormality.

REFERENCES

1. Allan WC, Holt PJ, Sawyer LR, Tito AM, Meade SK. Ventricular dilation after neonatal periventricular-intraventricular hemorrhage. *Am J Dis Child* 1982;136:589–593.

2. Armstrong D, Norman MG. Periventricular leukomalacia in neonates: Complications and sequelae. *Arch Dis Child* 1974;49:367–375.
3. Atlas SW, Shkolnik A, Naidich TP. Sonographic recognition of agenesis of the corpus callosum. *AJR* 1985;145:167–173.
4. Babcock DS. Sonographic demonstration of lissencephaly (agyria). *J Ultrasound Med* 1983;2:465–466.
5. Babcock DS. The normal, absent, and abnormal corpus callosum: Sonographic findings. *Radiology* 1984;151:449–453.
6. Babcock DS. Sonography of congenital malformations of the brain. *Neuroradiology* 1986;28:428–439.
7. Babcock DS, Ball W Jr. Postasphyxial encephalopathy in full-term infants: Ultrasound diagnosis. *Radiology* 1983;148:417–423.
8. Babcock DS, Bove KE, Han BK. Intracranial hemorrhage in premature infants: Sonographic-pathologic correlation. *AJNR* 1982;3:309–317.
9. Babcock DS, Han BK. Cranial sonographic findings in meningomyelocele. *AJR* 1981;136:563–569.
10. Babcock DS, Han BK. Sonographic recognition of gyral infarction in meningitis. *AJR* 1985;144:833–836.
11. Babcock DS, Han BK, Weiss RG, Ryckman FC. Brain abnormalities in infants on extracorporeal membrane oxygenation: Sonographic and CT findings. *AJR* 1989;153:571–576.
12. Bada HS, Miller JE, Menke JA, et al. Intraventricular pressure and cerebral arterial pulsatile flow measurements in neonatal intraventricular hemorrhage. *J Pediatr* 1982;100:291–296.
13. Barkovich AJ, Chuang SH, Norman D. MR of neuronal migration anomalies. *AJR* 1988;150:179–187.
14. Barkovich AJ, Kjos BO, Norman D, Edwards MS. Revised classification of posterior fossa cysts and cystlike malformations based on the results of multiplanar MR imaging. *AJNR* 1989;10:977–988.
15. Barkovich AJ, Norman D. MR imaging of schizencephaly. *AJNR* 1988;9:297–302.
16. Barkovich AJ, Norman D. Anomalies of the corpus callosum: Correlation with further anomalies of the brain. *AJNR* 1988;9:493–501.
17. Berman PH, Banker BQ. Neonatal meningitis. A clinical and pathological study of 29 cases. *Pediatrics* 1966;38:6–24.
18. Bowerman RA, Donn SM, DiPietro MA, D'Amato CJ, Hicks SP. Periventricular leukomalacia in the pre-term newborn infant: Sonographic and clinical features. *Radiology* 1984; 151:383–388.
19. Bowerman RA, Donn SM, Silver TM, Jaffe MH. Natural history of neonatal periventricular/intraventricular hemorrhage and its complications: Sonographic observations. *AJNR* 1984;5:527–538.
20. Bowie JD, Kirks DR, Rosenberg ER, Clair MR. Caudothalamic groove: Value in identification of germinal matrix hemorrhage by sonography in preterm neonates. *AJR* 1983;141:1317–1320.
21. Brown BSJ, Thorp P. The ultrasonographic diagnosis of bacterial meningitis and ventriculitis in infancy: Six case reports. *J Can Assoc Radiol* 1984;35:47–51.
22. Carey BM, Arthur RJ, Houlsby WT. Ventriculitis in congenital rubella: Ultrasound demonstration. *Pediatr Radiol* 1987; 17:415–416.
23. Chow PP, Horgan JG, Taylor KJW. Neonatal periventricular leukomalacia: Real-time sonographic diagnosis with CT correlation. *AJR* 1985;144:155–160.
24. Chuang S, Harwood-Nash D. Tumors and cysts. *Neuroradiology* 1986;28:463–475.
25. Cremin BJ, Lamont AC. Neurosonography in full-term cerebral haemorrhage. *Br J Radiol* 1985;58:111–114.
26. Cubberley DA, Jaffe RB, Nixon GW. Sonographic demonstration of galenic arteriovenous malformations in the neonate. *AJNR* 1982;3:435–439.
27. Delaporte B, Labrune M, Imbert MC, Dehan M. Early echographic findings in non-hemorrhagic periventricular leukomalacia of the premature infant. *Pediatr Radiol* 1985;15:82–84.
28. DiPietro MA, Brody BA, Teele RL. Peritrigonal echogenic "blush" on cranial sonography: Pathologic correlates. *AJR* 1986;146:1067–1072.
29. Edwards MK, Brown DL, Chua GT. Complicated infantile meningitis: Evaluation by real-time sonography. *AJNR* 1982; 3:431–434.
30. Enzmann DR, Britt RH, Lyons B, Carroll B, Wilson DA, Buxton J. High-resolution ultrasound evaluation of experimental brain abscess evolution: Comparison with computed tomography and neuropathology. *Radiology* 1982;142:95–102.
31. Farruggia S, Babcock DS. The cavum septi pellucidi: Its appearance and incidence with cranial ultrasonography in infancy. *Radiology* 1981;139:147–150.
32. Fiske CE, Filly RA, Callen PW. The normal choroid plexus: Ultrasonographic appearance of the neonatal head. *Radiology* 1981;141:467–471.
33. Fitz CR. Midline anomalies of the brain and spine. *Radiol Clin North Am* 1982;20:95–104.
34. Fitz CR. Holoprosencephaly and related entities. *Neuroradiology* 1983;25:225–238.
35. Fleischer AC, Hutchison AA, Bundy AL, et al. Serial sonography of posthemorrhagic ventricular dilatation and porencephaly after intracranial hemorrhage in the preterm neonate. *AJR* 1983;141:451–455.
36. Frank JL. Sonography of intracranial infection in infants and children. *Neuroradiology* 1986;28:440–451.
37. Franze I, Forrest TS. Sonographic diagnosis of a subdural hematoma as the initial manifestation of hemophilia in a newborn. *J Ultrasound Med* 1988;7:149–152.
38. Funk KC, Siegel MJ. Sonography of congenital midline brain malformations. *Radiographics* 1988;8:11–25.
39. Gebarski SS, Gebarski KS, Bowerman RA, Silver TM. Agenesis of the corpus callosum: Sonographic features. *Radiology* 1984;151:443–448.
40. Goldstein RB, Filly RA, Toi A. Septal veins: A normal finding on neonatal cranial sonography. *Radiology* 1986;161:623–624.
41. Goodwin L, Quisling RG. The neonatal cisterna magna: Ultrasonic evaluation. *Radiology* 1983;149:691–695.
42. Grant EG. Sonography of the premature brain: Intracranial hemorrhage and periventricular leukomalacia. *Neuroradiology* 1986;28:476–490.
43. Grant EG, Borts FT, Schellinger D, McCullough DC, Sivasubramanian KN, Smith Y. Real-time ultrasonography of neonatal intraventricular hemorrhage and comparison with computed tomography. *Radiology* 1981;139:687–691.
44. Grant EG, Borts F, Schellinger D, McCullough DC, Smith Y. Cerebral intraparenchymal hemorrhage in neonates: Sonographic appearance. *AJNR* 1981;2:129–132.
45. Grant EG, Kerner M, Schellinger D, et al. Evolution of porencephalic cysts from intraparenchymal hemorrhage in neonates: Sonographic evidence. *AJR* 1982;138:467–470.
46. Grant EG, Schellinger D. Sonography of neonatal periventricular leukomalacia: Recent experience with a 7.5-MHz scanner. *AJNR* 1985;6:781–785.
47. Grant EG, Schellinger D, Richardson JD. Real-time ultrasonography of the posterior fossa. *J Ultrasound Med* 1983;2:73–87.
48. Grant EG, Schellinger D, Richardson JD, Coffey ML, Smirniotopoulous JG. Echogenic periventricular halo: Normal sonographic finding or neonatal cerebral hemorrhage. *AJNR* 1983;4:43–46.
49. Grant EG, White EM, Schellinger D, Rosenbach D. Low-level echogenicity in intraventricular hemorrhage versus ventriculitis. *Radiology* 1987;165:471–474.
50. Grant EG, White EM, Schellinger D, Choyke PL, Sarcone AL. Cranial duplex sonography of the infant. *Radiology* 1987;163:177–185.
51. Grant EG, Williams AL, Schellinger D, Slovis TL. Intracranial calcification in the infant and neonate: Evaluation by sonography and CT. *Radiology* 1985;157:63–68.
52. Grunnet ML, Shields WD. Cerebellar hemorrhage in the premature infant. *J Pediatr* 1976;88:605–608.
53. Hambleton G, Wigglesworth JS. Origin of intraventricular haemorrhage in the preterm infant. *Arch Dis Child* 1976;51:651–659.
54. Han BK, Babcock DS, McAdams L. Bacterial meningitis in infants: Sonographic findings. *Radiology* 1985;154:645–650.

55. Han BK, Babcock DS, Oestreich AE. Sonography of brain tumors in infants. *AJR* 1984;143:31–36.

56. Harwood-Nash DC, Flodmark O. Diagnostic imaging of the neonatal brain: Review and protocol. *AJNR* 1982;3:103–115.

57. Hecht ST, Filly RA, Callen PW, Wilson-Davis SL. Intracranial hemorrhage: Late onset in the preterm neonate. *Radiology* 1983;149:697–699.

58. Hernanz-Schulman M, Cohen W, Genieser NB. Sonography of cerebral infarction in infancy. *AJR* 1988;150:897–902.

59. Hill A. Ventricular dilatation following intraventricular hemorrhage in the premature infant. *Can J Neurol Sci* 1983;10:81–85.

60. Hill A, Martin DJ, Daneman A, Fitz CR. Focal ischemic cerebral injury in the newborn: Diagnosis by ultrasound and correlation with computed tomographic scan. *Pediatrics* 1983;71:790–793.

61. Hill A, Melson GL, Clark HB, Volpe JJ. Hemorrhagic periventricular leukomalacia: Diagnosis by real-time ultrasound and correlation with autopsy findings. *Pediatrics* 1982;69:282–284.

62. Hill A, Shackelford GD, Volpe JJ. Ventriculitis with neonatal bacterial meningitis: Identification by real-time ultrasound. *J Pediatr* 1981;99:133–136.

63. Hill A, Shackelford GD, Volpe JJ. A potential mechanism of pathogenesis for early posthemorrhagic hydrocephalus in the premature newborn. *Pediatrics* 1984;73:19–21.

64. Hill A, Volpe JJ. Normal pressure hydrocephalus in the newborn. *Pediatrics* 1981;68:623–629.

65. Hill A, Volpe JJ. Decrease in pulsatile flow in the anterior cerebral arteries in infantile hydrocephalus. *Pediatrics* 1982;69:4–7

66. Horbar JD, Leahy KA, Lucey JF. Ultrasound identification of lateral ventricular asymmetry in the human neonate. *JCU* 1983;11:67–69.

67. Horgan JG, Rumack CM, Hay T, Manco-Johnson ML, Merenstein GB, Esola C. Absolute intracranial blood-flow velocities evaluated by duplex Doppler sonography in asymptomatic preterm and term neonates. *AJR* 1989;152:1059–1064.

68. Johnson ML, Rumack CM, Mannes EJ, Appareti KE. Detection of neonatal intracranial hemorrhage utilizing real-time and static ultrasound. *JCU* 1981;9:427–433.

69. Jooma R, Kendall BE. Intracranial tumours in the first year of life. *Neuroradiology* 1982;23:267–274.

70. Kangarloo H, Gold RH, Benson L, Diament MJ, DiSessa T, Boechat MT. Sonography of extrathoracic left-to-right shunts in infants and children. *AJR* 1983;141:923–926.

71. Karnaze MG, Shackelford GD, Abramson CL. Atrial ventricular diverticulum: Sonographic diagnosis. *AJNR* 1987;8:721–723.

72. Keller MS, DiPietro MA, Teele RL, et al. Periventricular cavitations in the first week of life. *AJNR* 1987;8:291–295.

73. Kreusser KL, Schmidt RE, Shackelford GD, Volpe JJ. Value of ultrasound for identification of acute hemorrhagic necrosis of thalamus and basal ganglia in an asphyxiated term infant. *Ann Neurol* 1984;16:361–363.

74. Levene MI. Measurement of the growth of the lateral ventricles in preterm infants with real-time ultrasound. *Arch Dis Child* 1981;56:900–904.

75. Levene MI, Starte DR. A longitudinal study of post-haemorrhagic ventricular dilatation in the newborn. *Arch Dis Child* 1981;56:905–910.

76. Levene MI, Wigglesworth JS, Dubowitz V. Hemorrhagic periventricular leukomalacia in the neonate: A real-time ultrasound study. *Pediatrics* 1983;71:794–797.

77. London DA, Carroll BA, Enzmann DR. Sonography of ventricular size and germinal matrix hemorrhage in premature infants. *AJR* 1980;135:559–564.

78. Luisiri A, Sotelo-Avila C, Silberstein MJ, Graviss ER. Sonography of the Zellweger syndrome. *J Ultrasound Med* 1988;7:169–173.

79. Mack LA, Alvord EC Jr. Neonatal cranial ultrasound: Normal appearances. *Semin US* 1982;3:216–230.

80. Mack LA, Rumack CM, Johnson ML. Ultrasound evaluation of cystic intracranial lesions in the neonate. *Radiology* 1980;137:451–455.

81. Mack LA, Wright K, Hirsch JH, et al. Intracranial hemorrhage in premature infants: Accuracy of sonographic evaluation. *AJR* 1981;137:245–250.

82. Martin R, Roessmann U, Fanaroff A. Massive intracerebellar hemorrhage in low-birth weight infants. *J Pediatr* 1976;89:290–293.

83. Martin CG, Snider AR, Katz SM, Peabody JL, Brady JP, Chir B. Abnormal cerebral blood flow patterns in preterm infants with a large patent ductus arteriosus. *J Pediatr* 1982;101:587–593.

84. McMenamin JB, Shackelford GD, Volpe JJ. Outcome of neonatal intraventricular hemorrhage with periventricular echodense lesions. *Ann Neurol* 1984;15:285–290.

85. Mercker JM, Blumhagen JD, Brewer DK. Echographic demonstration of extracerebral fluid collections with the lateral technique. *J Ultrasound Med* 1983;2:265–269.

86. Mitchell DG, Merton D, Desai H, et al. Neonatal brain: Color Doppler imaging. Part II. Altered flow patterns from extracorporeal membrane oxygenation. *Radiology* 1988;167:307–310.

87. Mitchell DG, Merton DA, Mirsky PJ, Needleman L. Circle of Willis in newborns: Color Doppler imaging of 53 healthy full-term infants. *Radiology* 1989;172:201–205.

88. Mitchell DG, Merton D, Needleman L, et al. Neonatal brain: Color Doppler imaging. Part I. Technique and vascular anatomy. *Radiology* 1988;167:303–306.

89. Motte J, Gomes H, Morville P, Cymbalista M. Sonographic diagnosis of lissencephaly. *Pediatr Radiol* 1987;17:362–364.

90. Naidich TP, McLone DG, Fulling KH. The Chiari II malformation: Part IV. The hindbrain deformity. *Neuroradiology* 1983;25:170–197.

91. Naidich TP, Pudlowski RM, Naidich JB. Computed tomographic signs of Chiari II malformation. II: Midbrain and cerebellum. *Radiology* 1980;134:391–398.

92. Naidich TP, Pudlowski RM, Naidich JB. Computed tomographic signs of the Chiari II malformation. III: Ventricles and cisterns. *Radiology* 1980;134:657–663.

93. Naidich TP, Pudlowski RM, Naidich JB, Gornish M, Rodriguez FJ. Computed tomographic signs of the Chiari II malformation. Part I: Skull and dural partitions. *Radiology* 1980;134:65–71.

94. Naidich TP, Schott LH, Baron RL. Computed tomography in evaluation of hydrocephalus. *Radiol Clin North Am* 1982;20:143–167.

95. Newlin NS, Seeger JF, Stuck KJ. Vein of Galen aneurysm. Diagnosis by real-time ultrasound. *J Assoc Can Radiol* 1981;32:224–226.

96. Pape K, Armstrong D, Fitzhardinge P. Central nervous system pathology associated with mask ventilation in the very low birth weight infant: A new etiology for intracerebellar hemorrhage. *Pediatrics* 1976;58:473–483.

97. Papile L-A, Burstein J, Burstein R, Koffler H. Incidence and evolution of subependymal and intraventricular hemorrhage: A study of infants with birth weights less than 1,500 gm. *J Pediatr* 1978;92:529–534.

98. Peterson CM, Smith WL, Franken EA. Neonatal intracerebellar hemorrhage: Detection by real-time ultrasound. *Radiology* 1984;150:391–392.

99. Pigadas A, Thompson JR, Grube GL. Normal infant brain anatomy: Correlated real-time sonograms and brain specimens. *AJR* 1981;137:815–20.

100. Poland RL, Slovis TL, Shankaran S. Normal values for ventricular size as determined by real time sonographic techniques. *Pediatr Radiol* 1985;15:12–14.

101. Raju TNK, Zikos E. Regional cerebral blood velocity in infants: A real-time transcranial and fontanellar pulsed Doppler study. *J Ultrasound Med* 1987;6:497–507.

102. Reddy PSV, Wild SR, Hendry GMA. Ultrasonic diagnosis of a choroid plexus neoplasm in a child. *Br J Radiol* 1984;57:342–344.

103. Reeder JD, Kaude JV, Setzer ES. Choroid plexus hemorrhage in premature neonates: Recognition by sonography. *AJNR* 1982;3:619–622.

104. Reeder JD, Sanders RC. Ventriculitis in the neonate: Recognition by sonography. *AJNR* 1983;4:37–41.

105. Reeder JD, Setzer ES, Kaude JV. Ultrasonographic detection of perinatal intracerebellar hemorrhage. *Pediatrics* 1982; 70:385–386.

106. Richardson JD, Grant EG. Scanning techniques and normal anatomy. In: Grant EG, ed. *Neurosonography of the Pre-term Neonate*. New York: Springer-Verlag, 1986:1–24.

107. Rodemyer CR, Smith WL. Diagnosis of a vein of Galen aneurysm by ultrasound. *JCU* 1982;10:297–298.

108. Rosenberg HK, Levine RS, Stoltz K, Smith DR. Bacterial meningitis in infants: Sonographic features. *AJNR* 1983;4:822–825.

109. Rumack CM, Appareti K, Johnson ML. Neonatal scanning techniques. In: Rumack CM, Johnson ML, eds. *Perinatal and Infant Brain Imaging*. Chicago: Year Book Medical Publishers, Inc. 1984:3–37.

110. Rumack CM, Manco-Johnson ML, Manco-Johnson MJ, Koops BL, Hathaway WE, Appareti K. Timing and course of neonatal intracranial hemorrhage using real-time ultrasound. *Radiology* 1985;154:101–105.

111. Sauerbrei EE. Serial brain sonography in two children with leukomalacia and cerebral palsy. *J Can Assoc Radiol* 1984;35:164–167.

112. Sauerbrei EE, Cooperberg PL. Cystic tumors of the fetal and neonatal cerebrum: Ultrasound and computed tomographic evaluation. *Radiology* 1983;147:689–692.

113. Sauerbrei EE, Digney M, Harrison PB, Cooperberg PL. Ultrasonic evaluation of neonatal intracranial hemorrhage and its complications. *Radiology* 1981;139:677–685.

114. Schellinger D, Grant EG, Manz HJ, Patronas NJ. Intraparenchymal hemorrhage in preterm neonates: A broadening spectrum. *AJR* 1988;150:1109–1115.

115. Schellinger D, Grant EG, Richardson JD. Cystic periventricular leukomalacia: Sonographic and CT findings. *AJNR* 1984;5:439–445.

116. Seibert JJ, McCowan T, Chadduck WM, et al. Duplex pulsed Doppler US versus intracranial pressure in the neonate: Clinical and experimental studies. *Radiology* 1989;171:155–159.

117. Shackelford GD. Neurosonography of hydrocephalus in infants. *Neuroradiology* 1986;28:452–462.

118. Shackelford GD, Fulling KH, Glasier CM. Cysts of the subependymal germinal matrix: Sonographic demonstration with pathologic correlation. *Radiology* 1983;149:117–121.

119. Shackelford GD, Volpe JJ. Cranial ultrasonography in the evaluation of neonatal intracranial hemorrhage and its complications. *J Perinat Med* 1985;13:293–304.

120. Shankaran S, Slovis TL, Bedard MP, Poland RL. Sonographic classification of intracranial hemorrhage. A prognostic indicator of mortality, morbidity, and short-term neurologic outcome. *J Pediatr* 1982;100:469–475.

121. Shaw C, Alvord E. Cava septi pellucidi et vergae: Their normal and pathologic states. *Brain* 1969;92:213–224.

122. Shuman WP, Rogers JV, Mack LA, Alvord EC Jr, Christie DP. Real-time sonographic sector scanning of the neonatal cranium: Technique and normal anatomy. *AJNR* 1981;2:349–356.

123. Shuman RM, Selednik LJ. Periventricular leukomalacia. A one year autopsy study. *Neurology* 1980;37:231–235.

124. Siedler DE, Mahony BS, Hoddick WK, Callen PW. A specular reflection arising from the ventricular wall: A potential pitfall in the diagnosis of germinal matrix hemorrhage. *J Ultrasound Med* 1985;4:109–112.

125. Siegel MJ, Patel J, Gado MH, Shackelford GD. Cranial computed tomography and real-time sonography in full-term neonates and infants. *Radiology* 1983;149:111–116.

126. Siegel MJ, Shackelford GD, Perlman JM, Fulling KH. Hypoxic-ischemic encephalopathy in term infants: Diagnosis and prognosis evaluated by ultrasound. *Radiology* 1984;152:395–399.

127. Slovis TL, Shankaran S, Bedard MP, Poland RL. Intracranial hemorrhage in the hypoxic-ischemic infant: Ultrasound demonstration of unusual complications. *Radiology* 1984;151:163–169.

128. Smith AS, Weinstein MA, Quencer RM, et al. Association of heterotopic gray matter with seizures: MR imaging. *Radiology* 1988;168:195–198.

129. Stannard MW, Jimenez JF. Sonographic recognition of multiple cystic encephalomalacia. *AJR* 1983;141:1321–1324.

130. Stannard MW, Pearrow J. Ultrasound diagnosis of purulent ventriculitis. *J Ultrasound Med* 1984;3:143–144.

131. Strassburg HM, Sauer M, Weber S, Gilsbach J. Ultrasonographic diagnosis of brain tumors in infancy. *Pediatr Radiol* 1984;14:284–287.

132. Takashima S, Armstrong DL, Becker LE. Subcortical leukomalacia. Relationship to development of the cerebral sulcus and its vascular supply. *Arch Neurol* 1978;35:470–472.

133. Takashima S, Tanaka K. Development of cerebrovascular architecture and its relationship to periventricular leukomalacia. *Arch Neurol* 1978;35:11–16.

134. Taylor GA, Fitz CR, Kapur S, Short BL. Cerebrovascular accidents in neonates treated with extracorporeal membrane oxygenation: Sonographic-pathologic correlation. *AJR* 1989; 153:355–361.

135. Taylor GA, Sanders RC. Dandy-Walker syndrome: Recognition by sonography. *AJNR* 1983;4:1203–1206.

136. Teele RL, Hernanz-Schulman M, Sotrel A. Echogenic vasculature in the basal ganglia of neonates: A sonographic sign of vasculopathy. *Radiology* 1988;169:423–427.

137. Tessler FN, Dion J, Viñuela F, et al. Cranial arteriovenous malformations in neonates: Color Doppler imaging with angiographic correlation. *AJR* 1989;153:1027–1030.

138. Vachon L, Mikity V. Computed tomography and ultrasound in purulent ventriculitis. *J Ultrasound Med* 1987;6:269–271.

139. Volpe JJ. Normal and abnormal human brain development. *Clin Perinatol* 1977;4:3–30.

140. Volpe JJ. Hypoxic-ischemic encephalopathy: Clinical aspects. In: Volpe JJ, ed. *Neurology of the Newborn*, 2nd ed. Philadelphia: W.B. Saunders Co., 1987:236–279.

141. Volpe JJ. Intracranial hemorrhage: Subdural, primary subarachnoid, intracerebellar, intraventricular (term infant), and miscellaneous. In: Volpe JJ, ed. *Neurology of the Newborn*, 2nd ed. Philadelphia: W.B. Saunders Co., 1987:282–310.

142. Volpe JJ. Intracranial hemorrhage: Periventricular-intraventricular hemorrhage of the premature infant. In: Volpe JJ, ed. *Neurology of the Newborn*, 2nd ed. Philadelphia: W.B. Saunders Co., 1987:311–361.

143. Volpe JJ. Viral, protozoan, and related intracranial infections. In: Volpe JJ, ed. *Neurology of the Newborn*, 2nd ed. Philadelphia: W.B. Saunders Co., 1987:548–595.

144. Williams JL. Intracranial vascular pulsations in pediatric neurosonology. *J Ultrasound Med* 1983;2:485–488.

145. Winchester P, Brill PW, Cooper R, Krauss AN, Peterson H deC. Prevalence of "compressed" and asymmetric lateral ventricles in healthy full-term neonates: Sonographic study. *AJR* 1986;146:471–475.

146. Wolpert SM, Anderson M, Scott RM, Kwan ESK, Runge VM. Chiari II malformation: MR imaging evaluation. *AJNR* 1987;8:783–792.

147. Wong WS, Tsuruda JS, Liberman RL, Chirino A, Vogt JF, Gangitano E. Color Doppler imaging of intracranial vessels in the neonate. *AJR* 1989;152:1065–1070.

3

Neck

Marilyn J. Siegel

High-resolution sonography has greatly improved the ability of the radiologist to evaluate the soft tissue structures of the neck. With this imaging technique, it is possible to confirm the clinical impression of a neck mass as well as to demonstrate a lesion that is not detectable with physical examination. Moreover, sonography can provide valuable information about the nature of the lesion, its precise location, and its effect on adjacent structures (2,16,32,59).

TECHNIQUE

Patients for cervical sonography are examined in the supine position with the neck hyperextended so that the entire neck can be examined from the mandible to the thoracic inlet. Images are obtained in sagittal, transverse, and, if necessary, oblique positions. In cooperative patients with suspected thyroid or parathyroid disease, additional scans are obtained with the patient swallowing during the examination. As a result of this maneuver, masses located at the upper and lower poles of the thyroid are better detected.

Optimal demonstration of neck anatomy requires higher frequency transducers, either 7.5 or 10 MHz. The 10 MHz transducer improves the resolution of the superficial tissue layers, but penetration into the deeper soft tissues is limited. With the 7.5 MHz transducer, deeper penetration of the soft tissues is possible, but some degradation of the superficial soft tissues results. The use of real-time linear array transducers, rather than sector scanners, also facilitates maximal visualization of the neck structures. Linear array transducers produce a square or rectangular image and, therefore, include more of the area of interest. In contrast, the pie-shaped image of the sector scanner includes the area of interest only in the narrow apex portion of the scan. Duplex and color Doppler imaging are useful for evaluating the dynamics of blood flow in the large blood vessels.

NORMAL GROSS ANATOMY

An understanding of normal anatomy is important if correct diagnoses with sonography are to be made. The normal gross anatomy, therefore, will be reviewed prior to a discussion of pathology.

The neck spans the distance between the mylohyoid muscle superiorly and the first rib inferiorly. Traditionally, the neck has been divided into two paired triangles, anterior and posterior, by the sternocleidomastoid muscle (20) (Fig. 1).

Anterior Triangle

The anterior triangles meet in the midline and are bordered by the body of the mandible superiorly, the midline of the neck medially, and the sternocleidomastoid muscle posteriorly. The hyoid bone separates each anterior triangle into suprahyoid and infrahyoid divisions. The suprahyoid division is composed of the submental and submandibular triangles. The submental triangle, bordered by the anterior bellies of the digastric muscles and the hyoid bone, contains a few lymph nodes and branches of the facial artery and vein. The submandibular triangle, formed by the anterior and posterior bellies of the digastric muscles and the mandibular rami, contain lymph nodes and the submandibular gland.

The infrahyoid portion of the anterior triangle contains the visceral structures of the neck, namely the trachea, esophagus, thyroid and parathyroid glands, as well as the carotid sheath structures. The carotid sheath courses the entire length of the anterior triangle, lying adjacent to the anterior margin of the sternocleidomastoid muscle. Within this sheath, the common carotid artery lies medially, the internal jugular vein laterally, and the vagus nerve posteriorly, located between the two great vessels.

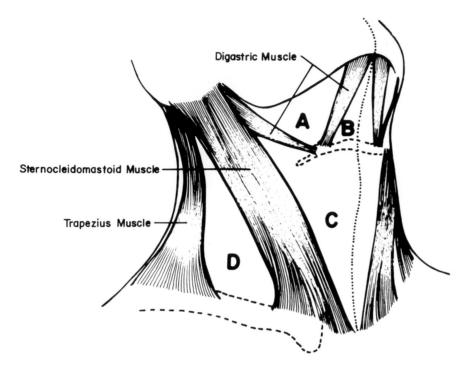

Digastric Muscle

Sternocleidomastoid Muscle

Trapezius Muscle

A B C D

FIG. 1. Triangles of the neck. The sternocleidomastoid muscle divides the neck into anterior and posterior triangles. The hyoid bone separates each anterior triangle into a suprahyoid and infrahyoid division. *A*, submandibular triangles; *B*, submental triangle of suprahyoid division; *C*, infrahyoid division of anterior triangle; *D*, posterior triangle. (From Glazer et al., ref. 15.)

Posterior Triangle

The borders of the posterior triangle are defined by the sternocleidomastoid muscle anteriorly, the trapezius muscle posteriorly, the deep cervical fascia superiorly, and the clavicle inferiorly. The posterior triangle is composed mainly of fat, but also contains small nerves (cutaneous branches of the cervical plexus and spinal accessory nerve), nutrient vessels, and lymph nodes. From a sonographic viewpoint, the anterior triangle, particularly the infrahyoid portion, is more important than the posterior triangle because of the major structures it contains.

The most important lymph nodes of the neck are those of the lateral cervical chain (Fig. 2). These nodes are divided into superficial (external jugular) and deep

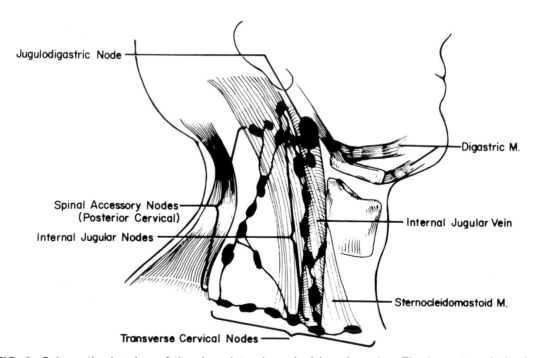

Jugulodigastric Node

Spinal Accessory Nodes (Posterior Cervical)

Internal Jugular Nodes

Digastric M.

Internal Jugular Vein

Sternocleidomastoid M.

Transverse Cervical Nodes

FIG. 2. Schematic drawing of the deep lateral cervical lymph nodes. The largest node in the upper portion of the internal jugular chain is the jugulodigastric node. (From Glazer et al., ref. 15.)

(internal jugular, spinal accessory, and transverse cervical) groups. The superficial group parallels the course of the external jugular vein from the base of the skull to its junction with the brachiocephalic vessels. The nodes of the internal jugular chain follow the course of the internal jugular vein; the spinal accessory chains are located lateral and posterior to the spinal accessory nerve; the transverse cervical nodes join the inferior jugular and spinal accessory chains and are seen in the supraclavicular area. The importance of these nodes is that they drain the major structures of the head and neck, including the nasopharynx, oropharynx, tonsils, hypopharynx, and larynx. In general, normal lymph nodes in children are not recognizable by sonography. When they become pathologically enlarged due to inflammation or tumor, they become visible around the carotid sheath or in the posterior triangle, appearing as somewhat flattened hypoechoic structures. Enlarged lymph nodes usually have a ho-mogeneous appearance on sonography, but they may appear inhomogeneous as a result of fatty changes (36).

SONOGRAPHIC ANATOMY

Landmarks seen on all sonograms of the neck are the strap muscles of the neck anteriorly, the anterior wall of the trachea in the midline, the carotid sheath laterally, and the thyroid gland. Review of the normal sonographic anatomy of the thyroid gland will be presented later in the chapter. The strap muscles (sternohyoid, sternothyroid, thyrohyoid, and omohyoid muscles) of the neck are located anterior and lateral to the vessels and the thyroid gland, and appear relatively hypoechoic compared to the gland. The anterior wall of the trachea is readily identified as a well-defined echogenic band. Air within the trachea, behind the anterior tracheal wall, reflects the sound beam and pro-

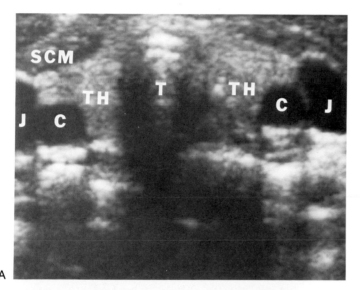

A

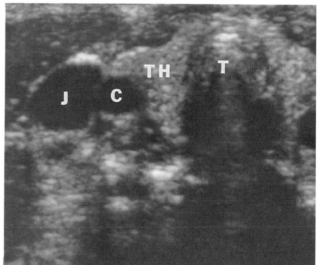

B

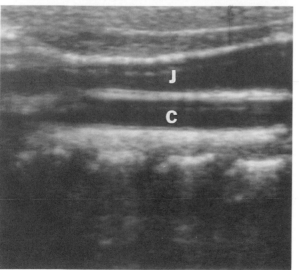

C

FIG. 3. Normal sonographic anatomy. **A**: Transverse sonogram through mid neck. **B**: Transverse sonogram through right side of neck. On each side of the trachea (*T*) are the lobes of the thyroid (*TH*). A small isthmus of thyroid tissue is seen anteriorly to the trachea. The anterior wall of the trachea posterior to the isthmus is strongly echogenic. Posterolateral to the thyroid gland and posterior to the sternocleidomastoid muscle (*SCM*) are the common carotid artery (*C*) and jugular vein (*J*). **C**: Longitudinal sonogram through the lateral neck. Both the carotid artery (*C*) and jugular vein (*J*) are entirely anechoic. **D** (see Colorplate 2): Color flow imaging shows flow in the common carotid artery (*CCA*) and internal jugular vein (*IJV*).

duces intense acoustic shadowing, thereby obliterating the posterior and lateral tracheal walls.

The carotid artery and jugular vein are normally echo-free structures, with the walls of the carotid artery more echogenic than those of the jugular vein. The jugular vein changes in size with respiration, reaching maximum caliber with a Valsalva maneuver. On images through the upper neck, the common carotid artery and internal jugular vein are positioned medially and posteriorly to the strap muscles. Images at the thyroid gland level usually show the carotid sheath structures posterior and lateral to the thyroid gland and posterior to the sternocleidomastoid muscle (Fig. 3). At this level, the sternocleidomastoid muscle has a more anterior position in the neck than on images obtained at higher levels, where it is more lateral.

PATHOLOGY

Cervical masses in infants and children are usually benign and predominantly anterior or lateral in location. Congenital lesions (cystic hygromas, thyroglossal duct cysts, branchial cleft cysts, teratomas, hemangiomas), lymphadenopathy caused by inflammatory disease, and thyroid tumors are the most common benign masses of the neck (13,32,46). Approximately 15% of the neck masses in childhood are malignant and usually lymphomas or rhabdomyosarcomas (40).

Sonography is the preferred imaging examination for evaluating neck masses in children and often can suggest the correct diagnosis, particularly in congenital lesions. If sonography can define the full extent of a lesion, no further imaging is required. However, if the lesion is large or malignancy is suspected, computerized tomography (CT) or magnetic resonance (MR) imaging is required to define the deep tissue extent, which facilitates complete surgical removal (23,51,61,62,68). The role of scintigraphy is currently limited to the evaluation of midline masses. The possibility that such a mass represents ectopic thyroid tissue or the only functioning thyroid tissue necessitates thyroid imaging prior to surgical intervention.

Congenital and Developmental Abnormalities

Cystic Hygromas

Cystic hygromas or lymphangiomas are congenital malformations of lymphatic channels and are believed to arise from sequestered embryonic lymphatic sacs (68). The three major types are: (a) simple, composed of capillary-sized lymphatics; (b) cavernous, containing minimally dilated lymphatic spaces; and (c) cystic hygroma, consisting of large lymphatic cysts (30). Radiologically, and often pathologically, it is difficult to

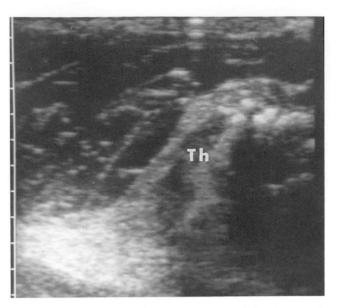

FIG. 4. Cystic hygroma. Transverse scan of the right neck of a newborn boy. A complex mass with multiple septations and through-transmission fills the right neck. *Th,* thyroid gland.

differentiate between the cavernous and cystic lymphangiomas, and for the purposes of this review these lesions will be termed cystic hygromas. Cystic hygromas frequently present at or shortly after birth as painless soft tissue masses posterior to the sternocleidomastoid muscle. Large ones may fill one side of the

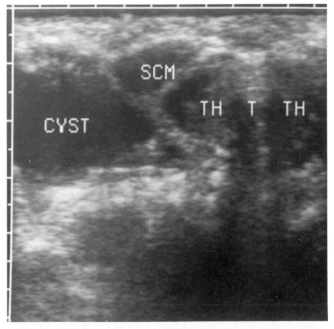

FIG. 5. Cystic hygroma. Transverse sonogram of the right neck shows a cystic mass with some posterior enhancement. *CYST,* cystic hygroma; *TH,* thyroid; *T,* trachea; *SCM,* sternocleidomastoid muscle.

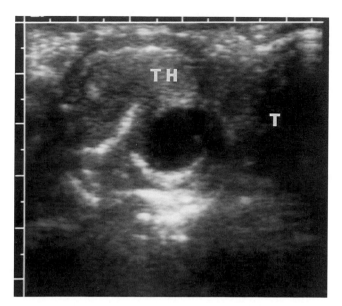

FIG. 6. Thyroglossal duct cyst. Transverse sonogram of a newborn with a cervical mass. An anechoic mass with acoustic enhancement is present posterior to the right lobe of the thyroid (*TH*) and lateral to the trachea (*T*).

neck and extend into the mediastinum, producing a significant degree of esophageal or airway compression (62,63).

Sonography usually shows a thin-walled, multiloculated, cystic mass containing septa of variable thickness (60) (Fig. 4). Rarely, cystic hygromas may appear as solitary cysts (Fig. 5) or they may contain echogenic fluid if recent hemorrhage is present. Because these lesions tend to infiltrate adjacent structures, the fascial planes adjacent to the lesions often are obliterated. The location of this lesion, as well as its multicystic appearance in an infant or young patient, usually allows the correct preoperative diagnosis.

Thyroglossal Duct Cysts

Thyroglossal duct cysts arise from remnants of the embryonic thyroglossal duct that connects the foramen cecum at the base of the tongue to the thyroid gland; the remnants enlarge secondary to secretions from the epithelial lining. Cysts may develop anywhere along the path of descent of the thyroglossal duct as well as within the hyoid bone. About 65% of thyroglossal duct cysts are located below the hyoid bone, 20% are suprahyoid, and 15% are at the level of the hyoid (41). Infrahyoid thyroglossal duct cysts characteristically are embedded within the strap muscles of the neck. Most thyroglossal duct cysts present during the first decade of life as asymptomatic masses in the anterior neck, in the midline, or slightly off midline.

On sonography, thyroglossal duct cysts appear as anechoic or hypoechoic, well-circumscribed masses with good-through transmission (Figs. 6,7). Fine or coarse echoes within the lesion and septations usually are associated with prior inflammation (Fig. 8). Those cysts that develop above or at the level of the hyoid bone typically are midline in location, whereas below the hyoid bone thyroglossal duct cysts often have both midline and off-midline components. The midline location is helpful in arriving at the correct diagnosis of a thyroid-related mass.

Branchial Cleft Cysts

The branchial network consists of a series of six mesodermal arches separated by ectodermal lined grooves. As the branchial apparatus develops, the first and second arches grow in a caudal direction. As a result, the third and fourth arches and their clefts become recessed in a deep pit, the cervical sinus, which normally is obliterated during subsequent develop-

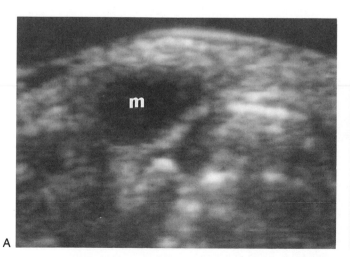
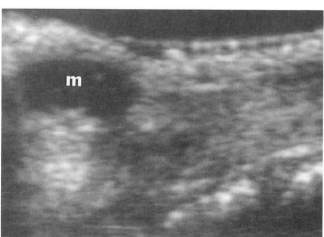

FIG. 7. Thyroglossal duct cyst. **A:** Transverse and **B:** longitudinal image of a 5-year-old boy with a neck mass. A hypoechoic mass (*m*) is identified slightly to the right of the midline of the neck.

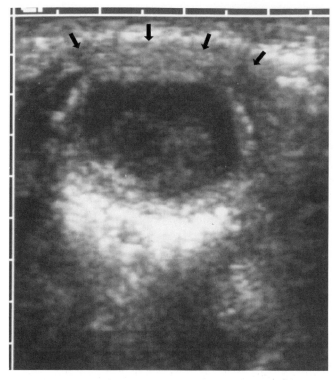

FIG. 8. Infected thyroglossal duct cyst. Transverse sonogram at the base of the tongue shows a midline, predominantly cystic mass with internal echoes, throughtransmission, and a thick wall (*arrows*).

ment (10,81). Persistence of these embryonic structures leads to the formation of a branchial cleft cyst. Second branchial cleft cysts account for 90% of branchial cleft abnormalities, first branchial cleft cysts for 8%, and third branchial cleft cysts for the remainder (10). Branchial cleft cysts can occur anywhere from the tonsillar fossa to the supraclavicular area, but most are located in the upper neck anterior to the sternocleidomastoid muscle (35). They generally become evident in later childhood and adulthood, presenting as recurrent, painless, fluctuant, nontender masses. On pathologic section, the cyst is usually thin-walled, lined with stratified squamous epithelium, and filled with yellowish fluid which may contain cholesterol products.

On sonography, the branchial cleft cyst characteristically appears as a well-defined, anechoic mass displacing the sternocleidomastoid muscle posteriorly or posterolaterally and the carotid artery and jugular vein medially or posteromedially (3) (Fig. 9). In the absence of infection, the cyst wall is smooth and thin and the surrounding fascial planes are well-defined. Wall thickness as well as the echogenicity of the fluid may increase if there is superimposed infection. The upperlateral neck location usually allows differentiation of branchial cleft cysts from other anterior triangle lesions.

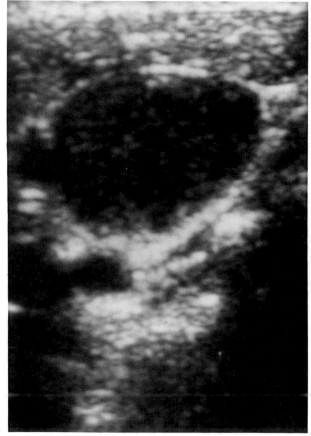

A

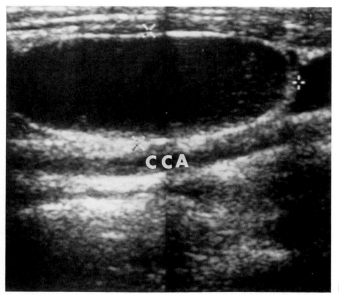

B

FIG. 9. Branchial cleft cyst. **A**: Transverse and **B**: longitudinal sonograms of an 18-year-old girl with a painless, left neck mass. A thin-walled, anechoic mass with low-level echoes is present anterior to the common carotid artery (*CCA*). An infected branchial cleft cyst was removed surgically.

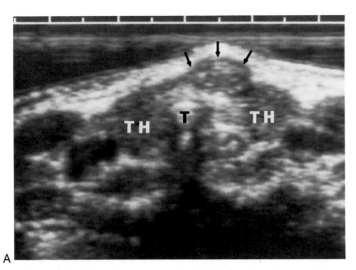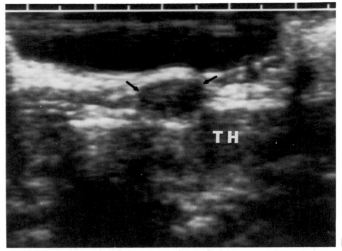

FIG. 10. Dermoid. **A**: Transverse view of the neck of a 15-month-old boy demonstrates a well-defined echogenic mass (*arrows*) slightly to the left of midline. *T*, trachea; *TH*, thyroid. **B**: Longitudinal image shows the mass just superior to the left lobe of the thyroid gland (*TH*).

Teratomas and Dermoid Cysts

Teratomas and dermoid cysts are developmental lesions arising from pluripotential embryonal cells. Dermoid cysts are composed of two germ cell layers (ectoderm and mesoderm), whereas teratomas contain elements from all three germ cell layers. They are most frequently seen in infants and are usually asymptomatic at the time of presentation (10,68).

The typical sonographic appearance of a dermoid or teratoma is a well-circumscribed, thin-walled mass that is either echogenic or complex, depending on the relative amounts of fat, calcification, and soft tissue (Fig. 10). Rarely, teratomas may be purely cystic and simulate thyroglossal duct or branchial cleft cysts. Most teratomas and dermoid cysts are midline in location, but occasionally they can be off-midline.

Hemangiomas

Hemangiomas are developmental vascular abnormalities that usually are found in infants under 6 months of age and frequently regress spontaneously later in childhood (10). The two major types of hemangiomas are capillary and cavernous. Capillary ones are composed of capillary-sized vascular spaces with few, if any, recognizable erythrocytes, whereas cavernous hemangiomas consist of larger, dilated, erythrocyte-filled vascular spaces. Both forms may be localized to the skin or involve the deeper soft tissues of the neck.

On sonography, cavernous hemangiomas typically are complex masses containing anechoic areas separated by echogenic tissue (Fig. 11). They usually have a thin wall and may be well-defined or may displace and infiltrate normal structures. Occasionally, hemangiomas appear echogenic because they contain nu-

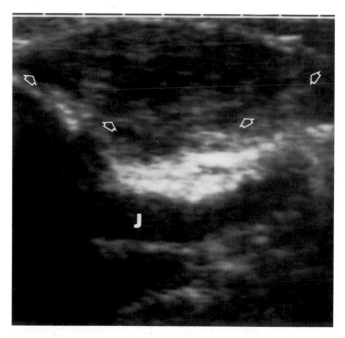

FIG. 11. Cavernous hemangioma. Longitudinal sonogram of a 6-month-old girl with a right-sided neck mass shows a complex lesion (*open arrows*) just anterior to the jugular (*J*) vein. The mass is predominantly hypoechoic but contains echogenic septations. Acoustic enhancement is present.

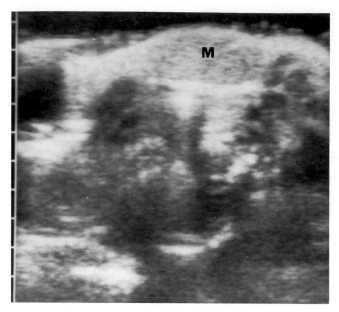

FIG. 12. Capillary hemangioma. Transverse sonogram of a newborn shows a homogeneous echogenic mass (*M*) in the midline of the lower neck. Histologically, the lesion contained multiple tiny vascular channels.

merous interfaces, proteinaceous material, or areas of thrombosis and fibrosis (Fig. 12).

Neoplasms

Neurogenic tumors are the most common primary neoplasms of the neck in childhood, occurring anywhere along the course of the cervical nerve roots. Approximately 90% of these are neuroblastomas, gan-glioneuroblastomas, or ganglioneuromas; 10% are neurofibromas. Neuroblastoma and ganglioneuroblastoma frequently present before 10 years of age. Most are incidental findings on chest radiographs, but they may present with dysphagia or respiratory distress.

On sonography, a neurogenic tumor appears as a solid mass with or without irregular hypoechoic areas due to necrosis (Fig. 13). These findings combined with the paraspinal location of the mass can suggest the diagnosis of a neural tumor, although differentiation among the various types of tumors requires tissue sampling. Other findings with neuroblastoma include infiltration of the soft tissues, irregular margins, vascular encasement, and intraspinal extension. Rarely, neuroblastomas can be entirely cystic and resemble a cystic hygroma or teratoma (14).

Lymphoma and rhabdomyosarcoma are the most frequent secondary tumors of the neck. These diseases produce enlarged nodes, over 5 mm in diameter, with a homogeneous or heterogeneous echo pattern (Figs. 14,15). Although it is possible to detect palpable as well as nonpalpable nodal disease using sonography, physical examination and computerized tomography have been primarily relied upon for the detection of nodal disease and determination of its extent.

Other Masses

Fibromatosis colli is an uncommon benign lesion of the sternocleidomastoid muscle. Affected patients usually present by 2 weeks of life with a mass in the anterior portion of the neck, often on the right side. A history of traumatic parturition associated with a

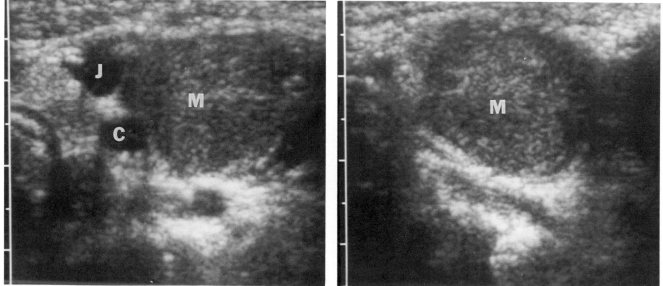

FIG. 13. Neuroblastoma. **A**: Transverse and **B**: longitudinal sonograms of the neck of a 3-year-old boy show a large echogenic mass (*M*) medial to the jugular vein (*J*) and carotid artery (*C*).

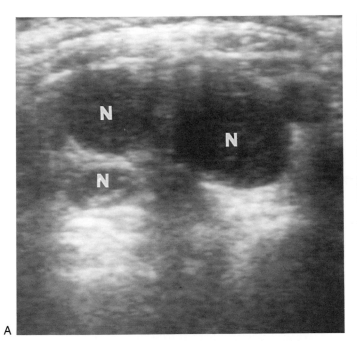

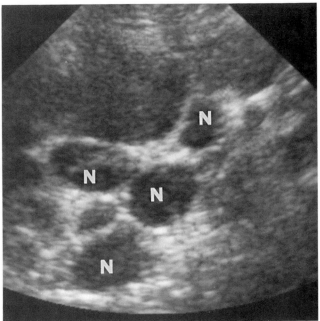

A   B

FIG. 14. Lymphoma. **A**: Transverse and **B**: longitudinal sonograms of the right neck of an 18-year-old girl with palpable neck masses show multiple enlarged hypoechoic lymph nodes (*N*). Biopsy confirmed nodal enlargement secondary to Hodgkin's lymphoma.

breech or forceps delivery is frequent. The lesion frequently regresses over 4 to 8 months with conservative therapy (21).

The sonographic findings of fibromatosis colli are either diffuse enlargement of the sternocleidomastoid muscle or a well-defined homogeneous mass within the sternocleidomastoid muscle with an echogenicity that is equal to or slightly lower than that of adjacent muscle (Fig. 16). With real-time sonography, the lesion can be noted to move synchronously with the sternocleidomastoid muscle (7,13,32).

Infection

Infections of the neck represent serious conditions that are often difficult to evaluate accurately by clinical methods. Sonography can be valuable in examining

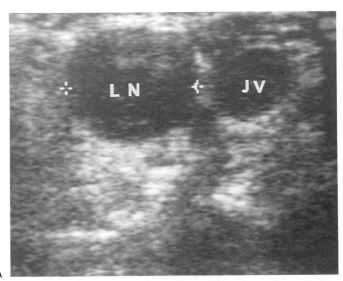

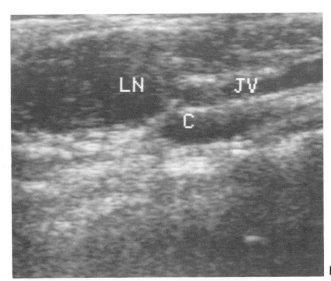

A   B

FIG. 15. Metastatic rhabdomyosarcoma. **A**: Transverse and **B**: longitudinal views demonstrate a 2.5 cm hypoechoic node (*LN*) lateral and anterior to the carotid sheath. *JV*, jugular vein; *C*, carotid artery.

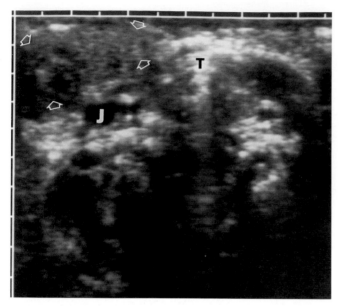

FIG. 16. Fibromatosis colli. A 2-month-old boy with torticollis. A transverse scan of the neck demonstrates a well-marginated, diffusely enlarged right sternocleidomastoid muscle (*open arrows*). The echogenicity of the enlarged muscle is normal. J, jugular vein; *T*, trachea.

cervical infections, especially for differentiating between nonsuppurative adenopathy and abscess. Moreover, sonography may be useful in guiding aspiration biopsy as well as in demonstrating the presence of venous thrombosis complicating infection.

Cervical adenitis usually results from tonsillar, pharyngeal, or dental infections. The submandibular and upper deep cervical nodes lying near the angle of the mandible are most frequently involved by infections of the oral cavity. These nodes drain to the deep cervical nodes that lie along the carotid sheath in the lateral neck.

Nonsuppurative lymphadenopathy appears on sonography as relatively hypoechoic, lateral neck masses, usually larger than 5 mm in diameter (22,59). Duplex Doppler or color flow imaging is useful for separating small nodes from vessels (Fig. 17). In contrast, an abscess appears as a well-defined, partially or totally fluid-filled mass with a thick wall (Figs. 18,19). Occasionally, increased echogenicity with shadowing may be apparent in the center of the abscess, secondary to gas bubbles. Distinguishing suppurative from nonsuppurative adenitis is important because nonsuppurative adenopathy can be treated with antibiotics, whereas abscesses often require surgical or percutaneous drainage.

Computerized tomography also is valuable in examining cervical infections and is superior to sonography in demonstrating important complications such as airway encroachment, osteomyelitis, and paranasal sinus and orbital involvement. In addition, CT has the capability of detecting posterior cervical, mediastinal, and intracranial extension (42).

Tuberculous Infection

Tuberculous adenitis is a granulomatous disease that should be included in the differential diagnosis of an

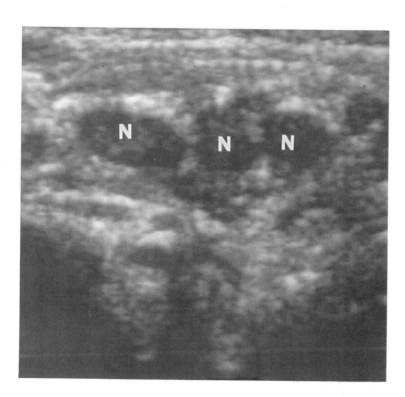

FIG. 17. Inflammatory lymphadenitis. **A:** Longitudinal sonogram of a 2-year-old boy with bilateral palpable masses show multiple enlarged nodes (*N*) measuring 8–10 mm in diameter. The nodes are slightly hypoechoic relative to surrounding tissues and muscle. **B** (see Colorplate 3): On color flow images, the avascular nodes are easily differentiated from arteries (*red*) and veins (*blue*).

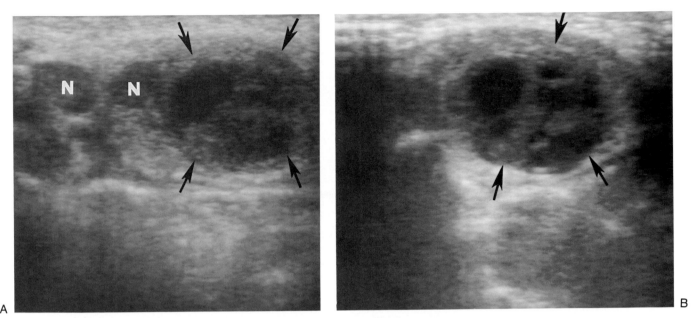

FIG. 18. Cervical abscess. **A**: Longitudinal and **B**: transverse sonograms demonstrate two hypoechoic nodes (*N*) and a well-defined mass (*arrows*) with multiple fluid-filled areas. At surgery, the mass was composed of multiple small suppurative nodes matted together. Cultures grew *S. aureus*.

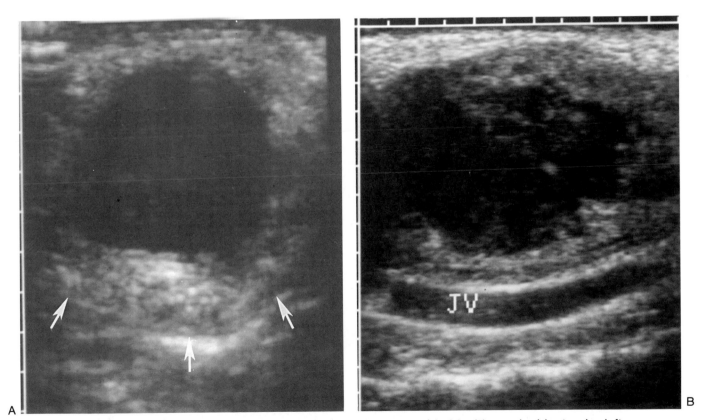

FIG. 19. Cervical abscess. **A**: Longitudinal scan of a 2-year-old girl with a palpable, tender left neck mass. The mass is well-defined with a large central anechoic component and thick wall (*arrows*). At operation, purulent fluid was aspirated. **B**: Longitudinal scan in another patient demonstrates an irregular, nearly anechoic mass superficial to the jugular vein (*JV*). *S. aureus* grew from a percutaneous aspirate.

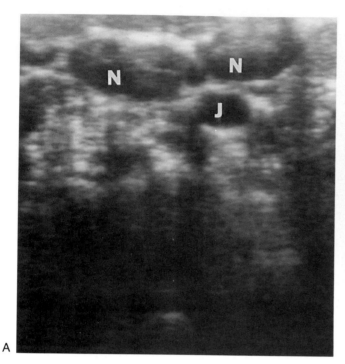
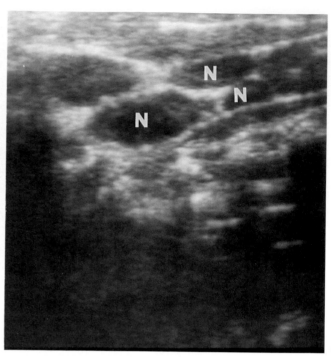

FIG. 20. Tuberculous adenopathy. **A**: Transverse and **B**: longitudinal sonograms of the right neck demonstrate several hypoechoic nodes (*N*) anterior to the jugular vein (*J*).

inflammatory neck mass, in the appropriate clinical setting. The clinical and sonographic findings of a tuberculous abscess are similar to those of pyogenic adenitis, except that associated cutaneous and subcutaneous inflammation is seen frequently in patients with tuberculous adenitis but not in patients with pyogenic infections (Fig. 20).

Vascular Abnormalities

Normal Variants

Recognition of the variations in the vasculature of the neck is important so that they are not mistaken for a mass lesion. The most common variation of normal neck anatomy is asymmetry in the size of the internal jugular veins. It is not unusual for the right internal jugular vein to be larger than the left, presumably due to the predominance of the right cerebral venous drainage.

Jugular Vein Thrombosis

Thrombosis of the internal jugular vein in childhood presents as swelling or a palpable cervical mass and is seen mainly as a complication of an indwelling cen-

tral venous line. Other predisposing conditions include neck surgery, intravenous drug abuse, neoplasms of the head and neck, and conditions such as lymphadenitis, abscess, or cellulitis. The classic sonographic appearance of acute venous thrombosis is a distended jugular vein with low-level intraluminal echoes (Fig. 21). Venous pulsation and a normal Valsalva-maneuver effect are absent or diminished on duplex and color Doppler imaging (1). With chronic thrombosis, the clot becomes hypoechoic due to lysis of red blood cells; collateral vessels also may be noted (82).

In most patients with jugular venous thrombosis, sonography can provide adequate diagnostic information. Although it cannot determine the extent of thrombus in the thorax, this information rarely influences therapeutic planning. Sonography also is a valuable means to evaluate the adjacent soft tissues for associated lymphadenopathy and to serially follow thrombi to document resolution.

Arterial Occlusion

Carotid artery occlusion occurs principally as a complication of extracorporeal membrane oxygenation. The procedure involves placement of two perfusion cannulas, one in the right atrium via the right jugular

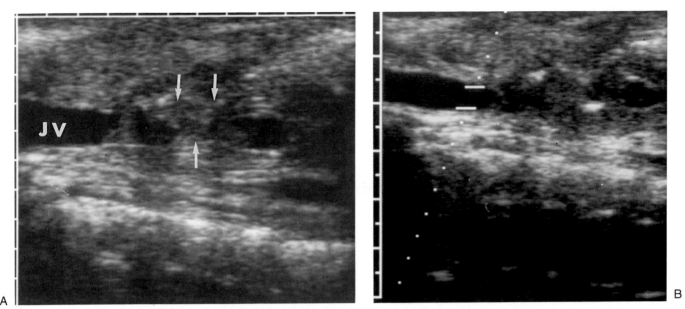

FIG. 21. Jugular vein thrombosis. A 2-year-old patient with a previous indwelling catheter. **A**: Longitudinal image shows distension of the left jugular vein (*JV*) above an area of echogenic, organizing thrombus (*arrows*). **B**: Doppler waveform demonstrates absence of venous pulsation.

vein and the second in the common carotid artery. After the cannulas are removed, the carotid and jugular vessels are ligated. The sonographic findings of arterial occlusion are lack of visualization of the lumen of the affected vessel (Fig. 22); retrograde flow in the distal internal carotid artery; and collateral flow patterns, seen as flow reversal in the right anterior cerebral artery and antegrade filling of the middle cerebral artery.

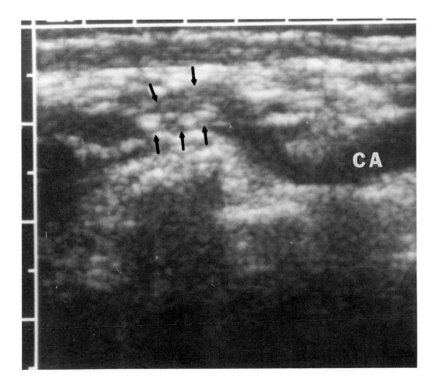

FIG. 22. Arterial occlusion. A 2-month-old boy who had been on extracorporeal membrane oxygenation. Longitudinal image shows distension and tortuosity of the inferior portion of the right carotid artery (*CA*). The lumen is interrupted proximally by thrombus (*arrows*).

THYROID GLAND

Normal Anatomy and Development

The normal thyroid gland is composed of two lateral lobes, one on each side of the trachea, connected by an isthmus of thyroid tissue that crosses the trachea anteriorly. Occasionally an extra lobe, the pyramidal lobe, extends superiorly from the isthmus in the midline. The gland is covered by a fibrous capsule that is fixed to the deep pretracheal fascia, causing it to move upward with deglutition. Size and weight of the thyroid vary with age (80). The lateral lobe measures between 1 and 1.5 cm in transverse diameter, 2 to 3 cm vertically, and 0.2 to 1.2 cm in anteroposterior diameter in infants and young children. In adolescents and adults, the lateral lobes measure 2 to 4 cm in transverse dimension, 5 to 8 cm vertically, and 1 to 2.5 cm in anteroposterior diameter (6). The right lobe usually is larger than the left.

Embryologically, the thyroid gland arises as a midline ventral outgrowth from the floor of the embryonic pharynx at the level of the first pharyngeal pouch. As the thyroid anlage migrates caudally to its cervical po-

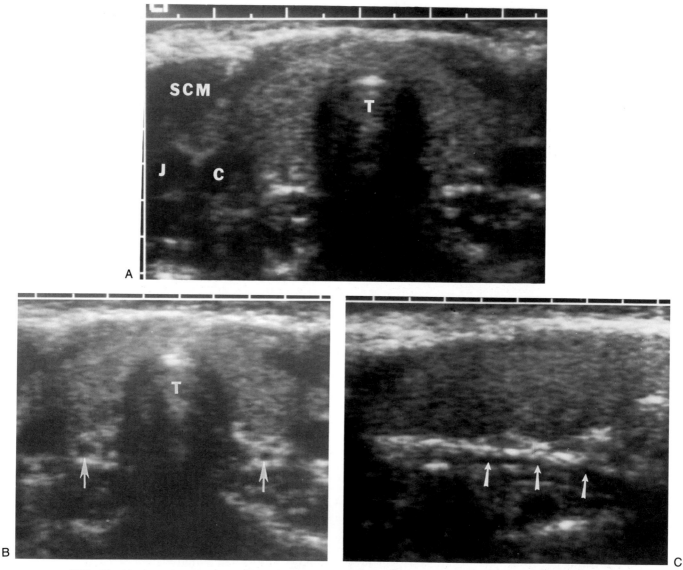

FIG. 23. Normal thyroid gland. **A:** On a transverse sonogram, the parenchyma of the lobes of the thyroid gland as well as the isthmus have a homogeneous echotexture. This uniform echogenicity makes detection of thyroid masses relatively easy in most cases. *C*, common carotid; *J*, internal jugular vein; *T*, trachea; *SCM*, sternocleidomastoid muscle. **B:** Transverse sonograms at a slightly lower level. Small hypoechoic structures posterior to the thyroid lobes represent the minor neurovascular bundles (*arrows*); *T*, trachea. **C:** A longitudinal sonogram shows the longus colli muscle (*arrows*) posterior to the thyroid gland.

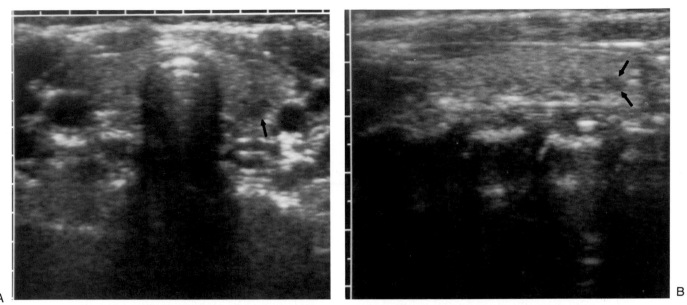

FIG. 24. Normal thyroid gland. **A**: Transverse and **B**: longitudinal scans of the thyroid of an 11-year-old girl demonstrate relatively homogeneous parenchyma in both lobes. In the inferior aspect of the left lobe, there is a small hypoechoic area (*arrows*) believed to represent a dilated colloid follicle, which is a normal variant.

sition in front of the larynx, it retains its connection with the base of the tongue via a tubular stalk, known as the thyroglossal duct. Once the gland reaches its final position in the neck, the duct atrophies and disappears.

Arrest in the development of the thyroid primordium produces total or partial absence of one or both lobes; abnormalities of migration result in ectopic tissue or thyroglossal duct remnants. Ectopic thyroid tissue may be found anywhere along the course of migration of the thyroid primordium. In most cases, the interruption is at the base of the tongue, producing a lingual thyroid. The ectopic thyroid may represent the only glandular tissue present and its secretion may or may not be adequate to maintain a euthyroid state. The most common anomaly is the thyroglossal duct cyst, which is due to the persistence of a portion of the embryonic stalk between the pharynx and thyroid gland.

The thyroid gland is easily recognized with sonography by its characteristic homogeneous echo texture, which is greater than that of the neck muscles (2,28) (Fig. 23). The thyroid is bordered posterolaterally by the common carotid artery and internal jugular vein and medially by the trachea on the right and esophagus on the left. Anterolateral to the thyroid gland are the sternocleidomastoid and strap muscles, which are hypoechoic relative to the thyroid. Posterolateral to the thyroid gland is the longus colli muscle, appearing as a sonolucent structure adjacent to the cervical vertebrae (28).

Small vessels coursing within the thyroid gland occasionally can be recognized by real-time imaging. At times, dilated colloid follicles are imaged within the normal gland, appearing as cystic areas under 3 mm in diameter without acoustic enhancement (Fig. 24). In some instances, the follicles contain echogenic foci, which represent inspissated colloid (4,29).

Indications

The major uses of thyroid sonography are to characterize thyroid nodules and to distinguish solitary from multiple thyroid nodules (2). Other uses include screening patients with histories of head and neck irradiation, guidance of fine-needle aspiration biopsy of a nodule, and follow-up evaluation of changes in the size of the nodules or the thyroid overall during suppressive therapy (4,65,74,77).

An application of high-resolution real-time sonography in neonates is the evaluation of congenital thyroid disease (2,8,39). Hypothyroidism is one of the most frequent endocrine disorders in neonates and usually results from thyroid agenesis or dysgenesis. Less frequent causes include defective thyroxine synthesis, also known as goitrous hypothyroidism, end-organ unresponsiveness to thyrotropin or thyroid hormone, and maternal ingestion of medications. The role of sonography in infants with congenital hypothyroidism is to identify the presence or absence of the thyroid gland and to distinguish rudimentary glands from anatomically normal thyroid glands. This information can be useful in clarifying the type of thyroid defect. Hyperthyroidism may be found in neonates but it is a rare condition, even in infants born to mothers with Graves' disease.

Benign Thyroid Nodules

Thyroid nodules are relatively rare in children, compared to adults, and are estimated to occur in 0.2% to 1.5% of the pedatric population (47,77). Although the majority of these are benign, a 14% to 40% incidence of malignancy has been reported (26,53,57). Most thyroid nodules are detected by palpation of the neck. Sonography complemented by radionuclide scintigraphy are the primary imaging techniques for confirming suspected thyroid disease. The principal value of sonography is the differentiation of solid from cystic nodules. Cystic lesions should be aspirated and the fluid examined, whereas solid lesions should be excised. Sonography can be used to guide the aspiration in difficult cases. At present, the role of CT and MR imaging seems to be limited to depicting the extent of very large thyroid masses or intrathoracic goiters (25).

Adenomas

Adenomas (follicular, embryonal, Hürthle cell) are the most frequently encountered benign neoplasms in the thyroid gland and are a result of hyperplasia and involution of a thyroid lobule. Pathologically, adenomas tend to be solitary, well-encapsulated, and noninvasive, and arise in glands that are otherwise entirely normal. Since the anatomic appearance is similar to that found in the late stage of multinodular goiter, the terms "adenomatous goiter," "adenomatous nodule," and "nodular adenomatous goiter" also have been applied to adenomas (27,29).

On sonography, the majority of adenomas are hypoechoic relative to the normal thyroid, although some demonstrate increased echogenicity and a few have the same echogenicity as the normal gland (28,32,54,64). A thin (1 to 2 mm) capsular "halo" or sonolucent rim surrounding the lesion has been seen in approximately 60% of adenomas (64) and may represent the fibrous capsule, compressed thyroid parenchyma, or pericapsular inflammatory infiltrate (45,54) (Fig. 25). Many adenomas also contain small cystic areas due to internal hemorrhage and necrosis (Fig. 26). Calcifications in benign adenomas are rare. They tend to occur at the periphery of the nodule and when present, appear as bright echogenic foci with associated acoustic shadowing. The presence of the halo sign, cystic changes, and calcifications are not specific indicators of benign disease and occasionally have been reported in malignant nodules (28,45).

Hemorrhagic Cysts

A hemorrhagic thyroid cyst may be the result of trauma to the neck or may develop spontaneously;

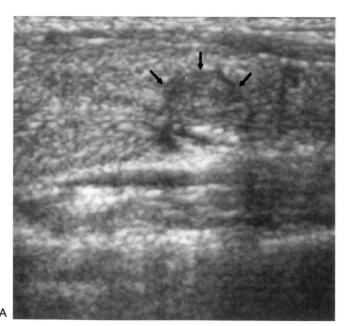
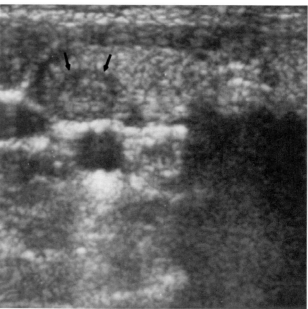

FIG. 25. Thyroid adenoma. **A**: Transverse and **B**: longitudinal images of the left lobe of the thyroid of a 13-year-old girl show an ovoid, slightly hypoechoic mass (*arrows*) with a sonolucent rim.

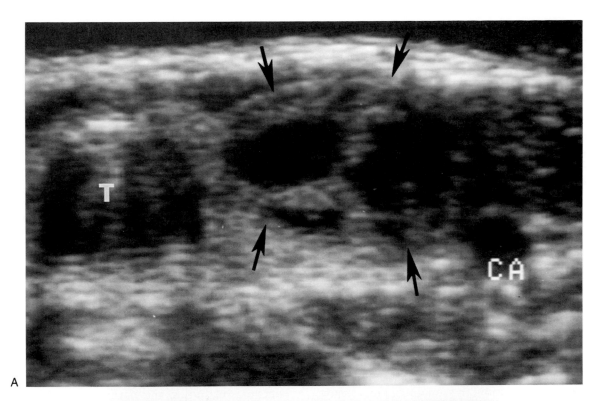

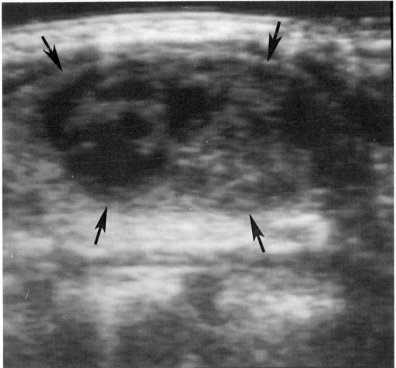

FIG. 26. Thyroid adenoma. **A**: Transverse and **B**: longitudinal sonograms of the left lobe of the thyroid show a 1.5 × 3.0 cm ovoid, complex mass (*arrows*) with multiple fluid-filled areas. At operation, a necrotic adenoma was found in the left thyroid lobe. *T*, trachea; *CA*, carotid artery.

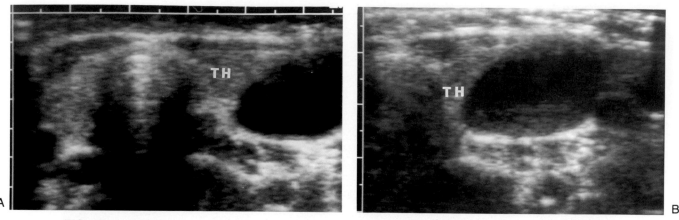

FIG. 27. Hemorrhagic cyst. A 14-year-old girl with a painless left thyroid mass. **A**: Transverse and **B**: longitudinal sonograms demonstrate a well-defined anechoic lesion contiguous with the left lobe of the thyroid (*TH*). A fluid debris level is present within the mass. At surgery, an adenoma with extensive hemorrhage was found in the lower pole of the left thyroid lobe.

most are believed to be the result of acute hemorrhage into follicular adenomas. The sonographic appearance of the acute lesion is that of a sonolucent mass with irregular borders and occasional internal septations or debris (4,65). With evolution, the sonolucent mass may develop a more circumscribed border; the septations may or may not persist, and a fluid-fluid level occasionally can develop (Fig. 27).

Simple Cysts

A true epithelial-lined simple cyst of the thyroid is rare and accounts for about 1% of benign thyroid masses. Most thyroid cysts are probably the result of cystic degeneration of a follicular adenoma rather than a true cyst. Sonographically, the appearance of a thyroid cyst is similar to that of cysts elsewhere in the body.

Malignant Thyroid Nodules

Carcinoma

Carcinoma of the thyroid gland accounts for about 1.5% of all malignancies before the age of 15 years. Two-thirds of these tumors occur in girls between 7 and 12 years and present as a palpable nodule in the thyroid or in the neck, an enlarging goiter, hoarseness, and pain (5). Enlarged anterior cervical lymph nodes may be present if there is tumor extension beyond the thyroid capsule. The major types of thyroid cancer in childhood are papillary (70%), follicular (20%), and medullary (5–10%) (5). Rarely, anaplastic carcinomas, lymphomas, and sarcomas are found. Metastases are primarily to regional lymph nodes and lung. Follicular

carcinomas may spread to bone or become endocrinologically functional.

The most common sonographic appearance of thyroid cancer is a predominantly solid mass that is hypoechoic relative to the normal thyroid parenchyma (28,65) (Fig. 28). Occasionally the lesion can be isoechoic relative to the normal gland and be unrecognized unless it alters the contour of the gland. The margins between the tumor and normal parenchyma vary from irregular to well-delineated with a sonolucent rim. Calcifications also may be found in thyroid carcinomas, particularly in association with papillary carcinomas. On sonography, they appear as focal, intensely echogenic areas, often associated with acoustic shadowing, either within the primary tumor or within metastases in lymph nodes (18).

Sonographic examination also has been used to detect recurrent thyroid carcinoma in patients who have been treated previously for thyroid malignancy. Because of scarring, clinical examination is often difficult in these patients. In detecting recurrent thyroid carcinoma, sonography has a sensitivity of 96% and a specificity of 83%. Scintigraphy with I^{131} has a similar sensitivity and a specificity of 100% (64). On sonography, recurrent carcinoma appears as hypoechoic masses in the bed of the excised thyroid gland and in the lateral neck. Needle biopsy using sonographic guidance is an accurate method for diagnosing recurrence (74).

Lymphoma

Lymphoma of the thyroid is an unusual condition that has been described almost exclusively in elderly adults; however, recent reports indicate that the dis-

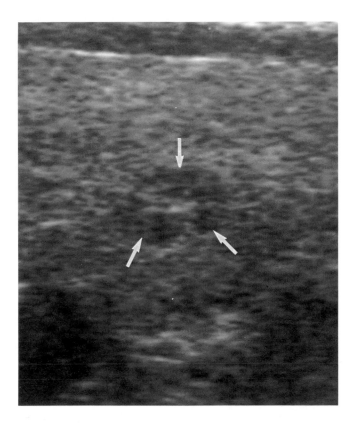

FIG. 28. Thyroid cancer. Transverse sonogram shows a 6 mm hypoechoic focus (*arrows*) within the right lobe of the thyroid. A papillary carcinoma was removed at operation.

ease can be found in children and adolescents (12,78). The sonographic findings vary from those of a solitary, inhomogeneous, hypoechoic mass to multiple hypoechoic and anechoic masses replacing the thyroid gland (43,76).

Thyroid Disease Following Irradiation

Irradiation of the head and neck region results in an increased frequency of thyroid, parathyroid, and salivary gland tumors. A latent period of 10 to 25 years following irradiation precedes the appearance of the tumors, both in children and adults. About 30% of patients with a history of radiation therapy to the head and neck will develop nodular thyroid disease (11) and between 6% to 9% of patients will have thyroid cancer (11,52). Radiation-induced cancers have a high frequency of multicentricity (55%) and bilaterality (35%) (56).

The irradiated thyroid gland can have a spectrum of abnormalities on sonography, including unilateral or bilateral atrophy; multiple hypoechoic lesions smaller than 0.75 cm in size; and dominant cystic, solid, or complex lesions larger than 0.75 cm in size (73). Although sonography cannot separate benign from malignant lesions, it can be used to identify nonpalpable nodules and look for changes in the echotexture of the thyroid gland in patients who have undergone cervical irradiation, to follow the course of parenchymal abnormalities, and to direct the site of biopsy (4,73).

Diffuse Thyroid Disease

Thyroid imaging is rarely indicated in patients with diffuse thyroid enlargement, but occasionally can be requested to examine patients who are obese or who have had prior surgery. The most likely cause of diffuse thyroid enlargement in childhood or adolescence is Hashimoto's thyroiditis. The next most likely etiologies include simple sporadic goiter, congenital dyshormonogenesis syndromes, iodine deficiency, and Graves' disease.

Hashimoto's Thyroiditis

Hashimoto's thyroiditis or lymphocytic thyroiditis is an organ-specific autoimmune disease primarily affecting adolescent girls. Histologically, the disorder is characterized by lymphocytic infiltration of the thyroid gland and by atrophy and fibrosis of the follicles. Most affected children are euthyroid with normal thyroid function tests.

Sonographically the thyroid gland is diffusely enlarged, often with a coarse, hypoechoic echotexture (24,28,34,65). This appearance may reflect the marked infiltration of the parenchyma with lymphoid tissue and severe degeneration of thyroid follicles (24,34). Occasionally, the echogenicity is almost normal and greater than that of adjacent muscle, presumably reflecting fibrotic tissue (34). About half of affected patients have discrete hypoechoic nodules (65) (Fig. 29). These areas of sonolucency may represent either areas of relatively normal tissue or aggregates of lymphoid tissue interspersed in fibrotic tissue. Multiple nodules in the lateral neck, reflecting lymphadenopathy, also can be seen in Hashimoto's thyroiditis.

Other Goiters

Simple goiter is a condition of unknown etiology that is characterized histologically by variable follicular size and dense colloid. Patients are euthyroid with normal or low levels of thyroid-stimulating hormone. Goiters associated with congenital defects in hormonogenesis or with iodine deficiency result from increased pituitary secretion of thyroid-stimulating hormone in response to decreased circulatory levels of thyroid hormones. Over a long time, repeated cycles of hyperplasia and involution lead to a multinodular goiter (27). Patients may be euthyroid or hypothyroid.

Sonographically, the enlarged thyroid gland is inhomogeneous, often with no recognizable thyroid parenchyma. Well-defined sonolucent areas, representing colloid cysts, may be present in a multinodular goiter due to congenital dyshormonogenesis or iodine deficiency (28,65) (Fig. 30). Hemorrhage and necrosis, manifested as fluid-filled areas, or calcifications may be found within the nodules (29,54).

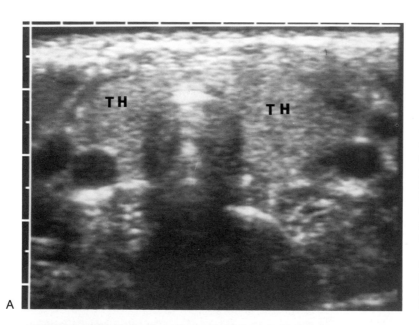

A

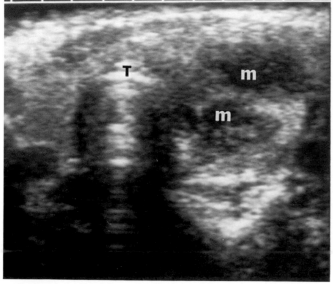

B

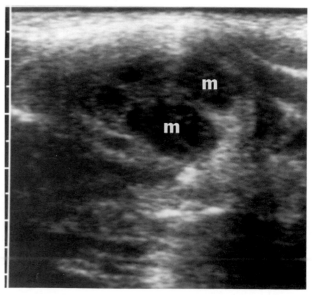

C

FIG. 29. Hashimoto's thyroiditis. A 12-year-old euthyroid girl with an enlarged thyroid gland. **A:** A transverse scan through the superior portion of the thyroid (*TH*) shows normal homogeneous echotexture, but the left lobe is noted to be larger than the right. **B, C:** On transverse and longitudinal images at a lower level, multiple hypoechoic masses (*m*) are noted within the enlarged left lobe. *T*, trachea. In this case, thyroiditis cannot be differentiated from a multinodular goiter based on the sonographic findings alone. Clinical history and aspiration are necessary for the correct diagnosis.

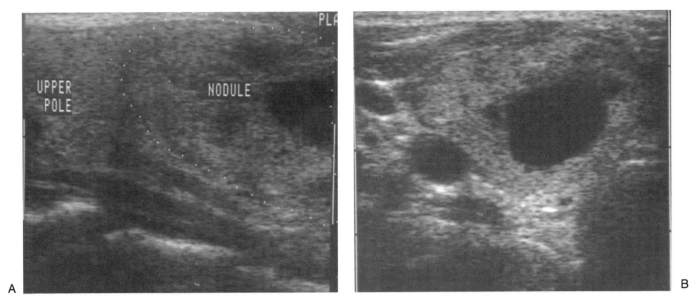

FIG. 30. Multinodular goiter. **A**: Longitudinal and **B**: transverse scans demonstrate a large nodule in the lower pole of the right lobe of the thyroid. Within the nodule are multiple anechoic nodules.

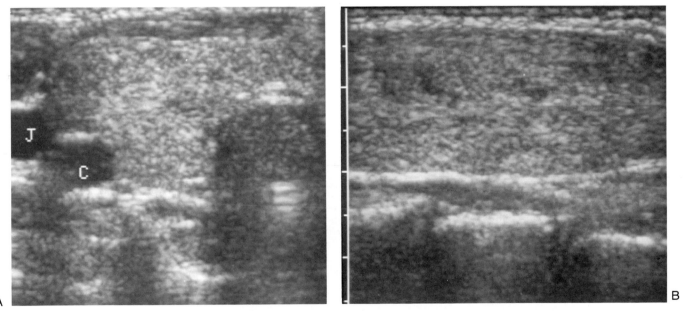

FIG. 31. Graves' disease. **A**: Transverse and **B**: longitudinal scans of the thyroid show an enlarged right lobe with a normal echotexture. *J*, jugular vein; *C*, carotid artery.

Graves' Disease

Thyroid enlargement in patients with thyrotoxicosis is caused by thyroid-stimulating immunoglobulin which binds to the receptors for thyroid-stimulating hormone. On sonography, the thyroid gland is diffusely enlarged, often with a normal echotexture (Fig. 31).

PARATHYROID GLANDS

Normal Anatomy

The parathyroid glands are derived from the third and fourth pharyngeal pouches. There are usually four glands. The paired superior glands arise from the fourth branchial pouch and have a fairly constant position near the upper surface of the thyroid lobes. The inferior parathyroid glands arise from the third branchial pouch and are found in close proximity to the lower pole of the thyroid gland (79). As in the case of thyroid development, the parathyroid glands also may arrest in their migration or migrate below the thyroid gland into the mediastinum. Fewer than 5% will be found in ectopic locations in the neck or in a substernal position (79). Occasionally, there may be more than four parathyroid glands. These supernumerary glands are frequently found in the mediastinum in association with the thymus.

Normal parathyroid glands are not visualized routinely by sonography because of their small size (less than 5 mm in length) and echotexture similar to that of overlying thyroid parenchyma. On occasion, however, the echogenicity may be slightly less than the thyroid's, and a discrete parathyroid gland may be demonstrated as an elongated mass between the posterior longus colli muscle and the anterior thyroid lobe.

Indications

High-resolution sonography of the parathyroid gland is useful in the preoperative evaluation of patients with primary hyperparathyroidism, in the guidance of fine-needle aspiration biopsy, in the postoperative evaluation of persistent or recurrent hyperparathyroidism, and in the percutaneous ethanol ablation of parathyroid tumors (67,71,72).

Benign adenomas account for approximately 80% of cases of primary hyperparathyroidism in children, with multiglandular hyperplasia occurring in 20% of cases, and carcinoma and parathyroid cysts in a few cases

(5). Surgical intervention is currently favored in all cases of primary hyperparathyroidism. An experienced surgeon can successfully treat 90% to 95% of patients without the routine use of preoperative imaging procedures. Preoperative localization is useful, however, if the surgeon wants to perform a unilateral neck exploration and does not insist on exploring all four glands. Preoperative imaging also is important in patients with persistent or recurrent hyperparathyroidism who have had previous neck surgery. In these patients, postoperative scarring and adhesions make reoperation more difficult and there is a higher complication rate. Preoperative localization of a missed adenoma or gland reduces operation time, decreases the risk of complications, and provides more favorable technical conditions for reexploration. This is especially important if the missing gland is located in the mediastinum since thoracic, rather than cervical, exploration would be required for removal (79).

Diseases of the Parathyroid Glands

Adenoma

About 90% of parathyroid adenomas are situated posterior to the thyroid gland; the remainder are located ectopically in the neck or mediastinum (79). Adenomas usually are discrete, well-marginated, solid masses varying in length from 6 to 42 mm (71). They may be round, but usually tend to be oval or teardrop-shaped due to dissection between the longitudinally oriented tissue planes. The majority have an echogenicity that is lower than that of the thyroid gland (66,71) (Fig. 32). Rarely, adenomas may be entirely cystic,

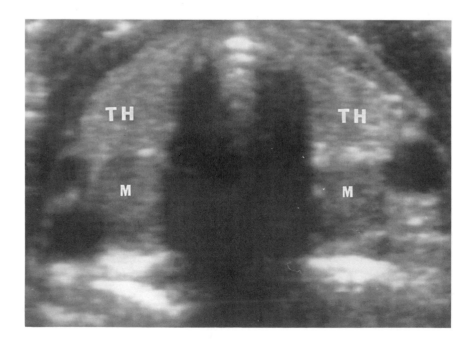

FIG. 32. Parathyroid adenoma. Transverse sonogram shows bilateral hypoechoic round masses (*M*) behind the thyroid (*TH*) gland. The lesions are relatively hypoechoic compared to thyroid parenchyma. Parathyroid adenomas were confirmed surgically.

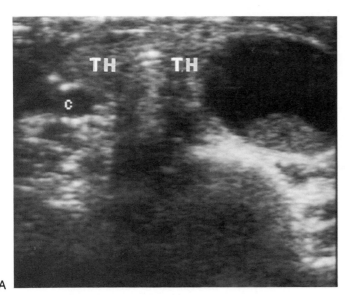 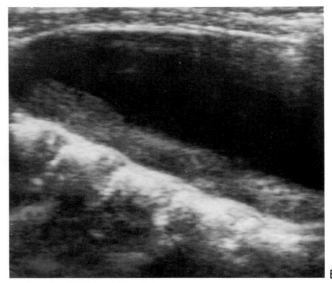

A   B

FIG. 33. Parathyoid cyst. **A**: Transverse and **B**: longitudinal sonograms of the left neck show a large cyst with dependent debris adjacent to the left lobe of the thyroid (*TH*). *C*, carotid artery.

contain calcifications, or have a multilobulated configuration (48).

Hyperplasia

Multiglandular hyperplasia accounts for very few cases of primary hyperparathyroidism, although it is the cause of nearly all cases of secondary hyperparathyroidism. In most cases all the glands are involved in hyperplasia. The hyperplastic glands range from 5 mm to 25 mm in length (71,72). On sonography, hyperplastic glands may appear as solid nodules with homogeneous low-level echoes, but more often they are diffusely enlarged with an echogenicity less than that of adjacent thyroid tissue (75). The enlarged glands are separated from the thyroid by a highly echogenic line, believed to represent the fibrous capsule.

There are no entirely reliable sonographic characteristics to distinguish adenoma and hyperplasia. The presence of a single nodule or enlarged gland favors the diagnosis of an adenoma. If multiple glands are enlarged, hyperplasia is a more likely explanation of hyperparathyroidism. However, adenomas can occasionally be multiple and produce bilateral glandular enlargement. The definitive diagnosis requires tissue sampling.

Parathyroid Cysts

Parathyroid cysts are rare in childhood. Most are associated with the inferior parathyroid glands, but they can occur anywhere from the angle of the mandible to the mediastinum. They are usually nonfunc-tioning and present as palpable masses; rarely, signs of hyperparathyroidism are present (9,33). On sonography, the cysts are unilocular, fluid-filled lesions, lying lateral to the thyroid gland (Fig. 33). Because of their relationship to the thyroid gland, separating parathyroid from thyroid cysts may be impossible without analysis of the cyst fluid. Percutaneous aspiration of the cyst and determination of hormone levels is an effective method to establish the diagnosis (9).

Comparative Imaging Techniques

The sensitivity of high-resolution sonography for detecting abnormal parathyroid glands in patients with and without prior surgery is 65% to 88% (16,17,19, 49,50,55,66,71,72,83). The presence of concurrent nodular thyroid disease or lymph nodes can result in false-positive diagnoses, while false-negative results are associated with lesions that are ectopic, very cephalad or caudad in the neck, extremely small, or entirely intrathyroid (17,19,38,83). In addition, retrotracheal or mediastinal tumors cannot be detected by sonography because acoustic transmission is blocked by overlying bone and lung.

If the sonographic study of the neck is negative, other localizing studies such as thallium scintigraphy and CT or MR imaging are indicated to evaluate the presence of ectopic glands. The sensitivity of thallium scintigraphy for detecting abnormal glands in patients with initial and recurrent hyperparathyroidism is approximately 60% to 87% (17,44,83). Likewise, CT has a sensitivity of 50% to 87% (69,72,75) and MR imaging a sensitivity of 64% to 79% (31,44,70). The advantage of these techniques over sonography is their increased ability to depict ectopic parathyroid adenomas. As with sonography, intrathyroid masses or lymph nodes may be difficult to distinguish from parathyroid adenoma.

PAROTID GLAND

Normal Anatomy

The parotid gland, the largest of the salivary glands, lies between the ramus of the mandible anteriorly and the mastoid process and sternocleidomastoid muscle posteriorly. It is subdivided into a lateral or superficial and medial or deep lobe, separated by the facial nerve. The superficial lobe is the larger portion of the parotid, accounting for 80% of the gland; the deep lobe accounts for 20%. The parotid, or Stensen's duct, drains the parotid gland and is found along the anterior border of the parotid below the zygoma, crosses the masseter muscle, and then pierces the muscle to enter the oral cavity. Branches of the external carotid artery supply the parotid gland and the retromandibular vein drains it.

The salivary glands are superficial structures and are best evaluated by high frequency, 7 or 10 MHz transducers (58,84). Transverse or cross-sectional views are obtained initially with the transducer perpendicular and inferior to the earlobe. In this plane, the mandible anteriorly, masoid tip posteriorly, and posterior facial vein and external carotid artery within the substance of the parotid can be identified. In addition, coronal

views are obtained. Coronal views, parallel and anterior to the ear, best display the substance of the parotid gland. The normal gland is seen just below the skin surface and is elliptical with an echogenic homogeneous texture (Fig. 34).

Pathology

Parotid gland neoplasms are rare in children, accounting for about 1% of all tumors in the general population. The vast majority of malignant tumors are pleomorphic adenomas or mixed tumors; benign lesions are usually hemangiomas and lymphangiomas. Patients typically present with a slow-growing, painless mass.

Sonography is useful for differentiating an intraparotid lesion from a superficial lesion extrinsic to the gland. If the lesion is deep, CT is the method of choice for further evaluation since sonography cannot visualize the entire deep lobe. On sonography, most parotid tumors are hypoechoic relative to the adjacent parotid and are inhomogeneous.

Inflammatory diseases are more common than tumors in the parotid gland. Acute inflammation of the gland is usually secondary to mumps and does not require imaging studies. Acute suppurative sialadenitis is rare, but involves the parotid gland more than other glands and tends to occur in dehydrated, debilitated patients. Sonography can be useful in identifying the presence of infection and the extent of abscess formation (84).

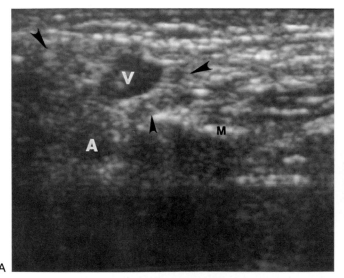
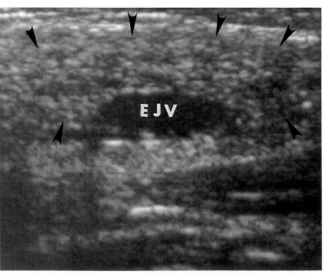

A

B

FIG. 34. Normal parotid gland. **A**: Cross-sectional scan perpendicular to the ear shows the posterior facial vein (*V*) and external carotid artery (*A*) in the substance of the parotid (*arrowheads*). *M*, mandible. **B**: Coronal scan parallel to ear shows the elliptical echogenic parotid gland (*arrowheads*). *EJV*, external jugular vein.

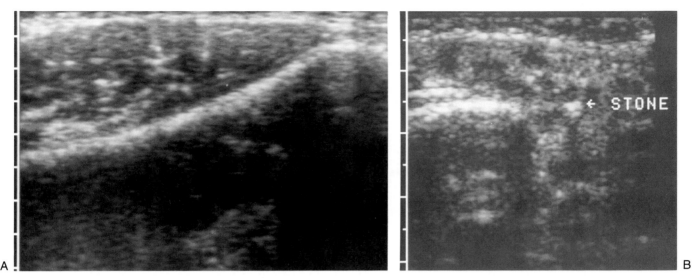

FIG. 35. Sialadenitis with sialolithiasis. **A**: Coronal and **B**: transverse scans of the parotid demonstrate parotid enlargement and inhomogeneous parenchyma. Also noted is an echogenic focus (*stone*) casting an acoustic shadow consistent with a calculus.

Calculi predominate in the submandibular and parotid glands. Approximately 80% to 90% occur in the submandibular gland and most of the remainder occur in the parotid gland. The majority of calculi are opaque, but up to 40% may not be seen on plain radiographs because they are superimposed on bone (37). In these instances, sonography may be helpful by demonstrating an echogenic focus with acoustic shadowing (Fig. 35). Associated sialectasis may be noted.

REFERENCES

1. Albertyn LE, Alcock MK. Diagnosis of internal jugular vein thrombosis. *Radiology* 1987;162:505–508.
2. Bachrach LK, Daneman D, Daneman A, Martin DJ. Use of ultrasound in childhood thyroid disorders. *J Pediatr* 1983; 103:547–552.
3. Badami JP, Athey PA. Sonography in the diagnosis of branchial cysts. *AJR* 1981;137:1245–1248.
4. Butch RJ, Simeone JF, Mueller PR. Thyroid and parathyroid ultrasonography. *Radiol Clin North Am* 1985;23:57–71.
5. Chrousos GP. Endocrine tumors. In: Pizzo PA, Poplack DG, eds. *Pediatric Oncology*. Philadelphia: J.B. Lippincott, 1989; 741–744.
6. Cole-Beuglet C. Ultrasonography of thyroid, parathyroid and neck masses. In: Sarti, DA, ed. *Diagnostic Ultrasound: Text and Cases*. Chicago: Year Book Medical Publishers, 1987;608–618.
7. Crawford SC, Harnsberger HR, Johnson L, Aoki JR, Giley J. Fibromatosis colli of infancy: CT and sonographic findings. *AJR* 1988;151:1183–1184.
8. Dammacco F, Dammacco A, Cavallo T, et al. Serum thyroglobulin and thyroid ultrasound studies in infants with congenital hypothyroidism. *J Pediatr* 1985;106:451–453.
9. DeRaimo AJ, Kane RA, Katz JF, Rolla AP. Parathyroid cyst: Diagnosis by sonography and needle aspiration. *AJR* 1984;142:1227–1228.
10. Donegan JO. Congenital neck masses. In: Cummings CW, Fredrickson JM, Harker LA, Krause CJ, Schuller DE, eds. *Otolar-yngology—Head and Neck Surgery*. St. Louis: Mosby, 1986;1597–1608.
11. Favus MJ, Schneider AB, Stachura ME, et al. Thyroid cancer occurring as a late consequence of head-and-neck irradiation. Evaluation of 1056 patients. *N Engl J Med* 1976;294:1019–1025.
12. Fiorillo A, Migliorati R, Fiore M, Caldore M, Menna G, Celentano L. Non-Hodgkin's lymphoma in childhood presenting as thyroid enlargement. *Clin Pediatr* 1987;26:152–154.
13. Friedman AP, Haller JO, Goodman JD, Nagar H. Sonographic evaluation of non-inflammatory neck masses in children. *Radiology* 1983;147:693–697.
14. Ganick DJ, Kodroff MB, Marrow HG, Holbrook CT, Pories WJ. Thoracic neuroblastoma presenting as a cystic hygroma. *Arch Dis Child* 1988;63:1270–1271.
15. Glazer HS, Balfe DM, Sagel SS. Neck. In: Lee KTL, Sagel SS, Stanely RJ, eds. *Computed Body Tomography with MRI Correlation*. New York: Raven Press, 1989;1009–1067.
16. Gooding GAW, Herzog KA, Laing FC, McDonald EJ, Jr. Ultrasonographic assessment of neck masses. *JCU* 1977;5:248–252.
17. Gooding GAW, Okerlund MD, Stark DD, Clark OH. Parathyroid imaging: Comparison of double-tracer (T1-201, Tc-99m) scintigraphy and high-resolution US. *Radiology* 1986;161:57–64.
18. Gorman B, Charboneau JW, James EM, et al. Medullary thyroid carcinoma: Role of high-resolution US. *Radiology* 1987;162: 147–150.
19. Graif M, Itzchak Y, Strauss S, Dolev E, Mohr R, Wolfstein I. Parathyroid sonography: Diagnostic accuracy related to shape, location and texture of the gland. *Br J Radiol* 1987;60:439–443.
20. Graney DO. Neck anatomy. In: Cummings CW, Fredrickson JM, Harker LA, Krause CJ, Schuller DE, eds. *Otolaryngology—Head and Neck Surgery*. St. Louis: Mosby, 1986;1573–1586.
21. Gruhn J, Hurwitt ES. Fibrous sternomastoid tumor of infancy. *Pediatrics* 1951;8:522–526.
22. Hajek PC, Salomonowitz E, Turk R, Tscholakoff D, Kumpan W, Czembirek H. Lymph nodes of the neck: Evaluation with US. *Radiology* 1986;158:739–742.
23. Harnsberger HR, Mancuso AA, Muraki AS, Byrd SE, Dillon WP, Johnson LP, Hanafee WN. Branchial cleft anomalies and their mimics: Computed tomographic evaluation. *Radiology* 1984;152:739–748.
24. Hayashi N, Tamaki N, Konishi J, et al. Sonography of Hashimoto's thyroiditis. *JCU* 1986;14:123–126.

25. Higgins CB, Auffermann W. MR imaging of thyroid and parathyroid glands: A review of current status. *AJR* 1988;151:1095–1106.

26. Hung W, August GP, Randolph JG, Schisgall RM, Chandra R. Solitary thyroid nodules in children and adolescents. *J Pediatr Surg* 1982;17:225–229.

27. Ingbar SH. The thyroid gland. In: Wilson JD, Foster DW, eds. *Textbook of Endocrinology*, 7th ed. Philadelphia: WB Saunders. 1985;682–815.

28. James EM, Charboneau JW. High-frequency (10 MHz) thyroid ultrasonography. *Sem US, CT, MR* 1985;6:294–309.

29. Katz JF, Kane RA, Reyes J, Clarke MP, Hill TC. Thyroid nodules: Sonographic-pathologic correlation. *Radiology* 1984;151: 741–745.

30. Kittredge RD, Finby N. The many facets of lymphangioma. *AJR* 1965;95:56–66.

31. Kneeland JB, Krubsack AJ, Lawson TL, et al. Enlarged parathyroid glands: High-resolution local coil MR imaging. *Radiology* 1987;162:143–146.

32. Kraus R, Han BK, Babcock DS, Oestreich AE. Sonography of neck masses in children. *AJR* 1986;146:609–613.

33. Krudy AG, Doppman JL, Shawker TH, et al. Hyperfunctioning cystic parathyroid glands: CT and sonographic findings. *AJR* 1984;142:175–178.

34. Mailloux G, Bertrand M, Stampfler R, Ethier S. Computer analysis of echographic textures in Hashimoto disease of the thyroid. *JCU* 1986;14:521–527.

35. Maran ADG, Buchanan DR. Branchial cysts, sinuses and fistulae. *Clin Otolaryngol* 1978;3:77–92.

36. Marchal G, Oyen R, Verschakelen J, Gelin J, Baert AL, Stessens RC. Sonographic appearance of normal nodes. *J Ultrasound Med* 1985;4:417–419.

37. Miglets AW. Infections. In: Cummings CW, Fredrickson JM, Harker LA, Krause CJ, Schuller DE. *Otolaryngology—Head and Neck Surgery*. St. Louis: Mosby, 1986;999–1006.

38. Miller DL, Doppman JL, Shawker TH, et al. Localization of parathyroid adenomas in patients who have undergone surgery. Part I. Noninvasive imaging methods. *Radiology* 1987;162:133–137.

39. Miller JH. Lingual thyroid gland: Sonographic appearance. *Radiology* 1985;156:83–84.

40. Moussatos GH, Baffes TG. Cervical masses in infants and children. *Pediatrics* 1963;32:251–256.

41. Noyek AM, Friedberg J. Thyroglossal duct and ectopic thyroid disorders. *Otolaryngol Clin North Am* 1981;14:187–201.

42. Nyberg DA, Jeffrey RB, Brant-Zawadski MB, Federle M, Dillon W. Computed tomography of cervical infections. *J Comput Assist Tomogr* 1985;9:288–296.

43. Parulekar SG, Katzman RA. Primary malignant lymphoma of the thyroid: Sonographic appearance. *JCU* 1986;14:60–62.

44. Peck WW, Higgins CB, Fisher MR, Ling M, Okerlund MD, Clark OH. Hyperparathyroidism: Comparison of MR imaging with radionuclide scanning. *Radiology* 1987;163:415–420.

45. Propper RA, Skolnick ML, Weinstein BJ, Dekker A. The non-specificity of the thyroid halo sign. *JCU* 1980;8:129–132.

46. Putney FJ. The diagnosis of head and neck masses in children. *Otolaryngol Clin North Am* 1970;3:277–294.

47. Rallison ML, Dobyns BM, Keating FR, Jr, Rall JE, Tyler FH. Thyroid nodularity in children. *JAMA* 1975;233:1069–1072.

48. Randel SB, Gooding GAW, Clark OH, Stein RM, Winkler B. Parathyroid variants: US evaluation. *Radiology* 1987;165:191–194.

49. Reading CC, Charboneau JW, James EM, Karsell PR, Grant CS, van Heerden JA, Purnell DC. Postoperative parathyroid high-frequency sonography: Evaluation of persistent or recurrent hyperparathyroidism. *AJR* 1985;144:399–402.

50. Reading CC, Charboneau JW, James EM, Karsell PR, Purnell DC, Grant CS, van Heerden JA. High-resolution parathyroid sonography. *AJR* 1982;139:539–546.

51. Reede DL, Bergeron T, Som PM. CT of thyroglossal duct cysts. *Radiology* 1985;157:121–125.

52. Refetoff S, Harrison J, Karanfilski BT, Kaplan EL, DeGroot LJ, Bekerman C. Continuing occurrence of thyroid carcinoma after irradiation to the neck in infancy and childhood. *N Engl J Med* 1975;292:171–175.

53. Rojeski MT, Gharib H. Nodular thyroid disease. Evaluation and management. *N Engl J Med* 1985;313:428–436.

54. Scheible W, Leopold GR, Woo VL, Gosink B. High-resolution real-time ultrasonography of thyroid nodules. *Radiology* 1979;133:413–417.

55. Scheible W, Deutsch AL, Leopold GR. Parathyroid adenoma: Accuracy of preoperative localization by high-resolution real-time sonography. *JCU* 1981;9:325–330.

56. Schneider AB, Pinsky S, Bekerman C, Ryo UY. Characteristics of 108 thyroid cancers detected by screening in a population with a history of head and neck irradiation. *Cancer* 1980;46:1218–1227.

57. Scott MD, Crawford JD. Solitary thyroid nodule in childhood: Is the incidence of thyroid carcinoma declining? *Pediatrics* 1976;58:521–525.

58. Seibert RW, Seibert JJ. High resolution sonography of the parotid gland in children. *Pediatr Radiol* 1986;16:374–379.

59. Sherman NH, Rosenberg HK, Heyman S, Templeton J. Ultrasound evaluation of neck masses in children. *J Ultrasound Med* 1985;4:127–134.

60. Sheth S, Nussbaum AR, Hutchins GM, Sanders RC. Cystic hygromas in children: Sonographic-pathologic correlation. *Radiology* 1987;162:821–824.

61. Siegel MJ, St. Amour TE. Neck. In: Siegel MJ, ed. *Pediatric Body CT*. New York: Churchill Livingstone Inc., 1988;293–312.

62. Siegel MJ, Glazer HS, St. Amour TE, Rosenthal DD. Lymphangiomas in children: MR imaging. *Radiology* 1989;170:467–470.

63. Siegel MJ, McAlister WH, Askin FN. Lymphangiomas in children: Report of 121 cases. *J Can Assoc Radiol* 1979:30:99–102.

64. Simeone JF, Daniels GH, Hall DA, et al. Sonography in the follow-up of 100 patients with thyroid carcinoma. *AJR* 1987;148:45–49.

65. Simeone JF, Daniels GH, Mueller PR, et al. High-resolution real-time sonography of the thyroid. *Radiology* 1982;145:432–435.

66. Simeone JF, Mueller PR, Ferrucci JT, et al. High-resolution real-time sonography of the parathyroid. *Radiology* 1981;141:745–751.

67. Solbiati L, Giangrande A, de Pra L, Bellotti E, Cantù P, Ravetto C. Percutaneous ethanol injection of parathyroid tumors under US guidance: Treatment for secondary hyperparathyroidism. *Radiology* 1985;607–610.

68. Som PM, Sacher M, Lanzieri CF, et al. Parenchymal cysts of the lower neck. *Radiology* 1985;157:399–406.

69. Sommer B, Welter HF, Spelsberg F, Scherer U, Lissner J. Computed tomography for localizing enlarged parathyroid glands in primary hyperparathyroidism. *J Comput Assist Tomogr* 1982;6:521–526.

70. Spritzer CE, Gefter WB, Hamilton R, Greenberg BM, Axel L, Kressel HY. Abnormal parathyroid glands: High-resolution MR imaging. *Radiology* 1987;162:487–491.

71. Stark DD, Gooding GAW, Clark OH. Noninvasive parathyroid imaging. *Sem US, CT, MR* 1985;6:310–320.

72. Stark DD, Gooding GAW, Moss AA, Clark OH, Ovenfors C-O. Parathyroid imaging: Comparison of high-resolution CT and high-resolution sonography. *AJR* 1983;141:633–638.

73. Stewart RR, David CL, Eftekhari F, et al. Thyroid gland: US in patients with Hodgkin's disease treated with radiation therapy in childhood. *Radiology* 1989;172:159–163.

74. Sutton RT, Reading CC, Charboneau JW, James EM, Grant CS, Hay ID. US-guided biopsy of neck masses in postoperative management of patients with thyroid cancer. *Radiology* 1988; 168:769–772.

75. Takebayashi S, Matsui K, Onohara Y, Hidai H. Sonography for early diagnosis of enlarged parathyroid glands in patients with secondary hyperparathyroidism. *AJR* 1987;148:911–914.

76. Takashima S, Morimoto S, Ikezoe J, et al. Primary thyroid lymphoma: Comparison of CT and US assessment. *Radiology* 1989;171:439–443.

77. Van Vliet G, Glinoer D, Verelst J, Spehl M, Gompel C, Delange

F. Cold thyroid nodules in childhood: Is surgery always necessary? *Eur J Pediatr* 1987;146:378–382.

78. Wallace JHK. Ultrasonography in the diagnosis of thyroid lymphoma. *J Can Assoc Radiol* 1985;36:317–319.

79. Wang C-A. The anatomic basis of parathyroid surgery. *Ann Surg* 1976;183:271–275.

80. Williams RH, ed. *Textbook of Endocrinology*. Philadelphia: W. B. Saunders Co., 1981;117–247.

81. Wilson DB. Embryonic development of the head and neck: Part 2, the branchial region. *Head and Neck Surg* 1974;2:59–66.

82. Wing V, Scheible W. Sonography of jugular vein thrombosis. *AJR* 1983;140:333–336.

83. Winzelberg GC, Hydovitz JD, O'Hara KR, et al. Parathyroid adenomas evaluated by T1-201/Tc-99m pertechnetate subtraction scintigraphy and high-resolution ultrasonography. *Radiology* 1985;155:231–235.

84. Wittich GR, Scheible WF, Hajek PC. Ultrasonography of the salivary glands. *Radiol Clin North Am* 1985;23:29–36.

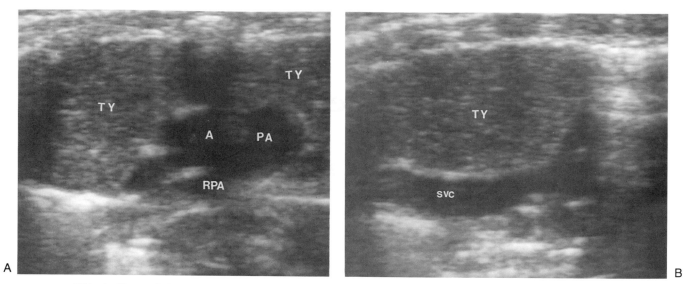

FIG. 1. Normal thymus. **A:** Transverse and **B:** longitudinal scans of the upper mediastinum in an infant show a homogeneously echogenic thymus (*TY*). The aorta (*A*), pulmonary artery (*PA*), right pulmonary artery (*RPA*), and superior vena cava (*SVC*) are seen.

oval shape on longitudinal scans (Fig. 1). The echogenicity is homogeneous and slightly less than that of the thyroid gland (18). Rarely, the thymus may extend into the posterior mediastinum or superiorly above the brachiocephalic vessels (Fig. 2) (53). The abnormally positioned thymus can be recognized on sonography by its pliability, direct continuity with the anterior mediastinal thymic tissue, and echogenicity similar to that of normal thymic tissue (5). Detection of the thymus decreases with increasing age, because of aerated lung in the anterior mediastinum which interferes with sound transmission and a relative decrease in size of the organ.

Trachea

The anterior wall of the trachea appears as an echogenic curvilinear midline band (Fig. 3). The posterior

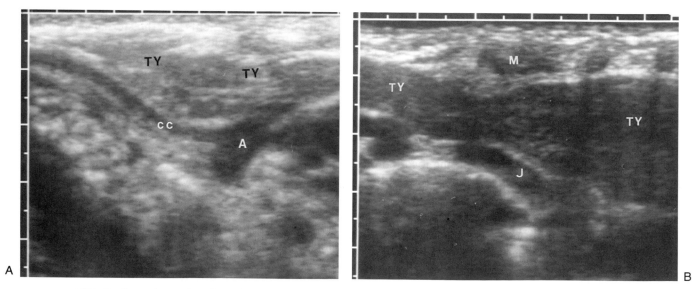

FIG. 2. Superior extension of normal thymus into the neck. **A:** Longitudinal scan to the left of midline shows normally echogenic thymus (*TY*) anterior to the aortic arch (*A*) and left common carotid artery (*CC*). **B:** Longitudinal scan of another infant shows a normal thymus (*TY*) in the anterior mediastinum with superior extension above the manubrium (*M*). The left internal jugular (*J*) is seen posterior to the thymus.

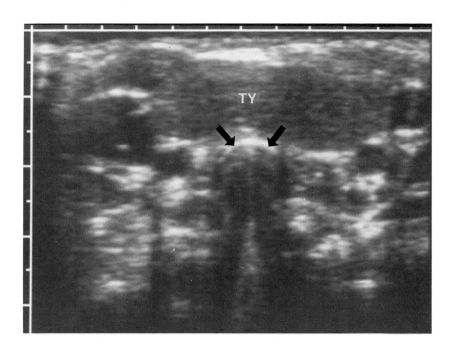

FIG. 3. Anterior wall of trachea. Transverse scan of the thoracic inlet demonstrates the highly echogenic curved midline band of the trachea (*arrows*) posterior to the thymus (*TY*).

wall, however, is not routinely visualized by sonography because of reverberation artifacts from air. Because of this limitation, sonography has minimal or no value in the evaluation of tracheal abnormalities.

Esophagus

The esophagus is difficult to image by sonography because it is normally collapsed. Visualization of the esophagus can be improved by having the patient swallow fluid. In general, evaluation of the esophagus in the neonate or children is of limited practical value. Occasionally, however, the diagnosis of gastroesophageal reflux can be made by seeing echogenic reflections within the esophageal contents (see Chapter 7). The diagnosis of esophageal atresia in the neonate also can be made by sonography by demonstration of a distended proximal esophageal segment. The distal esophageal segment may be dilated if there is both esophageal and gastric atresia (8).

Great Vessels

Transverse and sagittal sections through a suprasternal approach are useful for imaging the aortic arch and brachiocephalic arteries and veins (Figs. 1,2,4). The ascending and descending aorta and main pulmonary artery are best seen with longitudinal parasternal scans. Duplex or color flow Doppler sonography are useful adjuncts to cross-sectional imaging when it is uncertain whether a vascular structure is arterial or venous. In normal patients, the vessels have sharp, echogenic walls and anechoic lumina. The luminal diameter varies with the respiratory cycle as do the Doppler waveforms, increasing during inspiration and decreasing during expiration (13).

Diaphragm

The diaphragm is the chief muscle of respiration. It is composed of a central tendon and peripheral muscle leaflets. The anterior portion is attached to the posterior surfaces of the sternum and lower six costal cartilages. The posterior or lumbar portion arises from two crura that attach the diaphragm to the front of the upper lumbar vertebral bodies. The right crus is attached to the bodies of the upper three lumbar vertebrae and the left crus to the bodies of the upper two. The posterior portion also is adherent to the anterior surface of the quadratus lumborum and psoas major muscles. This area is important because it represents a potential site for herniation.

The right hemidiaphragm is easily imaged through the right lobe of the liver, which provides an acoustic window. The left hemidiaphragm is more difficult to image because of adjacent gas in the stomach and splenic flexure of the colon. Scanning may be successful if the spleen can be used as an acoustic window. In some instances, distention of the stomach with fluid, administered orally or through a nasogastric tube, and scanning with the patient in the supine Trendelenburg position may be useful in providing an acoustic window. Sonographically, the diaphragm is seen as an ech-

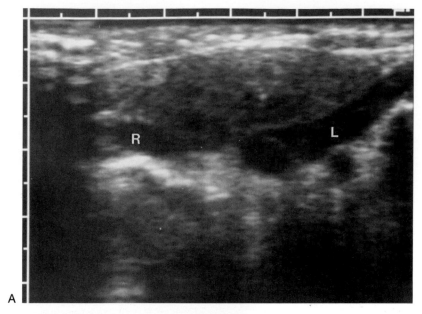

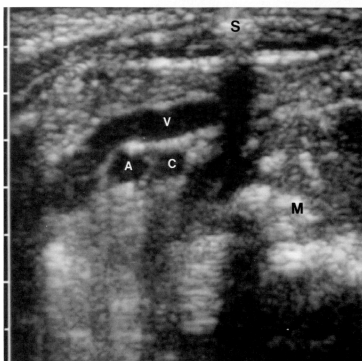

FIG. 4. Mediastinal vessels. A: Transverse scan of the upper mediastinum shows the left (*L*) and right (*R*) brachiocephalic veins posterior to the thymus. B: Transverse scan of another patient shows the left brachiocephalic vein (*V*), right brachiocephalic artery (*A*), and left common carotid artery (*C*). The ossified sternum (*S*) obscures the left subclavian artery. The vessels are displaced to the right by a large calcified neuroblastoma (*M*). C: (see Colorplate 4) Color flow imaging of mediastinal vessels. *LBC*, left brachiocephalic vein; *RBC*, right brachiocephalic vein; *SVC*, superior vena cava; *RBA*, right brachiocephalic artery.

ogenic band on both longitudinal and transverse scans (Fig. 5). The echogenicity represents a combination of echoes produced by the diaphragm-lung interface and the liver-diaphragm or spleen-diaphragm junction (30). The crura are seen as sonolucent structures near the midline on both longitudinal and transverse planes. The right crus tends to be larger than the left.

Diaphragm motion can be examined in both the longitudinal and transverse planes. The examination of the right diaphragm is easier because of the acoustic window provided by the liver. On the left, it is slightly more difficult unless there is a prominent left lobe of the liver or a spleen that can be used as an acoustic window. Motion is best assessed on transverse images which allow simultaneous identification of both hemidiaphragms. Measurements have been established for normal diaphragmatic excursion (29). On longitudinal views, the anterior, middle, and posterior thirds of the right diaphragm move 2.6 ± 0.1, 3.6 ± 0.2, and 4.5 ± 0.2 mm, respectively. The middle and

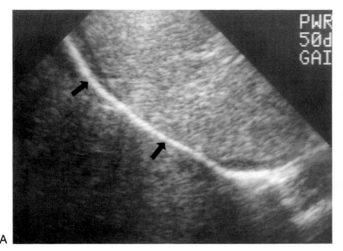

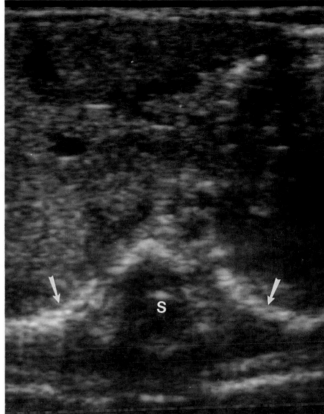

FIG. 5. Normal diaphragm. **A:** Longitudinal subcostal and **B:** transverse subxiphoid scans demonstrating the echogenic diaphragm (*arrows*). Portions of the right and left hemidiaphragms (*arrows*) are seen on the transverse scan on each side of the spine (*S*).

posterior thirds of the right diaphragm have a greater excursion than the anterior portion of the diaphragm.

INDICATIONS

The major indications for chest sonography include (a) identification of an anomalous vessel associated with pulmonary sequestration (16,17), (b) separation of pleural from parenchymal disease in a child with a partially or totally opacified hemithorax on chest radiography (3,17,39,53,55), (c) localization of pleural fluid for aspiration, (d) evaluation of diaphragmatic motion and masses (43), and (e) assessment of vascular abnormalities (42). Less often, sonography is used to evaluate mediastinal and chest wall lesions and endotracheal tube positioning.

PATHOLOGY

Lung Parenchyma

Although the normal air-filled lung limits the utility of chest sonography in evaluating parenchymal abnormalities, peripheral lesions adjacent to the chest wall or diaphragm or those next to the heart can be evaluated through an acoustic window created by con-tiguous soft tissue structures. The role of sonography in diagnosing parenchymal disease is limited, but occasionally sonography can identify a sequestration in an infant with recurrent infiltrates or a solid mass in a neonate with pleural fluid or an opaque hemithorax.

Sequestration

A persistent density, mass, or chronic recurrent segmental or subsegmental pneumonia, especially at a lung base, or a massive pleural effusion in a neonate are plain radiographic findings that suggest sequestration (14,59,60). Pathologically, bronchopulmonary sequestration is a mass of nonfunctioning lung tissue that has no normal connection with the bronchial tree and is supplied by an anomalous systemic vessel, usually arising from the aorta (26). When the sequestered lung is contained within the normal visceral pleura and has venous drainage to pulmonary veins, it is termed "intralobar." When the sequestered lung has a separate pleural investment and venous drainage into the azygos or hemiazygos system or portal vein, it is referred to as "extralobar (32). Occasionally, intralobar sequestration will drain into the azygos system, whereas extralobar sequestration will drain through pulmonary veins. Intralobar sequestration is more common (75% of cases) and is located in the left lower lobe in 90%

of cases (50). Sixty percent of extralobar sequestrations occur in the lower lobes. The remainder are found in an upper lobe, interlobar fissure, mediastinum, and abdomen. Sixty-five percent of extralobar sequestrations are associated with diaphragmatic or gastrointestinal anomalies, most often a diaphragmatic hernia (9). Other anomalies include bronchogenic cysts (37), and scimitar syndrome (9).

Sonography is more sensitive than chest radiography for identifying anomalous vessels and may obviate contrast-enhanced CT or MRI in neonates and young infants (26,63). Duplex or color flow Doppler sonography is especially useful in demonstrating the anomalous vessel and tracing it from the aorta to the sequestered lung. The sonographic appearance of the abnormal lung depends on whether the sequestered lung is aerated. When the sequestration acquires a bronchial communication with the remainder of the lung, usually after being infected, it appears echogenic with reverberation artifacts. A sequestration that does not communicate with the airway appears as a solid, echogenic homogeneous mass, usually in the posterior portion of the lower lobe (Fig. 6). Occasionally cystic fluid-filled bronchi are seen. In older patients in whom there are not good acoustic windows, the sequestered lung, feeding arteries, and draining veins are difficult

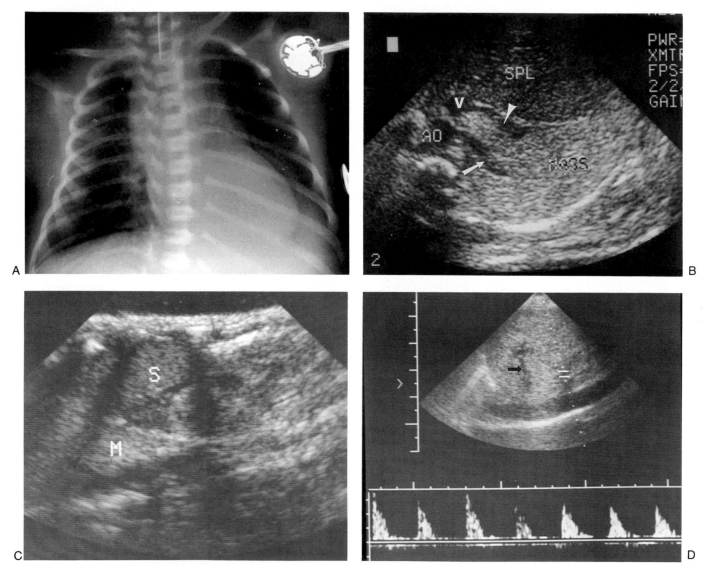

FIG. 6. Sequestrations. **A:** Chest radiograph in a newborn shows a left lower lobe density. The density had been present on several examinations. **B:** Transverse subcostal scan shows an echogenic mass posterior to the spleen (*SPL*) with a large feeding artery (*arrow*) from the aorta (*AO*) and a large vein (*arrowhead*) draining into the hemiazygos vein (*V*). Extralobar sequestration proven at operation. **C:** In another patient a longitudinal scan shows an echogenic mass (*M*) posterior and superior to the spleen (*S*). **D:** Duplex Doppler shows the arterial supply from the aorta. A draining vein (*arrow*) is seen leading into the hemiazygos vein. Proven intralobar sequestration.

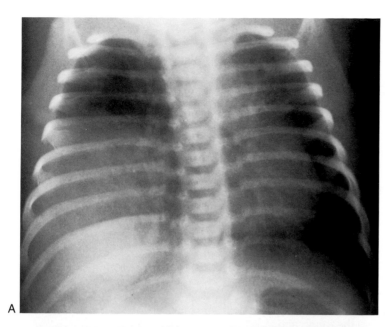

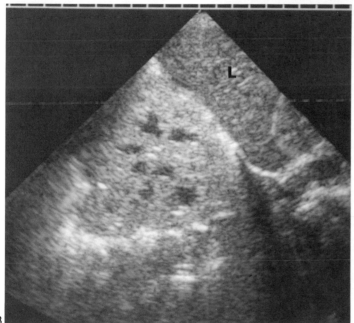

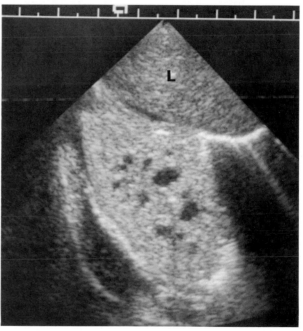

FIG. 7. Congenital cystic adenomatous malformation, type II. **A:** Chest radiograph of a newborn infant shows a large mass in the right lower lung field. **B:** Longitudinal and **C:** transverse scans of the right lower chest demonstrate an echogenic mass containing cystic cavities under 1 cm in diameter. The mass is adjacent to liver (*L*).

to visualize with sonography, and CT or MR imaging may be required. The main differential consideration of intralobar sequestration is cystic adenomatoid malformation. Visualization of anomalous vessels is more suggestive of sequestration, since such vessels are rare in patients with cystic adenomatoid malformation (41).

Cystic Adenomatoid Malformation

Congenital cystic adenomatoid malformation is a rare hamartomatous lesion that is believed to result from an overgrowth of distal bronchial tissue. Communication with the bronchial tree, vascular supply, and venous drainage is normal (34). Pathologically,

three types are recognized: type I, with one or more cysts greater than 2 cm in diameter (50% of cases); type II, with multiple small cysts under 1 cm in diameter (40%); and type III, a solid mass of tissue with microscopic cysts (10%) (31). Involvement is typically restricted to all or part of one lobe, without preference for either side or a particular lobe. The vast majority of cystic adenomatoid malformations are discovered shortly after birth because of respiratory distress or associated anomalies. On chest radiography, the lesions can be fluid-filled and mimic a pleural effusion (7). The sonographic findings are those of an echogenic or complex mass with variable sized fluid-filled spaces, multiple septations, and areas of solid tissue (Fig. 7)

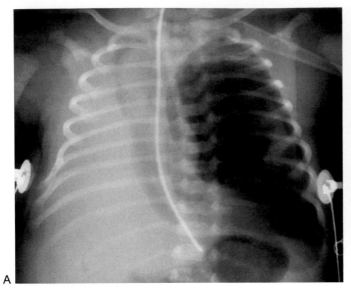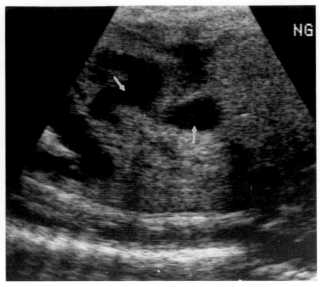

FIG. 8. Bronchial atresia. **A:** Chest radiograph in a newborn shows opacification of the right hemithorax with shift of the mediastinum to the right and a left pneumothorax. An air-filled esophagus with a nasogastric tube is seen. **B:** Anterior longitudinal scan of the opacified hemithorax demonstrates hypoechoic, branching, dilated bronchi (*arrows*) in the right lung parenchyma. At autopsy, there was atresia of the right main stem bronchus and multiple, large, dilated, mucus-filled bronchi occupying the right lung.

(19). Duplex Doppler or color flow Doppler imaging establishes that the cystic areas are not vascular. Marked shadowing occurs when the cysts contain air.

Bronchogenic Cyst

Intrapulmonary bronchogenic cyst is a developmental anomaly resulting from abnormal development of lung buds that fail to incorporate into the primitive lung tissue. Pathologically, these cysts are unilocular, lined by columnar epithelium, and contain either serous or mucoid material (1). The majority are located in the lower lobes. The sonographic appearance of the cyst varies depending on the fluid composition. Fluid-filled cysts are hypoechoic, whereas cysts containing air or thick mucus are echogenic.

Bronchial Atresia

Bronchial atresia is the result of failure of a segmental or lobar bronchus to develop or maintain communication with the central airway, probably the result of a vascular insult occurring after bronchial branching is complete (36). The bronchus distal to the atresia is

dilated and contains mucus plugs. Sonography can provide the diagnosis in a neonate with an opacified lung on chest radiography by demonstrating an echogenic lobe with dilated hypoechoic branching bronchi (Fig. 8). It may not be possible, however, to distinguish bronchial atresia from a congenital cystic adenomatoid malformation since both may be characterized by echogenic lungs with hypoechoic areas.

Pleura

Pleural Fluid

Conventional chest radiographs can detect the majority of pleural effusions, but when these are equivocal or nondiagnostic, sonography can be used to differentiate effusion from consolidation or a parenchymal or pleural mass (43,48). Sonography also can separate subpulmonic from subphrenic fluid collections (Fig. 9) in patients with apparently large livers or elevated hemidiaphragms on plain chest radiographs, and can distinguish between pleural and pericardial effusions (12,30). This has important implications for percutaneous aspiration and drainage.

Pleural fluid collections may be anechoic, hypoechoic, or complex. Anechoic effusions represent exu-

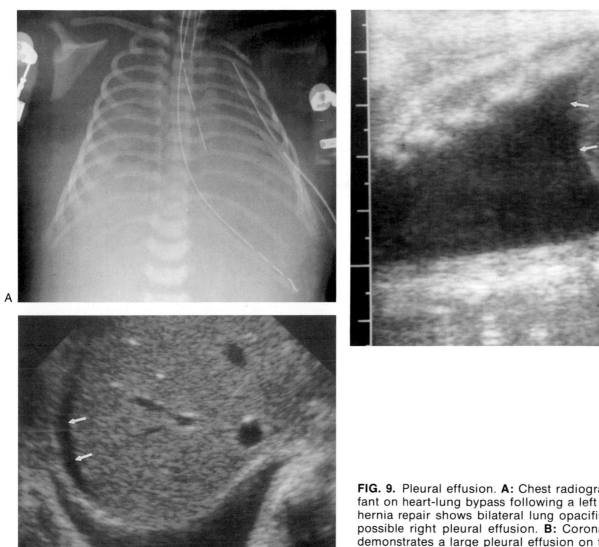

FIG. 9. Pleural effusion. **A:** Chest radiograph in an infant on heart-lung bypass following a left Bochdalek's hernia repair shows bilateral lung opacification and a possible right pleural effusion. **B:** Coronal sonogram demonstrates a large pleural effusion on the right. *Arrows*, diaphragm. Aspiration revealed serous fluid. **C:** Subcostal transverse scan in another patient showing fluid above (*arrows*) and below (*arrowheads*) the right diaphragm.

dative and transudative processes with almost equal frequency, while complex collections with septations and loculations are usually exudative (Fig. 10) (22). Small effusions occupy the inferior pleural space in patients scanned in the erect position. As effusions increase in size, they track to the lateral chest wall. On occasion, large effusions may invert the diaphragm or cause mediastinal shift (57). When there is need to differentiate pleural fluid from thickening or fibrosis, scans obtained with the patient in the lateral decubitus position may be helpful. Free pleural effusion is confirmed when the fluid shifts in response to a change in patient positioning. Echogenicity of the fluid is not a particularly useful feature in separating fluid amenable

to aspiration from organized or loculated pleural effusion (Fig. 11). Approximately 20% of anechoic pleural lesions will not yield free fluid, whereas complex-appearing lesions often yield fluid at thoracentesis (22,28). Unsuccessful taps of hypoechoic or anechoic areas are believed to be the result of malpositioning of the needle or the presence of fluid too viscous to pass through the needle. More reliable criteria for predicting whether fluid can be aspirated are changes in shape of the pleural fluid with respiration, and the presence of septations within the lesion that move with respiration (35). Septations or fibrin strands that demonstrate to-and-fro motion indicate a relatively low viscosity fluid collection. Septated or multilocular pleural

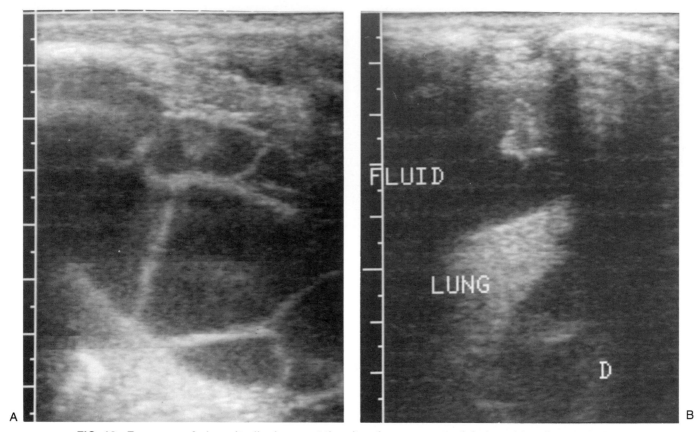

FIG. 10. Empyema. **A:** Longitudinal scan at the site of an unsuccessful pleural tap demonstrates multiple loculations of pleural fluid. **B:** Longitudinal scan more inferiorly shows a nonloculated collection of hypoechoic fluid, which was aspirated under sonographic guidance. *D*, diaphragm.

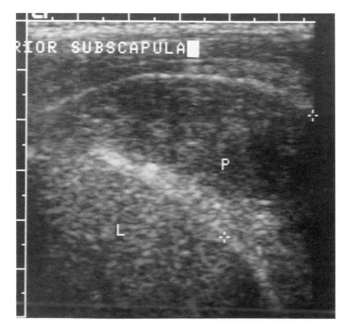

FIG. 11. Echogenic free pleural fluid. Transverse posterior scan through the thorax demonstrates echogenic pleural fluid (*P*) that was successfully removed by percutaneous aspiration. *L*, liver.

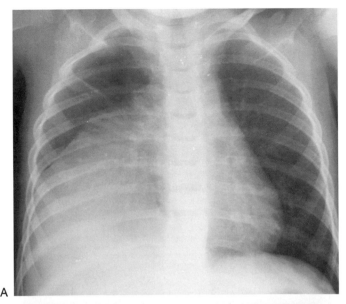

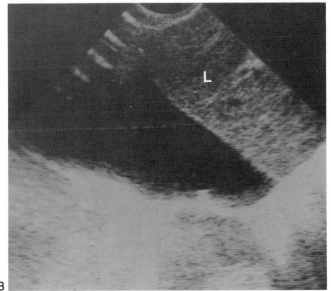

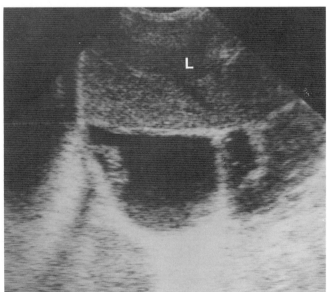

FIG. 12. Pleural lymphangioma. **A:** Frontal chest radiograph of a 2-year-old showing a soft tissue density adjacent to the right cardiac border. **B:** Longitudinal and **C:** transverse scans of the mass show hypoechoic fluid collections with multiple septations. A cystic lymphangioma in the right pleural space was found at operation. It was attached to, but did not communicate with, the pericardium. *L,* liver.

effusions may be indistinguishable from pleural lymphangiomas (Fig. 12).

Parenchymal or Pleural Disease

Consolidated lung can be differentiated from hypoechoic effusion by recognition of the sonographic air or fluid bronchogram (61). Consolidated lung is usually poorly defined, wedge-shaped, and hypoechoic when compared to the highly reflective normal lung and the liver and spleen (61). Air-filled bronchi within consolidated lung produce strong nonpulsatile linear reflections that converge toward the lung root, seen best when the scanning is parallel to the long axis of the bronchi (Fig. 13). Reverberations and acoustic shad-

owing are observed posterior to proximal large bronchi. When the bronchi are fluid-filled, they are seen as branching, anechoic, tubular structures (10,52,61). Absence of pulsations on Duplex or color flow Doppler can separate fluid-filled bronchi from pulmonary vessels. With large effusions causing partial atelectasis of the consolidated lung, the air bronchograms are still present, but are crowded together toward the lung root (61).

Although sonography is the method of choice for depicting pleural effusions, interpretative pitfalls exist. When an air bronchogram is absent, differentiation between a pulmonary lesion and pleural effusion may not be possible. In addition, consolidation or atelectasis adjacent to the heart may, at times, be mistaken for a pericardial effusion (12). In these instances, CT can be

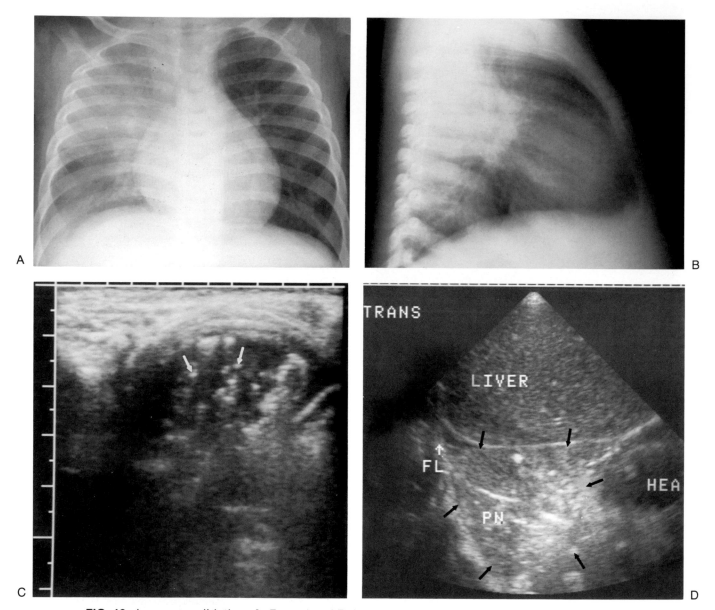

FIG. 13. Lung consolidation. **A:** Frontal and **B:** lateral chest radiographs demonstrate a partially opacified right hemithorax. Sonography was performed to separate parenchymal from pleural disease. **C:** Transverse scan of superior segment of the right lower lobe shows hypoechoic lung with multiple echogenic densities representing air bronchograms (*arrows*) and no pleural fluid. **D**: Transverse subcostal scan in another patient shows a consolidated, wedge-shaped, right lower lobe (*arrows*) with multiple echogenic densities representing air bronchograms. The appearance is consistent with pneumonia (*PN*). A small amount of pleural fluid is seen (*FL*). *HEA*, heart.

used to supplement or complement sonography to differentiate between parenchymal, pleural, and pericardial disease.

Diaphragm

Diaphragmatic Hernias

Diaphragmatic abnormalities in children include hernia, eventration, paralysis, and paresis. The diagnosis of a diaphragmatic hernia is usually easy by chest radiography when the herniation contains bowel. When the herniation does not contain bowel, it may be misdiagnosed as an elevated hemidiaphragm, pleural effusion, or mass. In these instances, sonography can provide the correct diagnosis (2,44,46,64). Diaphragmatic hernias are more often congenital than acquired. Of the congenital hernias, the Bochdalek's type is more common than the Morgagni type. In Bochdalek's hernia, a posterolateral defect in the diaphragm represents a persistent pleuroperitoneal canal. Bochdalek's hernias occur five times more commonly on the left than the right. Most present in neonates as the result of symptoms related to pulmonary hypoplasia. However, when the hepatic veins are occluded by the free edge of the diaphragmatic defect or by torsion caused by rotation of the liver, Budd-Chiari syndrome can occur.

Herniation usually involves the stomach, spleen, large or small bowel, omentum, or kidney. Associated anomalies are not uncommon with Bochdalek's hernia, and include congenital heart disease and malrotation.

Morgagni hernia is caused by failure of fusion between the fibrotendinous elements of the costal and xiphoid components of the diaphragm. It is most often right-sided since the heart and pericardium cover defects in the left hemidiaphragm, and it usually presents as a mass in the right anterior cardiophrenic angle on chest radiographs. The hernia typically contains omentum, transverse colon, and liver, but small bowel and stomach also can herniate.

Acquired hernias are caused by either penetrating or blunt abdominal trauma (2). Left-sided herniation predominates, probably because the liver protects the right side. Most tears involve the peripheral portion of the diaphragm at the junction of the tendon and posterior leaves.

Regardless of whether the hernia is congenital or acquired, posterior or anterior, sonography can accurately demonstrate the extent of the diaphragmatic defect and identify abdominal contents, including liver, spleen, kidney, and omental fat, and vessels passing through the discontinuity in the diaphragm (Fig. 14) (25). With real-time sonography the patency of the hepatic veins can be determined (38). The sonographic appearance of diaphragmatic hernias varies

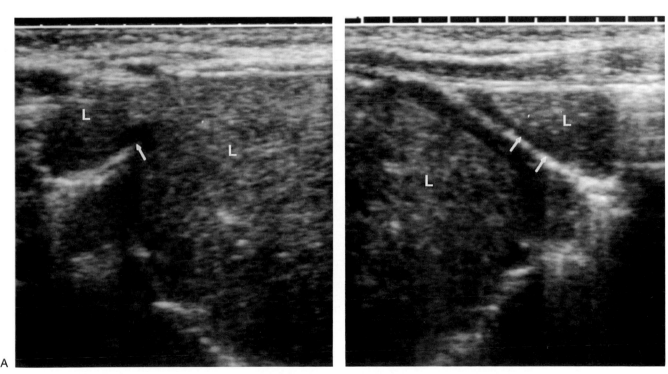

FIG. 14. Morgagni hernia in a 4-month-old boy. **A:** Longitudinal and **B:** transverse scans demonstrate a right Morgagni hernia containing liver (*L*). *Arrows,* diaphragm defect.

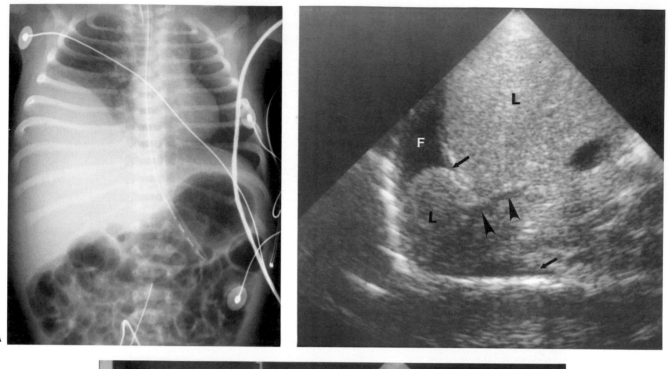

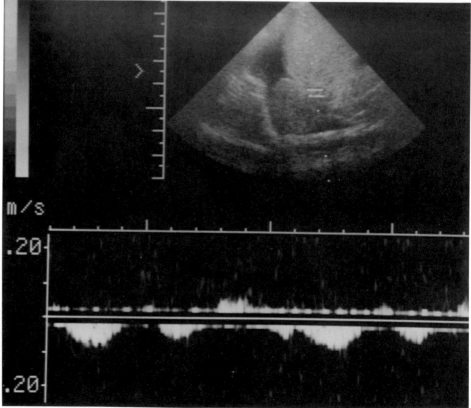

FIG. 15. Right Bochdalek's hernia covered by fluid-containing peritoneal sac. **A:** Frontal radiograph of the chest and abdomen shows a mass in the right lower chest. **B:** Longitudinal sonogram of the right upper quadrant shows liver (*L*) with hepatic vein (*arrowheads*) herniated through a posterior diaphragmatic defect (*arrows*). The covering peritoneal sac contains fluid (*F*). **C:** Duplex Doppler demonstrates flow in the hepatic veins within the herniated liver.

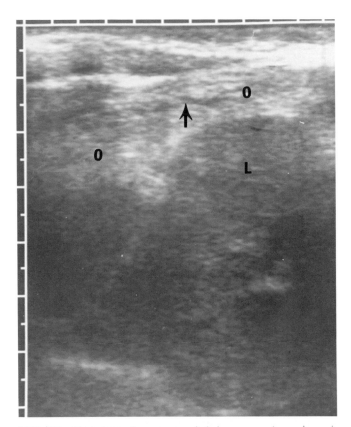

FIG. 16. Morgagni hernia containing omentum. Longitudinal scan demonstrates echogenic omentum (O) anterior and superior to the liver (L). Hypoechoic tubular structures represent vessels (*arrow*) within the omentum. The echogenicity of the omentum is slightly greater than that of the adjacent liver (L).

with their contents. If the hernia contains solid organs, the lesion appears echogenic. If the hernia contains fluid-filled bowel, it will appear hypoechoic. Occasionally a Bochdalek's hernia consists of herniated liver surrounded by a peritoneal sac that contains fluid. A hypoechoic component also is expected in these circumstances (Fig. 15). Herniated omentum may be hyper-, iso-, or hypoechoic relative to liver. When it is isoechoic it may be difficult to distinguish from liver by sonography (Fig. 16). Occasionally, pleural fluid or ascites resulting from lymphatic obstruction may be seen (15).

Eventration

Eventration of the diaphragm is more common than diaphragmatic hernia and is due to congenital weakness or thinness of the muscle. It may be focal, usually in the anteromedial portion of the right diaphragm, or total and more often left-sided (Fig. 17). In some cases, the thinned area of muscle is replaced by fibrous tissue. Large diaphragmatic eventrations, particularly when they are bilateral, can be associated with respiratory distress, but usually eventrations are of no clinical significance. Sonography can demonstrate the eventrated diaphragm and underlying liver or spleen (40). Sonography usually cannot distinguish between eventration and true diaphragmatic herniation.

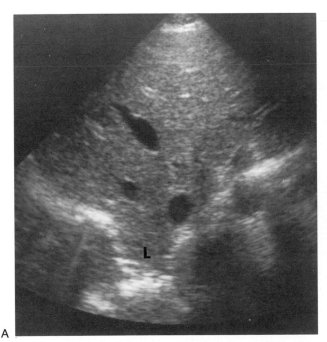
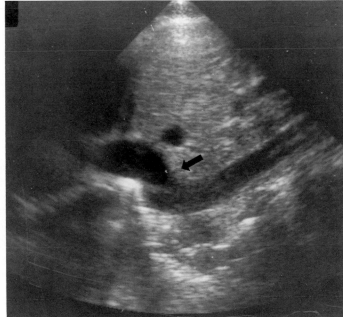

FIG. 17. Eventration. **A:** Transverse scan of the right diaphragm demonstrates herniation of the liver (L) into the chest. The diaphragm is intact. **B:** Longitudinal scan shows acute angulation of the inferior vena cava (*arrow*) associated with the eventration.

Paralysis

Diaphragmatic paralysis or paresis results from phrenic nerve injury, subpulmonic effusion, subphrenic abscess, pneumonia, and diaphragmatic hernias or eventration. With paralysis, the affected hemidiaphragm usually fails to change position with inspiration and expiration. Occasionally there is paradoxical diaphragmatic motion. With paradoxical motion, the paralyzed diaphragm elevates in inspiration and descends in expiration, in contrast to the normal diaphragm which moves inferiorly during inspiration and superiorly during expiration. In infants on mechanical ventilation and pharmacologic paralysis, the excursion of the anterior, middle, and posterior portions of the diaphragm is equal, in contrast to the normal situation where the middle and posterior parts move more than the anterior portion.

Paresis is a weakness of the muscular activity of the diaphragm. This is usually transient and occurs postoperatively. Sonography confirms decreased mobility of the diaphragm.

Miscellaneous Conditions

Mass lesions of the diaphragm are rare and include lipomas, hemangiomas, and rhabdomyosarcomas. Juxtadiaphragmatic abnormalities, such as subphrenic abscess, subpulmonic effusion, and hepatic or retroperitoneal tumors, are more common than diaphragmatic tumors. Sonography can easily identify these conditions and separate them from diaphragmatic herniation or disruption (30,44).

Great Vessels

Duplex or color Doppler sonography is a noninvasive method for demonstrating clinically suspected abnormality involving the great vessels. It is particularly valuable for detecting intraluminal thrombus, usually due to an indwelling catheter in the superior vena cava or right atrium (13). On sonography, acutely thrombosed vessels have poorly defined walls and echogenic lumens with absent Doppler signals (Fig. 18) (13). Collateral circulation can be seen with chronic thrombosis.

Abnormalities of the intrathoracic vessels, including the superior vena cava and its tributaries, the aorta and its branches, and the pulmonary arteries can alter the mediastinal contours on plain chest radiographs and be confused with a mass (20). Sonography can readily demonstrate the nature of these findings. In cases of aneurysms, sonography can demonstrate the lumen of the dilated vessel, its wall, and the presence or absence of thrombus. Anomalies of arch position can be detected by sonography. Similarly, idiopathic dilatation of the pulmonary artery can be recognized. Occasionally, anomalous pulmonary venous drainage in association with scimitar syndrome (Fig. 19) and pulmonary artery sling can be diagnosed if the abnormalities are near an acoustic window (24). Following surgery for repair of congenital heart disease, sonography can be used to evaluate vascular patency and complications such as inadvertent ligation of mediastinal vessels (23).

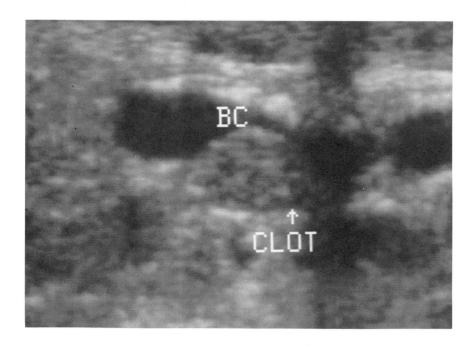

FIG. 18. Thrombus in the superior vena cava. Transverse scan at thoracic inlet shows an echogenic clot at the junction of the right and left brachiocephalic (*BC*) veins in a patient with a prior central line.

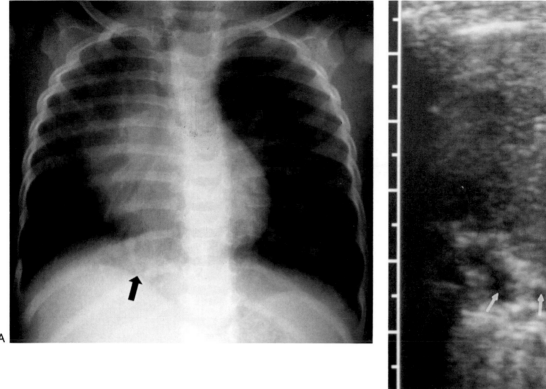

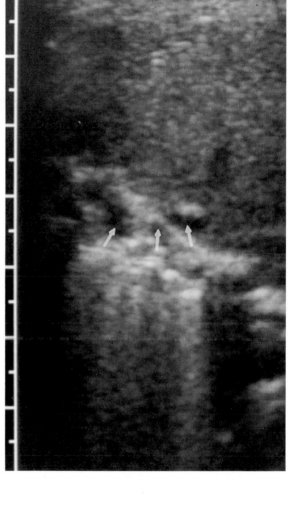

FIG. 19. Scimitar syndrome. **A:** Frontal chest radiograph in a patient with a heart murmur demonstrates dextroposition of the heart, a smaller right lung, and tubular densities at the right lung base (*arrow*). **B:** Transverse subcostal scan demonstrates sonolucent vessels (*arrows*) in the right lung base. Color flow Doppler imaging confirmed that the veins drained into the inferior vena cava and hepatic veins.

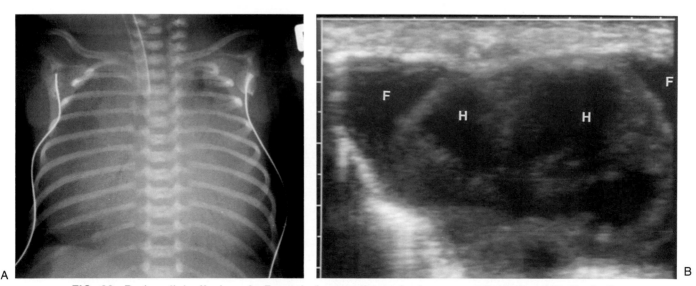

FIG. 20. Pericardial effusion. **A:** Frontal chest radiograph shows an enlarged mediastinal silhouette. **B:** Transverse scan demonstrates the mass to be pericardial fluid (*F*) and heart (*H*).

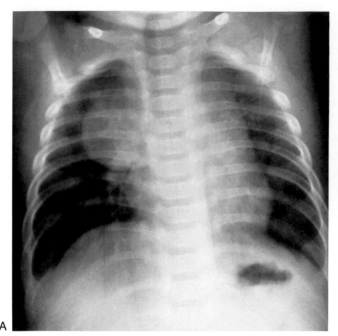

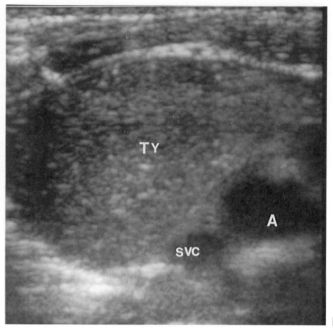

FIG. 21. Normal thymus simulating a mediastinal mass. **A:** Frontal chest radiograph in an infant referred for evaluation of a mediastinal mass shows a density in the right superior mediastinum. **B:** Transverse scan of the mass demonstrates a normal homogeneous thymus (TY). *A*, aorta; *SVC*, superior vena cava.

Mediastinum

Mediastinal Masses

The mediastinum is the most common site of primary thoracic masses in childhood (6,27). Patients often present with signs of airway compression, but occasionally the lesions are detected antenatally or are incidental findings on plain chest radiographs (4). Fol-

lowing chest radiography, CT usually is the procedure of choice in children for further evaluation of the nature, site of origin, and extent of a mediastinal lesion. However, sonography has been used as a supplementary or problem-solving technique when the etiology, nature, or precise location of a mass cannot be determined by CT. Using sonography, determination of the cystic, solid, or vascular nature of a suspected or known mediastinal mass and its relationship to sur-

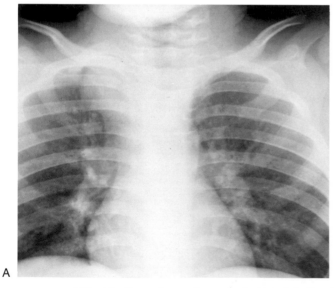

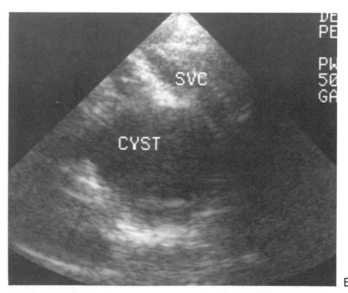

FIG. 22. Bronchogenic cyst. **A:** Frontal chest radiograph in a 3-year-old demonstrates a right paratracheal mass. **B:** Longitudinal scan shows the mass to be cystic with increased through-transmission. The superior vena cava (*SVC*) is bowed anteriorly by the cyst.

rounding vessels and heart is possible (Fig. 20). Sonography also can be used to help guide mediastinal biopsies and to monitor the treatment of mediastinal tumors.

The most common cause of a mediastinal mass in infancy is a normal thymus. As noted earlier, sonography has proven useful in noninvasively establishing the diagnosis of normal thymic tissue by demonstrating a homogeneous echogenic mass draping over the great vessels (Fig. 21). An abnormal mediastinum in infants often is due to a neuroblastoma or cystic lesion such as a bronchogenic, enteric, or neurenteric cyst. Hodgkin's disease, germ cell tumors, and thymoma are seen in older children (6,27).

Congenital Cysts

Congenital mediastinal cysts include foregut, pericardial, and thymic cysts. Foregut cysts may be clas-sified further as bronchogenic, esophageal duplication, and neurenteric cysts (37).

Bronchogenic cysts are lined by respiratory epithelium and result from abnormal budding of the tracheobronchial tree (11). Most mediastinal bronchogenic cysts are found in the subcarinal or right paratracheal region. On sonography, the cysts are well-defined hypoechoic lesions with thin walls and increased through-transmission, reflecting their serous nature (Fig. 22) (21). Occasionally, the lesions have internal echoes because of mucoid contents, debris, or air (47).

Esophageal duplication or enteric cysts are lined by gastrointestinal mucosa and arise either as a diverticulum from the dorsal bud of the foregut or from abnormal recanalization of the esophagus. They typically are located adjacent to or within the esophageal wall. Their appearance on sonograms can be identical to that of bronchogenic cysts (Fig. 23). Occasionally, an echogenic lining representing mucosa can be identified.

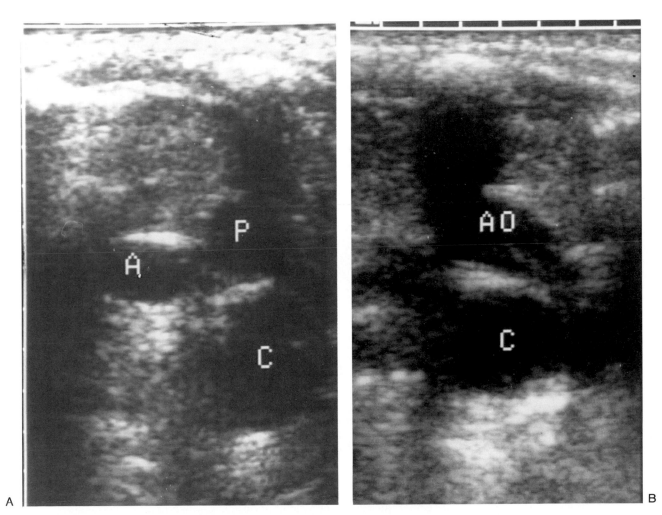

FIG. 23. Enteric cyst. Chest radiograph showed a mass in the region of the left hilum and emphysema of the left lung. **A:** Transverse and **B:** longitudinal scans demonstrate a cystic lesion with increased through-transmission. The cyst (C) is posterior to the aorta (A, AO) and pulmonary artery (P). Enteric cyst attached to the esophagus was proven at operation.

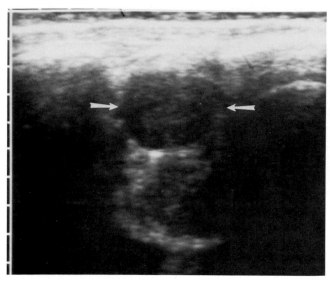

FIG. 24. Hodgkin's disease. Longitudinal parasternal scan of a patient with a widened superior mediastinum on chest radiograph demonstrates an enlarged anterior mediastinal node (*arrows*).

Neurenteric cysts are rare posterior mediastinal anomalies connected to the meninges through a midline defect in one or more vertebral bodies. They are lined by gastrointestinal mucosa. Associated vertebral anomalies on plain radiographs suggest the diagnosis.

Pericardial cysts are most frequently found in the right cardiophrenic angle. Sonographically, the cysts are sharply marginated and anechoic or hypoechoic. When they maintain a patent communication with the pericardial sac, they may decrease in size with the patient in the left lateral decubitus position.

Congenital thymic cysts are caused by persistence of the thyropharyngeal duct. Except for their location in the anterior mediastinum, their appearance on sonography is similar to that of the other mediastinal cysts. Hemorrhage into the cyst can increase the echogenicity. Rarely, thymic cysts may be bilobed, multiple, contain septations, or replace the entire thymus (49).

Neoplasms

Hodgkin's disease is the most common tumor involving the mediastinum. Typically, the disease presents in adolescents as an anterior mediastinal widening or a mass, reflecting either thymic infiltration by tumor or lymph node enlargement. On sonography, the enlarged thymus appears as an inhomogeneous lobulated mass. Enlarged lymph nodes appear as multiple sonolucent masses (Fig. 24). Internal mammary nodes are seen best on a parasternal approach, while supraaortic nodes are best demonstrated by a suprasternal approach (51,62). The differential diagnosis of anterior mediastinal masses also should include thymomas (Fig. 25) and germ cell tumors, as well as non-neoplastic lesions such as aneurysms and thymic hemorrhage or cysts, although these lesions are much rarer than Hodgkin's disease. Solid tumors appear as ho-

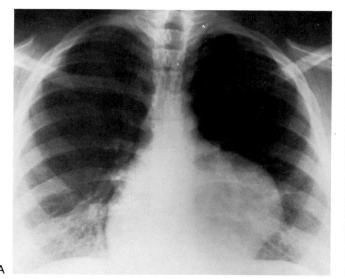

A

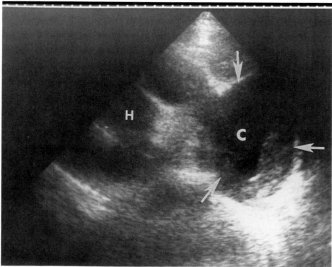

B

FIG. 25. Cystic thymoma. A: Chest radiograph shows an abnormal cardiac contour suggesting a pericardial mass. B: Transverse scan shows a mass with thick walls (*arrows*) and cystic center (*C*) adjacent to the heart (*H*). At operation the tumor arose from the left lobe of the thymus and was separable from the pericardium.

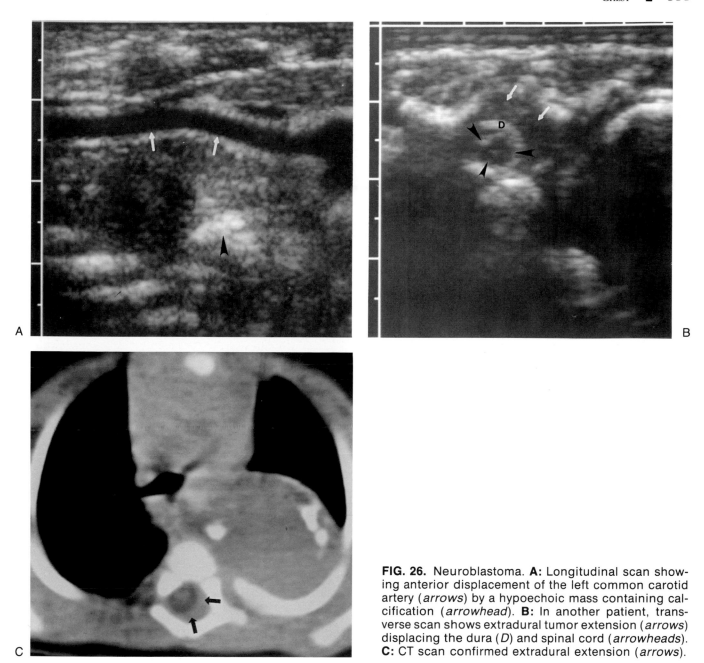

FIG. 26. Neuroblastoma. **A:** Longitudinal scan showing anterior displacement of the left common carotid artery (*arrows*) by a hypoechoic mass containing calcification (*arrowhead*). **B:** In another patient, transverse scan shows extradural tumor extension (*arrows*) displacing the dura (*D*) and spinal cord (*arrowheads*). **C:** CT scan confirmed extradural extension (*arrows*).

mogeneous or heterogeneous masses. Hemorrhage produces a heterogeneous gland with scattered echogenic foci (33).

Neurogenic tumors are the most frequent causes of posterior mediastinal masses and are usually neuroblastomas, ganglioneuroblastomas, or ganglioneuromas. They are typically paravertebral in location and may invade the spinal canal. On sonography, neural tumors appear as soft tissue masses that are hypoechoic relative to thymus or cardiac muscle. Sonolucent

or cystic areas due to necrosis or degeneration and brightly echogenic areas due to calcification may be present within the tumor. Sonography can recognize vessel displacement or invasion. Intraspinal extension can be recognized by sonography if it causes cord displacement. Tumor that invades the canal but does not displace the cord cannot be detected. Although sonography can demonstrate intraspinal tumor, CT or MR imaging is the preferred noninvasive technique to demonstrate extent of mass (Fig. 26).

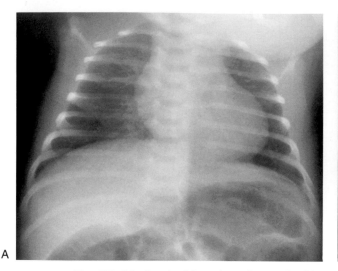
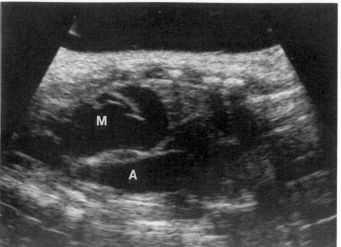

Fig. 27. Mediastinal lymphangioma. **A:** Chest radiograph demonstrates a large left neck mass with probable extension into the upper mediastinum. **B:** Longitudinal scan demonstrates a multicystic mass (*M*) in the anterior mediastinum. *A*, aorta.

Lymphangioma

Lymphangiomas are congenital malformations of lymphoid tissue. Pathologically, the lesions contain variably sized fluid-filled spaces ranging from capillary size to large cystic spaces which are separated by connective tissue. Most are detected in children under 1 year of age and appear as cervical masses posterior to the sternocleidomastoid muscle. Approximately 10% of these extend into the mediastinum; mediastinal lymphangiomas arising *de novo* in the mediastinum are extremely rare (54). Typically, they are multilocular, hypoechoic masses (Fig. 27) (58). Solid areas may be noted in the presence of hemorrhage, infection, or abundant connective tissue. Most lymphangiomas are well-defined, but they may infiltrate soft tissues and displace adjacent structures (Fig. 28).

Inflammatory Processes

Sonography can be useful in patients with tenderness or swelling over the sternum following sternotomy to identify a substernal fluid collection. However, differentiation of an abscess from an uninfected postoperative seroma or hematoma is not possible by sonography and requires percutaneous needle aspiration.

Chest Wall

Most soft tissue tumors of the chest wall are benign and include lymphangiomas, hemangiomas, and lipomas; the most frequent malignant soft tissue tumors are rhabdomyosarcomas and Askin tumors. Sonog-

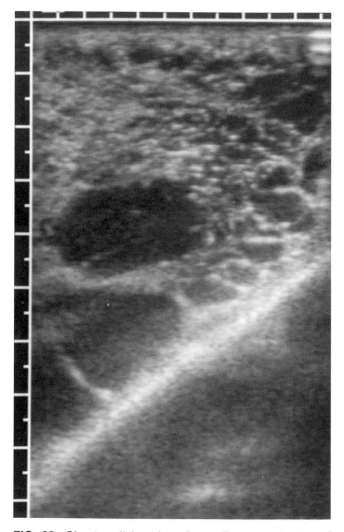

FIG. 28. Chest wall lymphangioma. Transverse scan of the chest wall demonstrates a multicystic mass infiltrating soft tissues. An echogenic rib is seen below the mass.

raphy can provide information about the cystic, solid, or vascular nature of a soft tissue mass (Fig. 28). If the lesion is cystic or vascular, it is more likely to be benign; if the lesion is solid, it is more likely to be malignant, especially if associated with pleural fluid (39). Sonography is less useful in determining the extent of a lesion than is MR imaging or CT.

Miscellaneous

Endotracheal intubation is a common procedure used in neonates with respiratory distress. Plain radiographs are the standard imaging examination used to evaluate endotracheal tube positioning, although there has been a report of the use of sonography for this determination. With the use of sonography, the distal tip of the endotracheal tube can be identified. Optimal tube position is present when the tip is 1 cm above the aortic arch (56).

Both the true and false cords can be imaged and abnormalities of motion detected. The true cords are hypoechoic while the false cords are echogenic, presumably due to fibrofatty tissue (45). Since sonography is time-consuming and does not provide detailed anatomic data, it has not gained widespread acceptance for diagnosing either vocal cord lesions or endotracheal tube malpositioning.

REFERENCES

1. Albright EA, Crane JP, Shackelford GD. Prenatal diagnosis of a bronchogenic cyst. *J Ultrasound Med* 1988;7:91–95.
2. Ammann AM, Brewer WH, Maull KI, Walsh JW. Traumatic rupture of the diaphragm: Real-time sonographic diagnosis. *AJR* 1983;140:915–916.
3. Amodio J, Abramson S, Berdon W, Stolar C, Markowitz R, Kasznica J. Iatrogenic causes of large pleural effusions in the premature infant: Ultrasonic and radiographic findings. Pediatr Radiol 1987;17:104–108.
4. Avni EF, Vanderelst A, Gansbeke DV, Schils J, Rodesch F. Antenatal diagnosis of pulmonary tumour: report of two cases. *Pediatr Radiol* 1986;16:190–192.
5. Bar-Ziv J, Barki Y, Itzchak Y, Mares AJ, Posterior mediastinal accessory thymus. *Pediatr Radiol* 1984;14:165–167.
6. Bower RJ, Kiesewetter WB. Mediastinal masses in infants and children. *Arch Surg* 1977;112:1003–1009.
7. Claiborne AK, Martin CM, McAlister WH, Gast MJ. Antenatal diagnosis of cystic adenomatoid malformation: Effect on patient management. *Pediatr Radiol* 1985;15:337–339.
8. Claiborne AK, Blocker SH, Martin CM, McAlister WH. Prenatal and postnatal sonographic delineation of gastrointestinal abnormalities in a case of the Vater syndrome. *J Ultrasound Med* 1986;5:45–47.
9. Collin PP, Desjardins JG, Khan AH. Pulmonary sequestration. *J Pediatr Surg* 1987;22:750–753.
10. Dorne HL. Differentiation of pulmonary parenchymal consolidation from pleural disease using the sonographic fluid bronchogram. *Radiology* 1986;158:41–42.
11. DuMontier C, Graviss ER, Silberstein MJ, McAlister WH. Bronchogenic cysts in children. *Clin Radiol* 1985;36:431–436.
12. Erasmie U, Lundell B. Pulmonary lesions mimicking pericardial effusion on ultrasonography. *Pediatr Radiol* 1987;17:447–450.
13. Falk RL, Smith DF. Thrombosis of upper extremity thoracic inlet veins: Diagnosis with duplex Doppler sonography. *AJR* 1987;149:677–682.
14. Felker RE, Tonkin ILD. Imaging of pulmonary sequestration. *AJR* 1990;154:241–249.
15. Gilsanz V, Emons D, Hansmann M, et al. Hydrothorax, ascites, and right diaphragmatic hernia. *Radiology* 1986;158:243–246.
16. Glasier CM, Leithiser RE, Jr, Williamson SL, Seibert JJ. Extracardiac ultrasonography in infants and children. Radiographic and clinical indications. *J Pediatr* 1989;114:540–544.
17. Haller JO, Schneider M, Kassner EG, Friedman AP, Waldroup LD. Sonographic evaluation of the chest in infants and children. *AJR* 1980;134:1019–1027.
18. Han BK, Babcock DS, Oestreich AE. The normal thymus in infancy: Sonographic characteristics. *Radiology* 1989;170:471–474.
19. Hartenberg MA, Brewer WH. Cystic adenomatoid malformation of the lung: Identification by sonography. *AJR* 1983;140:693–694.
20. Helund GL, Bisset GS. Esophageal duplication cyst and aberrant right subclavian artery mimicking a symptomatic vascular ring. *Pediatr Radiol* 1989;19:543–544.
21. Hendry PJ, Hendry GMA. Ultrasonic diagnosis of a bronchogenic cyst in a child with persistent stridor. *Pediatr Radiol* 1988;18:338.
22. Hirsch JH, Rogers JV, Mack LA. Real-time sonography of pleural opacities. *AJR* 1981;136:297–301.
23. Jaffe RB, Orsmond GS, Veasy LG. Inadvertent ligation of the left pulmonary artery. *Radiology* 1986;161:355–357.
24. Kangarloo H, Gold RH, Benson L, Diament MJ, DiSessa T, Boechat MT. Sonography of extrathoracic left-to-right shunts in infants and children. *AJR* 1983;141:923–926.
25. Kangarloo H, Sukov R, Sample WF, Lipson M, Smith L. Ultrasonographic evaluation of juxta diaphragmatic masses in children. *Radiology* 1977;125:785–787.
26. Kaude JV, Laurin S. Ultrasonographic demonstration of systemic artery feeding extrapulmonary sequestration. *Pediatr Radiol* 1984;14:226–227.
27. King RM, Telander RL, Smithson WA, Banks PM, Han MT. Primary mediastinal tumors in children. *J Pediatr Surg* 1982;17:512–520.
28. Laing FC, Filly RA. Problems in the application of ultrasonography for the evaluation of pleural opacities. *Radiology* 1978;126:211–214.
29. Laing IA, Teele RL, Stark AR. Diaphragmatic movement in newborn infants. *J Pediatr* 1988;112:638–643.
30. Landay M, Harless W. Ultrasonic differentiation of right pleural effusion from subphrenic fluid on longitudinal scans of the right upper quadrant: Importance of recognizing the diaphragm. *Radiology* 1977;123:155–158.
31. Landing BH, Dixon LG. Congenital malformations and genetic disorders of the respiratory tract (larynx, trachea, bronchi, and lungs). *Am Rev Respir Dis* 1979;120:151–185.
32. Leijala M, Louhimo I. Extralobar sequestration of the lung in children. *Prog Pediatr Surg* 1987;21:98–106.
33. LeMaitre L, Leclerc F, Dubos JB, Marconi V, Lemaire D. Thymic hemorrhage: A cause of symptomatic mediastinal widening in an infant with late hemorrhagic disease. Sonographic findings. *Pediatr Radiol* 1989;19:128–129.
34. Madewell JE, Stocker JT, Korsower JM. Cystic adenomatoid malformation of the lung. Morphologic analysis. *AJR* 1975;124:436–448.
35. Marks WM, Filly RA, Callen PW. Real-time evaluation of pleural lesions: New observations regarding the probability of obtaining free fluid. *Radiology* 1982;142:163–164.
36. McAlister W, Wright JR, Crane JP. Main-stem bronchial atresia: Intrauterine sonographic diagnosis. *AJR* 1987;148:364–366.
37. McMullin N, Osamu D, Kent M. The spectrum of bronchopulmonary foregut malformations. A case of combined bronchogenic cyst and sequestration. *Pediatr Surg Int* 1987;2:304–306.
38. Merten DF, Bowie JD, Kirks DR, Grossman H. Anteromedial diaphragmatic defects in infancy: Current approaches to diagnostic imaging. *Radiology* 1982;142:361–365.
39. Miller JH, Reid BS, Kemberling CR. Water-path ultrasound of chest disease in childhood. *Radiology* 1984;152:401–408.

40. Moccia WA, Kaude JV, Felman AH. Congenital eventration of the diaphragm. Diagnosis by ultrasound. *Pediatr Radiol* 1981; 10:197–200.
41. Morin C, Filiatrault D, Russo P. Pulmonary sequestration with histologic changes of cystic adenomatoid malformation. *Pediat Radiol* 1989;19:130–132.
42. O'Laughlin MP, Huhta JC, Murphy DJ. Ultrasound examination of extracardiac chest masses in children. *J Ultrasound Med* 1987;6:151–157.
43. O'Moore PV, Mueller PR, Simeone JF, et al. Sonographic guidance in diagnostic and therapeutic interventions in the pleural space. *AJR* 1987;149:1–5.
44. Pery M, Kaftori JK, Rosenberger A. Causes of abnormal right diaphragmatic position diagnosed by ultrasound. *JCU* 1983;11:269–275.
45. Raghavendra BN, Horii SC, Reede DL, et al. Sonographic anatomy of the larynx, with particular reference to the vocal cords. *J Ultrasound Med* 1987;6:225–230.
46. Rao KG, Woodlief RM. Grey scale ultrasonic demonstration of ruptured right hemidiaphragm. *Br J Radiol* 1980;53:812–814.
47. Ries T, Currarino G, Nikaidoh H, Kennedy L. Real-time ultrasonography of subcarinal bronchogenic cysts in two children. *Radiology* 1982;145:121–122.
48. Rosenberg HK. The complementary roles of ultrasound and plain film radiography in differentiating pediatric chest abnormalities. *Radiographics* 1986;3:427–445.
49. Rudick MG, Wood BP. The use of ultrasound in the diagnosis of a large thymic cyst. *Pediatr Radiol* 1980;10:113–115.
50. Savic B, Birtel FV, Tholen W, et al. Lung sequestration: Report of seven cases and review of 540 published cases. *Thorax* 1979;34:96–101.
51. Scatarige JC, Hamper UM, Sheth S, Allen HA. Parasternal sonography of the internal mammary vessels: Technique, normal anatomy, and lymphadenopathy. *Radiology* 1989;172:453–457.
52. Seibert RW, Seibert JJ, Williamson SL. The opaque chest: When to suspect a bronchial foreign body. *Pediatr Radiol* 1986;16:193–196.
53. Shackelford GD, McAlister WH. The aberrantly positioned thymus—A cause of mediastinal or neck masses in children. *AJR* 1974;120:291–296.
54. Siegel MJ, Sagel SS, Reed K. The value of computed tomography in the diagnosis and management of pediatric mediastinal abnormalities. *Radiology* 1982;142:149–155.
55. Slovis TL, Sell LL, Bedard MP, Klein MD. Ultrasonographic findings (CNS, thorax, abdomen) in infants undergoing extracorporeal oxygenation therapy. *Pediatr Radiol* 1988;18:112–117.
56. Slovis TL, Poland RL. Endotracheal tubes in neonates: Sonographic positioning. *Radiology* 1986;160:262–263.
57. Subramanyam BR, Raghavendra BN, LeFleur RS. Sonography of the inverted right hemidiaphragm. *AJR* 1981;136:1004–1006.
58. Sumner TE, Volberg FM, Kiser PE, Shaffner LdeS. Mediastinal cystic hygroma in children. *Pediatr Radiol* 1981;11:160–162.
59. Thomas CS, Leopold GR, Hilton S, Key T, Coen R, Lynch F. Fetal hydrops associated with extralobar pulmonary sequestration. *J Ultrasound Med* 1986;5:668–671.
60. Vade A, Kramer L. Extralobar pulmonary sequestration presenting as intractable pleural effusion. *Pediatr Radiol* 1989; 19:333–334.
61. Weinberg B, Diakoumakis EE, Kass EG, Seife B, Zvi ZB. The air bronchogram: Sonographic demonstration. *AJR* 1986; 147:593–595.
62. Wernecke K, Peters PE, Galanski M. Mediastinal tumors: Evaluation with suprasternal sonography. *Radiology* 1986;159: 405–409.
63. West MS, Donaldson JS, Shkolnik A. Pulmonary sequestration: Diagnosis by ultrasound. *J Ultrasound Med* 1989;8:125–129.
64. Worthen NJ, Worthen WF. Disruption of the diaphragmatic echoes: A sonographic sign of diaphragmatic disease. *JCU* 1982;10:43–45.

5

Liver and Biliary Tract

Marilyn J. Siegel

Prior to the advent of sonography, plain radiography, excretory urography, barium studies, and oral cholecystography were the standard, noninvasive imaging examinations for investigating suspected liver and gallbladder disease. However, with the development of gray-scale and subsequently real-time sonography and the improvements in image quality, sonography has largely replaced these other examinations as the primary method for evaluating diseases of the liver and biliary tract. Sonography is preferred due to its ease of performance and ability to image the entire upper abdomen at the time of the examination (51,88).

This chapter will address the use of sonography in diagnosing focal and diffuse liver disease and biliary tract abnormalities. A discussion of the clinical and pathologic features of the various diseases also is included to provide a basis for understanding the sonographic features.

SCANNING TECHNIQUE

When examining the liver, a systematic approach with standard views is required so that the entire liver will be imaged and subtle abnormalities will not be missed. A 5 MHz real-time transducer provides optimal visualization of the liver in most children. Generally, the liver is evaluated in both longitudinal and transverse scans with the patient in the supine position. The gain setting is adjusted so that the hepatic parenchyma appears homogeneous throughout. During the examination, all portions of the hepatic parenchyma, the hepatic and portal veins, common hepatic artery and common bile duct, and the gallbladder fossa should be examined.

Examination of the gallbladder requires adequate fasting to ensure satisfactory gallbladder distention. Eating or drinking produces physiologic contraction and a small, thick-walled gallbladder that may be mistaken for a pathologic process. For most children, a 5.0 MHz transducer provides excellent resolution, but in larger or obese patients a 3.5 MHz transducer is preferable. In patients who can cooperate, the gallbladder should be examined during suspended respiration. The gallbladder usually is examined by transverse and longitudinal scans with the patient in the supine, left lateral decubitus, and left posterior oblique positions. Occasionally, an erect position or even prone position will be required to confirm the presence or absence of calculi.

The extrahepatic ducts are examined at the same time the gallbladder is evaluated. Longitudinal and transverse views of the common duct are performed with the patient in the same supine, oblique, and decubitus positions used to image the gallbladder. Although these positions are acceptable for imaging the common hepatic duct or proximal common bile duct, they are not satisfactory for visualizing the distal common bile duct. In the supine and left lateral decubitus or left posterior oblique position, the distal duct is frequently obscured by an overlying, gas-filled duodenum. Visualization of the distal duct is improved by placing the patient in a semi-erect, slight right posterior oblique position, and obtaining transverse instead of longitudinal scans. The semierect position allows air in the gastric antrum and duodenum to rise and gastric fluid to empty into the duodenum. In addition, in this position the left lobe of the liver descends, permitting it to be used as an acoustic window. With this technique, the distal duct can be seen in approximately 90% of cases (81).

NORMAL ANATOMY

Lobar Anatomy

The liver is divided into right and left lobes. The right lobe generally is larger than the left and usually extends inferiorly to the level of the renal fossa, although occasionally a more caudal bulbous extension, labeled Riedel's lobe, is found. The left lobe is particularly inconsistent in size and position and may be found entirely on the right side of the abdomen or may cross the midline as far as the left lateral abdominal wall, occasionally wrapping around the spleen. Rarer variations include situs inversus, in which the liver is on the left side, and polysplenia or asplenia, in which the liver is transverse and symmetric. Knowledge of these variations in anatomy is important so that they are not mistaken for pathologic processes.

Each lobe of the liver has two segments, with the right lobe having anterior and posterior segments and the left lobe having medial and lateral segments. Additionally, there is a separate caudate lobe that is anatomically distinct because it receives its blood supply from both the right and left hepatic arteries and portal veins; hepatic venous blood drains directly into the inferior vena cava (42).

Sonography provides an easy method of visualizing the anatomic structures that divide the liver into lobes and segments. Typically, major hepatic veins run within the fissures between lobes and segments and may be used as boundary markers. In contrast, major portal vessels cross through segments but never across fissures.

Several fissures define the segmentation of the liver (Fig. 1). The main or interlobar fissure divides the right from left hepatic lobes. A portion of this fissure contains fat and is visible in many patients, appearing as a linear echodensity extending from the gallbladder fossa to the right portal vein. Even though the fissure is generally difficult to identify, there are anatomic landmarks that make it possible to define its location. These anatomic landmarks are the middle hepatic vein coursing within the superior portion of the fissure, and the gallbladder fossa located within the posterior-inferior portion of the fissure.

The right intersegmental fissure divides the right lobe into anterior and posterior segments (Fig. 2). This fissure can be recognized on sonographic images by identification of the right hepatic vein which courses within it. The left intersegmental fissure defines the inferior boundary between the medial and lateral segments of the left hepatic lobe. This fissure contains two visible anatomic markers: the left hepatic vein superiorly and the portion of the falciform ligament that contains the ligamentum teres caudally. On longitudinal scans, the falciform ligament appears as a linear echodensity extending from the anterior aspect of the liver toward the umbilicus, and on transverse scans as an echodense structure extending between the anterior abdominal wall and left portal vein.

The ligamentum teres appears as a rounded echogenic area to the right of midline on transverse scans, and as an echogenic line extending from the anterior

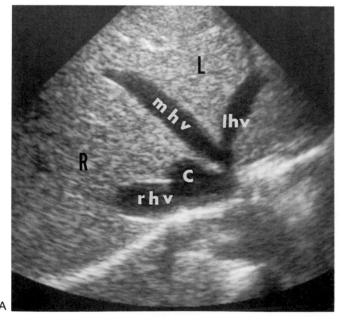 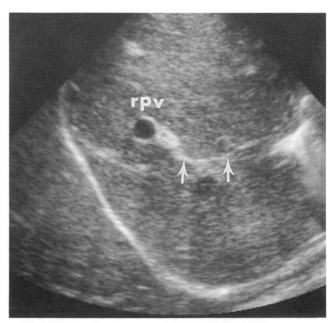

FIG. 1. Normal lobar anatomy: **A:** Transverse scan. In the cephalic portion of the liver, the middle hepatic vein (*mhv*) courses within the main lobar fissure, dividing the liver into the right (*R*) and left (*L*) lobes; *rhv*, right hepatic vein; *lhv*, left hepatic vein; *C*, inferior vena cava. **B:** Longitudinal scan at a lower level shows a linear echodensity (*arrow*) extending from the gallbladder fossa to the right portal vein (*rpv*). This band represents a visible portion of the main lobar fissure.

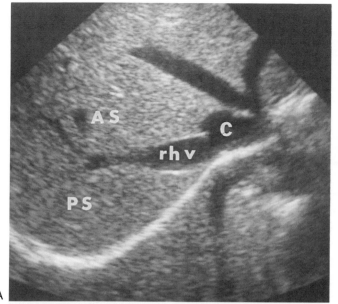

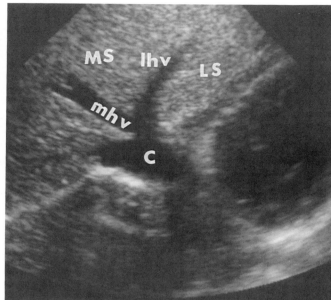

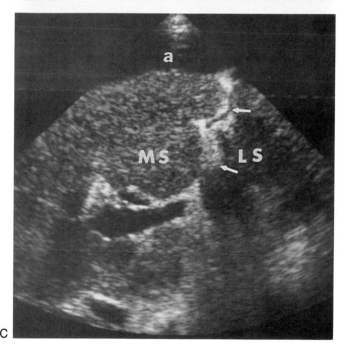

FIG. 2. Normal segmental anatomy. Transverse images. **A:** The right hepatic lobe is divided along a horizontal plane into anterior (*AS*) and posterior (*PS*) segments by the longest branch of the right hepatic vein (*rhv*). *C,* inferior vena cava. **B:** On an image through the superior aspect of the liver, the left hepatic vein (*lhv*) forms the border between the medial (*MS*) and lateral (*LS*) segments of the left lobe; *mhv,* middle hepatic vein; *C,* inferior vena cava. **C:** A more caudal level in another patient shows the falciform ligament (*arrows*) extending from the anterior aspect of the liver to the left portal vein, separating the medial (*MS*) and lateral (*LS*) segments. Ascites (*a*) is present anteriorly.

surface of the liver to the porta hepatis on longitudinal scans. When the ligamentum teres leaves the liver ventrally, it is located in the free edge of the falciform ligament, a peritoneal reflection arising from the anterior-superior surface of the left lobe. The ligamentum teres is continuous caudally with the fissure for the ligamentum venosum. The fissure for the ligamentum venosum separates the anterior margin of the caudate lobe from the medial segment of the left lobe (42,103). This fissure has a right-left orientation on transverse views, in contrast to the fissure for the ligamentum teres which runs in an anteroposterior direction (Fig.

3). By recognizing these fissures, it is possible to define segmental anatomy. Understanding hepatic segmental anatomy is helpful in assessing the extent of hepatic malignancies and in determining the feasibility of surgical resection. Even when the fissures are not visible, imaginary lines may be drawn in the expected location of the fissures to help define segmental boundaries.

Accessory fissures occasionally are recognized on sonography. The inferior accessory hepatic fissure extends inferiorly from the porta hepatis through the posterior segment of the right lobe, dividing the posterior segment into anterolateral and posteromedial parts.

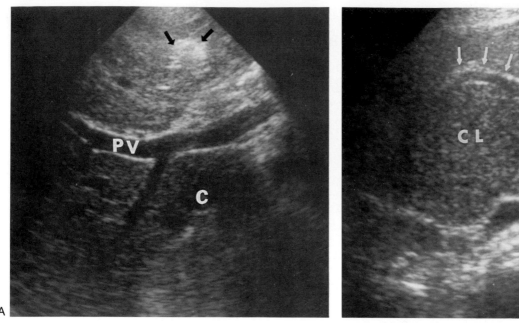

FIG. 3. Ligaments. Transverse scans. **A:** Ligamentum teres (*arrows*) appears as a round echogenic area. It courses between the medial and lateral segments of the left lobe. *C*, inferior vena cava; *PV*, portal vein. **B:** Ligamentum venosum appears as an echogenic line (*arrows*) anterior to the caudate lobe (*CL*).

When present the fissure is seen as a thin, echogenic membrane within the right lobe posteriorly (87).

Portal Veins

Portal veins carry blood from the splenic and mesenteric circulations to the liver. The main portal vein, formed by the junction of the splenic and superior mesenteric veins, courses cephalad and to the right to enter the liver at the porta hepatis. Within the porta hepatis, the main portal vein divides into a more caudad and posterior right portal vein and a more cephalad and anterior left portal vein (Fig. 4). The right portal vein divides in the substance of the liver into anterior and posterior branches which supply the corresponding segments of the right hepatic lobe. The left portal vein courses horizontally over the anterior surface of the caudate lobe through the ligamentum teres to supply the medial and lateral segments of the left hepatic lobe.

On sonography portal veins are easily recognized in the area of the porta hepatis because they are large and have an echogenic rim, caused by surrounding fibrofatty tissue. The mean diameter of the main portal vein is 8.5 ± 2.7 mm in patients under 10 years of age and 10 ± 2 mm in patients 10 to 20 years of age (150).

The portal veins within the liver are too small to be seen individually. Rather, they appear as small, rounded echogenic areas because of the surrounding fibrofatty tissue.

Hepatic Veins

The right, middle, and left hepatic veins transport blood from the hepatic parenchyma into the systemic circulation, draining into the inferior vena cava. As mentioned earlier, the main hepatic veins are found between hepatic segments. The right hepatic vein lies between the anterior and posterior segments of the right lobe, the middle hepatic vein is in the main lobar fissure between the right and left lobes, and the left hepatic vein lies in the intersegmental fissure between the medial and lateral segments of the left lobe. Hepatic veins are easily recognized on sonography by their location in the cephalad portion of the liver. They become larger as they approach their junction with the inferior vena cava, in contrast to portal veins which increase in diameter as they approach the porta hepatis (Fig. 5). Additionally, hepatic veins do not have the prominent peripheral echogenicity that is associated with portal veins, and they frequently appear to have no walls at all.

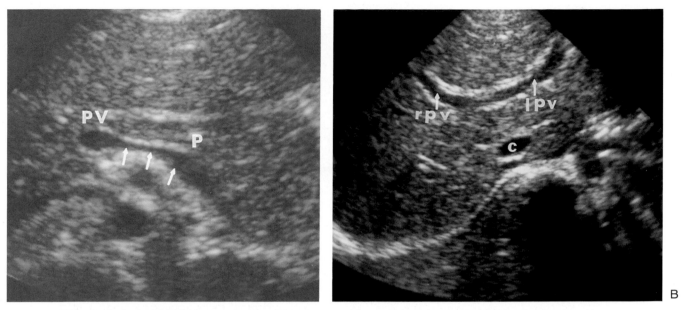

FIG. 4. Portal vein anatomy. **A:** Transverse scan. The main portal vein (*PV*) is formed by the junction of the splenic (*arrows*) and superior mesenteric veins in the region of the body of the pancreas (*P*). **B:** On a transverse scan, at a more cephalad level the portal vein divides into right (*rpv*) and left (*lpv*) branches. The walls of the portal veins are more echogenic than those of the vena cava (*C*). The tiny hyperechoic areas within the hepatic parenchyma represent portal triads surrounded by fatty tissue.

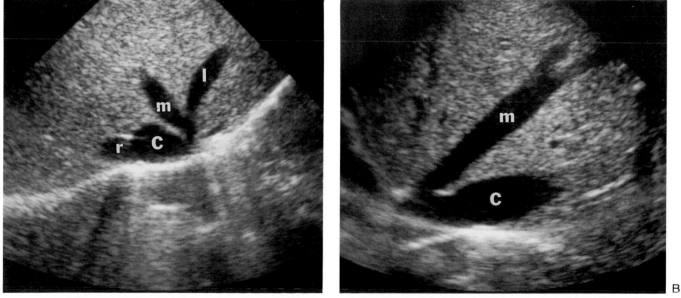

FIG. 5. Hepatic vein anatomy. **A:** Transverse section of the liver demonstrates the right (*r*), middle (*m*), and left (*l*) hepatic veins at their confluence with the inferior vena cava (*C*). **B:** Longitudinal sonogram demonstrates the middle (*m*) hepatic vein draining into the inferior vena cava (*C*).

Arterial and Biliary Anatomy

Arteries and bile ducts within the liver travel with the portal vein branches and together form the portal triads. Only the extrahepatic portions of these structures are seen relatively frequently on sonography. The normal size intrahepatic arterial structures and bile ducts are not large enough to be imaged sonographically.

The common hepatic artery arises from the celiac axis and runs to the right to enter the porta hepatis. At times, an anomalous right hepatic artery will arise separately from the superior mesenteric artery and pass behind, rather than anterior to, the portal vein. Within the porta hepatis, the hepatic artery is normally located anterior and slightly medial to the main portal vein, whereas the common hepatic duct is anterior and lateral to the portal vein (Fig. 6). The hepatic artery and bile duct usually can be differentiated by their relative positions within the porta hepatis and by the presence of intrinsic pulsations of the artery, but in problem cases duplex or color flow Doppler imaging can aid in differentiation (14,59,115).

After leaving the porta hepatis, the common hepatic duct joins the cystic duct to form the common bile duct which descends vertically and posteriorly within the hepatoduodenal ligament to reach the head of the pancreas (Fig. 7). Occasionally the course of the extrahepatic bile duct may be more transverse than vertical and may be mistaken for the portal or splenic vein (68). In these cases, the use of pulsed Doppler or color Dop-

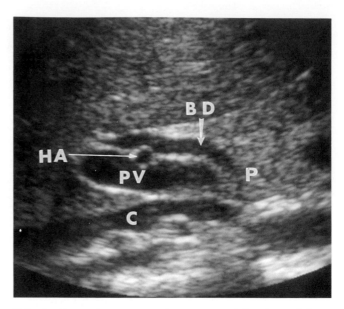

FIG. 7. Normal extrahepatic common bile duct. A longitudinal sonogram in another patient demonstrates the normal distal segment of the common bile duct (*BD*) as it enters the pancreas (*P*). *HA*, hepatic artery; *PV*, portal vein; *C*, inferior vena cava.

pler sonography usually allows the correct diagnosis to be made.

The size of the extrahepatic bile duct is the most sensitive indicator for distinguishing medical from surgical jaundice. Normally, the diameter of the common bile duct should not exceed 2 mm in infants under 1 year of age, 4 mm in older children, and 7 mm in adolescents and adults (93). If the common duct is larger, biliary obstruction is probably present. The size of the common duct may be somewhat larger in patients who have undergone prior biliary surgery. Measurements of the bile duct should be made from internal wall to internal wall. They are usually obtained in the most proximal extrahepatic portion of the bile duct just as it emerges from the liver. In the transverse plane the duct is measured just anterior to the portal vein in the area of the porta hepatis, whereas in the sagittal plane, the duct is measured just anterior to the hepatic artery and portal vein. The portion of the bile duct measured is actually the common hepatic duct, but it has been referred to as the common duct or common bile duct in the sonographic literature. Care should be taken not to mistake a folded gallbladder neck for a common bile duct (79).

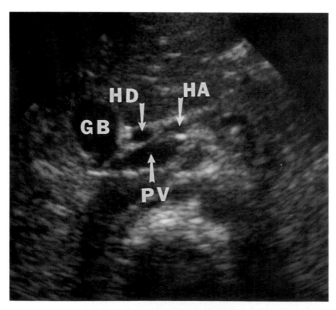

FIG. 6. Normal arterial and biliary anatomy at the level of the porta hepatis. Transverse sonogram through the porta hepatis demonstrates the common hepatic duct (*HD*) anterolateral to the main portal vein (*PV*). A small part of the hepatic artery (*HA*) is also seen anteromedially to the vein. *GB*, gallbladder.

Normal Doppler Waveform in the Porta Hepatis

Duplex Doppler and color flow imaging are useful techniques in evaluating the patency of the hepatic vasculature. Each of the major hepatic vessels possesses a unique Doppler signal (Fig. 8) (139). The portal vein

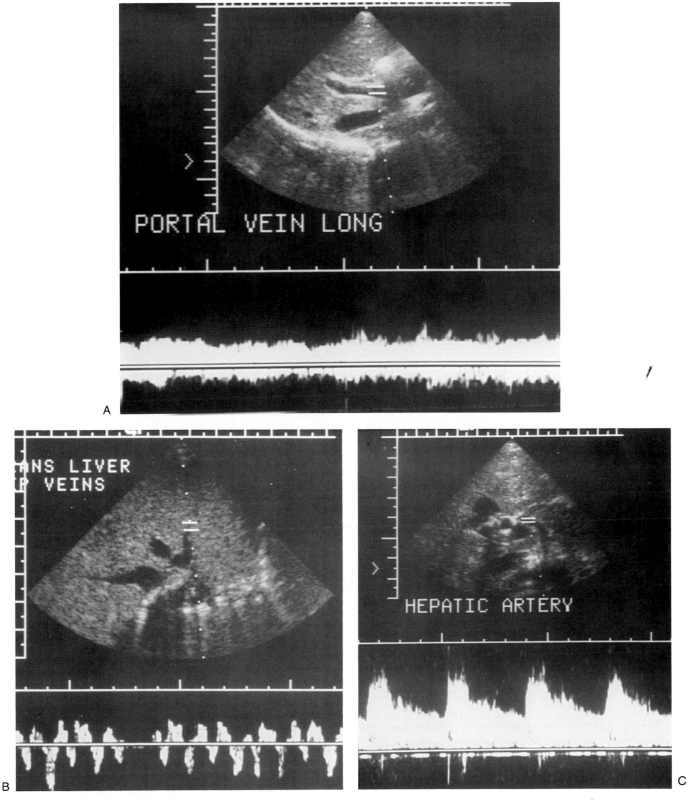

FIG. 8. Normal Doppler waveform. **A:** Portal vein waveform has a nearly continuous waveform with minimal variation with respirations. **B:** Waveform of the hepatic vein is irregular with variations in flow velocity and direction corresponding to changes in the respiratory and cardiac cycles. **C:** Hepatic artery waveform is characterized by high diastolic flow.

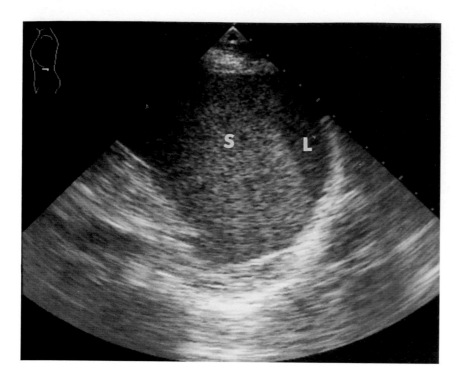

FIG. 9. Parenchymal echogenicity. Transverse view of left upper quadrant shows a hypoechoic left lobe of the liver (*L*) anterior and lateral to the spleen (*S*). The liver is normally lower in echogenicity than the spleen.

displays low velocity flow with a continuous waveform that diminishes slightly during inspiration. The inferior vena cava and hepatic veins, on the other hand, demonstrate an irregular complex waveform with wide variations in flow velocity and direction because of the regurgitation of blood from the right atrium secondary to systole and the variations in respiration and intraabdominal pressure. The hepatic artery typically demonstrates high diastolic flow due to low impedance. Other veins around the liver, such as the splenic and superior mesenteric veins, have waveforms similar to that of the portal vein. One exception to the normal pattern is found in patients with severe right heart failure. In these patients, the elevated systemic venous pressures may be transmitted into the portal venous system, producing a waveform similar to that of the hepatic veins.

Hepatic Parenchyma

The normal liver has a homogeneous, median-level echotexture. In the neonate and young infant, the hepatic parenchyma and renal cortex are equally echogenic. By 6 months of age, the liver is more echogenic than the kidney in virtually all patients. Normally, the liver is hypoechoic relative to the spleen (Fig. 9). Interspersed throughout the hepatic parenchyma are small, rounded echogenic areas due to periportal fibrofatty tissue and echogenic linear structures representing fissures and ligaments.

Occasionally, the caudate lobe appears more hy-

poechoic than the rest of the liver, presumably because of acoustic shadowing from fat or fibrous tissue along the fissure of the ligamentum venosum (Fig. 10). The use of a lower frequency transducer or a decubitus position may eliminate the shadowing effect of the fissure and establish the presence of a normal caudate lobe (97).

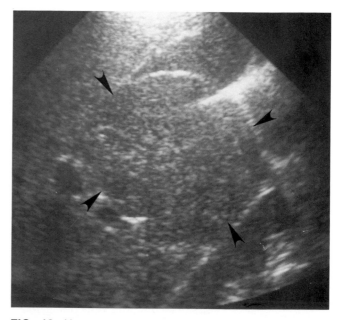

FIG. 10. Hypoechoic caudate lobe. On a longitudinal scan of the upper abdomen, the caudate lobe (*arrowheads*) is slightly hypoechoic compared with adjacent hepatic parenchyma.

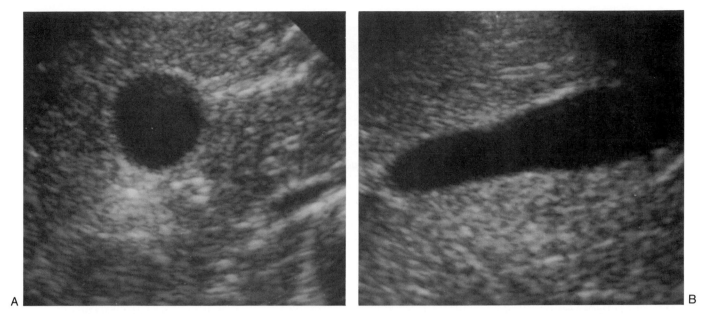

FIG. 11. Normal gallbladder. **A:** On a transverse scan, the gallbladder appears as a round anechoic structure with nearly imperceptible walls. **B:** Longitudinal image shows an oval-shaped gallbladder.

Gallbladder

The normal gallbladder is an oval or elliptical, anechoic structure located in a fossa on the undersurface of the liver between the right and left lobes (Fig. 11). Its segments include the fundus, body, and neck. The fundus is situated anterior, lateral, and caudad to the body and neck and often projects beyond the caudal margin of the liver parenchyma. The body and neck are oriented posteromedially toward the porta hepatis and to the left of the fundus. The neck of the gallbladder usually is in contact with the main segment of the right portal vein or the main portal vein near its origin with the left portal vein. Occasionally the neck is redundant and folded and may be mistaken for a septation or a dilated common bile duct (Fig. 12). Folds and kinks also occur in the body and fundus. The most common are the phrygian cap, representing a fold in

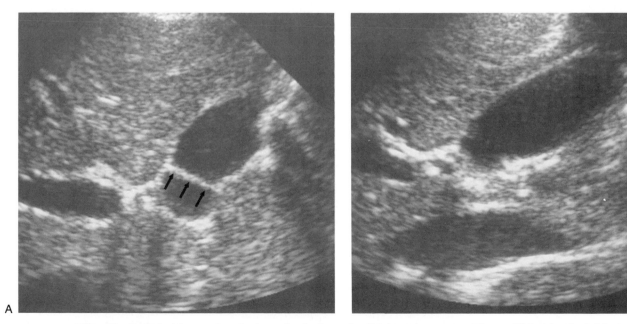

FIG. 12. Gallbladder, redundant neck. **A:** Longitudinal supine scan. The gallbladder is folded upon itself in the region of the neck, creating the appearance of a septum (*arrows*). **B:** On a longitudinal left posterior oblique view, the gallbladder is unfolded and clearly normal.

the distal portion of the fundus, and the incisura between the body and neck. Care must be taken not to confuse folds for septations or calculi; scanning in multiple planes usually allows the correct diagnosis to be made.

Rarely, the gallbladder lies in an ectopic position, below the left lobe of the liver or between the liver and diaphragm. It may also extend intrahepatically, deep into the interlobar fissure. Other rare anatomic variations include duplications, triplications, and multiseptate gallbladder.

The size and shape of the gallbladder are variable. When distended, the gallbladder has a smooth wall, with a thickness of 3 cm or less (93). In infants under 1 year the gallbladder is usually between 1.5 and 3 cm in length. In older children, the length is between 3 and 7 cm. Smaller diameters after adequate fasting indicate an abnormally contracted gallbladder. Conversely, a larger gallbladder with a round, rather than ovoid shape, on longitudinal scans suggests the diagnosis of hydrops (93).

PATHOLOGY

Hepatic Mass Lesions

Hepatic masses in children are most commonly malignant tumors or abscesses. Cysts and benign neoplasms are rarer in children. Because of its ease of performance, sonography is the initial examination of choice in determining the presence, site, and extent of a mass (95,96,133). In addition, sonography has the capability of differentiating among lesions composed of water, soft tissue, and calcification and hence, it can narrow the differential diagnostic considerations. However, sonography provides little or no information concerning the function or vascularity of the mass. Computerized tomography (CT) or magnetic resonance (MR) imaging can help delineate the vascular nature of the lesion and its relationship to the interlobar fissure and the intersegmental fissure of the left lobe (130). This knowledge can be important in determining resectability. More invasive diagnostic studies, such as hepatic arteriography and CT arteriography, are limited to patients who are being considered for partial hepatic resections for primary or metastatic neoplasms.

Primary Malignant Neoplasms

Hepatoblastoma and Hepatocellular Carcinoma

Hepatic tumors are the third most frequent neoplasm in children, following Wilms' tumor and neuroblastoma. Malignant lesions account for about two-thirds of all primary hepatic tumors in children; these are usually hepatoblastomas or hepatocellular carcinomas, and rarely embryonal sarcomas (30,40,43, 47,121,148). Pathologically, hepatoblastoma contains small, primitive epithelial cells resembling fetal liver, and hepatocellular carcinoma is composed of large, pleomorphic, multinucleated cells with variable degrees of differentiation. The former is slightly more common in infants and young children under 3 years of age, whereas hepatocellular carcinoma is most frequent after 3 years of age. Both tumors usually produce findings of an upper abdominal mass, occasionally associated with anorexia and weight loss. Jaundice and acute abdominal symptoms due to bleeding into the mass or spontaneous rupture are less frequent presentations. Alpha-fetoprotein levels are elevated in at least 80% of patients.

A number of conditions have been associated with hepatoblastoma in children, including Beckwith-Weidemann syndrome (characterized by hypoglycemia, macroglossia, visceromegaly, and umbilical hernias), isosexual precocity, and osteopenia. Diseases that have been associated specifically with hepatocellular carcinomas include type I glycogen storage disease, cystinosis, tyrosinemia, Wilson's disease, alpha-1-antitrypsin deficiency, extrahepatic biliary atresia, and giant cell hepatitis (159). Although cirrhosis is commonly associated with primary carcinoma of the liver in adults, such an association is rare in children.

Treatment of hepatoblastoma and hepatocellular carcinoma is surgical resection of the tumor. Determination of resectability depends on the extent of involvement, particularly the presence or absence of vascular invasion and extrahepatic spread. Distant sites of metastases for both tumors are the lungs, lymph nodes, brain, and skeleton (47). Sonography is valuable in detecting local tumor extent and venous vascular invasion. The sonographic appearances of hepatoblastoma and hepatocellular carcinoma in childhood are similar. Most commonly the tumors are confined to a single lobe, with the right lobe affected twice as often as the left, but the lesions may also involve both lobes of the liver or be multicentric in origin. On sonography, both tumors may appear as solitary masses or as diffusely abnormal parenchyma (Fig. 13) (34). When presenting as solitary masses, the tumors often are echogenic. Occasionally they are complex with hypoechoic areas reflecting the presence of partial necrosis and hemorrhage. Diffuse infiltration produces parenchymal inhomogeneity and distorted vascular anatomy. Calcifications are found in 50% of hepatoblastomas and in 10% to 25% of hepatomas, and appear as punctate or linear echogenic foci with acous-

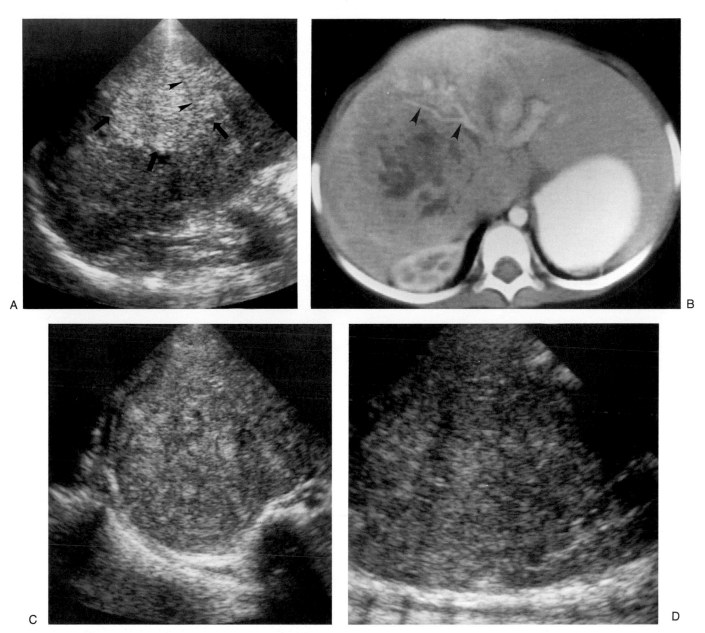

FIG. 13. Hepatoblastoma. **A:** Transverse scan shows a fairly well-defined echogenic mass (*arrows*) occupying the anterior segment of the right lobe and medial segment of the left lobe. The hypoechoic tubular structure (*arrowheads*) represents encased middle hepatic vein. **B:** CT scan confirms a large mass surrounding the middle hepatic vein (*arrowheads*). **C:** Transverse and **D:** longitudinal scans in another patient demonstrate diffusely heterogeneous parenchyma in the anterior segment of the right lobe of the liver. The margins are not well-defined, indicating that the tumor is more infiltrative. At operation, hepatoblastoma replaced the entire right lobe.

tic shadowing (Fig. 14). Intravascular invasion appears as an echogenic intraluminal thrombus. On duplex Doppler sonography, primary hepatic malignancies have Doppler shifts of 5 KHz or greater.

The sonographic findings of a large, complex mass replacing a large portion of the liver are nonspecific and can be seen with primary malignant lesions as well as metastatic disease, abscess, and benign vascular le-

sions (71). However, demonstration of invasion of the portal or hepatic veins strongly suggests the diagnosis of malignancy (23). The presence of high-velocity Doppler signals within a lesion also supports the diagnosis of malignancy, whereas no or minimal Doppler shift suggests a vascular tumor (141). The definitive diagnosis ultimately requires tissue sampling. Although percutaneous biopsy under sonographic guidance may

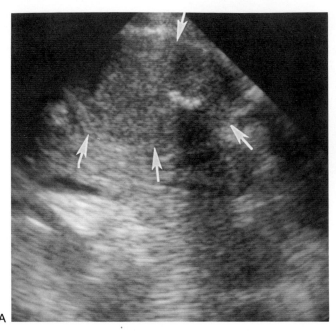
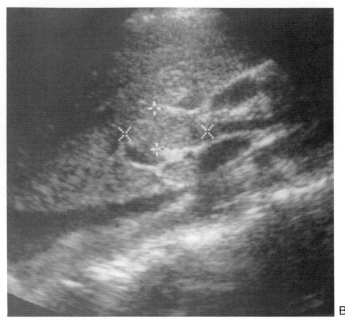

A   B

FIG. 14. Hepatocellular carcinoma. **A:** A transverse sonogram demonstrates a large, slightly hypoechoic mass (*arrows*) in the left lobe of the liver. Focal areas of increased echogenicity with associated shadowing represent calcifications within the tumor. **B:** Longitudinal scan through the porta hepatis shows an echogenic lymph node (*cursors*).

be performed, caution is needed because of the highly vascular nature of these lesions.

Secondary Hepatic Neoplasms

Metastases

In childhood, metastatic tumors of the liver are more common than primary tumors. The malignant tumors that most frequently metastasize to the liver are Wilms' tumor, neuroblastoma, and lymphoma. Neuroblastoma may affect the liver in either stage IV or IV-S disease. Stage IV disease is defined as the presence of retroperitoneal mass extending beyond the midline in association with distant disease to skeleton, visceral organs, and/or distant nodes. Stage IV-S neuroblastoma occurs in a subset of patients, usually infants under 1 year of age, whose primary lesions often

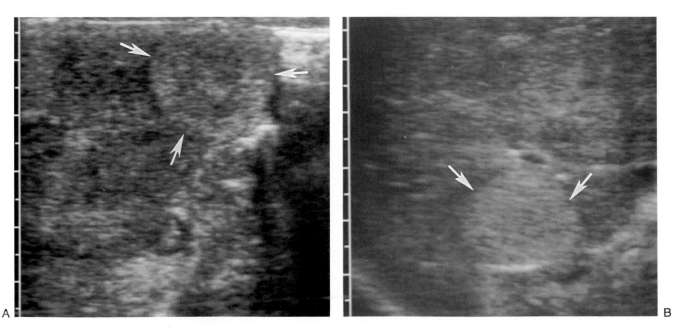

A   B

FIG. 15. Metastatic neuroblastoma. **A:** Transverse and **B:** longitudinal images display a solitary, sharply defined, slightly echogenic mass (*arrows*) within the right lobe.

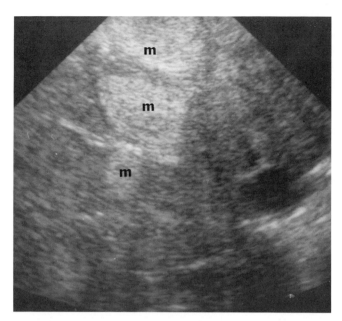

FIG. 16. Metastatic neuroblastoma in a 2-year-old girl. Transverse scan: Multiple hyperechoic masses (*m*) are present within the right lobe.

are small and do not cross the midline and who have metastases to liver, skin, and bone marrow, but not to bone. Clinically, patients may present with hepatomegaly, jaundice, pain, abdominal mass, or an abnormal liver function test.

Hepatic metastases have a variable sonographic appearance ranging from diffuse parenchymal inhomogeneity to multiple hypo-, iso-, or hyperechoic lesions

(Figs. 15, 16). Occasionally a large solitary metastasis or calcified lesion may be found. Calcified lesions are particularly echogenic and also demonstrate acoustic shadowing. The sonographic findings of hepatic metastases are not specific, but in the appropriate clinical setting, the correct diagnosis usually is not difficult. Diffuse involvement of the liver by metastases may be difficult to recognize by sonography. Computerized tomography scans or MR imaging can help confirm multiple lesions in such patients with diffusely altered echotexture.

Lymphoma

Hepatic involvement by lymphoma is rarely detected clinically, but is present at autopsy in over 50% of individuals. Recognition of hepatic involvement at the time of diagnosis or during follow-up studies is important because it indicates stage IV disease and a poorer prognosis. The sonographic diagnosis is based on the demonstration of diffuse parenchymal inhomogeneity or single or multiple hypoechoic lesions (Fig. 17). In some cases, these lesions appear entirely cystic, with poor or minimal through-transmission (129). Rarely, echogenic lesions surrounded by a hypoechoic rim are observed (154). Hepatosplenomegaly also may be observed, but it is a nonspecific finding. Almost 50% of patients with hepatomegaly have no histologic evidence of lymphoma. On the other hand, patients with normal size livers can have extensive involvement by lymphoma.

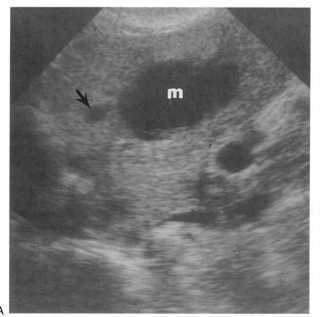

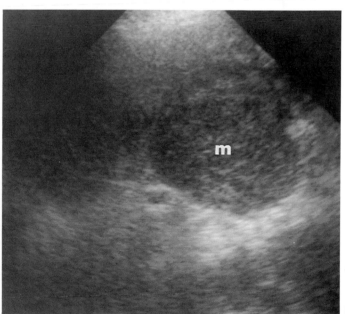

A   B

FIG. 17. Hepatic lymphoma in a 14-year-old girl. **A:** A longitudinal sonogram demonstrates a large anechoic area (*m*) within the right lobe of the liver. A smaller sonolucent mass (*arrow*) also can be noted. **B:** Hepatic lymphoma in a 16-year-old boy. Transverse scan demonstrates a well-defined, slightly hypoechoic mass (*m*) on the inferior surface of the left lobe.

Benign Neoplasms

Angiomatous Lesions

The majority of benign hepatic neoplasms in children are of vascular origin, usually hemangioendothelioma or cavernous hemangioma (39,44,148). Hemangioendothelioma occurs less frequently than cavernous hemangioma, but it is more often symptomatic. More than 85% are diagnosed under 6 months of age, presenting as asymptomatic hepatomegaly or an abdominal mass. Occasionally the tumor may present as high output congestive heart failure due to arteriovenous shunting within the lesion, a bleeding diathesis secondary to platelet sequestration, or massive hemoperitoneum due to spontaneous rupture. One or more cutaneous hemangiomas are found in about 50% of patients with hemangioendothelioma and support its diagnosis (39,40). In contrast, cavernous hemangioma affects older children and generally is an incidental postmortem finding. When present, symptoms are most commonly hepatomegaly or an enlarging abdomen. Congestive heart failure is rarely a feature of cavernous hemangioma.

On gross examination, hemangioendothelioma is a relatively bloodless tumor containing multiple, rounded, discrete nodules ranging from 2 to 15 cm (mean, 4 cm) in diameter. On microscopic examination, however, the tumor is quite vascular and typically contains variably sized vascular channels lined by plump endothelial cells that are supported by reticulin fibers. Rarely, an aggressive histologic subtype demonstrating irregular branching channels lined by more immature, bigger pleomorphic cells has been reported. This form has some limited malignant potential and rarely metastasizes (35,39,40). In contrast, cavernous hemangioma has a grossly vascular appearance. Histologically, it contains multiple, dilated, blood-filled spaces lined by mature, flat endothelial cells and separated by fibrous septa. Malignant potential is absent (148).

There is a spectrum of sonographic findings in hemangioendotheliomas and cavernous hemangiomas. Both lesions typically are solitary with a slight predilection for the posterior segment of the right lobe, but multiple lesions with a random distribution may occur. The echotexture of the mass is variable, and ranges from highly echogenic relative to liver to hypoechoic or anechoic with echogenic septa (Figs. 18,19) (22,71,102). The increased echogenicity is presumably due to the multiple interfaces between the walls of the vascular spaces and the blood within them (21). Acoustic enhancement has been associated with hypo- and hyperechoic lesions (21). Decreased size of the aorta at its junction with the celiac artery and a large celiac artery also have been observed.

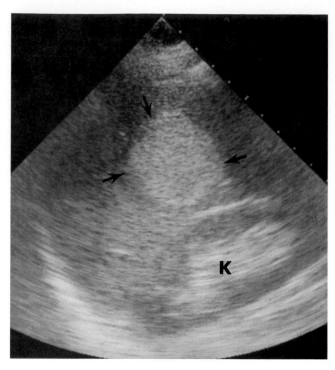

FIG. 18. Cavernous hemangioma in an 18-year-old girl. Longitudinal sonograms through the upper abdomen demonstrate a sharply marginated hyperechoic mass (*arrows*) within the right lobe. Slight distal acoustic enhancement is present. The diagnosis was confirmed by CT scanning. *K*, kidney.

Mesenchymal Hamartoma

After the vascular lesions, cystic mesenchymal hamartoma is the next most common benign hepatic tumor in childhood. Pathologically, mesenchymal hamartoma is a well-circumscribed, encapsulated mass lesion measuring in excess of 8 to 10 cm. Characteristically it contains multiple cysts ranging from 1 to 6 cm in diameter. This cystic spaces typically contain mucoid or gelatinous material and are separated by a fibrous stroma (40,148). Mesenchymal hamartoma usually is found in children under 2 years of age and affects boys twice as commonly as girls. Most children present with an asymptomatic abdominal mass. Rarely, the hamartoma has a large vascular component producing arterial venous shunting and congestive heart failure (1,120).

On sonography, the lesion appears as a well-circumscribed, multilocular mass containing anechoic spaces separated by echogenic septa (Fig. 20) (1,39,41,58,73, 111,120,122,135). If the cystic spaces are small, the mass will appear predominantly solid. A dilated proximal aorta and large draining hepatic veins may be present when there is significant arteriovenous shunting.

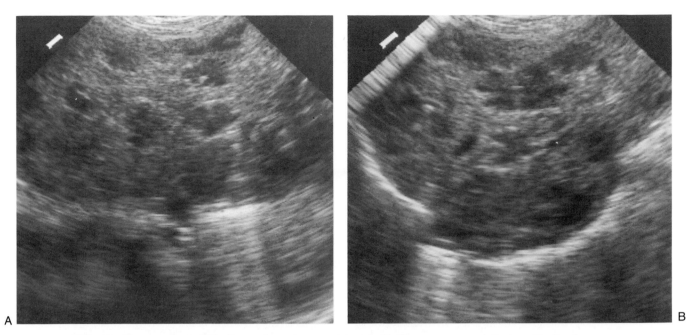

FIG. 19. Hemangioendothelioma in a 1-year-old girl. **A:** Transverse and **B:** longitudinal sonograms demonstrate multiple hypoechoic lesions replacing a large portion of the liver.

Epithelial Lesions

Focal nodular hyperplasia and hepatic adenoma are benign lesions that together account for approximately 2% of the hepatic tumors in children (40,41). A benign proliferation of hepatocytes characterizes both lesions. Pathologically, focal nodular hyperplasia is a well-circumscribed, unencapsulated mass, composed of an abnormal arrangement of normal hepatocytes, Kupffer's cells, and bile ducts. A central fibrous stellate scar is a distinctive feature of this tumor. Hepatic adenoma is a well-defined, encapsulated tumor, composed entirely of hepatocytes and devoid of Kupffer's cells, bile ducts, or a central fibrous scar (40). Hepatic

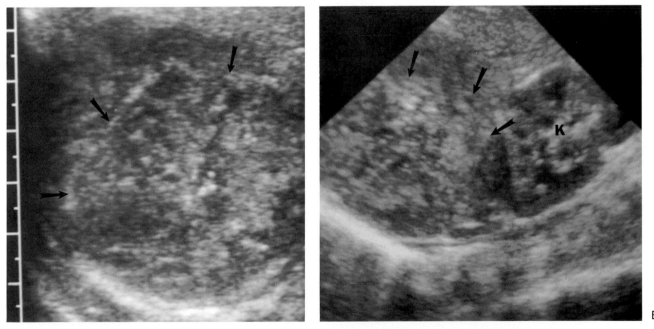

FIG. 20. Mesenchymal hamartoma in a 2-year-old boy. **A:** Transverse and **B:** Longitudinal sonograms reveal a complex mass (*arrows*) containing multiple tiny hypoechoic areas surrounded by echogenic parenchyma or septa. *K*, kidney.

adenomas in childhood have been associated with glycogen storage disease, Fanconi's anemia, and galactosemia (24), whereas focal nodular hyperplasia has no strong association with preexisting abnormalities. Both tumors tend to present as abdominal masses or hepatomegaly, although hepatic adenoma may present with abdominal pain from spontaneous hemorrhage (41).

The sonographic findings of hepatic adenomas and focal nodular hyperplasia are similar and indistinguishable from primary or metastatic tumors. Both lesions usually are well-circumscribed and may be iso-, hypo-, or hyperechoic or have a mixed echo pattern (6,24, 62,119,151,152). Demonstration of a central scar or linear echo would favor focal nodular hyperplasia, whereas sonolucent areas, reflecting hemorrhage or necrosis, would be more suggestive of hepatic adenoma.

Cysts

Cystic lesions of the liver are rare in children and can be congenital or acquired in origin, as well as single or multiple in number. Congenital cysts arise from intrahepatic biliary ducts which fail to involute and are more common than acquired ones which are the result of inflammation, trauma, or parasitic disease. The majority of hepatic cysts are solitary. Multiple hepatic

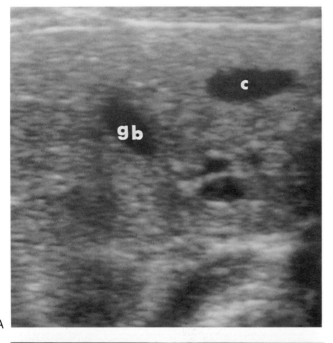

A

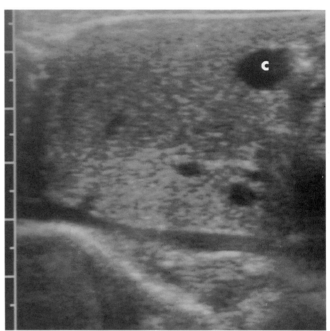

B

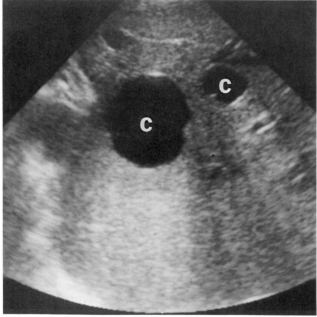

C

FIG. 21. Benign hepatic cyst. **A:** Transverse and **B:** longitudinal scans in a 12-year-old girl. An incidentally found, sharply defined, anechoic mass in the lateral aspect of the right lobe was proven surgically to be a benign cyst (*c*). *gb*, gallbladder. **C:** Longitudinal scan in another patient shows two round cysts (*C*). The largest one has marked acoustic enhancement.

cysts usually are seen with polycystic renal disease, and are found in one-third of affected patients. Hepatic cysts are generally incidental findings, although large ones may present as abdominal masses or hepatomegaly, or produce abdominal pain.

The sonographic appearance of benign cysts is usually characteristic, whether the lesions are single or multiple. They are anechoic, sharply delineated, and round or oval lesions with thin walls and variable degrees of through-transmission (see Fig. 21). Most cysts are unilocular, but occasionally internal septations can be seen. Differentiation of hepatic cysts from other hepatic mass lesions is usually not difficult because the sonographic appearance is so characteristic. Rarely, however, an echinococcal cyst, hematoma, or abscess may have a similar appearance. Atypical features such as a thick wall, mural nodules, septations, or inhomogeneous internal contents should suggest the possibility that something other than a benign cyst is present. In some cases, the correct diagnosis may be suspected on the basis of the clinical history, especially the patient's nationality or travel history in cases of hydatid disease. In problem cases, a percutaneous needle aspiration may be indicated for diagnosis (118).

Inflammatory Lesions

Viral Hepatitis

Hepatitis is a diffuse inflammatory process of the liver parenchyma, usually of viral origin. The most common causes of viral hepatitis are the hepatitis A, hepatitis B, and hepatitis non-A, non-B viruses. Cy-tomegalovirus, herpes, and Epstein-Barr viruses are less common etiologies. Hepatitis may also follow ingestion, inhalation, or parenteral administration of drugs or toxins.

Sonography is not necessary to provide the diagnosis of hepatitis, but may be useful when there is clinical uncertainty whether the patient's jaundice is cholestatic or obstructive in nature. In most patients, the sonographic appearance of the liver is normal (57). However, in acutely severe disease, sonography may show hepatomegaly, hypoechoic parenchyma due to edematous liver cells and increased periportal echogenicity (17), or very echogenic portal vein walls (77). The gallbladder wall also may be thick and edematous early in the course of the disease (85). With chronic hepatitis, the liver increases in echogenicity and becomes inhomogeneous secondary to cirrhosis and periportal fibrosis. The gallbladder becomes smaller and may contain thick bile, sludge, or stones.

Pyogenic Abscess

Pyogenic hepatic abscesses in children are rare and usually are associated with systemic sepsis, hematogeneous spread from distant sites of infection such as appendicitis or inflammatory bowel disease, omphalitis, thrombophlebitis after umbilical vein catheterization, and trauma (132). Children with depressed immunity, especially those with chronic granulomatous disease of childhood, also are at risk of developing hepatic abscesses (29). In the older infant and child, *Staphylococcus aureus* is the most common etiologic agent, and in the neonatal period gram-negative or-

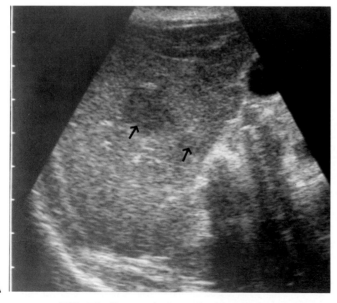
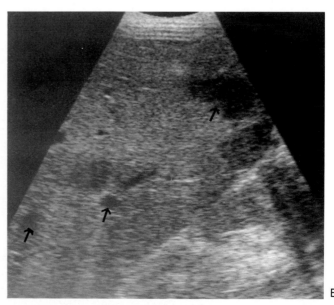

FIG. 22. Pyogenic hepatic abscesses. **A:** Transverse and **B:** longitudinal scans through the right lobe of the liver demonstrates multiple, poorly defined hypoechoic lesions (*arrows*).

ganisms are more frequent. Clinical manifestations of hepatic abscesses include fever, upper abdominal pain or tenderness, hepatomegaly, and leukocytosis.

Sonography is the examination of choice in patients with suspected hepatic abscesses who have localizing signs of disease (136). Pyogenic abscesses can occur in any part of the liver, but the majority are found in the posterior portion of the right lobe for reasons not clearly established, but thought to be due to the pattern of portal venous flow. Other sonographic findings include: (a) variable size; (b) irregular, ill-defined walls; (c) anechoic or hypoechoic center; and (d) through-transmission (53,83,101,157) (Fig. 22). Occasionally, the central contents are highly echogenic because gas is present within the abscess (32). Septations, debris, and fluid-fluid levels also can be seen (Fig. 23).

Included in the differential of entities that mimic pyogenic abscesses are certain stages of hydatid disease, old intrahepatic hematoma, and, rarely, cystic metastases. When the diagnosis of hepatic abscess is not certain from the clinical history, percutaneous needle aspiration of a lesion can help resolve the question. The therapy of hepatic abscess is based on drainage of the localized lesion and long-term antibiotic therapy. Sonography can be used to guide drainage of the abscess if this is accomplished percutaneously (138,145).

Fungal Abscess

Fungal abscesses are almost always found in patients with compromised immune systems. Abscesses due to *Candida albicans* are particularly common in this clinical setting. Although large, single fungal ab-

scesses may be observed, more often there are multiple lesions, 1 to 2 cm in diameter, with irregular walls. These are scattered throughout both lobes of the liver and often involve the spleen and occasionally the kidneys as well. Four sonographic patterns of hepatic abscesses from candidiasis have been described (105). The most frequent appearance is a nonspecific hypoechoic nodule. Other sonographic patterns include a uniformly echogenic lesion and a "target" appearance characterized by a central echogenic area surrounded by a hypoechoic zone (Fig. 24) (28). The fourth pattern is a "wheel within a wheel" appearance, consisting of a central hypoechoic area surrounded by an echogenic ring and outer hypoechoic ring (105). Patients with fungal abscesses represent special management problems, since size and multiplicity of the abscesses make percutaneous and surgical drainage difficult or impossible.

Hydatid Disease

Hydatid liver disease (echinococcosis) is a parasitic infestation caused by the larval stage of the tapeworm *Echinococcus granulosus* or *E. alveolaris*, the former being the more common in the United States. Pathologically, *E. granulosus* produces well-defined, cystic lesions, whereas *E. alveolaris* produces poorly defined infiltrating lesions. Three main sonographic patterns have been defined; these patterns are more characteristic of *E. granulosus* than of *E. alveolaris* (86). Type I refers to a simple anechoic cyst which may be homogeneous or contain detached membranes. Type II lesions contain daughter cysts and/or echogenic ma-

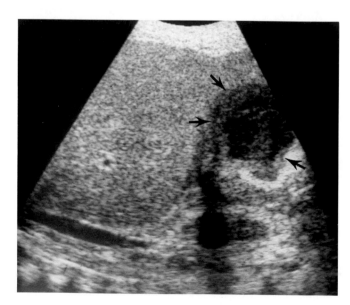

FIG. 23. Pyogenic abscess. Longitudinal scan demonstrates a hypoechoic lesion (*arrows*) with central debris in the inferior aspect of the right hepatic lobe.

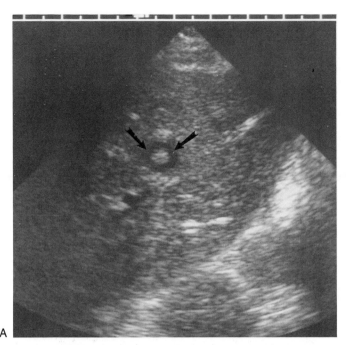
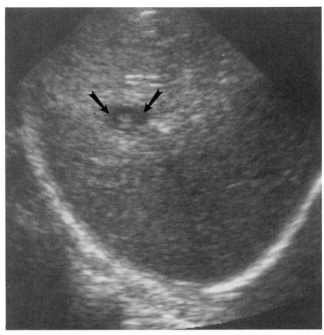

FIG. 24. *Candida albicans* abscess. **A:** Transverse and **B:** longitudinal images show a hypoechoic lesion (*arrows*) with a central echogenic focus (bull's-eye or target lesion).

trix, and type III cysts are densely calcified lesions. Children tend to demonstrate a propensity for type I cysts, whereas older patients show type II and III lesions (Fig. 25). Demonstration of daughter cysts is pathognomonic of hydatid disease. Hydatid disease may be treated surgically or medically. The response to medical treatment is significantly higher in those lesions without daughter cysts (16).

Amebic Abscesses

Amebiasis most commonly occurs in tropical or subtropical climates and is the result of infection by the protozoan *Entamoeba histolytica*. Amebic abscesses are solitary in about 80% of patients and have a propensity to localize peripherally, often involving the right lobe (15). On sonography, they may

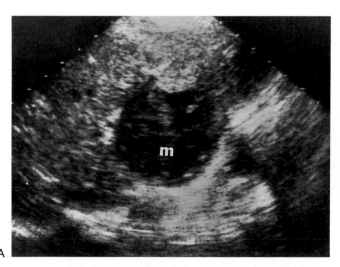
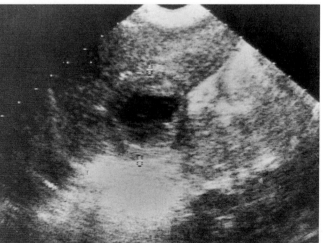

FIG. 25. Hydatid disease. **A:** Longitudinal sonogram shows a complex mass (*m*) containing detached membranes, typical of hydatid disease in childhood. **B:** At a higher level the cyst has a thick wall. (Courtesy of Dr. Maria Ines Boechat, Los Angeles, California)

be anechoic or hypoechoic with thin or thick walls (22,112,113,116). Other findings are internal debris and a "target" appearance (65) (Fig. 26). Because the sonographic features are similar to those of pyogenic abscesses, surgical or percutaneous aspiration is required for diagnosis and treatment. When aspiration is performed, the fluid is extremely thick and sometimes referred to as "anchovy paste."

The majority (72%) of hepatic amebic abscesses resolve over several months without sequelae. Early in treatment the lesions may decrease, remain unchanged, or increase in size. Eventually the abscess shrinks and the internal contents increase in echogenicity and acquire a pattern indistinguishable from normal hepatic parenchyma. A smaller subgroup of patients with amebic abscesses have persistent cystic lesions that mimic benign, simple cysts. Occasionally the lesions show only slightly increased or decreased echogenicity after treatment (112,116,117).

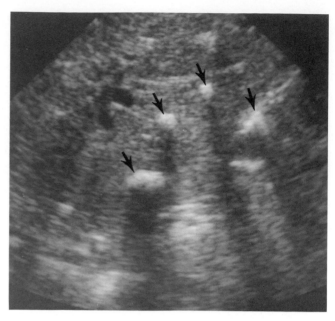

FIG. 27. Chronic granulomatous disease. Transverse sonogram shows multiple calcifications (*arrows*) with distal acoustic shadowing. Previous scans had shown multiple hypoechoic hepatic abscesses.

Chronic Granulomatous Disease

Chronic granulomatous disease is an X-linked recessive disorder characterized by inability of leukocytes to lyse phagocytized bacteria. Patients present with recurrent infections of the lung, bones, lymph nodes, or liver often due to *S. aureus*. Abdominal sonography shows multiple, poorly defined hepatic abscesses. With treatment, the lesions may resolve or become more echogenic due to calcification (Fig. 27).

Diffuse Liver Disease

Neoplasm

Tumors that diffusely involve the hepatic parenchyma include lymphoma, metastatic neuroblastoma, and rarely hepatoma in patients with cirrhosis. Sonographic features of diffuse hepatic neoplasm include hepatomegaly and parenchymal inhomogeneity. Compression and distortion of normal vascular anatomy also may be noted.

Fatty Infiltration

Fatty infiltration is the result of an excessive accumulation of triglycerides within hepatocytes. It appears to be a nonspecific response of the hepatocytes to injury and occurs in association with numerous disorders, including obesity, Cushing's disease or syn-

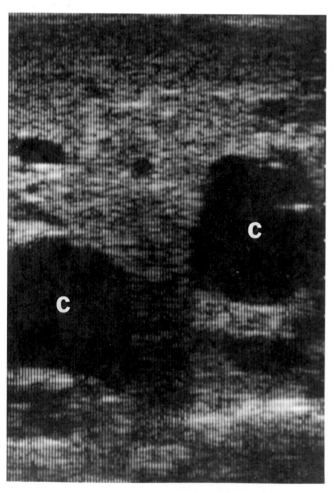

FIG. 26. Amebic hepatic abscess. Transverse scan of the liver demonstrates two well-defined, cystic masses (*C*) in the right lobe of the liver. (Courtesy of Dr. Maria Ines Boechat, Los Angeles, California)

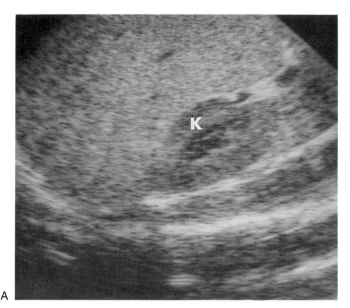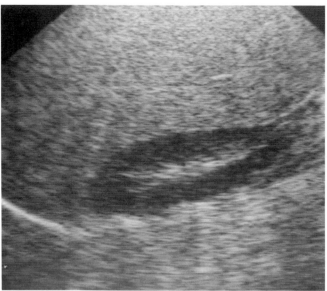

A   B

FIG. 28. Fatty infiltration in cystic fibrosis. **A:** On a transverse view the liver is slightly echogenic relative to the right kidney (*K*). **B:** A longitudinal scan in another patient shows more severe fatty infiltration. The kidney is markedly hypoechoic relative to the liver secondary to increased attenuation of the sound beam.

drome, chemotherapy, hyperalimentation, severe protein malnutrition, cystic fibrosis, metabolic liver disorders, and congenital generalized lipodystrophy.

Fatty infiltration is generally diffuse throughout the liver, but it can be focal. The diffuse form produces hepatomegaly, parenchymal homogeneity or heterogeneity, and increased echogenicity that varies from mild to marked (125,142). With diffuse fatty infiltra-

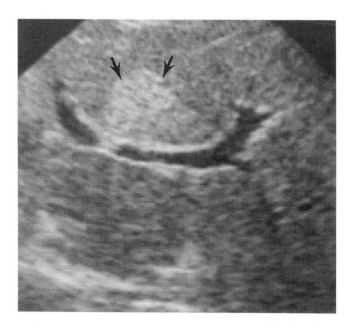

FIG. 29. Focal fatty infiltration. Transverse sonogram demonstrates a focal area (*arrows*) of increased echogenicity anterior to the portal vein, which corresponded to fat on a CT scan.

tion, there is increased attenuation of the sound beam so that the adjacent renal cortex appears sonolucent relative to the liver (Fig. 28) (66). Focal fatty infiltration appears as a lobar, segmental, or wedge-shaped area of increased echogenicity with sharp, angulated margins, predominantly involving the right lobe (127) (Fig. 29). Occasionally, a hypoechoic mass may be present and may be mistaken for a mass lesion. This "pseudotumor" is caused by the presence of normal areas of liver in a background of fatty changes.

Cirrhosis

Cirrhosis is a diffuse process characterized by chronic destruction of the normal hepatic parenchyma with replacement by fibrosis and nodular regeneration. Diseases that have been associated with cirrhosis in childhood include chronic hepatitis, congenital hepatic fibrosis, biliary atresia, cystic fibrosis, metabolic disease (Wilson's disease, glycogen storage disease, tyrosinemia, galactosemia, alpha-1-antitrypsin deficiency), Budd-Chiari syndrome, and drugs. Rarely, cirrhosis can occur in newborns receiving prolonged total parenteral nutrition (128).

Characteristic features of cirrhosis include: (a) a small right hepatic lobe and medial segment of the left lobe, with compensatory hypertrophy of the lateral segment of the left lobe and the caudate lobe; (b) irregular margins of the liver; (c) heterogeneity of the parenchyma; and (d) increased echogenicity with decreased beam penetration secondary to fatty infiltration or decreased echogenicity secondary to fibrosis and regenerating nodules (Fig. 30) (38,106,142,147). Hepatic and portal vein radicals within the liver usually are compressed and difficult to visualize, and the gallbladder often is small or not visualized. Secondary signs of cirrhosis, namely ascites, splenomegaly, and multiple varices, are common when portal hypertension develops. Although sonography is useful in detecting diffuse parenchymal disease, it is unable to differentiate cirrhosis from fatty infiltration or chronic hepatitis.

Disorders of Hepatic Vessels

Portal Hypertension

Portal hypertension usually results when there is increased resistance to hepatopetal blood flow. The obstruction may be intrahepatic secondary to cirrhosis or extrahepatic at the level of the portal or hepatic veins. In children, the incidence of extrahepatic obstruction is relatively higher than it is in adults and in some series it is more frequent than intrahepatic obstruction as a cause of portal hypertension (11). Rarely, portal venous hypertension is caused by increased blood flow due to an arteriovenous fistula. Clinical signs include splenomegaly, ascites, promi-

nent abdominal veins (capat medusae), hematemesis due to esophageal varices, hepatic encephalopathy, and hypersplenism.

Real-time and duplex Doppler sonography can be helpful in diagnosing portal hypertension (4,6,59, 109,147). Sonographic findings of portal hypertension include spontaneous portosystemic shunts, reversal of flow to a hepatofugal direction in the portal or splenic vein (Fig. 31), splenomegaly, abnormal hepatic parenchyma, and a thick lesser omentum.

Portal Vein Abnormalities

The portal vein often is large in patients with severe portal hypertension (Fig. 32). The size of the vein, however, is related to the size and number of varices and if shunts are present, the caliber tends to diminish. When portal vein dilatation is used alone as a criteria for portal hypertension, a sensitivity of about 40% is found (18). When variations in caliber of the portal vein and its branches during respiration are assessed, the sensitivity for sonography in the diagnosis of portal hypertension is 80% with a specificity of 100% (18). With portal hypertension, the normal variations in caliber (i.e., increase during inspiration and decrease during expiration) in the portal and splenic veins are absent.

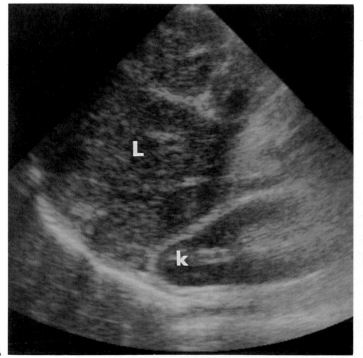
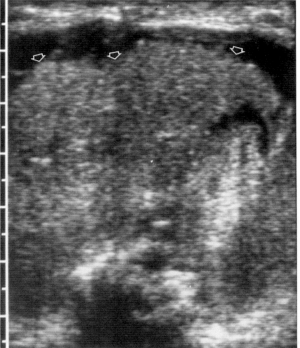

A   B

FIG. 30. Hepatic cirrhosis. **A:** A longitudinal sonogram demonstrates heterogeneity of the hepatic parenchyma. The echogenicity of the liver (*L*) is decreased secondary to fibrosis and is equal to that of the kidney (*k*). **B:** In another patient with cirrhosis, the margins of the liver (*open arrows*) are irregular. A small amount of hypoechoic ascites is present anteriorly.

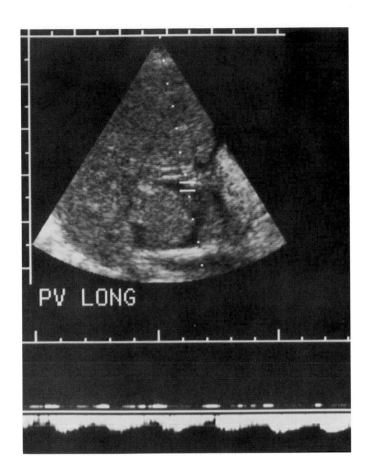

FIG. 31. Reverse flow in the portal vein in a patient with portal hypertension. Longitudinal Doppler interrogation of the portal vein demonstrates flow directed away from the transducer consistent with reversed flow.

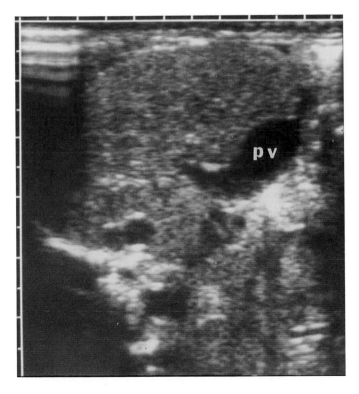

FIG. 32. Portal hypertension. Transverse scan. Large portal vein (*pv*), measuring 1.8 cm in diameter, in a patient with severe portal hypertension.

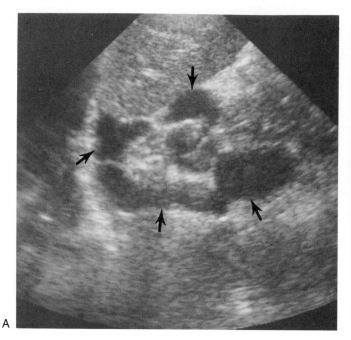

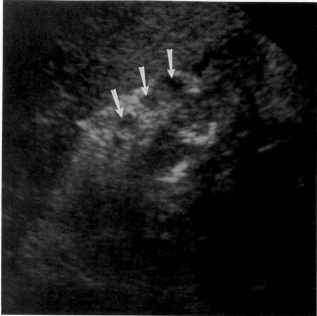

FIG. 33. Varices in portal hypertension. **A:** Longitudinal scan shows a dilated and markedly tortuous vessel (*arrows*) beneath the left lobe of the liver, compatible with coronary varices. **B:** Transverse scan shows multiple, round hypoechoic gastroesophageal varices (*arrows*).

Portosystemic Collaterals

The major collateral veins in portal hypertension are the coronary-gastroesophageal and paraumbilical veins. Less frequently visualized channels include anastomoses between the splenic and renal veins and between the superior mesenteric vein and inferior vena cava. The coronary vein arises from the portal vein and runs cephalad between the two layers of the lesser omentum to drain into the esophageal veins. When dilated, it appears as a tortuous vessel beneath the left lobe of the liver, best seen on a longitudinal scan obtained near the junction of the splenic vein and portal vein (137). Gastroesophageal varices formed by enlargement of the coronary vein and branches of the splenic vein appear as tortuous anechoic or hypoechoic structures near the gastroesophageal junction. Esophageal varices are best seen on a transverse scan with the transducer angled cranially through the left lobe of the liver. Coronary-gastroesophageal varices can be detected by sonography in about 90% of children with varices (25) (Fig. 33).

The patent paraumbilical vein originates from the left portal vein and extends through the ligamentum teres to the abdominal wall, terminating at the umbilicus. On transverse sonograms, it appears as an anechoic, round, or oval structure (usually greater then 3 mm in diameter) within the falciform ligament (126). Its origin from the left portal vein and termination near the umbilicus are best seen on parasagittal views (124) (Fig. 34). The presence of portal venous flow within a

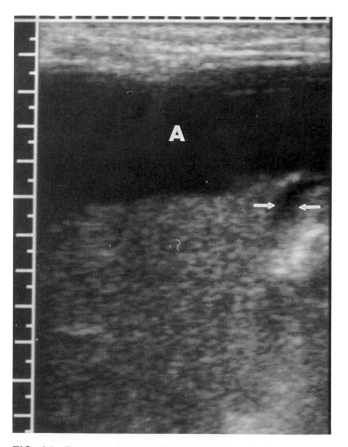

FIG. 34. Patent paraumbilical vein. A parasagittal scan shows a patent vessel (*arrows*) beneath the anterior abdominal wall. A large amount of ascites (*A*) surrounds the liver.

patent paraumbilical view is a valuable finding to support the diagnosis of portal hypertension.

Hepatic and Splenic Abnormalities

The liver may be small and shrunken with an irregular margin in end-stage liver disease, or it may be enlarged due to significant fatty infiltration. Increased echogenicity and attenuation of the sound beam are seen with fatty infiltration. In contrast, the spleen is almost always enlarged in portal hypertension and often there are multiple distended veins in the splenic hilum (Fig. 35). Splenic echotexture usually is normal and homogeneous.

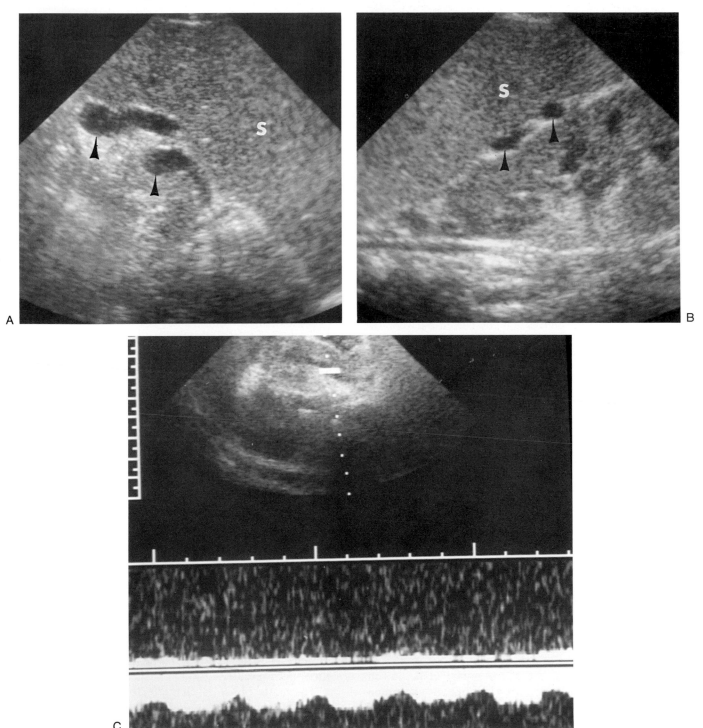

FIG. 35. Splenic varices. **A:** Transverse and **B:** coronal views of the spleen (*S*) demonstrate dilated splenic vein collaterals (*arrowheads*). **C:** Longitudinal Doppler waveform of the splenic vein collaterals shows reversed flow. The waveform is similar to that of the portal vein.

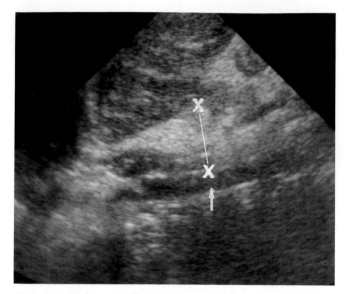

FIG. 36. Thickened lesser omentum. Lesser omental thickness is the distance (X—X) between the origin of the celiac axis and the inferior hepatic surface. Ratio of this measurement to the anteroposterior diameter of aorta at same level is 3.8. *Arrow*, posterior wall of aorta.

Thickened Omentum

Lesser omentum thickness is measured between the celiac axis and inferior surface of the liver on the sagittal view and should not exceed 1.7 times the diameter of the aorta at the same level. Measurements greater than 1.7 have been seen in the majority of children with portal hypertension (Fig. 36). The increased thickness of the lesser omentum is due to the presence of tortuous coronary and omental varices and lymphatic congestion (25,107). Besides portal hypertension, increased thickness of the lesser omentum has been associated with fatty infiltration due to obesity or systemic steroid therapy, and with lymphadenopathy (107).

Evaluation of Surgical Shunt Procedures

Sonography also is valuable in the follow-up evaluation of surgically created portosystemic shunts performed to relieve portal hypertension. Signs of patency include a decrease in the thickness of the lesser omentum, diminution or disappearance of the collateral veins, decreased diameter of the portal vein, and increased diameter of the inferior vena cava when compared to preoperative sonograms (19,25). Duplex or color flow Doppler can facilitate the evaluation of shunts that are difficult to visualize because the postsurgical anatomy is inconstant or bowel gas obscures anatomic detail (60). In addition to demonstrating flow

at the anastomotic site, the Doppler study provides an easy way to assess shunt patency. Reversed flow in the portal veins almost always indicates a patent shunt, even if the anastomotic site cannot be directly visualized (78).

Portal Vein Thrombosis

Partial or complete portal vein thrombosis in childhood has been associated with perinatal omphalitis, sepsis, appendicitis, acute dehydration, and umbilical vein catheterization (8,132). Tumor, a major cause of portal vein thrombosis in adults, in an infrequent etiology in children. The clinical presentation is variable depending on etiology and chronicity of occlusion, and ranges from occult symptoms to a fulminant clinical course with septicemia and signs of infarction.

The acute stage is characterized by focal enlargement of the involved vein, or more definitively, an echogenic intraluminal thrombus. Doppler flow is absent when venous occlusion is complete (Fig. 37). Serial sonography may demonstrate a change in the extent of thrombus, recanalization of part of the vessel, and enlargement of collateral veins such as the umbilical, superior mesenteric, and splenic veins. The thrombus also becomes more hypoechoic. Portal vein thrombosis may cause marked dilatation of periportal collaterals, which has been termed "cavernous transformation of the portal vein" or "portal cavernoma." The collaterals permit continued hepatopetal blood flow. Sonographic findings of portal cavernoma include failure to visualize the extrahepatic portal vein, visualization of multiple vascular channels in the porta hepatis, and typical portal venous waveforms in the dilated vessels (153) (Fig. 38).

Hepatic Veno-occlusive Disease

Hepatic veno-occlusive disease (Budd-Chiari syndrome) is a rare disorder that may involve the hepatic venules, major hepatic veins, or intrahepatic vena cava. The causes of obstruction include polycythemia, lupus erythematosus, sickle cell anemia, congenital webs or diaphragms of the inferior vena cava or hepatic veins, and tumor masses invading or compressing the lumen. The etiology, however, is unknown in more than half the cases.

The acute phase is characterized by hepatomegaly and ascites. At least one major hepatic vein usually is visualized; the vein or veins may be filled with thrombi, stenotic, or thick-walled. Extrahepatic collaterals and narrowing of the intrahepatic portion of the inferior vena cava are other findings. In chronic

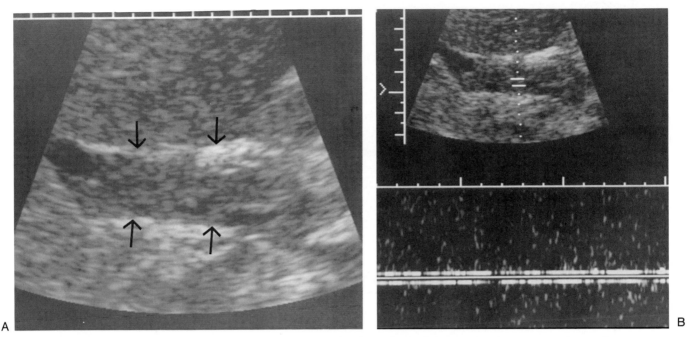

FIG. 37. Acute portal vein thrombus. **A:** Longitudinal view of the porta shows an echogenic thrombus in the portal vein (*arrows*). **B:** Doppler confirms absent flow.

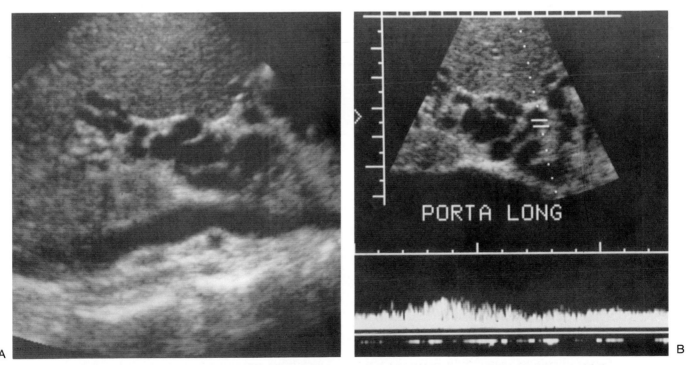

FIG. 38. Cavernous transformation of the portal vein. **A:** Longitudinal scan demonstrates multiple dilated vessels in the porta hepatis. A normal portal vein cannot be identified. **B:** Duplex Doppler sonography of the porta shows portal venous waveforms.

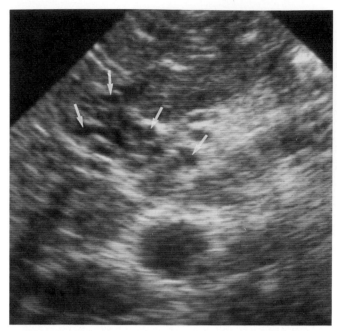

FIG. 39. Chronic hepatic vein occlusion (Budd-Chiari syndrome). A transverse sonogram through the porta hepatis demonstrates a network of multiple collateral channels (*arrows*).

cases, hepatic veins are not visualized and numerous collateral venous channels can be identified within the porta hepatis (Fig. 39). Caudate lobe hypertrophy is usually present (94).

Doppler examination can be used to assess the patency of the hepatic veins, although the diagnosis of venous occlusion is complicated by transmitted cardiac pulsations which can simulate hepatic venous flow. In addition, hepatomegaly alone can result in compression of the hepatic veins and render them difficult to localize with duplex Doppler. Color flow Doppler imaging appears to be significantly better in determining the status of the hepatic veins, direction of flow, and sites of occlusion (60).

Hepatic Infarcts

Hepatic arterial infarcts are rare since the liver is protected by its dual blood supply from the portal veins. The majority of cases in childhood are related to decreased arterial perfusion secondary to surgery. On sonography, areas of infarction are often hypoechoic lesions that are peripherally located within the liver. Increased echogenicity within the lesion may be present if the infarct contains gas. After hepatic infarction, cystic collections of bile (bile lakes) may develop.

Other Hepatic Lesions

Trauma

Hepatic injuries occur in approximately 25% of all children with blunt abdominal trauma (134). Injuries of the right lobe occur in about 80% of pediatric patients with hepatic trauma and are four times more common than injuries of the left lobe. The posterior segment of the right lobe is injured in about 65% of patients, the dome of the right lobe in about 30%, and the anterior segment in approximately 20%. In the left lobe, injuries are evenly divided between the medial and lateral segments (134). Traumatic lesions include hepatic parenchymal hematomas, lacerations, and fractures with varying degrees of capsular disruption and associated hemoperitoneum. Hepatic hematomas are focal collections of blood that may be round or have irregular margins. Hepatic lacerations appear as linear or branching parenchymal defects. Hepatic fractures traverse the entire extent of a lobe or segment. Subcapsular collections appear as lenticular collections that flattened the lateral aspect of the liver. The associated hemoperitoneum is variable in size and may be small, confined to the right subphrenic and subhepatic spaces, or more extensive, accumulating in the paracolic gutter and the pelvic cul-de-sac.

Hepatic injuries have a variable sonographic appearance related to the age of the hematoma. Acutely, parenchymal or subcapsular fluid collections appear hyperechoic or nearly isoechoic with normal liver due to the presence of fibrin or clot formation. Within 2 to 3 days, the hematoma becomes more hypoechoic and cystic as the blood undergoes liquefaction with resorption of hemoglobin (Fig. 40).

Although sonography can detect hepatic injury, it generally is not the initial examination of choice since it is impaired by paralytic ileus, which usually accompanies abdominal trauma, open wounds, and dressings. Moreover, false negative sonographic results are common if the injury involves the dome of the liver. Hence, CT is the preferred method to determine the presence and extent of liver injury. However, sonography is valuable to follow the healing of a known hepatic injury (82).

Most intrahepatic hematomas resolve spontaneously within weeks to several months, but posttraumatic bile pseudocysts or pseudoaneurysms may develop in some patients. Pseudocysts or bilomas appear as large, homogeneous, thin-walled, anechoic collections with through-transmission (46). Focal fatty infiltration, presumably related to local vascular injury, or calcifications are other late sequelae of hepatic trauma (Fig. 41).

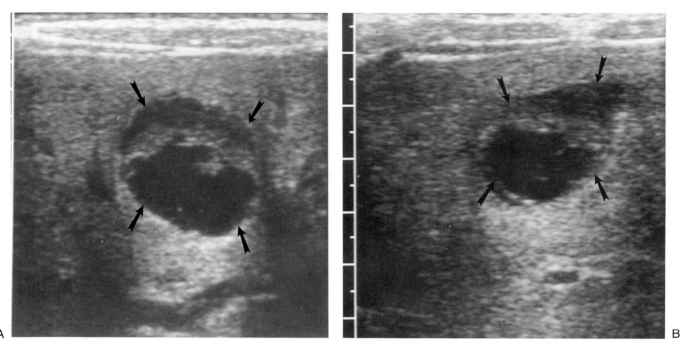

FIG. 40. Intrahepatic hematoma. **A:** Transverse and **B:** longitudinal scans 7 days after injury demonstrate a well-defined, predominantly hypoechoic lesion (*arrows*) with through-transmission.

Radiation Effects

The liver usually is not directly irradiated for therapeutic purposes, but it may be incidentally included in radiation ports designed to encompass tumors in adjacent organs or bony structures. Clinically and pathologically, the effects of radiation may be classified into acute and chronic stages. The acute phase has its onset 2 to 6 weeks after the completion of radiation therapy. During that time patients may present with

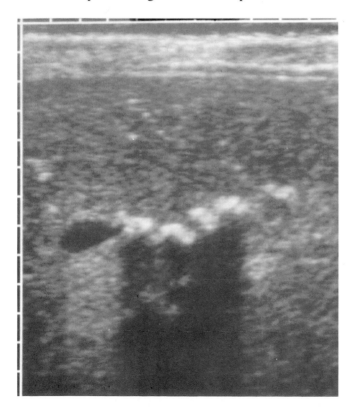

FIG. 41. Hepatic calcification. A longitudinal scan shows a linear echogenic band with acoustic shadowing. Patient had a history of a hepatic laceration.

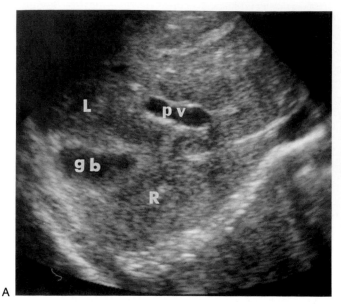

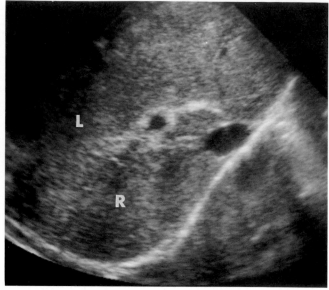

FIG. 42. Chronic radiation injury. **A:** Transverse and **B:** longitudinal sonograms of the liver at the level of the kidney show a small right lobe of the liver and heterogeneity of the parenchyma. The gallbladder (*gb*) and portal vein (*pv*) are displaced posteriorly because of the volume loss. The small, fibrotic right lobe corresponds to radiation portals. *R*, right lobe; *L*, left lobe.

sudden enlargement of the liver, jaundice, and ascites. Histologically, there is a spectrum of changes varying from mild panlobar congestion to severe congestion and hemorrhagic necrosis (49,143). In the chronic stage, the irradiated liver is typically small, contracted, and fibrotic (143).

On sonography, acute radiation-induced hepatic injury produces a sharply demarcated area of decreased echogenicity reflecting edema and hepatic congestion. The sharp, straight line of demarcation between the normal and abnormal liver corresponds to the predetermined radiation port in each patient (54). Sonographic findings in the chronic stage are those of decreased hepatic volume or cirrhosis (Fig. 42).

Liver Transplantation

Preoperative Evaluation

Sonography plays an important role in the evaluation of patients before and after liver transplantation. Before liver transplantation, sonography, especially duplex Doppler or color flow sonography, is important in determining patency of the extrahepatic portal vein because marked narrowing or occlusion makes surgical anastomosis difficult or impossible. If normal antegrade flow is demonstrated in the extrahepatic portal vein and no collateral vessels are detected, angiography is not required. However, when portal flow is absent or markedly diminished or when multiple collateral venous channels are found, angiography is indicated to precisely define anatomy.

The patency of the inferior vena cava, hepatic veins, and hepatic artery also should be evaluated prior to transplant. This evaluation is particularly important in patients with thrombosis or occlusion of the hepatic vein, since the suprahepatic portion of the inferior vena cava must be patent for transplant. In addition, sonography can detect other anomalies, especially in patients with biliary atresia. Up to 25% of patients with biliary atresia have associated anomalies including partial or complete malrotation of the bowel, polysplenia, and vascular anomalies such as absent inferior or superior vena cava as well as absence of the hepatic artery (2).

Postoperative Evaluation

Postoperative sonography is valuable in assessing patency of the hepatic artery (Fig. 43, Colorplate 5). Hepatic artery thrombosis is the most common vascular complication of hepatic transplantation and has been reported in about 40% of children. Hepatic artery stenosis at the anastomotic site or in the donor hepatic artery is a rarer complication (158). Although the hepatic artery has a small role in maintaining the viability of the normotopic liver, the transplant liver is highly dependent on the hepatic artery for its perfusion. Since arterial occlusion leads to hepatic necrosis and death, the sonographic detection of hepatic artery thrombosis is an indication for immediate retransplantation.

Portal vein complications, specifically thrombosis and stenosis, are not as frequent as arterial compli-

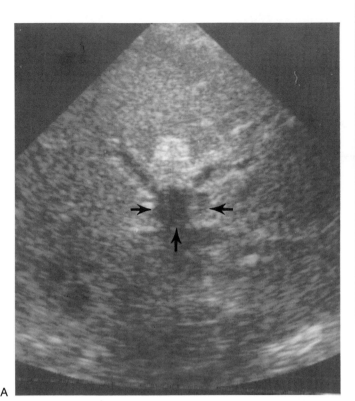
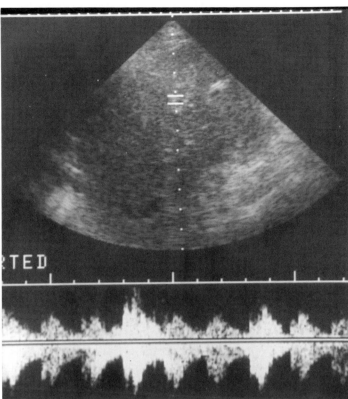

A   B

FIG. 44. Arteriovenous fistula. **A:** A longitudinal sonogram through the left lobe of the liver shows a hypoechoic fluid collection (*arrows*). **B:** Doppler waveforms show turbulent arterial flow. **C** (see Colorplate 6): Transverse color flow image shows an admixture of arterial and venous blood in the lesion. Arteriovenous fistula was confirmed by angiography.

cations, occurring in about 15% of children (158). Doppler examination demonstrates no evidence of flow in portal venous thrombosis. In portal vein stenosis, there is a high-velocity jet at the stenotic site, with distal turbulence. Other postoperative complications recognizable by sonography include biliary obstruction, intra- and extrahepatic fluid collections, abnormal hepatic echotexture secondary to rejection, ischemia, infection or drug toxicity, abscesses, and vascular complications, including aneurysms and arteriovenous fistulas (84). Duplex Doppler or color flow sonography is especially important in evaluating the vascular or nonvascular nature of abnormal fluid collections prior to biopsy (Fig. 44, and Colorplate 6) (140). Sonography, including duplex scanning, appears to be of no value in aiding the diagnosis of acute rejection (91).

DISEASES OF THE BILIARY TRACT

Jaundice is the most common clinical problem leading to examination of the biliary tract in childhood. In newborns, biliary atresia and neonatal hepatitis are the most common causes of jaundice and account for 70% to 80% of neonatal cholestasis cases (10,11). Occasionally, choledochal cyst, inspissated bile, metabolic defects (alpha 1-antitrypsin deficiency, galactosemia, glycogen storage disease) cystic fibrosis, or total parenteral nutrition may lead to cholestasis (10,11, 37,92,110). In older children jaundice is most frequently due to hepatocellular disease, but it can be the result of biliary tract obstruction. The common lesions producing obstructive jaundice are neoplasm, particularly rhabdomyosarcoma, lymphoma or neuroblastoma, biliary calculi, and choledochal cyst (92).

In evaluation of the patient with clinical or biochemical evidence of jaundice, the correct etiology often can be predicted by the appropriate utilization of a variety of laboratory tests of liver function in conjunction with the pertinent historical and physical findings. Nevertheless, imaging examinations, such as sonography and CT, are used often to confirm or alter the clinical impression (61,74). Besides demonstrating the presence of biliary tract obstruction, these studies can show the level and cause of obstruction (81). When both studies are available, sonography is the preferred procedure because of its lower cost and lack of ionizing radiation. If the extrahepatic ducts are well visualized by sonography and are normal in caliber and there is no evidence of intraductal dilatation, no further radiologic evaluation is needed. Computerized tomography plays a role only in those children in whom sonographic studies indicate ductal dilatation but do not clearly establish an etiology of the obstruction. Hepatobiliary scintigraphy currently is used primarily to study suspected choledochal cysts and biliary atresia.

Biliary Tract Obstruction

Sonographic Features

The sonographic diagnosis of biliary obstruction is based on demonstration of dilated intrahepatic or extrahepatic bile ducts. Normally, no intrahepatic bile ducts are visible within the portal triads on sonography. If sonolucencies are seen, biliary dilatation needs to be considered. The sonographic findings of intrahepatic duct dilatation include circular or tubular anechoic structures which are tortuous, have irregular walls, and demonstrate acoustic enhancement (Fig. 45). In the presence of moderate biliary tract dilatation, several ducts may converge and have a stellate branching appearance. Another finding is the "parallel-channel" sign. This refers to the simultaneous imaging of the dilated common hepatic duct and adjacent main portal vein branch.

Level and Cause of Obstruction

The level of biliary obstruction can be at three sites: the porta hepatis, suprapancreatic common duct, or intrapancreatic common duct. Tumors most often cause obstruction at the porta hepatis level. The intrahepatic bile ducts are typically dilated. Tumors, calculi, and distal bile duct strictures are causes of suprapancreatic or intrapancreatic common duct obstruction. Rarely, pancreatitis or inspissated bile may cause distal bile duct obstruction (37,110). With distal obstruction, the extrahepatic bile duct should be dilated throughout its course. Depending on the severity and duration of the obstruction, the intrahepatic bile ducts may or may not be dilated.

The sensitivity of sonography for establishing a diagnosis of biliary tract obstruction in children has not been established in large series, but in adults it is about 95%, while accuracy for determining the level and cause of obstruction is about 90% and 70%, respectively (81). With optimal scanning techniques, calculi in the proximal common bowel duct can be demonstrated in about 90% of patients (80), and distal bile duct calculi can be identified in 70% of patients. The diagnosis of ductal calculi is based on the presence of echogenic material within the dilated duct with associated acoustic shadowing (Fig. 46) (144). Calculi in the distal common bile duct are more difficult to detect because they are often obscured by overlying bowel gas. Visualization may be improved by placing the patient in a semierect right posterior oblique position and

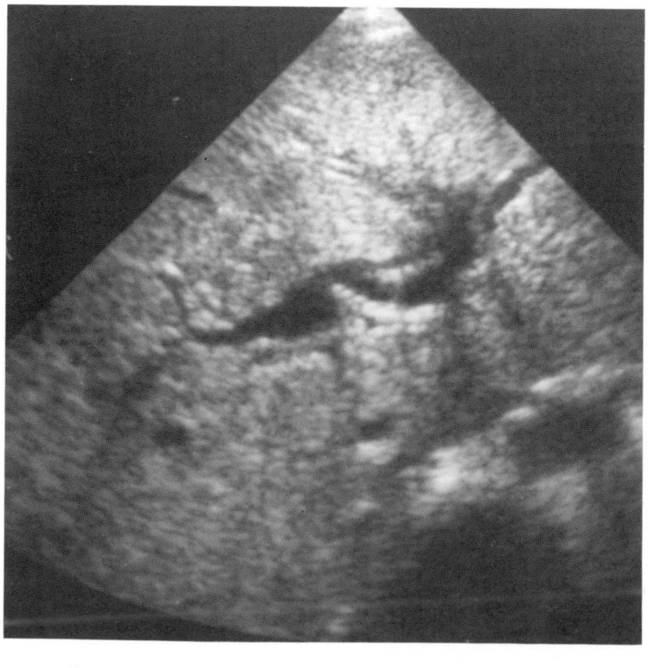

FIG. 45. Intrahepatic bile duct dilatation. A transverse scan through the dome of the liver demonstrates dilated intrahepatic bile ducts which exhibit an irregular branching pattern.

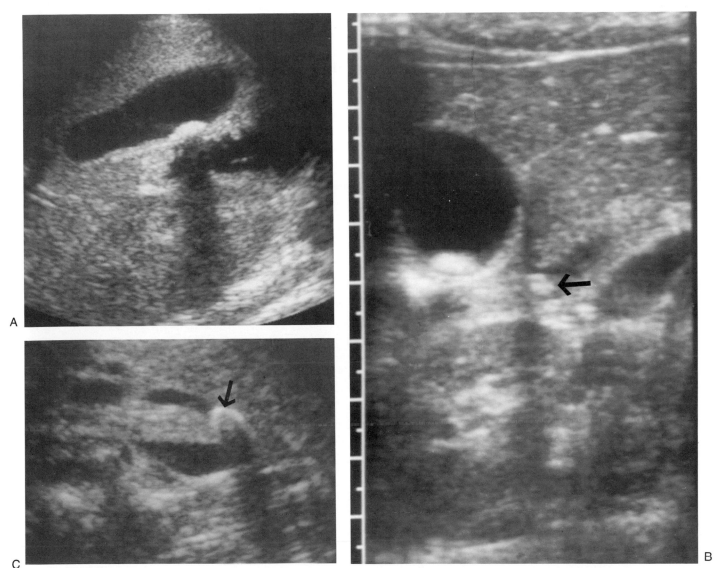

FIG. 46. Choledocholithiasis. **A:** Longitudinal scan through the upper abdomen demonstrates an echogenic stone within the gallbladder lumen. **B:** Longitudinal and **C:** transverse scans through the distal common bile duct show another small echogenic stone (*arrow*). Note the presence of acoustic shadowing created by the stone. At operation, calcium bilirubinate stones were found in the gallbladder and distal common bile duct.

scanning in a transverse plane. Occasionally, a stone in the distal common duct may move more cephalad and hence become visible with the patient in the Trendelenburg position. The diagnosis of choledocholithiasis is also difficult if the duct is not dilated, because the absence of surrounding bile make the stones less visible.

The sonographic features of both primary and secondary neoplasms include hypoechoic masses around the common duct or in the region of the porta hepatis, intraluminal soft-tissue echoes without shadowing, and marked biliary tract dilatation (5,55,156). Strictures, an uncommon cause of distal obstruction, are difficult to detect sonographically. However, the diagnosis needs to be considered in patients with biliary obstruc-

tion in whom no calculus or other obstructing lesion can be visualized. Often there is an abrupt transition from a dilated duct to one of normal caliber. In this situation, an endoscopic retrograde cholangiogram or percutaneous cholangiogram can provide more precise anatomic detail (Fig. 47).

Although sonography can separate medical from surgical jaundice in most patients, atypical cases occasionally will be encountered. Infrequently, patients with obstructive jaundice fail to manifest bile duct dilatation or conversely, some patients will have dilatation of the biliary tree without jaundice. Partial or intermittent obstruction from choledocholithiasis or strictures of the extrahepatic ducts usually are responsible for these cases. In nonjaundiced patients with equivocal or mild ductal dilatation, repeating the scans after a fatty meal can be helpful. If obstruction is present, the duct should increase in size (36). When the clinical course, including liver function tests, suggests the possibility of obstruction while sonography demonstrates normal caliber ducts, CT or an endoscopic retrograde examination may be necessary to provide a diagnosis. Conversely, percutaneous cholangiography may be required in patients with anicteric dilatation to determine how readily bile passes from the dilated bile duct into the duodenum. Radionuclide imaging using technetium-labeled biliary agents also can be used to assess physiology and gross anatomic patency of the biliary system.

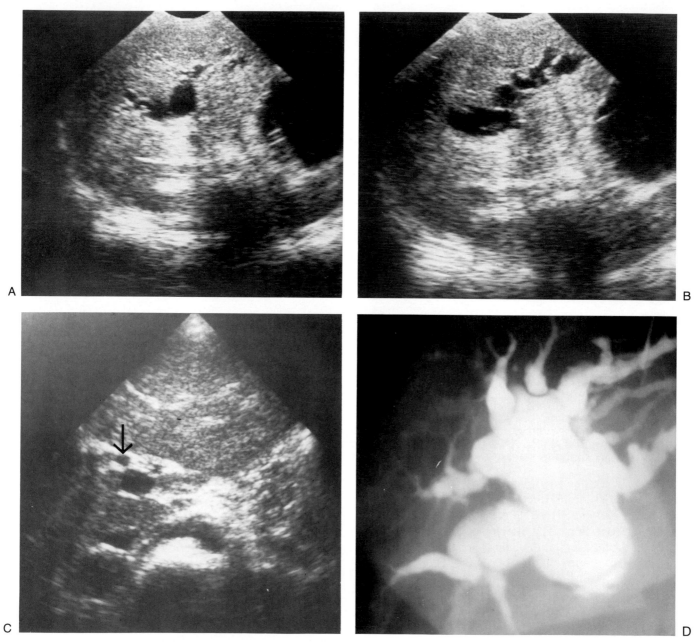

FIG. 47. Common bile duct stricture. **A,B:** Two transverse images through the liver show dilatation of intrahepatic ducts with acoustic enhancement. **C:** A scan through the porta demonstrates a normal caliber distal bile duct (*arrow*). **D:** Percutaneous cholangiography shows obstruction at the porta hepatis due to stricture.

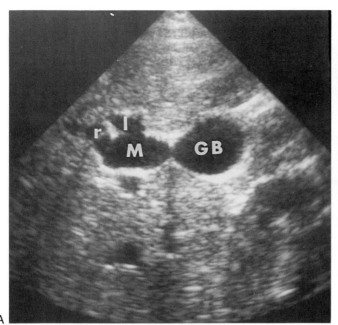 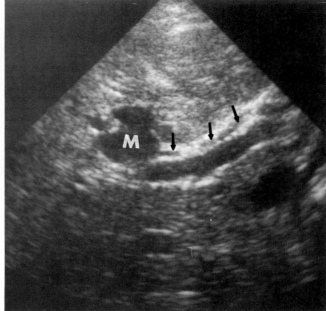

FIG. 48. Choledochal cyst. **A:** Transverse scan through the liver demonstrates dilatation of the right (*r*) and left (*l*) hepatic ducts and a cystic mass (*M*) in the porta hepatis. *GB*, gallbladder. **B:** On a longitudinal sonogram, the mass (*M*) is continuous with a normal caliber distal common bile duct (*arrows*). Hepatobiliary scintigraphy confirmed communication of the cystic structure, representing a dilated common bile duct, with the biliary system.

Cystic Disease of the Biliary Tree

Choledochal Cyst

Choledochal cyst is characterized by cystic dilatation of the common bile duct and is usually found in children between 1 and 10 years of age, although it may present in the neonate and young child (7). Classically, the cyst produces jaundice, pain, and a palpable abdominal mass, although the complete triad is present in less than one-third of patients (13). Three patterns of cystic dilatation have been described: (a) cystic or fusiform dilatation of the common bile duct, with or without intrahepatic biliary dilatation (classic choledochal cyst); (b) eccentric dilatation of the common duct, also referred to as a diverticulum; and (c) focal dilatation of the duodenal portion of the common bile duct or choledochocele.

Sonography supplemented by hepatobiliary scintigraphy usually is sufficient to provide the diagnosis of choledochal cyst. On sonography, a choledochal cyst appears as a well-defined, fluid-filled mass in the porta hepatis, separate from the gallbladder (64,69). Dilatation of intrahepatic biliary ducts is present in about half of affected patients and is limited to the central portions of the left and right main hepatic ducts (Fig.

48). Generalized ductal dilatation typical of acquired obstruction is absent. In most cases, scintigraphy with hepatobiliary agents confirms that the cystic mass communicates with the biliary system.

Caroli's Disease

Congenital cystic dilatation of the intrahepatic ducts, referred to as Caroli's disease, is a rare abnormality which is believed to be transmitted as an autosomal recessive trait. Two extreme types of the disease exist. One is a pure form characterized by sacular dilatation of the intrahepatic bile ducts, calculus formation, and cholangitis. The second form is associated with congenital hepatic fibrosis and portal hypertension with minimal dilatation of the large intrahepatic ducts. Stone formation and cholangitis are absent or occur late in the patient's course. Intermediate forms of disease may exist in some patients. All forms of biliary ductal dilatation have been associated with renal tubular ectasia or cysts in the medulla, cortex, and corticomedullary junction.

Sonography characteristically demonstrates multiple, dilated tubular structures typical of biliary radicals, extending to the periphery of the liver. These

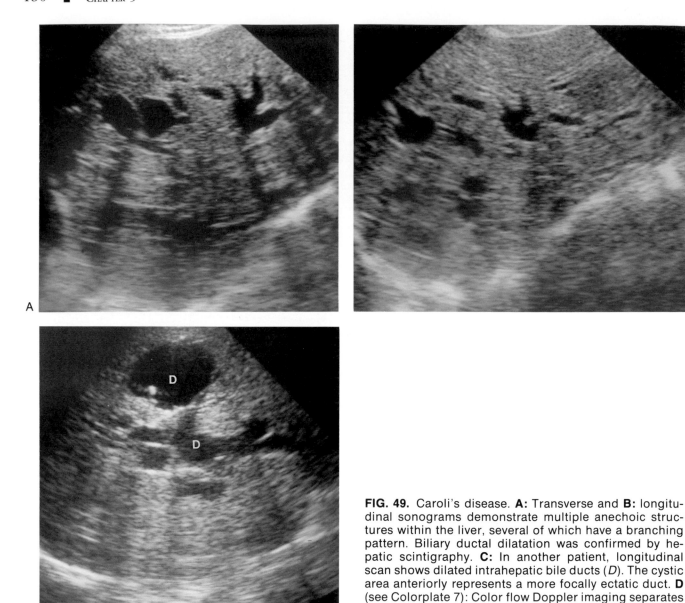

FIG. 49. Caroli's disease. **A:** Transverse and **B:** longitudinal sonograms demonstrate multiple anechoic structures within the liver, several of which have a branching pattern. Biliary ductal dilatation was confirmed by hepatic scintigraphy. **C:** In another patient, longitudinal scan shows dilated intrahepatic bile ducts (*D*). The cystic area anteriorly represents a more focally ectatic duct. **D** (see Colorplate 7): Color flow Doppler imaging separates the dilated bile ducts (*D*) from vessels.

communicate with cystic areas (Fig. 49) which represent more focally ectatic portions of the biliary tree (98). Irregular walls with nodular protrusions and echogenic bands or bridges within the lumina of the dilated ducts also have been described (90).

Perforation of the Extrahepatic Bile Ducts

Spontaneous perforation of the extrahepatic bile ducts almost always occurs at the junction of the cystic and common hepatic ducts. Rarely the site of perforation is in the common hepatic or common bile duct or the gallbladder. The cause is unknown, although a localized developmental weakness of the wall of the bile duct has been postulated. In association with an increase in the pressure within the biliary tract secondary to calculi, inspissated bile, or a congenital stenosis, the weakened part of the wall perforates. Affected infants typically present within the first 3 months of life with jaundice and ascites (50). Except for mildly elevated serum bilirubin levels, liver function test results are normal, a feature that can help separate this condition from biliary atresia, with which it may be confused clinically.

On sonography, the extravasated bile appears as free fluid in the peritoneal cavity. Thin septations with finely echogenic debris may be present within the ascitic fluid. Occasionally a loculated fluid collection or pseudocyst, secondary to a walled-off perforation, is found in the region of the porta hepatis (Fig. 50) (9,63).

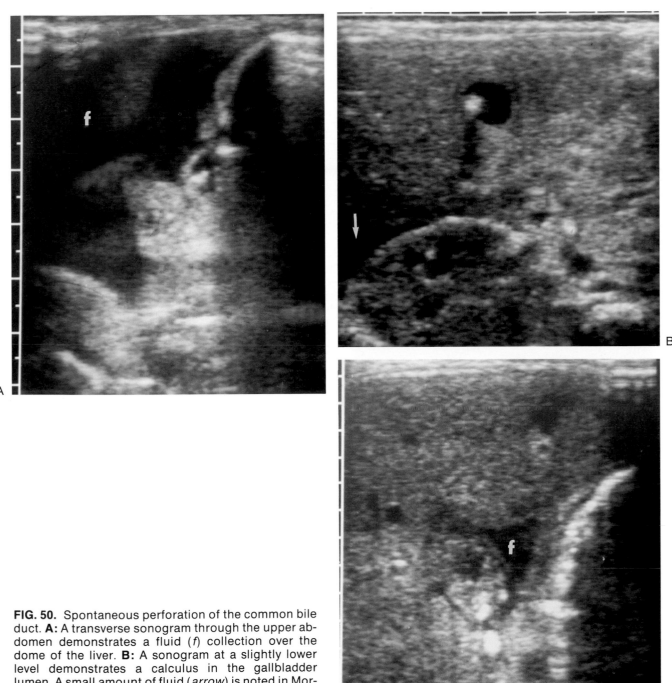

FIG. 50. Spontaneous perforation of the common bile duct. **A:** A transverse sonogram through the upper abdomen demonstrates a fluid (*f*) collection over the dome of the liver. **B:** A sonogram at a slightly lower level demonstrates a calculus in the gallbladder lumen. A small amount of fluid (*arrow*) is noted in Morrison's pouch. **C:** More caudad, a loculated fluid (*f*) collection is noted in the porta hepatis. At surgery, this patient had perforation of the common bile duct at its junction with the cystic duct.

Gallbladder Disease

Hydrops

Acute hydrops, characterized by massive distention of the gallbladder by serous fluid, is believed to be the result of gallbladder stasis secondary to fasting or dehydration with the resultant tenacious bile causing transient obstruction. Affected patients usually have right upper quadrant pain or a palpable mass. Conditions reported to cause hydrops of the gallbladder include scarlet fever, Kawasaki disease (mucocutaneous lymph node syndrome), leptospirosis, ascariasis, typhoid fever, familial Mediterranean fever, sepsis, and total parenteral nutrition (12,31).

Sonography demonstrates a massively enlarged gall-

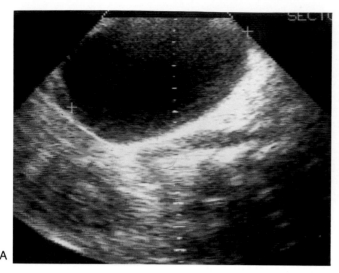

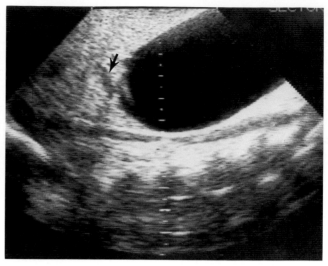

FIG. 51. Hydrops of the gallbladder in a patient with Kawasaki disease. **A:** Transverse and **B:** longitudinal sonograms show a markedly dilated gallbladder with an imperceptible wall. The large size and round shape are consistent with hydrops. *Arrow,* common hepatic duct.

bladder with a normal wall thickness and a biconvex appearance on longitudinal scans, in contrast to the normal ovoid shape (Fig. 51) (75,76). Sludge may or may not be present. The intra- and extrahepatic ductal structures are normal. Rehydration and resolution of the associated disease almost always result in spontaneous decompression of the gallbladder (12).

Inflammatory Conditions

Acute Cholecystitis

Acute cholecystitis is significantly less common in the pediatric patient than in the adult population. About half of cases in childhood are due to calculus obstruction of the gallbladder neck or cystic duct. In the remaining patients acalculous cholecystitis develops. Conditions predisposing to acalculous cholecystitis include recent surgery, burns, sepsis, and debilitation. In these patients prolonged bile stasis results in increased biliary viscosity and ultimately cystic duct obstruction. Clinical features of both calculous and acalculous disease are right upper quadrant pain, fever, and leukocytosis with or without jaundice.

Sonographic findings of acute calculous cholecystitis include cholelithiasis, gallbladder wall thickness greater than 3 mm, localized tenderness (sonographic Murphy's sign), and pericholecystic lucency (Fig. 52) (45). Each of these features alone is nonspecific, but the combination of sonographic signs in the appropriate clinical setting has a sensitivity of greater than 90% for the diagnosis of acute cholecystitis (114). The best

criteria for diagnosing acute cholecystitis are focal gallbladder tenderness in association with calculi (114). The sonographic criteria used to diagnose acalculous cholecystitis are similar to those of acute calculous cholecystitis except that calculi are absent. The sensitivity of sonography is less for acalculous cholecystitis than for calculous cholecystitis because one of the important diagnostic criteria (stones) is lacking.

A diffusely thickened gallbladder wall is seen in approximately 50% to 75% of patients with acute cholecystitis. Although originally thought to be a specific sign of acute cholecystitis, gallbladder wall thickening is now recognized as a nonspecific finding that may occur in many conditions unrelated to gallbladder disease, including hepatic dysfunction, congestive heart failure, renal disease, tumor, and sepsis (Fig. 53) (108). Besides wall thickening, a sonolucent rim or halo around the gallbladder has been reported in acute cholecystitis. The hypoechoic rim represents edema and cellular infiltration of the subserosa and adjacent liver. This halo is nonspecific and can be seen in patients with pancreatitis as well as in those with acute cholecystitis.

Emphysema, gangrene, and perforation are rare complications of acute cholecystitis. Emphysematous cholecystitis appears as hyperechoic foci with associated acoustic shadowing and reverberation in the region of the gallbladder bed (100,104,131). In gangrenous cholecystitis, the sloughed gallbladder mucosa produces an echogenic intraluminal membrane paralleling the wall of the gallbladder, while gallbladder perforation and abscess formation produce a localized pericholecystic fluid collection.

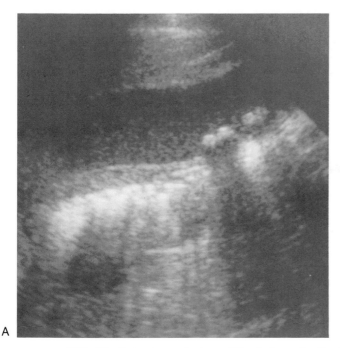

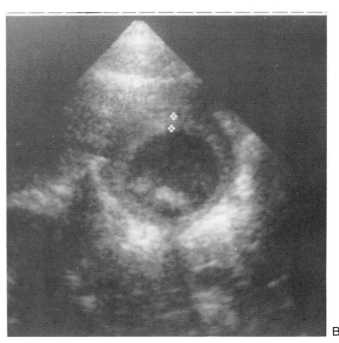

A   B

FIG. 52. Calculous cholecystitis. **A:** Longitudinal and **B:** transverse scans of the gallbladder demonstrate gallstones and wall thickening (*calipers*).

Chronic Cholecystitis

Chronic cholecystitis in childhood usually results from chronic irritation of the gallbladder secondary to gallstones or cystic fibrosis and rarely is caused by recurrent attacks of acute cholecystitis. Sonography may be normal or show sludge, gallstones, or a thickened gallbladder wall.

Noninflammatory Gallbladder Abnormalities

Noninflammatory abnormalities of the gallbladder in childhood are rare and usually are either adenomyomatosis or cholesterolosis. Adenomyomatosis is characterized by hyperplastic changes of the mucosa and muscular wall, resulting in outpouchings of mucosa into or through a thickened muscular layer (Rok-

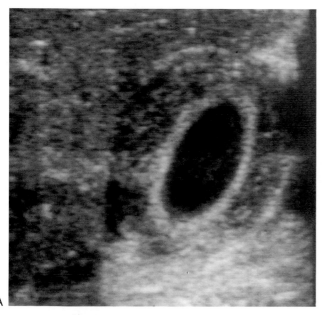

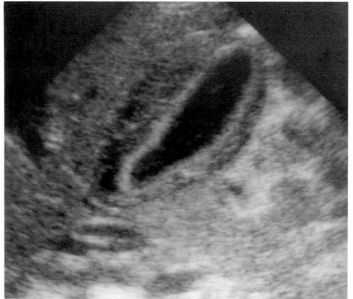

A   B

FIG. 53. Thickened gallbladder wall. **A:** Transverse and **B:** longitudinal sonograms of the gallbladder demonstrate a markedly thickened, hypoechoic wall in a patient with severe hypoproteinemia. There was no clinical evidence for primary gallbladder disease.

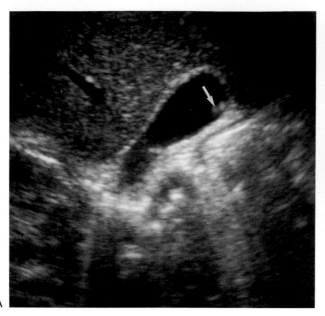
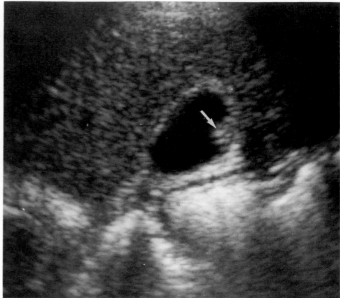

FIG. 54. Cholesterolosis. **A:** Transverse and **B:** longitudinal scans of the gallbladder demonstrate a polypoid mass (*arrow*) which remains attached to the wall with changes in patient position.

itansky-Aschoff sinuses). On sonography, adenomyomatosis is suspected when there is diffuse or segmental thickening of the gallbladder wall and intramural diverticula. Diverticula that contain bile appear anechoic, and diverticula that are small or contain sludge appear echogenic.

Cholesterolosis is characterized by abnormal accumulations of triglycerides and cholesterol esters or precursors in the lamina propria of the gallbladder wall. Sonography demonstrates single or multiple adherent nonshadowing echogenic masses protruding into the gallbladder lumen (Fig. 54). Sonographic findings of fixed lesions in the gallbladder wall or focal wall thickening are nonspecific and can be produced by other conditions including adenomas, papillomas, inflammatory polyps, mucus retention cysts, heterotopic pancreatic and gastric tissue, and carcinomas. These conditions are even rarer than adenomyomatosis and cholesterolosis.

Cholelithiasis

Cholelithiasis in infancy and childhood has been associated specifically with cystic fibrosis, malabsorption, total parenteral nutrition, furosemide therapy, bowel resection, and hemolytic anemia, but in most cases the cause is unknown (27,52,123,155). On sonography, calculi typically appear as movable, discrete echogenic foci with prominent posterior acoustic shadowing (Fig. 55). Normally, calculi layer in the depen-

dent portion of the gallbladder lumen, but they may float if they have a high cholesterol content or contain gas fissures. Rarely, stones can be adherent to the wall of the gallbladder and mimic a focal mass or calcification within the gallbladder wall.

The sensitivity of sonography for detecting gallstones is greater than 95% (33). Demonstration of posterior acoustic shadowing is important for diagnosis because it correlates with cholelithiasis in virtually all patients, whereas nonshadowing echogenic foci within the gallbladder correlate with gallstones in only 60% of cases (33). Acoustic shadowing is dependent on stone size and position within the sound beam, rather than stone composition. If the peripheral edge of the acoustic beam strikes the stone, no shadow is produced. If the stone is at the center or focal zone of the sound beam, an acoustic shadow will be easily seen. The ability to demonstrate an acoustic shadow also varies directly with the size of the stone. The smaller the stone, the more difficult it is to demonstrate acoustic shadowing. In these cases, repositioning the patient may cause small stones, which fail to demonstrate shadowing in standard projections, to pile up on one another. The result is an aggregate of small stones that behaves acoustically as a larger stone in its ability to produce posterior shadowing.

When the gallbladder is packed with calculi, it becomes more difficult to recognize. Instead of a well-defined, anechoic structure, a highly echogenic line with prominent acoustic shadowing is seen. The shadow that is cast prevents visualization of the in-

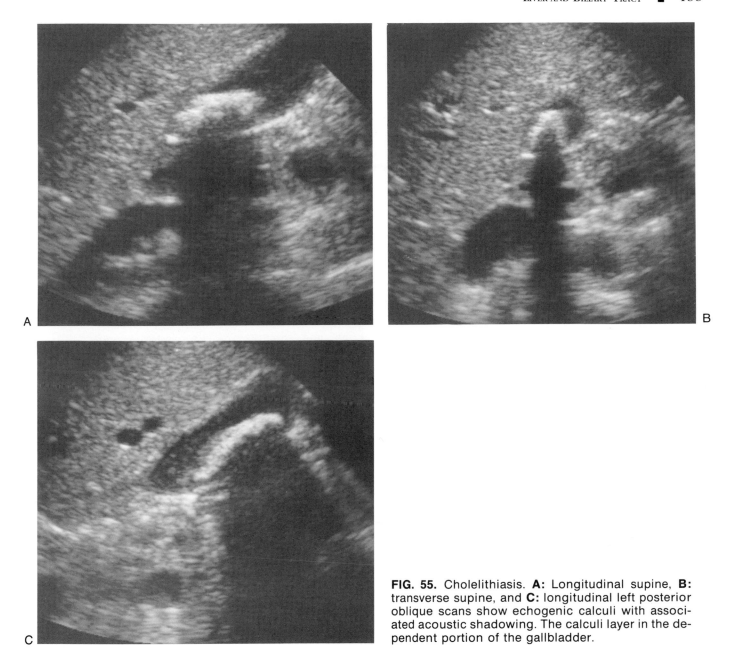

FIG. 55. Cholelithiasis. **A:** Longitudinal supine, **B:** transverse supine, and **C:** longitudinal left posterior oblique scans show echogenic calculi with associated acoustic shadowing. The calculi layer in the dependent portion of the gallbladder.

traluminal bile, more deeply positioned stones, and the posterior wall of the gallbladder. Recognition of the anterior gallbladder wall as well as the anterior layer of stones usually permits a diagnosis of cholelithiasis to be made.

Sludge

Biliary sludge or echogenic bile refers to the presence of particulate matter, usually calcium bilirubinate granules and occasionally cholesterol crystals, within bile. It is the result of bile stasis which can occur sec-

ondary to obstruction at the level of the gallbladder neck, cystic duct, or common bile duct, or following a prolonged fast or hyperalimentation (93,155). On sonography, sludge appears as nonshadowing low-to-medium–level echoes that layer in the dependent part of the gallbladder lumen (Fig. 56). Because of its viscous nature, the fluid-fluid level produced by the sludge moves very slowly with changes in patient position.

Blood seen with hematobilia or pus due to infection may cause echogenic bile and be indistinguishable from sludge. Differentiation of these conditions requires correlation with clinical history. Pseudosludge also is indistinguishable from true sludge and occurs

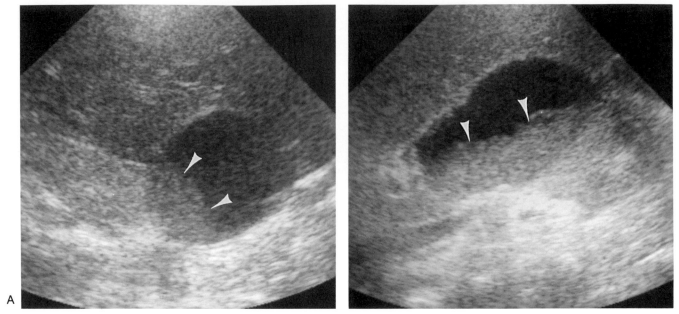

FIG. 56. Biliary sludge. **A:** Transverse and **B:** longitudinal scans through the gallbladder demonstrate a normal size gallbladder with low-level echoes representing sludge (*arrowheads*). There is no acoustic shadowing from the sludge, but there is acoustic enhancement behind the gallbladder.

as a result of the beam averaging effect at the diverging portion of the acoustic beam. This artifact occurs when a part of the beam interacts with normally anechoic bile while an adjacent part of the beam interacts with liver, producing an averaging of echoes. Changing the position of the patient or the angulation of the transducer eliminates the artifact.

Rarely, the particulate material in sludge does not form a fluid-fluid level but coalesces and appears as mobile masses within the gallbladder lumen, referred to as sludge balls or tumefactive biliary sludge. Sludge balls are not associated with posterior acoustic shadowing (Fig. 57). These lesions are transient and disappear spontaneously (48,72).

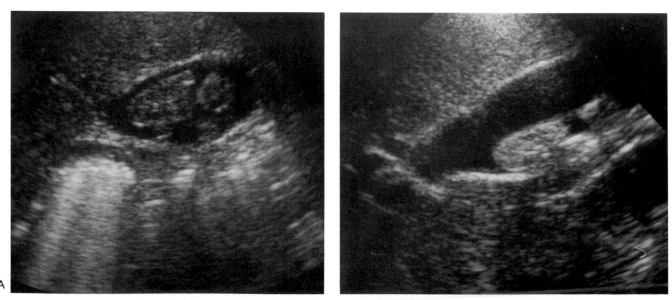

FIG. 57. Tumefactive biliary sludge. **A:** Longitudinal left lateral decubitus and **B:** longitudinal supine scans of the gallbladder in a patient with sickle cell anemia show several mobile echogenic masses without acoustic shadowing, consistent with sludge balls. An ultrasound 6 months earlier had shown biliary sludge. A follow-up study showed resolution of the masses.

Biliary Atresia and Neonatal Hepatitis

Biliary atresia and neonatal hepatitis are the most common causes of cholestasis in the neonate and are believed to be the result of an antenatal infection (99). Both conditions usually present as obstructive jaundice in infants 3 to 4 weeks of age who are not critically ill. Separation of the two conditions is important, because intrahepatic cholestatic jaundice secondary to hepatitis is managed medically, whereas infants with biliary atresia require surgical intervention. Surgical treatment varies with the level of obstruction. When the obstruction is in the distal common bile duct, a direct anastomosis between the patent portion of the extrahepatic bile duct and intestine is performed. Unfortunately this type of atresia occurs only in 15% to 25% of patients. In the remaining patients there is obliteration of all of the ducts in the porta hepatis (10,11). In these patients, hepatoportoenterostomy or the Kasai procedure (anastomosis of an intestinal conduit to transected ducts at the liver hilus) is the treatment of choice to provide bile drainage (70). The success rate is inversely proportional to the age of the patient and approaches 90% for infants under 2 months of age at the time of operation. For infants over 3 months of age at the time of operation, the success rate is less than 20% (10,11).

The sonographic findings of the hepatic parenchyma and intrahepatic bile ducts in neonatal hepatitis and biliary atresia are similar. In both conditions the liver echogenicity may be normal or increased. Both intra- and extrahepatic bile ducts are normal in caliber. The gallbladder in patients with neonatal hepatitis may be large, normal, small, or nonvisualized. Patients with biliary atresia usually have a small or absent gallbladder, although in about 10% of infants the gallbladder will be normal (1.5 cm or greater in diameter) (Fig. 58) (3,26,74). More recently it has been suggested that absence of gallbladder contractility after a feeding is evidence of biliary atresia. Conversely, if the gallbladder contracts, the diagnosis of atresia is unlikely since contraction is evidence of biliary tract patency (26,61, 67,149). Biliary atresia may coexist with a choledochal cyst. Other abnormalities associated with biliary atresia include polysplenia, preduodenal portal vein, azygos continuation of the inferior vena cava, diaphragmatic hernia, situs inversus, and hydronephrosis (2,26).

Radionuclide imaging with hepatobiliary agents usually can aid in differentiating biliary atresia and neonatal hepatitis (56,89) in the first 3 months of life. In biliary atresia, uptake of tracer by the liver is prompt, but excretion into the intestine is absent. In contrast, in neonatal hepatitis, extraction by the liver is poor, but tracer usually appears in the bowel (56). Ultimately, the final diagnosis requires percutaneous or surgical liver biopsy and cholangiography, possibly with sonographic guidance (146).

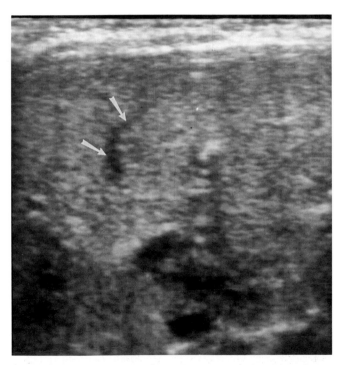

FIG. 58. Biliary atresia. Transverse scan shows a normal liver. The gallbladder (*arrows*) is visualized, but appears small. The patient had been fasting.

REFERENCES

1. Abramson SJ, Lack EE, Teele RL. Benign vascular tumors of the liver in infants: Sonographic appearance. *AJR* 1982; 138:629–632.
2. Abramson SJ, Berdon WE, Altman RP, Amodio JB, Levy J. Biliary atresia and noncardiac polysplenic syndrome: US and surgical considerations. *Radiology* 1987;163:377–379.
3. Abramson SJ, Treves S, Teele RL. The infant with possible biliary atresia: Evaluation by ultrasound and nuclear medicine. *Pediatr Radiol* 1982;12:1–5.
4. Alpern MB, Rubin JM, Williams DM, Capek P. Porta hepatis: Duplex Doppler US with angiographic correlation. *Radiology* 1987;162:53–56.
5. Arnaud O, Boscq M, Asquier E, Michel J. Embryonal rhabdomyosarcoma of the biliary tree in children: A case report. *Pediatr Radiol* 1987;17:250–251.
6. Atkinson GO, Kodroff M, Sones PJ, Gay BB. Focal nodular hyperplasia of the liver in children: A report of three new cases. *Radiology* 1980;137:171–174.
7. Babbitt DP, Starshak RJ, Clemett AR. Choledochal cyst: A concept of etiology. *AJR* 1973;119:57–62.
8. Babcock DS. Ultrasound diagnosis of portal vein thrombosis as a complication of appendicitis. *AJR* 1979;13:317–319.
9. Bahia JO, Boal DKB, Karl SR, Gross GW. Ultrasonographic detection of spontaneous perforation of the extrahepatic bile ducts in infancy. *Pediatr Radiol* 1986;16:157–159.
10. Balistreri WF. Neonatal cholestasis. *J Pediatr* 1985;106: 171–184.
11. Balistreri WF, Schubert WK. Liver diseases in infancy and childhood. In: Schiff L, Schiff ER, eds. *Diseases of the liver*, 6th ed. Philadelphia: JB Lippincott, 1987;1337–1426.

12. Barth RA, Brasch RC, Filly RA. Abdominal pseudotumor in childhood: Distended gallbladder with parenteral hyperalimentation. *AJR* 1981;136:341–343.
13. Bass EM, Cremin BJ. Choledochal cysts: A clinical and radiological evaluation of 21 cases. *Pediatr Radiol* 1976;5:81–85.
14. Berland LL, Lawson TL, Foley WD. Porta hepatis: Sonographic discrimination of bile ducts from arteries with pulsed Doppler with new anatomic criteria. *AJR* 1982;138:833–840.
15. Berry M, Bazaz R, Bhargava S. Amebic liver abscess: Sonographic diagnosis and management. *JCU* 1986;14:239–242.
16. Bezzi M, Teggi A, De Rosa F, Capozzi A, Tucci G, Bonifacino A, Angelini L. Abdominal hydatid disease: US findings during medical treatment. *Radiology* 1987;162:91–95.
17. Blane CE, Jongeward RH, Silver TM. Sonographic features of hepatocellular disease in neonates and infants. *AJR* 1983;141:1313–1316.
18. Bolondi L, Gandolfi L, Arienti V, Caletti GC, Corcioni E, Gasbarrini G, Labo G. Ultrasonography in the diagnosis of portal hypertension: Diminished response of portal vessels to respiration. *Radiology* 1982;142:167–172.
19. Boucher D, Brunelle F, Bernard O, Forel F, Autrel D, Hadchouel P, Chaumont P. Ultrasonic demonstration of portocaval anastomosis in portal hypertension in children. *Pediatr Radiol* 1985;15:307–310.
20. Boultbee JE, Simjee AE, Rooknoodeen F, Engelbrecht HE. Experiences with grey scale ultrasonography in hepatic amoebiasis. *Clin Radiol* 1979;30:683–689.
21. Bree RL, Schwab RE, Glazer GM, Fink-Bennett D. The varied appearances of hepatic cavernous hemangiomas with sonography, computed tomography, magnetic resonance imaging and scintigraphy. *Radiographics* 1987;7:1153–1175.
22. Bree RL, Schwab RE, Neiman HL. Solitary echogenic spot in the liver; Is it diagnostic of a hemangioma? *AJR* 1983;140: 41–45.
23. Brunelle F, Chaumont P. Hepatic tumors in children: Ultrasonic differentiation of malignant from benign lesions. *Radiology* 1984;150:695–699.
24. Brunelle F, Tammam S, Odievre M, Chaumont P. Liver adenomas in glycogen storage disease in children. Ultrasound and angiographic study. *Pediatr Radiol* 1984;14:94–101.
25. Brunelle F, Alagille D, Pariente D, Chaumont P. An ultrasound study of portal hypertension in children. *Ann Radiol (Paris)* 1981;24:121–130.
26. Brun P, Gauthier F, Boucher D, Brunelle F. Ultrasound findings in biliary atresia in children. *Ann Radiol* 1985;28:259–263.
27. Callahan J, Haller JO, Cacciarelli AA, Slovis TL, Friedman P. Cholelithiasis in infants: Association with total parenteral nutrition and furosemide. *Radiology* 1982;143:437–439.
28. Callen PW, Filly RA, Marcus FS. Ultrasonography and computed tomography in the evaluation of hepatic microabscesses in the immunosuppressed patient. *Radiology* 1980;136:433–434.
29. Chusid MJ. Pyogenic hepatic abscess in infancy and childhood. *Pediatrics* 1978;62:554–559.
30. Clatworthy W, Schiller M, Grosfeld JL. Primary liver tumors in infancy and childhood. *Arch Surg* 1974;109:143–147.
31. Cohen EK, Stringer DA, Smith CR, Daneman A. Hydrops of the gallbladder in typhoid fever as demonstrated by sonography. *JCU* 1986;14:633–635.
32. Conrad MR, Bregman R, Kilman WJ. Ultrasonic recognition of parenchymal gas. *AJR* 1979;132:395–399.
33. Crade M, Taylor KJW, Rosenfield AT, deGraff CS, Minihan P. Surgical and pathologic correlation of cholecystosonography and cholecystography. *AJR* 1978;131:227–229.
34. Dachman AH, Pakter RL, Ros PR, Fishman EK, Goodman ZD, Lichtenstein JE. Hepatoblastoma: Radiologic-pathologic correlation in 50 cases. *Radiology* 1987;164:15–19.
35. Dachman AH, Lichtenstein JE, Friedman AC, Hartman DS. Infantile hemangioendothelioma of the liver: A radiologic-pathologic-clinical correlation. *AJR* 1983;140:1091–1096.
36. Darweesh RMA, Dodds WJ, Hogan WJ, et al. Fatty-meal sonography for evaluating patients with suspected partial common duct obstruction. *AJR* 1988;151:63–68.
37. Davies C, Daneman A, Stringer DA. Inspissated bile in a neonate with cystic fibrosis. *J Ultrasound Med* 1986;5:335–337.
38. Day DL, Letourneau JG, Allan BT, Sharp HL, Ascher NA, Dehner LP, Thompson WM. Hepatic regenerating nodules in hereditary tyrosinemia. *AJR* 1987;149:391–393.
39. Dehner LP, Ishak KG. Vascular tumors of the liver in infants and children. A study of 30 cases and review of the literature. *Arch Pathol* 1971;92:101–111.
40. Dehner LP. Hepatic tumors in the pediatric age group: A distinctive clinicopathologic spectrum. *Perspect Pediatr Pathol* 1978;4:217–268.
41. Donovan AT, Wolverson MK, deMello D, Craddock T, Silberstein M. Multicystic hepatic mesenchymal hamartoma of childhood. *Pediatr Radiol* 1981;11:163–165.
42. Dodds WJ, Erickson SJ, Taylor AJ, Lawson TL, Stewart ET. Caudate lobe of the liver: Anatomy, embryology, and pathology. *AJR* 1990; 154:87–93.
43. Ein SH, Stephens CA. Malignant liver tumors in children. *J Pediatr Surg* 1974;9:491–494.
44. Ein SH, Stephens CA. Benign liver tumors and cysts in childhood. *J Pediatr Surg* 1974;9:847–851.
45. Engel JM, Deitch EA, Sikkema W. Gallbladder wall thickness: Sonographic accuracy and relation to disease. *AJR* 1980;134:907–909.
46. Essensten M, Ralls PW, Colletti P, Halls J. Posttraumatic intrahepatic biloma: Sonographic diagnosis. *AJR* 1983;140:303–305.
47. Exelby PR, Filler RM, Grosfeld JL. Liver tumors in children in the particular reference to hepatoblastoma and hepatocellular carcinoma: American Academy of Pediatrics Surgical Section Survey—1974. *J Pediatr Surg* 1975;10:329–337.
48. Fakhry J. Sonography of tumefactive biliary sludge. *AJR* 1982;139:717–719.
49. Fellows KE, Vawter GF, Tefft M. Hepatic effects following abdominal irradiation in children: Detection by Au[198] scan and confirmation by histologic examination. *AJR* 1968;103:422–431.
50. Fitzgerald RJ, Parbhoo K, Guiney EJ. Spontaneous perforation of bile ducts in neonates. *Surgery* 1978;83:303–305.
51. Franken EA, Smith WL, Siddiqui A. Noninvasive evaluation of liver disease in pediatrics. *Radiol Clin North Am* 1980;18:239–252.
52. Garel L, Lallemand D, Montagne J Ph, Forel F, Sauvegrain J. The changing aspects of cholelithiasis in children through a sonographic study. *Pediatr Radiol* 1981;11:75–79.
53. Garel LA, Pariente DM, Nezelof C, Barral VJ, Aboulker C, Sauvegrain JH. Liver involvement in chronic granulomatous disease: The role of ultrasound in diagnosis and treatment. *Radiology* 1984;153:117–121.
54. Garra BS, Shawker TH, Chang R, Kaplan K, White RD. The ultrasound appearance of radiation-induced hepatic injury. *J Ultrasound Med* 1988;7:605–609.
55. Geoffray A, Couanet D, Montagne JP, Leclère J, Flamant F. Ultrasonography and computed tomography for diagnosis and follow-up of biliary duct rhabdomyosarcomas in children. *Pediatr Radiol* 1987;17:127–131.
56. Gerhold JP, Klingensmith WC, Kuni CC. Diagnosis of biliary atresia with radionuclide hepatobiliary imaging. *Radiology* 1983;146:499–504.
57. Giorgio A, Amoroso P, Fico P, et al. Ultrasound evaluation of uncomplicated and complicated acute viral hepatitis. *JCU* 1986;14:675–679.
58. Giyanani VL, Meyers PC, Wolfson JJ. Mesenchymal hamartoma of the liver: Computed tomography and ultrasonography. *J Comp Assist Tomogr* 1986;10:51–54.
59. Grant EG, Tessler FN, Perrella RR. Clinical Doppler imaging. *AJR* 1989;152:707–717.
60. Grant EG, Perrella R, Tessler FN, Lois J, Busuttil R. Budd-Chiari syndrome: The results of duplex and color Doppler imaging. *AJR* 1989;152:377–381.
61. Green D, Carroll BA. Ultrasonography in the jaundiced infant: A new approach. *J Ultrasound Med* 1986;5:323–329.
62. Grossman H, Ram PC, Coleman RA, Gates G, Rosenberg ER,

Bowie JD, Wilkinson RH. Hepatic ultrasonography in type I glycogen storage disease (von Gierke disease). *Radiology* 1981;141:753–756.

63. Haller JO, Condon VR, Berdon WE, et al. Spontaneous perforation of the common bile duct in children. *Radiology* 1989;172:621–624.

64. Han BK, Babcock DS, Gelfand MH. Choledochal cyst with bile duct dilatation: Sonography and 99m-Tc IDA cholescintigraphy. *AJR* 1981;136:1075–1079.

65. Hayden CK, Toups M, Swischuk LE, Amparo EG. Sonographic features of hepatic amebiasis in childhood. *J Can Assoc Radiol* 1984;35:279–282.

66. Henschke CI, Goldman H, Teele RL. The hyperechogenic liver in children: Cause and sonographic appearance. *AJR* 1982;138:841–846.

67. Ikeda S, Sera Y, Akagi M. Serial ultrasonic examination to differentiate biliary atresia from neonatal hepatitis—Special reference to changes in size of the gallbladder. *Eur J Pediatr* 1989;148:396–400.

68. Jacobson JB, Brodey PA. The transverse common duct. *AJR* 1981;136:91–95.

69. Kangarloo H, Sarti DA, Sample WF, Amundson G. Ultrasonographic spectrum of choledochal cysts in children. *Pediatr Radiol* 1980;9:15–18.

70. Kasai M. Treatment of biliary atresia with special reference to hepatic porto-enterostomy and its modifications. *Progr Ped Surg* 1987;6:5–52.

71. Kaude JV, Felman AH, Hawkins IF, Jr. Ultrasonography in primary hepatic tumors in early childhood. *Pediatr Radiol* 1980;9:77–83.

72. Keller MS, Markle BM, Laffey PA, Chawla HS, Jacir N, Frank JL. Spontaneous resolution of cholelithiasis in infants. *Radiology* 1985;157:345–348.

73. Kenney IJ, Hendry GMA, Mackinlay GA. Spontaneous regression of mesenchymal hemartoma: Observations using ultrasound. *JCU* 1986;14:72–76.

74. Kirks DR, Coleman RE, Filston HC, Rosenberg ER, Merten DF. An imaging approach to persistent neonatal jaundice. *AJR* 1984;142:461–465.

75. Koss JC, Coleman BG, Mulhern CB, Arger PH, Tuchman DN. Mucocutaneous lymph node syndrome with hydrops of the gallbladder diagnosed by ultrasound. *JCU* 1981;9:477–479.

76. Kumari S, Lee WJ, Baron MG. Hydrops of the gallbladder in a child: Diagnosis by ultrasonography. *Pediatrics* 1979;63:295–297.

77. Kurtz AB, Rubin CS, Cooper HS, Nisenbaum HL, Cole-Beuglet C, Medoff J, Goldberg BB. Ultrasound findings in hepatitis. *Radiology* 1980;136:717–723.

78. Lafortune M, Patriquin H, Pomier G, et al. Hemodynamic changes in portal circulation after portosystemic shunts: Use of duplex sonography in 43 patients. *AJR* 1987;149:701–706.

79. Laing FC, Jeffrey RB. The pseudo-dilated common bile duct: Ultrasonographic appearance caused by the gallbladder neck. *Radiology* 1980;135:405–407.

80. Laing FC, Jeffrey RB, Wing VW. Improved visualization of choledocholithiasis by sonography. *AJR* 1984;143:949–952.

81. Laing FC, Jeffrey RB, Wing VW, Nyberg DA. Biliary dilatation: Defining the level and cause by real-time US. *Radiology* 1986;160:39–42.

82. Lam AH, Shulman L. Ultrasonography in the management of liver trauma in children. *J Ultrasound Med* 1984;3:199–203.

83. Laurin S, Kaude JV. Diagnosis of liver-spleen abscesses in children—With emphasis on ultrasound for the initial and follow-up examinations. *Pediatr Radiol* 1984;14:198–204.

84. Letourneau JG, Day DL, Ascher NL, et al. Abdominal sonography after hepatic transplantation; Results in 36 patients. *AJR* 1987;149:299–303.

85. Levine J, Seidman E, Teele RL, Walker WA. Gallbladder wall thickening in acute hepatitis. *J Pediatr Gastroenterol Nutr* 1986;5:147–149.

86. Lewall DB, McCorkell SJ. Hepatic echinococcal cysts: Sonography appearance and classification. *Radiology* 1985;155:773–775.

87. Lim JH, Ko YT, Han MC, Kim CW, Choi BI, Im JG. The inferior hepatic fissure: Sonographic appearance. *AJR* 1987;149:495–497.

88. Madigan SM, Teele RL. Ultrasonography of the liver and biliary tree in children. *Sem US, CT, MR* 1984;5:68–84.

89. Majd M. 99mTc-IDA scintigraphy in the evaluation of neonatal jaundice. *Radiographics* 1983;3:88–99.

90. Marchal GJ, Desmet VJ, Proesmans WC, Moerman PL, Van Roost WW. Van Holsbeeck MT, Baert AL. Caroli disease: High-frequency US and pathologic findings. *Radiology* 1986;158:507–511.

91. Marder DM, DeMarino GB, Sumkin JH, Sheahan DG. Liver transplant rejection: Value of the resistive index in Doppler US of hepatic arteries. *Radiology* 1989;173:127–129.

92. Markle BM, Potter BM, Majd M. The jaundiced infant and child. *Sem Ultrasound* 1980;2:123–133.

93. Matos C, Avni EF, Van Gansbeke D, Pardou A, Struyven J. Total parenteral nutrition (TPN) and gallbladder diseases in neonates. Sonographic assessment. *J Ultrasound Med* 1987; 6:243–248.

94. Menu Y, Alison D, Lorphelin JM, Valla D, Belghiti J, Nahum H. Budd-Chiari syndrome. *Radiology* 1985;157:761–764.

95. Miller JH, Greenspan BS. Integrated imaging of hepatic tumors in childhood. Part I: Malignant lesions (primary and metastatic). *Radiology* 1985;154:83–90.

96. Miller JH, Greenspan BS. Integrated imaging of hepatic tumors in childhood. Part II: Benign lesions (congenital, reparative, and inflammatory). *Radiology* 1985;154:91–100.

97. Mitchell SE, Gross BH, Spitz HB. The hypoechoic caudate lobe: An ultrasonic pseudolesion. *Radiology* 1982;144:569–572.

98. Mittelstaedt CA, Volberg FM, Fischer GJ, McCartney WH. Caroli's disease: Sonographic findings. *AJR* 1980;134:585–587.

99. Morecki R, Glaser JH, Cho S, Balistreri WF, Horwitz MS. Biliary atresia and reovirus type 3 infection. *N Engl J Med* 1982;307:481–484.

100. Nemcek AA, Jr., Gore RM, Vogelzang RL, Grant M. The effervescent gallbladder: A sonographic sign of emphysematous cholecystitis. *AJR* 1988;150:575–577.

101. Newlin N, Silver TM, Stuck KJ, Sandler MA. Ultrasonic features of pyogenic liver abscesses. *Radiology* 1981;139:155–159.

102. Pardes JG, Bryan PJ, Gauderer MWL. Spontaneous regression of infantile hemangioendotheliomatosis of the liver; Demonstration by ultrasound. *J Ultrasound Med* 1982;1:349–353.

103. Parulekar SG. Ligaments and fissures of the liver: Sonographic anatomy. *Radiology* 1979;130:409–411.

104. Parulekar SG. Sonographic findings in acute emphysematous cholecystitis. *Radiology* 1982;145:117–119.

105. Pastakia B, Shawker TH, Thaler M, O'Leary T, Pizzo PA. Hepatosplenic candidiasis: Wheels within wheels. *Radiology* 1988;166:417–421.

106. Patel PJ, Karrar AZ, Babiker MA, Hawass ND. Ultrasound findings in childhood chronic liver parenchymal diseases. An analysis of 41 patients. *Eur J Pediatr* 1987;146:565–567.

107. Patriquin H, Tessier G, Grignon A, Boisvert J. Lesser omental thickness in normal children: Baseline for detection of portal hypertension. *AJR* 1985;145:693–696.

108. Patriquin HB, DePietro M, Barber FE, Teele RL. Sonography of thickened gallbladder wall: Causes in children. *AJR* 1983; 141:57–60.

109. Patriquin H, Lafortune M, Burns PN, Dauzat M. Duplex Doppler examination in portal hypertension: Technique and anatomy. *AJR* 1987;149:71–76.

110. Pfeiffer WR, Robinson LH, Balsara VJ. Sonographic features of bile plug syndrome. *J Ultrasound Med* 1986;5:161–163.

111. Raffensperger JG, Gonzalez-Crussi F, Skeehan T. Mesenchymal hamartoma of the liver. *J Pediatr Surg* 1983;18:585–587.

112. Ralls PW, Barnes PF, Radin DR, Colletti P, Halls J. Sonographic features of amebic and pyogenic liver abscesses: A blinded comparison. *AJR* 1987;149:499–501.

113. Ralls PW, Colletti PM, Quinn MF, Halls J. Sonographic findings in hepatic amebic abscess. *Radiology* 1982;145:123–126.

114. Ralls PW, Colletti PM, Lapin SA, et al. Real-time sonography

in suspected acute cholecystitis: Prospective evaluation of primary and secondary signs. *Radiology* 1985;155:767–771.

115. Ralls PW, Mayekawa DS, Lee KP, Johnson MB, Halls J. The use of color Doppler sonography to distinguish dilated intrahepatic ducts from vascular structures. *AJR* 1989;152:291–292.

116. Ralls PW, Mikity VG, Colletti P, Boger D, Halls J, Quinn MF. Sonography in the diagnosis and management of hepatic amebic abscess in children. *Pediatr Radiol* 1982;12:239–243.

117. Ralls PW, Quinn MF, Boswell WD, Colletti PM, Radin DR, Halls J. Patterns of resolution in successfully treated hepatic amebic abscess: Sonographic evaluation. *Radiology* 1983; 149:541–543.

118. Roemer CE, Ferrucci JT, Jr., Mueller PR, Simeone JF, van Sonnenberg E, Wittenberg J. Hepatic cysts: Diagnosis and therapy by sonographic needle aspiration. *AJR* 1981;136:1065–1070.

119. Rogers JV, Mack LA, Freeny PC, Johnson ML, Sones PJ. Hepatic focal nodular hyperplasia: Angiography, CT, sonography, and scintigraphy. *AJR* 1981;137:983–990.

120. Ros PR, Goodman ZD, Ishak KG, Dachman AH, Olmsted WW, Hartman DS, Lichtenstein JE. Mesenchymal hamartoma of the liver: Radiologic-pathologic correlation. *Radiology* 1986; 158:619–624.

121. Ros PR, Olmsted WW, Dachman AH, Goodman ZD, Ishak KG, Hartman DS. Undifferentiated (embryonal) sarcoma of the liver: Radiologic-pathologic correlation. *Radiology* 1986; 160:141–145.

122. Rosenbaum DM, Mindell HJ. Ultrasonographic findings in mesenchymal hamartoma of the liver. *Radiology* 1981;138:425–427.

123. Roslyn JJ, Berquist WE, Pitt HA, Mann LL, Kangarloo H, DenBesten L, Ament ME. Increased risk of gallstones in children receiving total parenteral nutrition. *Pediatrics* 1983; 71:784–789.

124. Saddekni S, Hutchinson DE, Cooperberg PL. The sonographically patent umbilical vein in portal hypertension. *Radiology* 1982;145:441–443.

125. Scatarige JC, Scott WW, Donovan PJ, Siegelman SS, Sanders RC. Fatty infiltration of the liver: Ultrasonographic and computed tomographic correlation. *J Ultrasound Med* 1984;3:9–14.

126. Schabel SI, Rittenberg GM, Javid LH, Cunningham J, Ross P. The "bull's-eye" falciform ligament: A sonographic finding of portal hypertension. *Radiology* 1980;136:157–159.

127. Scott WW, Saunders RC, Siegelman SS. Irregular fatty infiltration of the liver: Diagnostic dilemmas. *AJR* 1980;135:67–71.

128. Sellier N, Adamsbaum C, Checoury A, Kalifa G. Sonographic hepatic arterialisation in newborns receiving parenteral nutrition. *Pediatr Radiol* 1988;18:471–473.

129. Siegel MJ, Melson GL. Sonographic demonstration of hepatic Burkitt's lymphoma. *Pediatr Radiol* 1981;11:166–167.

130. Siegel MJ. Liver and biliary tract. In: Siegel MJ, ed. *Pediatric Body CT*. New York: Churchill Livingstone, 1988:103–134.

131. Simeone JF, Brink JA, Mueller PR, et al. The sonographic diagnosis of acute gangrenous cholecystitis: Importance of the Murphy sign. *AJR* 1989;152:289–290.

132. Slovis TL, Haller JO, Cohen HL, Berdon WE, Watts FB. Complicated appendiceal inflammatory disease in children: Pylephlebitis and liver abscess. *Radiology* 1989;171:823–825.

133. Smith WL, Franken EA, Mitros FA. Liver tumors in children. *Sem Roentgenol* 1983;18:136–148.

134. Stalker HP, Kaufman RA, Towbin R. Patterns of liver injury in childhood. CT analysis. *AJR* 1986;147:1199–1205.

135. Stanley P, Hall TR, Woolley MM, Diament MJ, Gilsanz V, Miller JH. Mesenchymal hamartomas of the liver in childhood: Sonographic and CT findings. *AJR* 1986;147:1035–1039.

136. Sty JR, Starshak RJ. Comparative imaging in the evaluation of hepatic abscesses in immunocompromised children. *JCU* 1983;11:11–15.

137. Subramanyam BR, Balthazar EJ, Madamba MR, Raghavendra BN, Horii SC, Lefleur RS. Sonography of portosystemic venous collaterals in portal hypertension. *Radiology* 1983; 146:161–166.

138. Taguchi T, Ikeda K, Yakabe S, Kimura S. Percutaneous drainage for post-traumatic hepatic abscess in children under ultrasound imaging. *Pediatr Radiol* 1988;18:85–87.

139. Taylor KJW, Burns PN, Woodcock JP, Wells PNT. Blood flow in deep abdominal and pelvic vessels: Ultrasonic pulsed-Doppler analysis. *Radiology* 1985;154:487–493.

140. Taylor KJW, Morse SS, Weltin GG, Riely CA, Flye MW. Liver transplant recipients: Portable duplex US with correlative angiography. *Radiology* 1986;159:357–363.

141. Taylor KJW, Ramos I, Morse SS, Fortune KL, Hammers L, Taylor CR. Focal liver masses: Differential diagnosis with pulsed Doppler US. *Radiology* 1987;164:643–647.

142. Taylor KJW, Riely CA, Hammers L, et al. Quantitative US attenuation in normal liver and in patients with diffuse liver disease: Importance of fat. *Radiology* 1986;160:65–71.

143. Tefft M, Mitus A, Das L, Vawter GF, Filler RM. Irradiation of the liver in children: Review of experience in the acute and chronic phases, and in the intact normal and partially resected. *AJR* 1970;108:365–385.

144. Tomooka Y, Koga T, Onitsuka H, Hayashida Y, Kuroiwa T, Miyazaki S, Torisu M. Ultrasonic demonstration of a common bile duct calculus associated with congenital bile duct dilatation. *Pediatr Radiol* 1988;18:499–500.

145. Towbin RB, Strife JL. Percutaneous aspiration, drainage, and biopsies in children. *Radiology* 1985;157:81–85.

146. Treem WR, Grant EE, Barth KH, Kremers PW. Ultrasound guided percutaneous cholecystocholangiography for early differentiation of cholestatic liver disease in infants. *J Pediatr Gastroenterol Nutr* 1988;7:347–352.

147. Waller RM, Oliver TW, McCain AH, Sones PJ, Bernardino ME. Computed tomography and sonography of hepatic cirrhosis and portal hypertension. *Radiographics* 1984;4:677–715.

148. Weinberg AG, Finegold MJ. Primary hepatic tumors of childhood. *Hum Pathol* 1983;14:512–537.

149. Weinberger E, Blumhagen JD, Odell JM. Gallbladder contraction in biliary atresia. *AJR* 1987;149:401–402.

150. Weinreb J, Kumari S, Phillips G, Pochaczevsky R. Portal vein measurements by real-time sonography. *AJR* 1982;497–499.

151. Welch TJ, Sheedy PF II, Johnson CM, et al. Focal nodular hyperplasia and hepatic adenoma: Comparison of angiography, CT, US, and scintigraphy. *Radiology* 1985;156:593–595.

152. Welch TJ, Sheedy PF II, Johnson CM, et al. Radiographic characteristics of benign liver tumors: Focal nodular hyperplasia and hepatic adenoma. *Radiographics* 1985;5:673–682.

153. Weltin G, Taylor KJW, Carter AR, Taylor CR. Duplex Doppler: Identification of cavernous transformation of the portal vein. *AJR* 1985;144:999–1001.

154. Wernecke K, Peters PE, Kruger K-G. Ultrasonographic patterns of focal hepatic and splenic lesions in Hodgkin's and non-Hodgkin's lymphoma. *Br J Radiol* 1987;60:655–660.

155. Willi UV, Reddish JM, Teele RL. Cystic fibrosis: Its characteristic appearance on abdominal sonography. *AJR* 1980; 134:1005–1010.

156. Williams AG, Sheward SE. Ultrasound appearance of biliary rhabdomyosarcoma. *JCU* 1969;14:63–65.

157. Wilson SR, Arenson AM. Sonographic evaluation of hepatic abscesses. *J Can Assoc Radiol* 1984;35:174–177.

158. Wozney P, Zajko AB, Bron KM, Point S, Starzl TE. Vascular complications after liver transplantation: A 5-year experience. *AJR* 1986;147:657–663.

159. Zangeneh F, Limeck GA, Brown BI, Emch JR, Arcasoy MM, Goldenberg VE, Kelley VC. Hepatorenal glycogenosis (type I glycogenosis) and carcinoma of the liver. *J Pediatr* 1969;74:73–83.

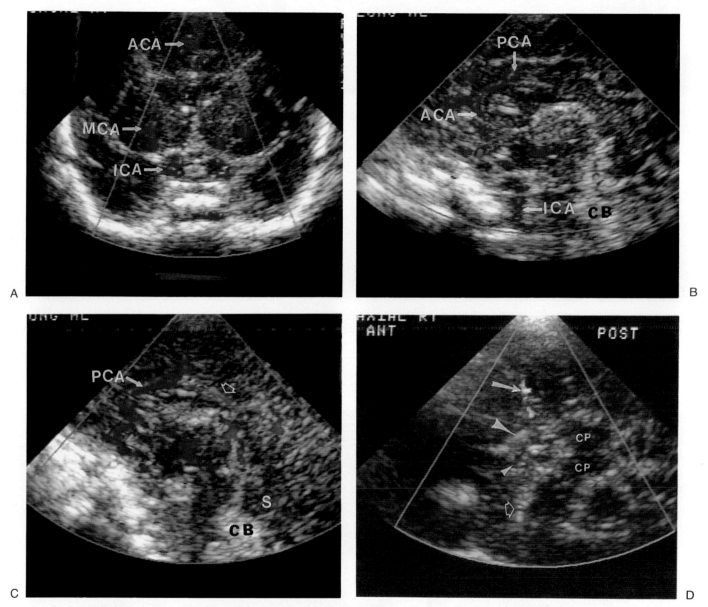

COLORPLATE 1. (Chapter 2, Fig. 12) Color Doppler. **A:** Coronal view through anterior fontanelle shows anterior cerebral (*ACA*), middle cerebral (*MCA*), and internal carotid (*ICA*) arteries. **B:** and **C:** Sagittal images demonstrate ACA, pericallosal artery (*PCA*), and *ICA*. Flow in the anterior portion of the PCA is red since it is toward the transducer; flow in the posterior part of the PCA (*open arrow*) is away from the transducer and is blue. It was noted to pulsate on real-time imaging. Flow in the straight sinus (*S*) is also blue but was nonpulsatile on real-time examination. *CB*, cerebellum. **D:** Axial image from the right lateral approach. Flow in the right MCA (*closed arrow*) is toward the transducer and is therefore red, whereas flow in the left MCA is away from the transducer and is blue (*open arrow*). Right ACA (*large arrowhead*), left ACA (*small arrowhead*), and cerebral peduncles (*CP*) are also seen.

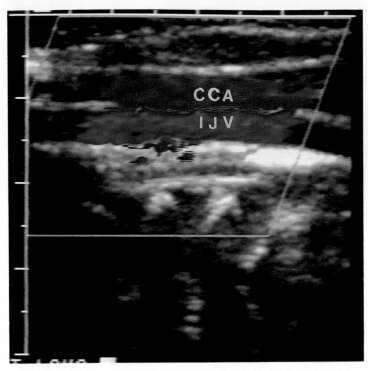

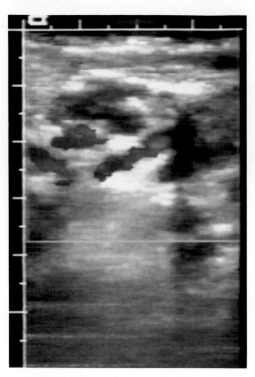

COLORPLATE 2. (Chapter 3, Fig. 3D) Color flow imaging shows flow in the common carotid artery (*CCA*) and internal jugular vein (*IJV*).

COLORPLATE 3. (Chapter 3, Fig. 17B) On color flow images, the avascular nodes are easily differentiated from arteries (*red*) and veins (*blue*).

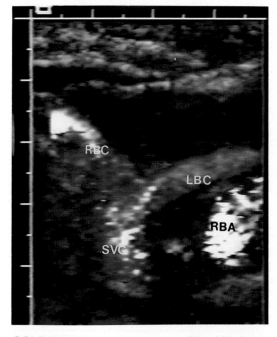

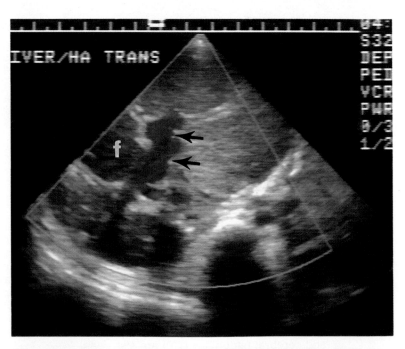

COLORPLATE 4. (Chapter 4, Fig. 4C) Color flow imaging of mediastinal vessels. *LBC,* left brachiocephalic vein; *RBC,* right brachiocephalic vein; *SVC,* superior vena cava; *RBA,* right brachiocephalic artery.

COLORPLATE 5. (Chapter 5, Fig. 43) Hepatic transplant. Color flow Doppler imaging reveals a patent hepatic artery with good flow (*arrows*). *f,* intrahepatic fluid collection.

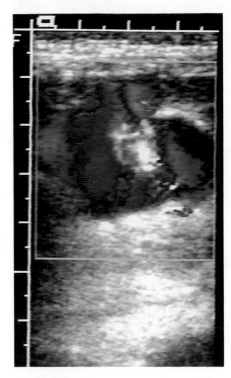

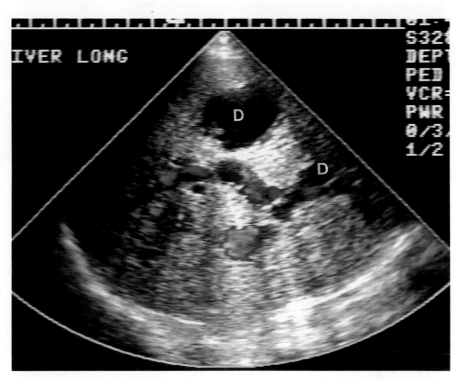

COLORPLATE 6. (Chapter 5, Fig. 44C) Transverse color flow image shows an admixture of arterial and venous blood in the lesion. Arteriovenous fistula was confirmed by angiography.

COLORPLATE 7. (Chapter 5, Fig. 49D) Color flow Doppler imaging separates the dilated bile ducts (*D*) from vessels.

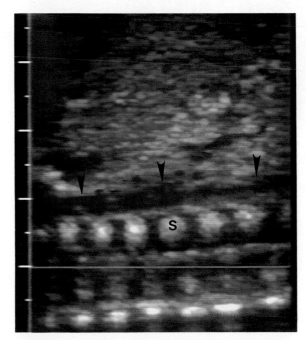

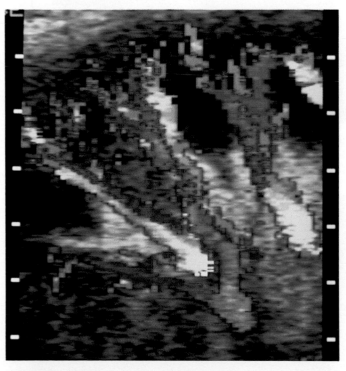

COLORPLATE 8. (Chapter 8, Fig. 30C) Aortic thrombus in a neonate with a history of umbilical arterial catheterization. Color Doppler image shows extensive thrombus in the abdominal aorta (*arrowheads*), with complete occlusion caudally. *S*, spine.

COLORPLATE 9. (Chapter 9, Fig. 47D) Normal Doppler waveform. Color Doppler imaging shows flow in the renal arteries (*red*) and veins (*blue*) throughout the allograft.

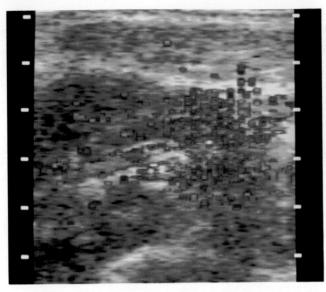

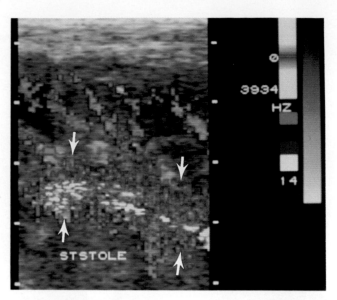

COLORPLATE 10. (Chapter 9, Fig. 52B) Transplant, main renal artery stenosis. Color flow imaging shows an admixture of red and blue colors, representing perivascular soft tissue vibrations, around the stenotic vessel. The underlying stenosis is obscured by the vibrations.

COLORPLATE 11. (Chapter 9, Fig. 53D) Transplant renal arteriovenous fistula. Color saturation is increased toward white in the artery supplying the fistula compared with flow in the normal interlobar arteries. *Arrows* indicate perivascular soft tissue vibrations.

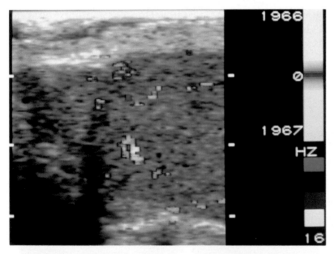

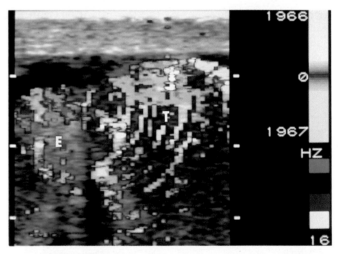

COLORPLATE 12. (Chapter 11, Fig. 2C) Normal testis. Color flow Doppler showing arteries (*red*) and veins (*blue*) within the testis.

COLORPLATE 13. (Chapter 11, Fig. 20) Acute epididymo-orchitis. Color flow Doppler longitudinal scan demonstrates increased testicular blood flow in the left testis (*T*) and epididymis (*E*).

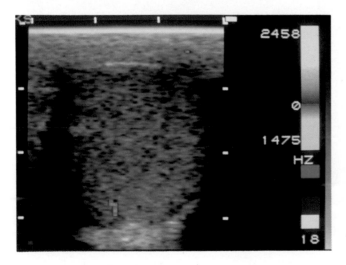

COLORPLATE 14. (Chapter 11, Fig. 25) Testicular torsion. Color flow imaging of the right testis shows lack of perfusion.

Spleen and Peritoneal Cavity

Marilyn J. Siegel

The normal spleen appears as a well-marginated ovoid or oblong organ in the left upper quadrant of the abdomen. The superior lateral surface of the spleen is convex beneath the left hemidiaphragm, while the inferior medial surface is often concave, conforming to the shape of the left kidney. The splenic artery and vein usually can be seen entering the splenic hilum on the medial aspect of the spleen. Typically, the splenic parenchyma is homogeneous and slightly more echogenic than the adjacent renal cortex (Fig. 1). Splenic volume increases proportionally with body length during childhood (10).

NORMAL VARIANTS AND CONGENITAL ANOMALIES

The spleen is sufficiently pliable that it can be deformed easily by adjacent masses. In addition, the spleen can change position when adjacent organs, particularly the left kidney, are surgically removed.

Wandering Spleen

The "wandering spleen" is a congenital variant characterized by abnormal splenic mobility. It develops when there is either incomplete fusion of the peritoneal leaves between the left kidney and spleen, resulting in a long, mobile splenic pedicle or failure of formation of splenic ligaments. The end result is an ectopic location of the spleen in the lower abdomen or pelvis. Clinically patients may present with an asymptomatic abdominal mass or an acute abdomen due to torsion of the splenic pedicle (4,37). Sonographic findings of a non-infarcted, ectopically located spleen consist of an echogenic abdominal "mass" with a size and shape appropriate for the spleen, plus absence of a

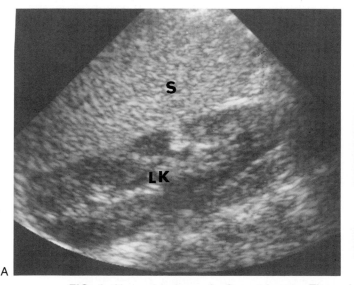
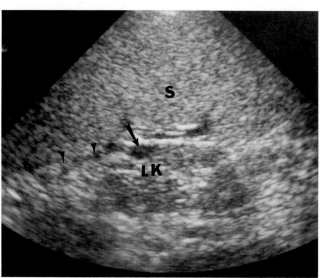

FIG. 1. Normal spleen. **A:** Coronal scan. The splenic parenchyma is homogeneous and more echogenic than the renal parenchyma. **B:** A more medial scan. The proximal splenic vein (*arrow*) is easily recognizable at the splenic hilum. Note the concave appearance (*arrowheads*) of the medial splenic surface. *S,* spleen; *LK,* left kidney.

spleen in the normal location (3,34). Occasionally, enlarged and tortuous vessels can be identified in the splenic hilum (43). In contrast, the torsed spleen is enlarged, as well as ectopic, with a course hypoechoic texture due to vascular congestion or infarction. In patients with mild abnormalities of splenic mobility, the initial transverse and longitudinal images of the spleen may appear normal. However, following dis-

tention of the stomach with fluid, inferior displacement of the spleen may be observed (Fig. 2) (44).

Accessory Spleens

Accessory spleens occur in approximately 15% of children and probably result from failure of some of the embryonic buds of splenic tissue in the dorsal me-

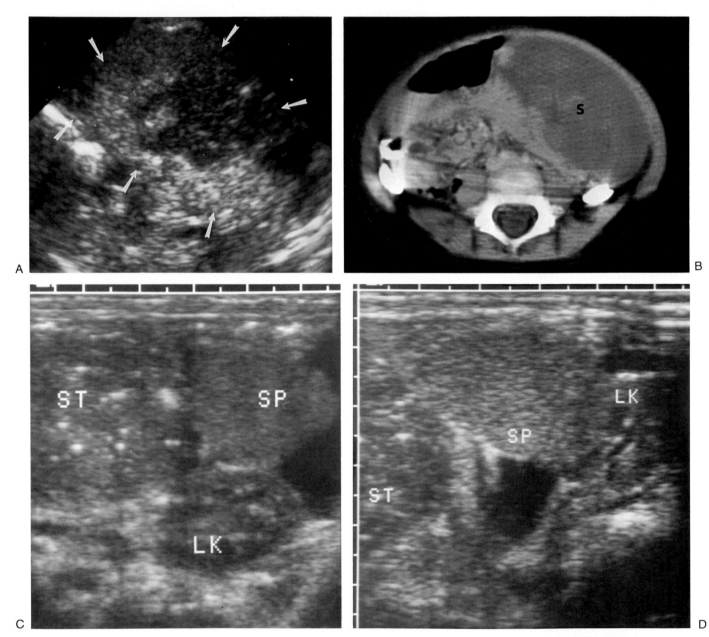

FIG. 2. Wandering spleen. **A:** Longitudinal sonogram in the midabdomen shows a solid mass (*arrows*) with a heterogeneous texture. **B:** CT scan through lower abdomen demonstrates an enlarged spleen (*S*). Note the reduced attenuation of the splenic parenchyma. At surgery, there was 270° torsion of the spleen on the pedicle. Splenic ligaments were absent. Pathologic examination demonstrated global infarction. Transverse scans in another patient. **C:** On initial images, the spleen lies superior to the left kidney and adjacent to the stomach. **D:** Following gastric distension, it is inferiorly displaced and medial to the left kidney. *SP*, spleen; *LK*, left kidney; *ST*, stomach.

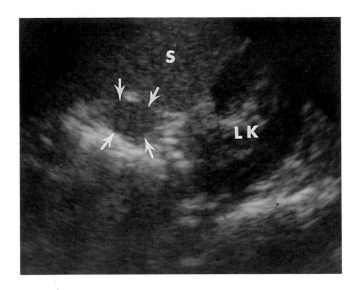

FIG. 3. Accessory spleen. A small nodule (*arrow*) of tissue is present adjacent to the splenic hilum. The echogenicity is equal to that of adjacent splenic (*S*) parenchyma and greater than that of renal parenchyma. *LK*, left kidney.

sogastrium to fuse (11). Most are found near the splenic hilum and tail of the pancreas, but they may be located in the greater omentum, gastrosplenic ligament, or along the splenic vessels. They are solitary in about 90% of cases, double in about 10%, and multiple in 3%. Their size varies, but typically they are about 1 cm in diameter. On sonography, they appear as round or oval, solid structures with an echogenicity similar to that of the main spleen (Fig. 3). A feeding splenic artery or draining vein can be seen near the splenic hilum by real-time imaging in 90% of cases (39).

Generally, accessory spleens remain small and are incidental findings of no clinical significance. However, accessory splenic tissue may undergo compensatory hypertrophy in previously splenectomized pa-

tients and be responsible for recurrent hematologic diseases or present as an abdominal mass. In these patients accessory spleens may reach a size of 5 cm or more (45).

Visceroatrial Anomalies

Visceroatrial abnormalities are associated with abnormalities of splenic number and location, including polysplenia, asplenia, and situs inversus. Polysplenia is a syndrome characterized by multiple aberrant nodules of splenic tissue in the right abdomen, a transverse liver, interruption of the inferior vena cava, and cardiac anomalies (Fig. 4). Asplenia is characterized by

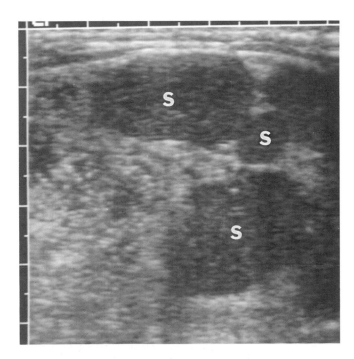

FIG. 4. Polysplenia. Multiple hypoechoic ovoid structures are noted in the left upper quadrant. The presence of multiple spleens (*S*) was confirmed by scintigraphy with TC-99m–labeled heat-damaged red blood cells.

the absence of splenic tissue, ambiguous abdominal situs, and cardiovascular anomalies. Situs inversus refers to mirror image positioning of the viscera and vascular structures (42). The spleen is located in the right upper quadrant and has a normal echogenicity.

PATHOLOGY

Splenomegaly

Sonography is rarely required to confirm the presence of splenomegaly apparent on physical examination. However, in cases where it is uncertain whether the mass palpable in the left abdomen is the spleen or a separate mass, sonography can provide a definite diagnosis. Although normal values of splenic size are available, measurements usually are not needed for the diagnosis of splenomegaly. In most instances the diagnosis is based on subjective criteria, including extension of the spleen below the left kidney and loss of the normal concavity of the spleen on its medial surface (Fig. 5).

Splenomegaly occurs with a variety of disease processes, including malignant, inflammatory, and infiltrative diseases. Although splenomegaly is a nonspecific feature, there often are other findings to suggest a specific diagnosis. The presence of abnormal mesenteric or retroperitoneal adenopathy in association with splenomegaly favors the diagnosis of lymphoma. Varices in the splenic hilum can suggest the diagnosis of portal hypertension or hepatic vein occlusion. Mass lesions producing splenic enlargement, including metastases, abscesses, cysts, and nodules of Gaucher's cells, also can be recognized (17).

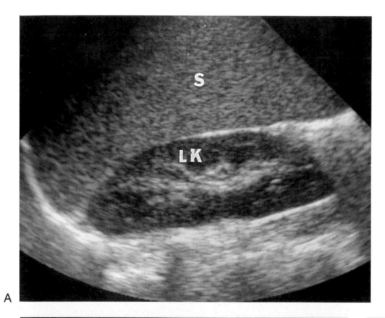

A

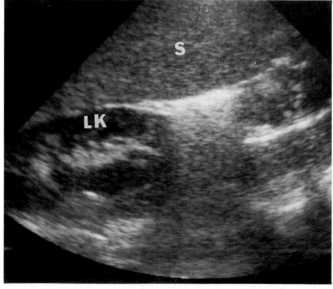

B

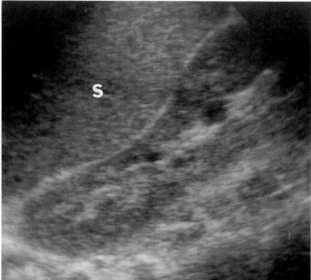

C

FiG. 5. Splenomegaly in a patient with lymphoma. **A,B:** Two coronal scans demonstrated extension of the spleen (*S*) below the inferior margin of the left kidney (*LK*). **C:** In another patient, a longitudinal scan shows a convex medial splenic border. *S*, spleen.

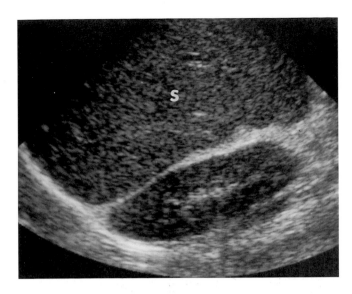

FIG. 6. Splenic involvement by lymphoma. Longitudinal scan shows an enlarged, hypoechoic spleen (*S*). Splenic echogenicity is equal to that of the kidney.

Neoplasm

Splenic involvement is found at staging laparotomy in approximately one-third of children with untreated Hodgkin's disease and in about 15% of children with non-Hodgkin's lymphoma. The affected spleen may or may not be enlarged, and conversely mild to moderate splenomegaly may be present in patients in whom no tumor is identified in the excised spleen. When splenomegaly is marked, however, there is a high likelihood of involvement by lymphoma (23). The splenic parenchyma may be normal, hypo-, or hyperechoic, and homogeneous or heterogeneous with focal hypoechoic nodules (Figs. 6,7).

The spleen frequently is involved by leukemia during active stages of the disease and often serves as a sanctuary during remission. Its appearance varies during the course of the disease and is modified by chemotherapy. Prior to therapy, it often is enlarged with homogeneous low-level echoes, while during and following treatment splenic size decreases and echogenicity increases (14).

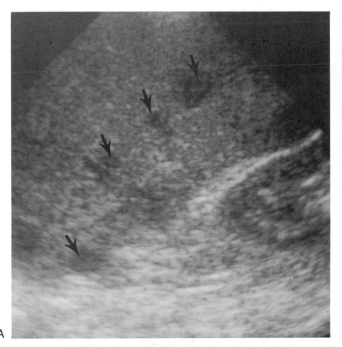

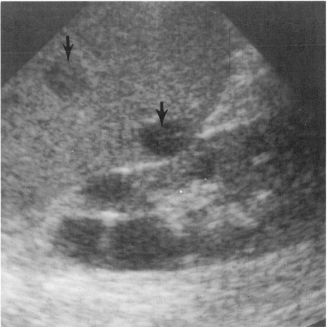

A

B

FIG. 7. Splenic involvement by lymphoma. **A,B:** Two longitudinal scans. Multiple hypoechoic masses (*arrows*) are noted within the splenic parenchyma. At operation, there were lymphomatous deposits in the spleen, retroperitoneal nodes, and mesentery.

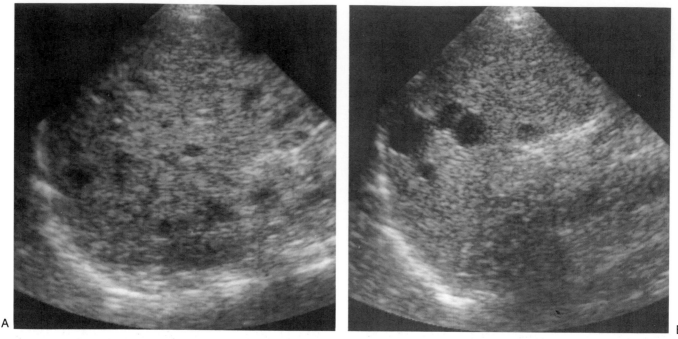

FIG. 8. Splenic hemangiomatosis in a patient with multiple cutaneous hemangiomas. **A,B:** Two longitudinal scans. The spleen is enlarged and contains multiple hypoechoic masses.

Primary tumors of the spleen are rare in children. The majority are benign and include lymphangiomatosis, cystic hamartoma, teratoma, and hemangioma (5,31). A rare malignant tumor is angiosarcoma. The appearance of these tumors ranges from minimal parenchymal inhomogeneity or multiple tiny lesions to a large, predominantly hypoechoic or echogenic mass (Fig. 8) (32,38). When splenic tumors are large or believed to be malignant, computerized tomography (CT) or magnetic resonance (MR) imaging are preferred over sonography to demonstrate the full extent of disease.

Cysts

Splenic cysts may be congenital, parasitic, or posthemorrhagic in origin. Symptoms produced by the cysts are nonspecific and include epigastric fullness, a palpable left upper quadrant mass, or chronic, low-grade pain due to compression of adjacent organs. Rarely, acute pain may occur because of infection or rupture of the cyst (6). Congenital cysts, also referred to as epidermoid or true cysts, are lined by epithelium and surrounded by fibrous walls. They usually are unilocular and rarely contain calcifications. The fluid within the cyst may be clear or viscous and may contain protein, blood, fat, or cholesterol crystals. Parasitic cysts, due to hydatid disease, and posthemorrhagic cysts, due to trauma or infarct, are classified as pseudocysts or false cysts since they are not epithelial-lined. They may or may not calcify.

On sonography, the three types of cyst usually are indistinguishable from each other. Most are well-circumscribed, spherical lesions that are sonolucent with good through-transmission (Fig. 9). A rib of splenic tissue usually is visible around part of the cyst (20).

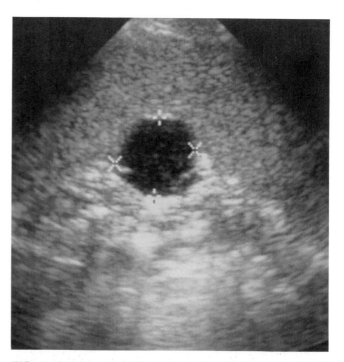

FIG. 9. Splenic cyst. Transverse image shows a round, sharply marginated, anechoic mass (*calipers*) with increased through-transmission at the splenic hilum. Epidermoid cyst was confirmed at operation.

Occasionally the cyst contains low-level internal echoes or is echogenic due to cholesterol crystals or breakdown products of hemoglobin (7). Daughter cysts and septations may be present in parasitic cysts.

The differential diagnostic considerations of a cystic splenic lesion include a large solitary abscess, hematoma, and cystic neoplasm. When clinical or laboratory data are inconclusive, fine needle aspiration of the cyst contents under sonographic guidance can be helpful for diagnosis and drainage (38). In some cases treatment can be facilitated by injection of a sclerosing agent (18).

Inflammatory Disease

Pyogenic Abscess

Most pyogenic splenic abscesses are solitary and the result of (a) infection, presumably of hematogeneous origin, in a spleen damaged by trauma or infarction; or (b) systemic bacteremia causing infection in a previously normal spleen. Less commonly, splenic abscess results from direct extension of a contiguous inflammatory process, such as a subphrenic abscess. The most common infecting organisms are staphylo-cocci, streptococci, and gram-negative rods such as salmonella.

The sonographic appearance of a pyogenic splenic abscess is similar to that of abscesses in other solid organs. Typically, the lesion is an irregular, poorly defined, hypoechoic mass with a variable amount of enhanced transmission and internal echoes (Fig. 10). Increased echogenicity with distal acoustic shadowing is seen if the abscess cavity contains gas (22,29,30,33,38). In contrast to the well-defined acoustic shadow caused by calcification, the shadow caused by gas is ill-defined. Occasionally, fluid-debris levels and multiple septations may be observed.

Fungal Abscess

Fungal abscesses are most often due to *Candida albicans* infection, occurring primarily in immunosuppressed patients, typically those with acute leukemia (40). The sonographic patterns of splenic candidiasis are similar to those of hepatic candidiasis and include: a "wheel within a wheel" appearance (hypoechoic center surrounded by alternating hyperechoic and hypoechoic rings), bull's-eye lesion (central echogenic

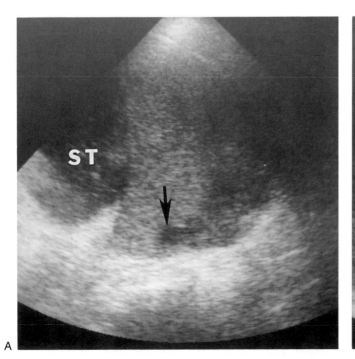 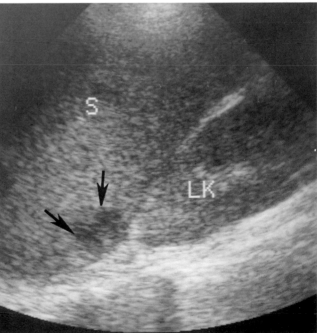

FIG. 10. Pyogenic splenic abscess. **A:** Transverse and **B:** longitudinal scans show an irregular hypoechoic area (*arrows*) near the splenic tip. *S. aureus* was obtained by cytologic examination of aspirated material. *S*, spleen; *LK*, left kidney; *ST*, stomach.

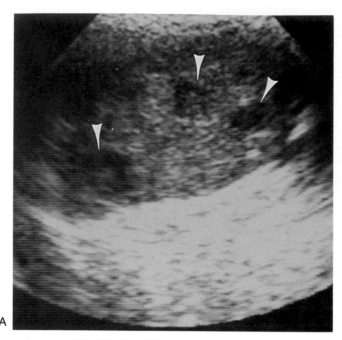

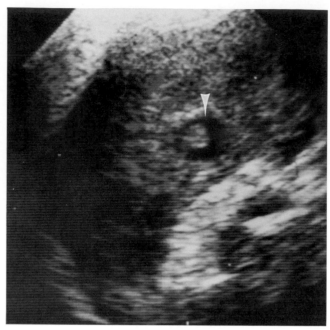

A   B

FIG. 11. Candida abscesses in a 5-year-old boy with acute lymphocytic leukemia. **A,B:** Two coronal scans of the spleen demonstrate several small hypoechoic lesions (*arrowheads*) with central echogenic foci, suggesting bull's-eye lesions. (From Sumner et al., ref. 40, with permission.)

area with a sonolucent rim) (Fig. 11), uniformly hypoechoic lesion, and echogenic focus with acoustic shadowing (28). Occasionally the splenic parenchyma may be diffusely hypoechoic (27).

Infarction

Splenic infarction results from occlusion of the splenic artery or its branches. In children, homoglobinopathies such as sickle cell disease or sickle thalassemia are the primary causes of splenic infarction. Less common etiologies include bland or septic emboli associated with bacterial endocarditis and angiographic embolization (24). Splenomegaly alone also increases the risk of infarction.

The sonographic appearance varies depending on the chronicity of the infarct. Acutely, the infarct appears as a wedge-shaped hypoechoic lesion located

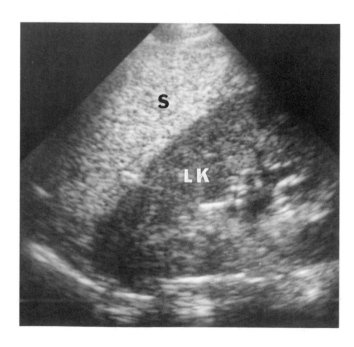

FIG. 12. Chronic splenic infarcts in a patient with sickle cell anemia. A longitudinal scan demonstrates a small, intensely echogenic spleen. *S,* spleen; *LK,* left kidney.

near the periphery of the spleen. Multiple, tiny, linear echoes sometimes may be noted within the infarcted tissue representing nonsuppurative gas formation (24). A chronic infarct appears as an area of increased echogenicity with retraction of the splenic contour, secondary to scarring and fibrosis. Occasionally the end result of infarction is a splenic cyst or a small, diffusely echogenic spleen (Fig. 12) (36).

The sonographic appearance of an acute splenic infarct is nonspecific and indistinguishable from abscess, hematoma, or tumor. Percutaneous needle aspiration may be needed for definitive diagnosis if the clinical setting does not suggest infarct.

Trauma

The spleen is the intraabdominal organ most commonly injured as a result of blunt abdominal trauma. Splenic injuries are classified as intraparenchymal hematomas, lacerations, and fractures, or as subcapsular fluid collections. Intraparenchymal hematomas generally are focal rounded or oval fluid collections. Splenic parenchymal lacerations almost always involve part of the lateral margin of the spleen and are irregular linear lesions that may have a branching appearance (Fig. 13). In more subtle cases the lacerations may not be readily evident; instead the spleen may appear mottled or inhomogeneous, probably representing tiny collections of blood within disrupted splenic pulp. Splenic fractures are the result of deep lacerations that traverse the splenic parenchyma and extend to the splenic hilum. The upper and lower poles of the spleen may be avulsed. Virtually all parenchymal lacerations and fractures are associated with subcapsular hematomas. Subcapsular hematomas are crescentic lesions that flatten and compress the lateral margin of the spleen. With capsular disruption, hemoperitoneum in the left paracolic gutter may be observed.

As is observed in other organs, the echogenicity of the hemorrhage varies with age. Recent splenic hematomas, less than 24 hours old, appear hyper- or isoechoic relative to normal splenic parenchyma. At this stage, the lesion may be indistinguishable from normal splenic tissue and only splenomegaly may be appreciated on sonography. With time as the protein and hemoglobin are resorbed, the hematoma becomes complex or hypoechoic relative to adjacent spleen (25,38). Intrasplenic hematomas and lacerations usually resorb over a period of months. Small lesions may disappear within 2 months of the injury, while larger lesions can persist up to a year. When followed to complete resolution, the spleen may appear normal or a small linear echogenic focus may be present, probably representing scar tissue (25).

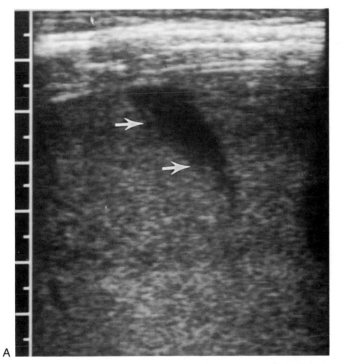
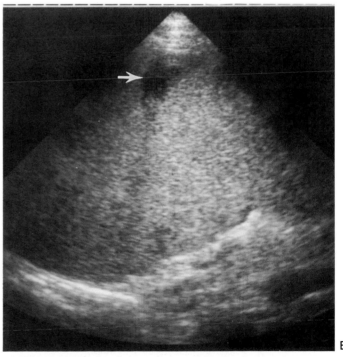

FIG. 13. Splenic laceration. **A:** Transverse and **B:** longitudinal images show a linear area of decreased echogenicity (*arrows*) in the lateral aspect of the spleen. The diagnosis of a splenic laceration was confirmed by CT.

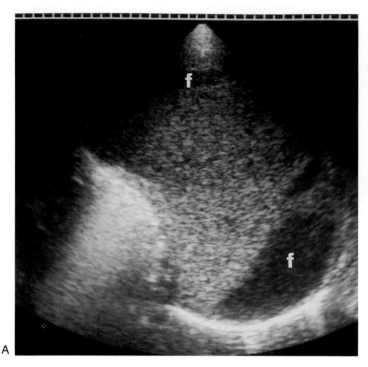
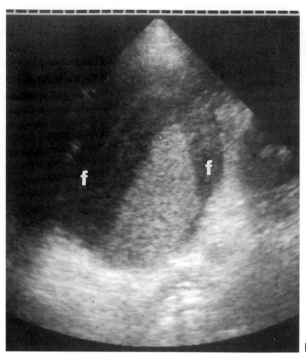

A   B

FIG. 14. Spontaneous splenic rupture in a patient with infectious mononucleosis. **A:** Transverse and **B:** longitudinal images show a crescentic, hypoechoic fluid (*f*) collection sharply demarcated from the adjacent spleen. The appearance is consistent with a subcapsular hematoma.

Occasionally the spleen spontaneously ruptures as a complication of infectious mononucleosis. Affected patients typically present with sudden onset of abdominal pain, which may be associated with shoulder pain. A history of significant trauma usually is absent. Sonographic findings in spontaneous trauma include splenomegaly, areas of decreased parenchymal echogenicity, subcapsular and pericapsular fluid collections, and free intraperitoneal fluid (Fig. 14) (19).

At the present time, CT is the preferred study for screening patients who have sustained blunt abdominal trauma. The sensitivity of CT in detecting splenic injury has been reported to be as high as 100% (21). The ability of this method to examine the entire abdomen and pelvis for the presence of associated injuries is an advantage over sonography. However, when the patient sustains only minimal trauma and an isolated splenic injury is suspected, sonography, because of its ease of performance, may be the screening procedure of choice (12). Sonography also can have a role in follow-up evaluation to demonstrate resolution of traumatic splenic lesions (1).

PERITONEAL CAVITY

Normal Anatomy

The peritoneal cavity contains a series of communicating spaces that usually are not visualized by sonography unless they are distended by fluid. Knowledge of the various compartments of the peritoneal cavity and of the ligaments and mesentery that limit them is essential for the recognition and localization of intraabdominal fluid and disease processes. The pathways of spread of intraabdominal disease processes have been elegantly described by Morton A. Meyers and his colleagues and the reader is referred to their works for further details (26). This section will discuss basic anatomy of the abdominal cavity before describing the sonographic manifestations of disease processes.

The peritoneal cavity is divided into various spaces and compartments by ligaments and mesentery. The transverse mesocolon divides the upper abdomen into supramesocolic and inframesocolic compartments. The supramesocolic compartment can be divided into left and right peritoneal spaces (2) (Fig. 15). The left peritoneal space can be further subdivided into four compartments: the anterior and posterior perihepatic spaces and the anterior and posterior subphrenic spaces. The right peritoneal space has two major divisions: the lesser sac and the right perihepatic space. The latter has a diaphragmatic or subphrenic surface coursing along the anterior and lateral surfaces of the liver and a subhepatic space underlying the visceral surface of the right lobe. The right subhepatic space is comprised of anterior and posterior compartments; the latter compartment is known as "Morrison's pouch" (Figs. 16,17).

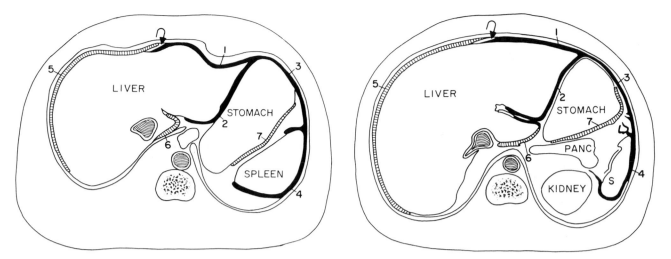

FIG. 15. Left (*heavy black lines*) and right (*vertical hatching*) peritoneal spaces of the upper abdomen. Four divisions of the left peritoneal space are present. Anterior to the liver and limited by the falciform ligament medially (*curved arrow*) is the left anterior perihepatic space (*1*). Posterior to the visceral hepatic surface is the left posterior perihepatic space (*2*). The anterior subphrenic space (*3*) lies between the stomach and diaphragm, while the posterior subphrenic (perisplenic) space (*4*) surrounds the spleen (*S*). The right peritoneal space consists of the perihepatic space and the lesser sac. The perihepatic space (*5*) is limited anteromedially by the falciform ligament and posteromedially by the hepatic bare area. The lesser sac has two components: the superior recess (*6*) and inferior recess (*7*). (Adapted from ref. 2.)

The inframesocolic compartment is subdivided by the obliquely oriented small bowel mesentery into a smaller right infracolic space and a larger left infracolic space. The left infracolic space is bordered laterally by the descending colon and inferiorly by the sigmoid colon and its peritoneal reflections. The right infracolic space is limited laterally by the ascending colon and inferiorly by the junction of the mesenteric root with the cecum.

The natural flow of intraperitoneal fluid is along pathways determined by the mesentery and peritoneal reflections (Fig. 18). Abscesses and metastases tend to grow in areas where fluid pools. Fluid within the inframesocolic compartment preferentially flows into the pelvis, where it accumulates in the posterior cul-de-sac and the lateral perivesical fossae. Fluid in the right infracolic space flows along the recesses of the small bowel mesentery before pooling at the junction

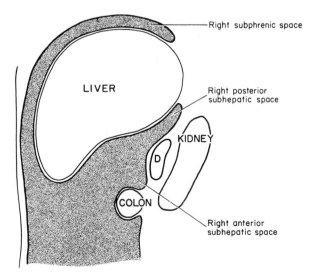

FIG. 16. Parasagittal diagram of right perihepatic spaces. The right subphrenic space is continuous with the right subhepatic space. The latter has an anterior space limited inferiorly by the transverse colon and a posterior space (Morrison's pouch) projecting superiorly in front of the kidney. *D*, duodenum.

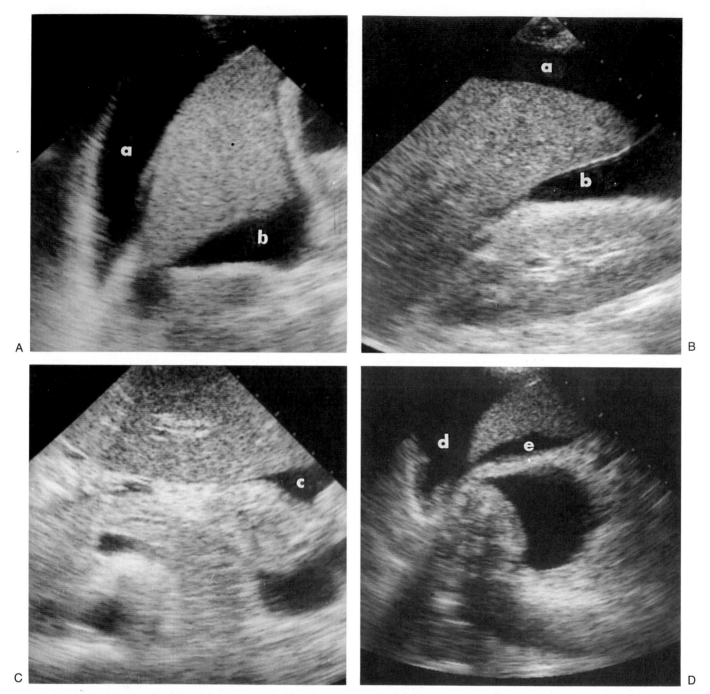

FIG. 17. Peritoneal spaces of the upper abdomen. Sonographic demonstration. **A,B:** Longitudinal and transverse scans shows ascites in the subphrenic (*a*) and subhepatic spaces (*b*) of the right perihepatic space. **C:** Transverse image through the upper mid abdomen shows fluid in the left posterior perihepatic (*c*) space. **D:** Coronal scan of the upper abdomen reveals fluid in the anterior (*d*) and posterior (*e*) subphrenic spaces around the spleen. Hepatic failure was the cause of the anechoic ascites.

of the mesentery with the cecum. Subsequently it spills into the cul-de-sac of the pelvis. Fluid in the left infracolic pools in the sigmoid mesocolon before overflowing into the pelvis. Once in the pelvis, fluid can flow via the right or left paracolic gutters into the upper abdomen. Flow occurs preferentially by way of the

right paracolic gutter into the posterior subhepatic space, also known as Morrison's pouch, of the supramesocolic compartment. From the right subhepatic space, fluid may extend to the right subphrenic space. Spread of fluid across the midline to the left subphrenic is prevented by the falciform and coronary ligaments

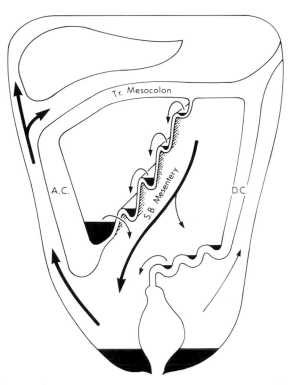

FIG. 18. Spread of peritoneal fluid. Natural flow of intraperitoneal fluid is directed along pathways determined by peritoneal reflections and recesses. *A.C.,* ascending colon; *D.C.,* descending colon. (Adapted from ref. 16.)

of the liver. Flow along the left paracolic gutter is slower and weaker than up the right paracolic gutter and is limited superiorly by the phrenicocolic ligament.

Pathologic Conditions

Ascites

Ascites refers to accumulation of fluid within the peritoneal cavity. The causes include transudate, exudate, blood, chyle, urine, and tumor implants. Sonography is a sensitive method for detecting peritoneal fluid. Ascites may appear anechoic or complex and may be loculated or free-flowing. Anechoic fluid collections usually are encountered with transudates resulting from hypoalbuminemia; hepatic, cardiac, or renal failure; or chyle, urine, or bile leakage. Complex ascites with internal echoes or septations is more often associated with hemorrhage, infection, or neoplasm. Omental or peritoneal nodules or hepatic masses may be recognized when the ascites is due to malignancy.

Localized or small amounts of ascites frequently are seen in the right perihepatic space, Morrison's pouch, or the cul-de-sac. Loculated ascites, secondary to postoperative or inflammatory adhesions, usually appears as a well-defined septated fluid collection displacing adjacent structures (Fig. 19). The sonographic

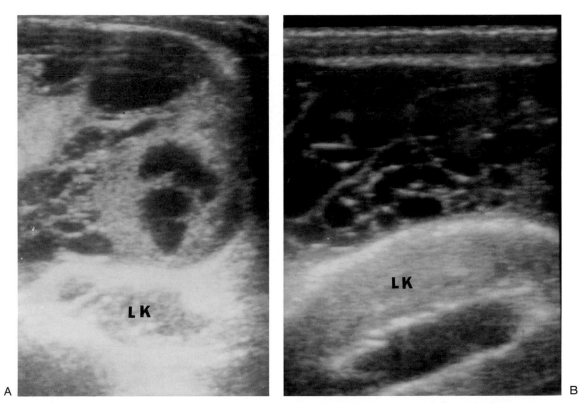

FIG. 19. Loculated ascites. **A:** Transverse and **B:** longitudinal scans of the left flank show a septated fluid collection in the left pericolic gutter surrounding the left kidney (*LK*).

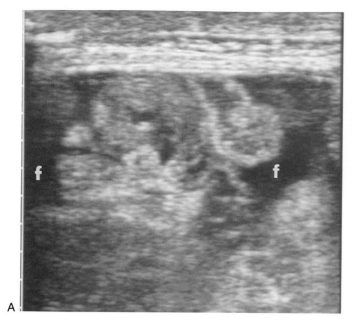

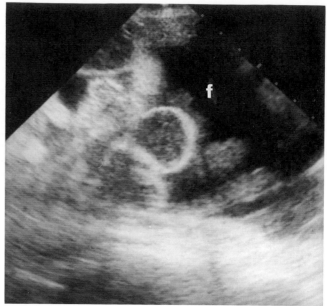

FIG. 20. Free ascites. **A:** Transverse and **B:** longitudinal scans of the pelvis show bowel loops floating within peritoneal fluid (*f*).

appearance is indistinguishable from a lymphocele, hematoma, or abscess. Differentiation requires clinical correlation and, in some instances, percutaneous needle aspiration. With a large amount of free ascites, the small bowel loops are displaced centrally within the abdomen, and fluid accumulates adjacent to and between bowel loops (Fig. 20). The leaves of the small bowel mesentery may be recognized as a series of linear echogenic structures radiating toward the center of the abdomen (9).

Intraperitoneal Abscess

Abdominal abscesses in children most often are the result of intestinal perforation secondary to appendicitis or Crohn's disease, but they may follow pelvic surgery or trauma or be a sequelae of pelvic inflammatory disease. Affected patients usually present with fever, leukocytosis, and abdominal pain, although patients with chronic walled-off abscesses may have few overt signs or symptoms. In the latter cases the combination of laboratory data and history usually indicates abscess as a possible source of the patient's symptoms.

The sonographic appearance of intraperitoneal abscess ranges from a fluid collection with low-level internal echoes and through-transmission to a solid lesion (Fig. 21). Most have a round or oval configuration. Occasionally, fluid-debris levels, septations, or gas may be encountered. Gas can be recognized as intensely echogenic foci, usually with acoustic shadowing.

The anatomic areas best suited for sonographic evaluation are the right upper quadrant and pelvis, because the liver and urinary bladder, respectively, serve as acoustic windows. If the spleen is present, the left upper quadrant and left subphrenic spaces also can be evaluated by sonography. Abscesses in the mid abdomen may be difficult to detect with sonography because of interruption of the ultrasonic beam by bowel gas. Moreover, gas containing abscesses may be con-

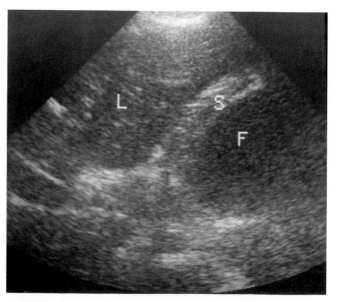

FIG. 21. Peritoneal abscess. A transverse scan of the upper abdomen demonstrates a poorly defined echogenic fluid collection (*F*) behind the stomach (*S*) in the lesser sac. *L*, Liver.

fused with a loop of gas-filled bowel. In addition, factors such as the presence of open wounds, drainage tubes, and large dressings may hamper the sonographic examination.

An approach to imaging a suspected intraabdominal abscess often involves more than one type of radiologic study. Sonography should be used as the initial examination if a right upper quadrant, left upper quadrant, or pelvic abscess is suspected. However, if an intraloop abscess is suspected or if the patient is immediately postoperative, CT is the examination of choice. Once identified, either sonography-, or CT-directed needle aspiration of the fluid collection can be performed.

Tumors of the Mesentery and Peritoneum

Various pathologic processes, both benign and malignant, may infiltrate the mesentery. As a general rule, benign inflammatory processes that cause thickening of the mesentery and peritoneal lining, such as pancreatitis, Crohn's disease, or peritonitis, are not seen by sonography. Computerized tomography is usually regarded as the method of choice in evaluating such lesions. Large mesenteric cysts, organized inflammatory lesions such as plasma cell granulomas, loculated

cerebrospinal fluid collections, and neoplasms, however, can be imaged by sonography (8,9), although CT may be a valuable ancillary examination to determine the extent of disease.

Cysts

Mesenteric cysts may be congenital or acquired secondary to a traumatic or infectious etiology. They usually present as asymptomatic abdominal masses or low grade pain, but can cause acute abdominal pain secondary to torsion. Generally, the cysts are single lesions that may be unilocular or multilocular, and contain fluid which ranges from a clear or straw-colored liquid to a thick viscous material. Calcifications occur, but are generally rare. Malignant changes are extremely infrequent, and are usually low-grade sarcomas, which have a good prognosis if properly excised.

Sonographically, mesenteric cysts may be anechoic or complex with fibrous septations or debris from infection or hemorrhage (Fig. 22) (13). Most are located in the small bowel mesentery, with the mesocolon and omentum being less common sites of origin (35). Omental cysts have a sonographic appearance similar to that of mesenteric cysts; they differ only by their location (15).

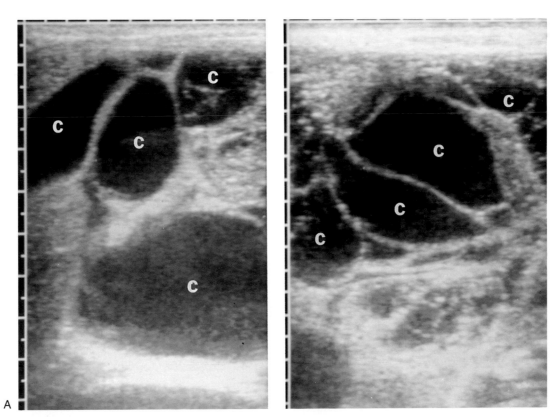

FIG. 22. Mesenteric cyst. **A,B:** Two longitudinal scans of the mid abdomen show a large complex mass with multiple cystic (C) spaces separated by fibrous septations in the anterior abdomen.

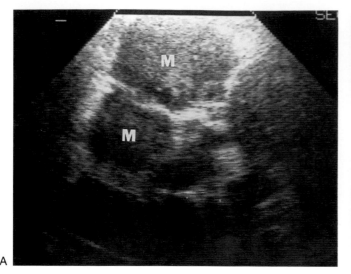
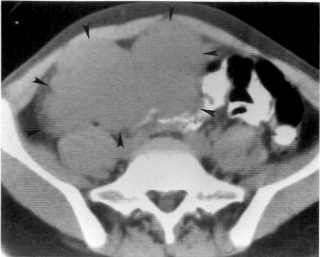

FIG. 23. Burkitt lymphoma. **A:** Transverse scan shows large hypoechoic masses (*M*) in the anterior pelvis. **B:** CT scan shows soft tissue masses (*arrowheads*) extending from the anterior abdominal wall to the retroperitoneum. The masses displace contrast-filled small bowel posteriorly.

Neoplasm

The most common malignant neoplasm of the mesentery in childhood is lymphoma. Mesenteric involvement is seen in approximately 50% of patients with non-Hodgkin's lymphoma and in about 5% of children with Hodgkin's lymphoma. On sonography, the appearance of mesenteric lymph nodes ranges from multiple, well-circumscribed, round masses to large, confluent masses infiltrating the mesentery and encasing the superior mesenteric artery and vein (Fig. 23). Characteristically, lymphomatous nodes are anechoic or hypoechoic.

Small mesenteric lymph nodes are a nonspecific finding and do not always indicate lymphoma. Nonneoplastic causes of mesenteric lymph node enlargement include inflammatory diseases such as Crohn's disease, tuberculosis, histoplasmosis, and acquired immunodeficiency syndrome. The demonstration of large, confluent, soft tissue masses in the mesentery

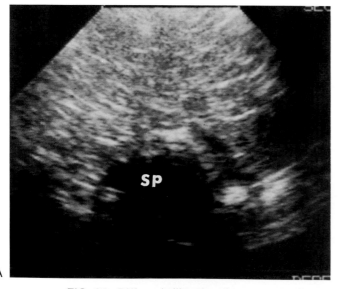
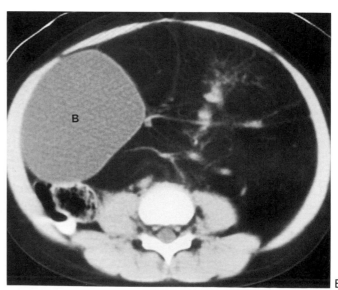

FIG. 24. Diffuse infiltrating lipomatosis. **A:** Transverse ultrasound shows diffuse increased echogenicity without distal shadowing throughout the abdomen. *SP,* spine. **B:** CT scan through lower abdomen reveals lipomatous tissue filling almost the entire abdomen and displacing the urinary bladder (*B*) to the right. Several linear soft tissue densities within the fatty mass represent vessels and fibrous septa.

should suggest lymphoma. Although metastatic disease and primary neoplasms, such as mesenteric desmoid tumor and mesothelioma, are causes of mesenteric masses in adults, they are rarely seen in children.

Primary mesenteric tumors are rare in childhood and are generally of lipomatous origin. Diffuse infiltrating lipomatosis is an invasive form of a simple lipoma. It occurs predominantly in young people and represents widespread overgrowth of fatty tissue (46). Like the lipoma this lesion is echogenic on sonography, but it is more extensive, growing along fascial planes and infiltrating muscle. Diffuse infiltrating lipomatosis may be difficult to distinguish from a lipogenic sarcoma on sonography. Computerized tomography can be helpful in confirming that the mesenteric abnormality is due to diffuse accumulation of fat (Fig. 24). Differentiation between benign lipomatosis and liposarcoma may be difficult on CT, although most sarcomas contain soft tissue components in addition to fatty tissue.

REFERENCES

1. Adler DD, Blane CE, Coran AG, Silver TM. Splenic trauma in the pediatric patient: The integrated roles of ultrasound and computed tomography. *Pediatrics* 1986;78:576–580.
2. Balfe DM, Peterson RR, Van Dyke JA. Normal abdominal and pelvic anatomy. In: Lee KTL, Sagel SS, Stanley RJ, eds. *Computed Body Tomography with MRI Correlation.* New York: Raven Press, 1989;415–475.
3. Barki Y, Bar-Ziv J. Wandering spleen in two children—The role of ultrasonic diagnosis. *Br J Radiol* 1984;57:267–270.
4. Bröker FHL, Fellows K, Treves S. Wandering spleen in three children. *Pediatr Radiol* 1978;6:211–214.
5. Cornaglia-Ferraris P, Perlino GF, Barabino A, Guarino C, Oliva L, Soave F, Massimo L. Cystic lymphangioma of the spleen. Report of CT scan findings. *Pediatr Radiol* 1982;12:94–95.
6. Dachman AH, Ros PR, Murari PJ, Olmsted WW, Lichtenstein JE. Nonparasitic splenic cysts: A report of 52 cases with radiologic-pathologic correlation. *AJR* 1986;147:537–542.
7. Daneman A, Martin DJ. Congenital epithelial splenic cysts in children. Emphasis on sonographic appearances and some unusual features. *Pediatr Radiol* 1982;12:119–125.
8. Day DL, Sane S, Dehner LP. Inflammatory pseudotumor of the mesentery and small intestine. *Pediatr Radiol* 1986;16:210–215.
9. Derchi LE, Solbiati L, Rizzatio G, De Fra L. Normal anatomy and pathologic changes of the small bowel mesentery: US appearance. *Radiology* 1987;164:649–652.
10. Dittrich M, Milde S, Dinkel E, Baumann W, Weitzel D. Sonographic biometry of liver and spleen size in childhood. *Pediatr Radiol* 1983;13:206–211.
11. Erkalis AJ, Filler RM. Splenectomy in childhood: A review of 1413 cases. *J Pediatr Surg* 1972;7:382–388.
12. Filiatrault D, Longpré D, Patriquin H, et al. Investigation of childhood blunt abdominal trauma: A practical approach using ultrasound as the initial diagnostic modality. *Pediatr Radiol* 1987;17:373–379.
13. Geer LL, Mittelstaedt A, Staab EV, Gaisie G. Mesenteric cyst: Sonographic appearance with CT correlation. *Pediatr Radiol* 1984;14:102–104.
14. Gore RM, Shkolnik A. Abdominal manifestations of pediatric leukemias: Sonographic assessment. *Radiology* 1982;143:207–210.
15. Haller JO, Schneider M, Kassner EG, Slovis TL, Perl LJ. Sonographic evaluation of mesenteric and omental masses in children. *AJR* 1978;130:269–274.
16. Heiken JP. Abdominal wall and peritoneal cavity. In: Lee KTL, Sagel SS, Stanley RJ, eds. *Computed Body Tomography with MRI Correlation.* New York: Raven Press, 1989:661–705.
17. Hill SC, Reinig JW, Barranger JA, Fink J, Shawker TH. Gaucher disease: Sonographic appearance of the spleen. *Radiology* 1986;160:631–634.
18. Jequier S, Guttman F, Lafortune M. Non-surgical treatment of a congenital splenic cyst. *Pediatr Radiol* 1987;17:248–249.
19. Johnson MA, Cooperberg PL, Boisvert J, Stoller JL, Winrob H. Spontaneous splenic rupture in infectious mononucleosis: Sonographic diagnosis and follow-up. *AJR* 1981;136:111–114.
20. Kaufman RA, Silver TM, Wesley JR. Preoperative diagnosis of splenic cysts in children by gray scale ultrasonography. *J Pediatr Surg* 1979;14:450–454.
21. Kaufman RA, Towbin R, Babcock DS, et al. Upper abdominal trauma in children: Imaging evaluation. *AJR* 1984;142:449–460.
22. Kay CJ, Pawar S, Rosenfield AT. Sonography of splenic abscesses. *Semin Ultrasound* 1983;4:91–101.
23. King DJ, Dawson AA, Bayliss AP. The value of ultrasonic scanning of the spleen in lymphoma. *Clin Radiol* 1985;36:473–474.
24. Kumpe DA, Rumack CM, Pretorius DH, Stoecker TJ, Stellin GP. Partial splenic embolization in children with hypersplenism. *Radiology* 1985;155:357–362.
25. Lupien C, Sauerbrei EE. Healing in the traumatized spleen: Sonographic investigation. *Radiology* 1984;151:181–185.
26. Meyers MA, ed. *Dynamic Radiology of the Abdomen. Normal and Pathologic Anatomy,* 3rd. ed. New York: Springer-Verlag, 1988.
27. Miller JH, Greenfield LD, Wald BR. Candidiasis of the liver and spleen in childhood. *Radiology* 1982;142:375–380.
28. Pastakia B, Shawker TH, Thaler M, O'Leary T, Pizzo PA. Hepatosplenic candidiasis: Wheels within wheels *Radiology* 1988;166:417–421.
29. Pawar S, Kay CJ, Gonzalez R, Taylor KJW, Rosenfield AT. Sonography of splenic abscess. *AJR* 1982;138:259–262.
30. Ralls PW, Quinn MF, Colletti P, Lapin SA, Halls J. Sonography of pyogenic splenic abscess. *AJR* 1982;138:523–525.
31. Rao BK, AuBuchon J, Lieberman LM, Polcyn RE. Cystic lymphangiomatosis of the spleen: A radiologic-pathologic correlation. *Radiology* 1981;141:781–782.
32. Rose SC, Kumpe DA, Manco-Johnson ML. Radiographic appearance of diffuse splenic hemangiomatosis. *Gastrointest Radiol* 1986;11:342–345.
33. Rudick MG, Wood BP, Lerner RM. Splenic abscess diagnosed by ultrasound in the pediatric patient. Report of three cases. *Pediatr Radiol* 1983;13:269–271.
34. Setiawan H, Harrell RS, Perret RS. Ectopic spleen. A sonographic diagnosis. *Pediatr Radiol* 1982;12:152–153.
35. Shackelford GD, McAlister WM. Cysts of the omentum. *Pediatr Radiol* 1975;3:152–155.
36. Shirkhoda A, Wallace S, Sokhandan M. Computed tomography and ultrasonography in splenic infarction. *J Can Assoc Radiol* 1985;36:29–33.
37. Smevik B, Monclair T. Torsion of a wandering spleen in an infant. Report of a case and a brief review of the literature. *Acta Radiol Diagnosis* 1986;27:715–717.
38. Solbiati L, Bossi MC, Bellotti E, Ravetto C, Montali G. Focal lesions in the spleen: Sonographic patterns and guided biopsy. *AJR* 1983;140:59–65.
39. Subramanyam BR, Balthazar EJ, Horii SC. Sonography of the accessory spleen. *AJR* 1984;143:47–49.
40. Sumner TE, Volberg FM, Chauvenet AR, Abramson JS, Turner CS, Young LW. Radiological case of the month. Hepatic and splenic candidiasis in acute leukemia. *Am J Dis Child* 1983;137:1193–1194.
41. Thurber LA, Cooperberg PL, Clement JG, Lyons FA, Gramiak R, Cunningham J. Echogenic fluid: A pitfall in the ultrasonographic diagnosis of cystic lesions. *JCU* 1979;7:273–278.
42. Tonkin IL, Tonkin AK. Visceroatrial situs abnormalities: Sonographic and computed tomographic appearance. *AJR* 1982;138:509–515.
43. Vermylen C, Lebecque P, Claus D, Otte JB, Cornu G. The wandering spleen. *Eur J Pediatr* 1983;140:112–115.

44. Vick CW, Hartenberg MA, Allen HA, Haynes JW. Abdominal pseudotumor caused by gastric displacement of the spleen: sonographic demonstration. *Pediatr Radiol* 1985;15:253–254.

45. Voet D, Afschrift M, Nachtegaele P, Delbeke MJ, Schelstraete K, Benoit Y. Sonographic diagnosis of an accessory spleen in recurrent idiopathic thrombocytopenic purpura. *Pediatr Radiol* 1983;13:39–41.

46. Waligore MP, Stephens DH, Soule EH, McLeod RA. Lipomatous tumors of the abdominal cavity: CT appearance and pathologic correlation. *AJR* 1981;137:539–545.

7

Gastrointestinal Tract

William H. McAlister

Barium examination has been the traditional study for evaluating gastrointestinal diseases, but recently, sonography has become an important addition in the study of the gastrointestinal tract (18,74,94). Barium studies remain the method of choice for the evaluation of the mucosal surface and contour of the bowel lumen, but these studies provide only limited information about the bowel wall or extrinsic abnormalities. Sonography has the advantage of being able to demonstrate the bowel wall as well as the bowel lumen, and can provide useful diagnostic information. In some instances, specifically in the diagnosis of pyloric stenosis and appendicitis, it is replacing conventional barium studies.

Knowledge of the sonographic appearance of the normal gastrointestinal tract is important in order to diagnose abnormalities. A discussion of the methods for examining each segment of the gastrointestinal tract is offered in appropriate sections of this chapter.

ORAL CAVITY, HYPOPHARYNX, AND ESOPHAGUS

Normal Anatomy

Most of the esophagus, when adequately distended, can be imaged by sonography through a suprasternal, parasternal, subcostal, or subxiphoid approach. The subcostal or subxiphoid approaches have been used most frequently because the liver provides an excellent acoustic window. These approaches allow for evaluation of the distal esophageal segment and the gastroesophageal junction. The examination is best performed with the patient supine or in the right lateral decubitus position. Scans are obtained in transverse and longitudinal planes.

The esophagus is recognized as a tubular structure with an echogenic center representing collapsed mucosa and submucosa, surrounded by a sonolucent outer wall representing muscle. Frequently, small amounts of fluid and gas are present in the lumen. The gastroesophageal junction appears as a bull's-eye or target structure. On longitudinal scans it lies anterior to the aorta, posterior to the left lobe of the liver, and adjacent to the diaphragm (Fig. 1). Sonography has been used to evaluate the tongue and swallowing mechanism, but it is difficult to perform and has limited applicability.

Gastroesophageal Reflux

Gastroesophageal reflux is the retrograde flow of gastric contents into the esophagus. Patients may be asymptomatic or present with vomiting, hematemesis, failure to thrive, weight loss, recurrent pneumonias, wheezing, and apnea (96). Barium esophagography has been the standard procedure for evaluating gastroesophageal reflux, but it may miss mild or intermittent reflux. Continuous pH monitoring and radionuclide scintigraphy are more sensitive in demonstrating reflux, and the scintigram also can record the presence of aspiration into the lungs.

More recently, real-time sonography has been used for the evaluation of gastrointestinal reflux in infancy (104). The sonographic technique is relatively straightforward. The infant is given the amount of fluid equivalent to a normal feeding. This is administered orally or via a nasogastric tube if necessary, 15 to 45 min before the start of the examination. With the transducer oriented in the longitudinal and transverse planes and positioned in the subxiphoid region, the distal esophagus, gastroesophageal junction, and abdominal portion of the esophagus are easily imaged. The sonographic appearance of gastroesophageal reflux varies with the amount of fluid and gas within the stomach. On sonography, the refluxed gastric contents are an admixture of hypoechoic fluid and echogenic gas

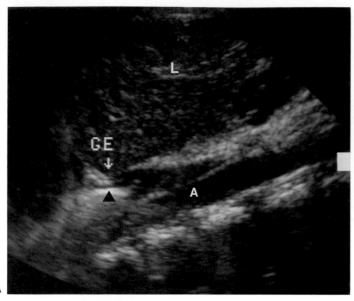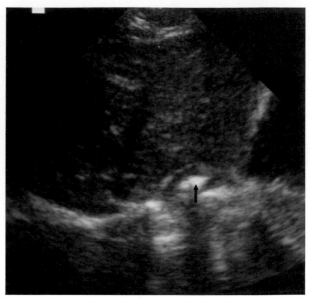

A   B

FIG. 1. Normal gastroesophageal junction. **A:** Longitudinal scan at the level of the gastroesophageal junction (*GE, arrow*) shows the esophagus with air bubbles (*arrowhead*) anterior to the
aorta (*A*) and posterior to the left lobe of the liver (*L*). **B:** Transverse scan shows the air-containing
esophagus (*arrow*) surrounded by a sonolucent wall.

bubbles (Fig. 2). Determination of the length of the
intraabdominal esophagus and the acuteness of the
angle of the gastroesophageal junction can be determined, although the clinical utility of these measurements is uncertain.

Several studies have shown that sonography is as
sensitive as pH monitoring in detecting reflux (114).
However, sonography is time consuming and difficult

to perform, particularly in the crying, uncooperative
child in whom it is not easy to obtain a good acoustic
window. Therefore, it is unlikely that sonography will
replace other methods of evaluation (75).

STOMACH

Normal Anatomy

The stomach can be evaluated if it is distended with
fluid, either by having the patient drink tap water or
by instilling fluid through a nasogastric tube. The body
and distal stomach are imaged through an epigastric
window with the patient supine or in a right lateral
decubitus position. The fundus may be imaged through
the left lobe of the liver or through the lower ribs or
spleen.

The antropyloric region is of particular interest in
pediatrics because of the number of disease processes
that affect this region. With the patient in a right lateral
decubitus position, a linear array transducer is positioned transversely slightly to the right of midline and
rotated slowly to visualize the long axis of the distal
stomach. The transducer is then rotated longitudinally,
approximately 90° perpendicular to the long axis of the
channel, to obtain cross-sectional views of the antropyloric region. The gastric antrum can be seen as a
target or bull's-eye structure on longitudinal scanning.
Three layers are often seen: an anechoic center representing fluid in the canal, an adjacent echogenic layer
representing mucosa and submucosa, and an outer hy-

FIG. 2. Gastroesophageal reflux. Longitudinal scan at
gastroesophageal junction shows fluid refluxing into the
esophagus (*arrows*). Echogenic foci within the fluid represent gas bubbles. *A*, aorta. *L*, liver.

poechoic rim representing muscle (Fig. 3). The normal thickness of the wall, measured from the inner edge of the echogenic mucosal layer to the outer edge of the hypoechoic wall, should be less than 4 mm in children (63,89,101). In adults, bowel wall thickness is between 4 and 6 mm (57). The hypoechoic muscle layer alone is 2 mm or less in diameter. It is important to obtain measurements of muscle wall thickness with the antrum distended by fluid to avoid confusing a contracted antrum with a thickened muscle (see Fig. 3) (105).

Evaluation of gastric peristalsis and emptying can be useful to diagnose conditions that obstruct the distal stomach, such as pyloric stenosis, or that delay gastric emptying, such as antral dyskinesia or peptic ulcer disease (97). Although sonographic measurements of gastric emptying time in response to predetermined amounts of gastric fluid are available, sonography probably will not replace scintigraphy for the evaluation of gastric emptying because scintigraphy has the advantage of providing quantitative measures and can determine residual volume in the stomach (62,101).

Microgastria

Microgastria is an unusual condition in which the stomach is midline in position. It often is seen with the polysplenia-asplenia syndrome and with malrotation. When distended with fluid, the midline tubular stomach can be easily recognized by sonography (5). Gastroesophageal reflux also is common.

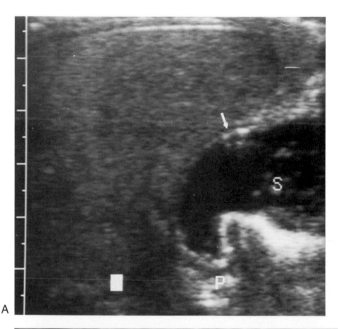

A

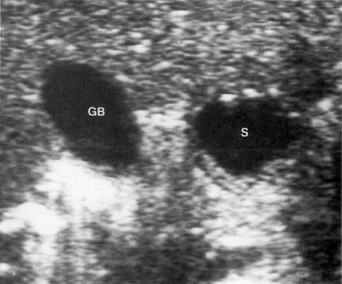

B

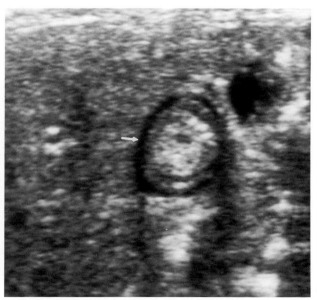

C

FIG. 3. Normal stomach. **A:** Scan along the long axis of the distal stomach (*S*) shows the fluid-filled lumen, echogenic mucosa, thin sonolucent muscle layer (*arrow*), and pyloroduodenal junction (*P*). **B:** Cross-sectional image with the stomach (*S*) distended. The wall is thin and barely visible. *GB*, gallbladder. **C:** Cross-sectional scan through a contracted distal stomach. Note that the antral wall appears slightly thickened and has a target or bull's eye appearance. *Arrow*, hypoechoic muscle.

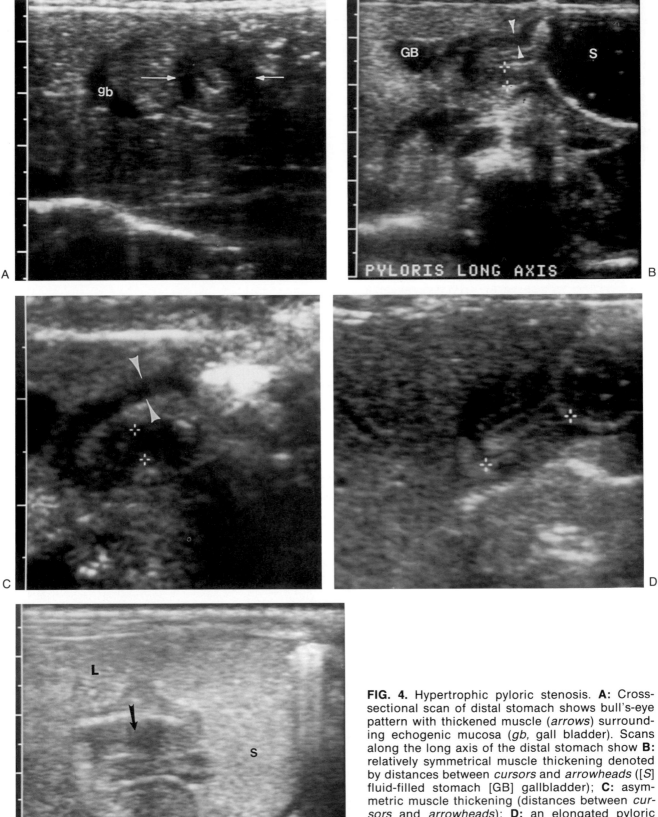

FIG. 4. Hypertrophic pyloric stenosis. **A:** Cross-sectional scan of distal stomach shows bull's-eye pattern with thickened muscle (*arrows*) surrounding echogenic mucosa (*gb,* gall bladder). Scans along the long axis of the distal stomach show **B:** relatively symmetrical muscle thickening denoted by distances between *cursors* and *arrowheads* ([*S*] fluid-filled stomach [GB] gallbladder); **C:** asymmetric muscle thickening (distances between *cursors* and *arrowheads*); **D:** an elongated pyloric channel (*cursors*); and **E:** double tract sign. The echogenicity of the muscle (*arrow*) is similar to the liver (*L*). The stomach (*S*) appears echogenic because it contains barium sulfate.

Obstruction

Hypertrophic Pyloric Stenosis

Hypertrophic pyloric stenosis (HPS) is a common abnormality of neonates and young infants characterized by hypertrophy of the circular muscle of the pylorus, which then proceeds to elongate and constrict the pyloric canal. The incidence of this disease is approximately 3 in 1000; boys are affected more than girls, and there is a familial pattern (98). Typically, patients present with projectile vomiting at 3 to 6 weeks of age, but symptoms may present at birth or as late as 5 months of age (89).

In patients in whom the diagnosis is clinically obvious, radiologic evaluation is unnecessary. When the clinical findings are unclear or equivocal, imaging studies are indicated. Recent series have shown that nearly 80% of patients with suspected HPS will have at least one imaging study (25). Until the advent of sonography, the upper gastrointestinal series was the examination of choice. Error rates of barium studies for diagnosing HPS range between 4.5% and 11% (16,48,49).

Currently, sonography is preferred for patients in whom there is a high clinical suspicion of HPS, because it can provide direct visualization of the pyloric muscle. When specifically examining for HPS, the procedure is begun with the patient in the supine position. Fluid administration may be unnecessary since the stomach is often filled with fluid due to the underlying obstruction. If, however, the distal stomach does not contain sufficient fluid (usually because the patient has been vomiting), fluid is administered in small amounts orally or through a nasogastric tube. It is important to avoid overdistention of the stomach, which in association with a posteriorly directed antrum may lead to a missed diagnosis of HPS (105). If fluid is placed in the stomach, it should be removed at the end of examination to prevent vomiting and potential aspiration. Because of the high incidence of associated renal anomalies, the kidneys should be examined when the diagnosis of HPS is made (8).

The findings of HPS include: (a) thickening of the pyloric muscle, which may be asymmetrical, (b) an elongated pyloric canal, (c) "double track" sign or linear echolucencies within the echogenic pyloric mucosa (31), (d) extension of the hypertrophied pyloric muscle into the fluid-filled antrum and the elongated narrow pyloric channel (11), (e) exaggerated peristaltic waves, and (f) delayed gastric emptying with failure to image the descending duodenum (Fig. 4). The hypertrophied pyloric muscle usually is hypoechoic relative to liver. Rarely, it is isoechoic (49).

Three objective measurements are available for evaluating HPS. These include the cross-sectional di-

ameter of the entire pylorus, muscle thickness of one wall, and length of the pyloric canal. The following measurements are characteristic of HPS: a diameter of 15 mm or greater, muscle thickness of 4 mm or greater, and a channel length equal to or greater than 18 mm. By contrast, normal muscle thickness is between 2.0 and 2.2 mm (63,89). Recent studies have suggested that of all measurements, muscle thickness is the most reliable and specific criteria for HPS (18). Although measurements of pyloric muscle volume have been established, they have not gained wide acceptance (113).

It is important to recognize that the size of the pyloric muscle mass is related to infant age. The diagnostic criteria that are appropriate for term infants may not be appropriate for premature infants. In these infants, the pliability and thickness of the pyloric muscle relative to the antrum are more important than specific dimensions (17). A diagnosis of HPS has been documented in premature infants with muscle thicknesses measuring 2.1 mm or less (15).

If the sonogram is positive, no additional imaging studies need to be performed and the patient requires surgery. If the stomach is well-distended and the sonogram is equivocal for HPS, a barium study should be performed for further evaluation.

Following surgery, 2 to 6 weeks are required for muscle hypertrophy to resolve (Fig. 5) (81). Therefore, sonography cannot be used in the early postoperative

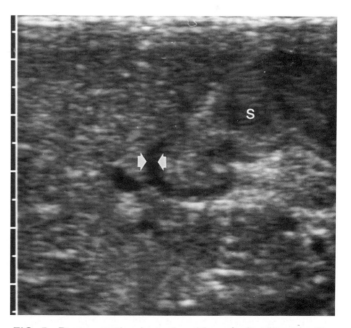

FIG. 5. Postoperative hypertrophic pyloric stenosis. Patient with persistent vomiting due to gastroesophageal reflux. Scan along the long axis of the distal stomach (*S*) shows residual muscle hypertrophy (*arrows*). Muscle thickness measures 3 mm. Four weeks earlier the wall thickness was 5.5 mm.

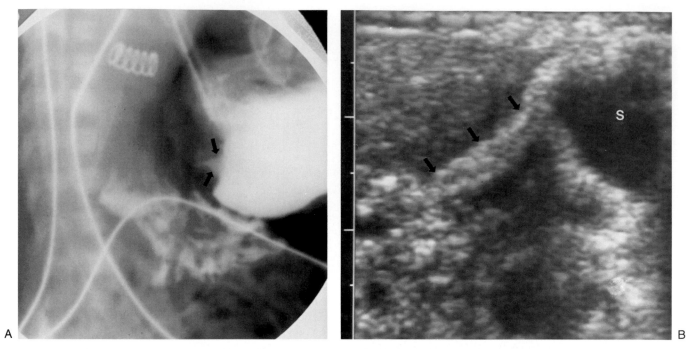

FIG. 6. Antral dyskinesia in a 10-day-old infant with persistent vomiting. **A:** An upper gastrointestinal series shows minimal filling of the pyloric channel suggestive of hypertrophic pyloric stenosis (*arrows*). **B:** Scan along long axis of the distal stomach (*S*) demonstrates an elongated contracted antrum (*arrows*) with echogenic mucosa and a normal muscle thickness of 2 mm. The patient did well on conservative management.

period to assess for incomplete pyloromyotomy in patients with persistent vomiting (55).

Antral Dyskinesia Syndrome

Infants with antral dyskinesia have recurrent non-bilious vomiting. Upper gastrointestinal series typically demonstrate a funnel-shaped antrum with absent peristalsis and delayed gastric emptying (105). If barium studies are equivocal and antral dyskinesia cannot be separated from pyloric stenosis, sonography can help to differentiate between the two conditions (41). Sonographic findings of antral dyskinesia include an elongated pyloric-antral channel without muscle hypertrophy, sluggish peristalsis, and delayed gastric emptying (Fig. 6).

Pyloric Atresia

Pyloric atresia is a rare congenital anomaly that presents with vomiting on the first or second day of life and may be isolated or associated with esophageal atresia or epidermolysis bullosa. Pathologically, the most common finding is an intraluminal diaphragm or web without an aperture. The distended stomach is easily recognized on sonography by its characteristic configuration and location (Fig. 7) (29).

Antral Membranes

Antral membranes usually are found in infants under 6 months of age. The majority are located 1 to 2 cm proximal to the pylorus and are incomplete with a central or eccentric aperture. If the opening is large, the diaphragm or web may be incompletely obstructing and the patient may be asymptomatic. If the aperture is small, the patient usually presents early with vomiting. Sonographically, the web appears as a linear echodensity extending into the fluid-filled gastric lumen.

Gastric Wall Thickening

Peptic Ulcer Disease and Gastritis

Peptic ulcer disease in children is relatively rare. Duodenal ulcers are more common than gastric ulcers in older children, whereas in neonates and young infants, gastric ulcers are more frequent. Affected patients typically present with vomiting or hematemesis. Sonographically, gastritis, secondary to peptic ulcer disease, produces elongation of the antropyloric canal

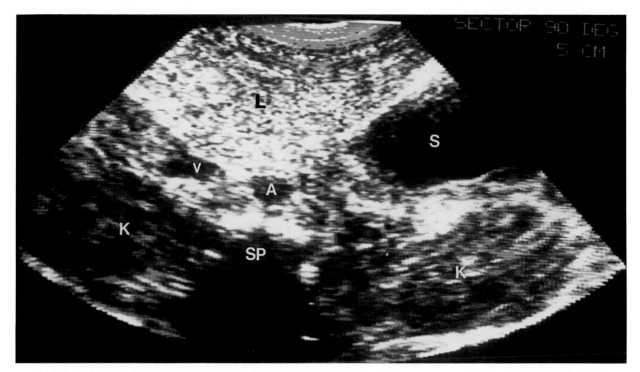

FIG. 7. Pyloric atresia. Transverse scan of the abdomen shows a fluid-filled stomach (*S*). This newborn infant had esophageal atresia without fistula and a gasless abdomen. *A*, aorta; *V*, inferior vena cava; *SP*, spine; *L*, liver; *K*, kidney.

with thickened echogenic mucosa (Fig. 8). Antropyloric wall thickening ranging between 4.5 and 7 mm may be present with gastric ulcers (52). Other findings include pylorospasm, delayed gastric emptying, and a visible ulcer crater (52).

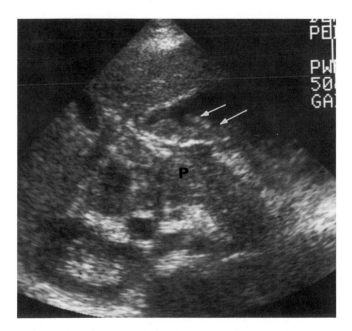

FIG. 8. Gastritis. Transverse scan of the abdomen shows polypoid thickening of the posterior surface of the stomach (*arrows*). The pancreas (*P*) is enlarged due to pancreatitis. Endoscopy confirmed gastric inflammation, presumably from the adjacent pancreatitis.

The complications of peptic ulcer disease include obstruction, wall penetration, and perforation. The latter two complications may be unapparent on contrast studies. With sonography, leaking gastric contents appear as a localized fluid collection which may be hypoechoic, complex, or echogenic. The fluid surrounds the site of the perforation and, in contrast to free peritoneal fluid, does not change shape or position when the patient's position is changed (69). Pneumoperitoneum secondary to perforation appears as an echogenic line with a posterior ring-down or reverberation artifact between the anterior abdominal wall and anterior surface of the liver (64). In addition to diagnosing ulcer craters and their complications, sonography can be used in the follow-up evaluation of patients with gastritis and peptic ulcer disease (108).

Ménétrier's Disease

Approximately 7% of all cases of Ménétrier's disease occur in childhood, usually affecting children under 15 years of age (12). Edema of the extremities or eyelids is the most common presenting symptom, although anorexia, abdominal pain, and vomiting are frequent also. Cytomegalovirus has been obtained from the gastric mucosa in some cases, suggesting that the disease process may have a viral etiology. Normally, the disease resolves spontaneously within a few weeks to a few months. Sonographic features of Ménétrier's disease are a thickened, echogenic, and tortuous mucosa.

Chronic Granulomatous Disease

Chronic granulomatous disease of childhood is an X-linked recessive disorder resulting from a defect in the bacteriolytic activity of polymorphonuclear leukocytes. Typically, patients present before 3 years of age with findings of lymphadenopathy, hepatosplenomegaly, pneumonia, and intermittent abdominal pain. Of the segments of the gastrointestinal tract, the distal stomach is the area characteristically involved. Pathologically, the wall is thickened and there are inflammatory and granulomatous changes in the lamina propria, submucosa, smooth muscle, and serosa. On sonography, there typically is circumferential antral thickening, although the proximal stomach can be involved (Fig. 9) (61). Such thickening is nonspecific and cannot be differentiated from eosinophilic enteritis, Crohn's disease, and acid ingestion. Clinical correlation or biopsy is required for the definitive diagnosis.

Mass Lesions

Gastric Duplication

Gastric duplications account for less than 5% of all gastrointestinal tract duplications. They usually occur along the greater curvature, measure less than 12 cm in diameter, and do not communicate with the stomach. On sonography a gastric duplication is a cystic mass with a thin echogenic lining representing mucosa, and a thick outer hypoechoic rim representing muscle (76). Internal contents occasionally may be echogenic due to hemorrhage and inspissated mucus.

Teratoma

Teratomas are the most common gastric neoplasms in patients under one year of age. Pathologically, these lesions are benign, large (5–20 cm in diameter), extraluminal masses that often contain calcification. Sonographically, teratomas are predominantly hypoechoic areas of intense echogenicity with associated shad-

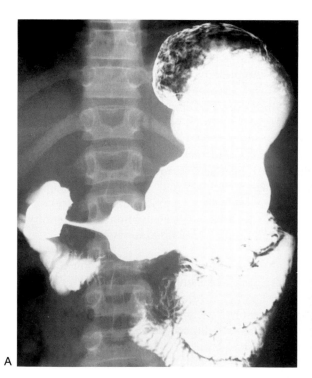
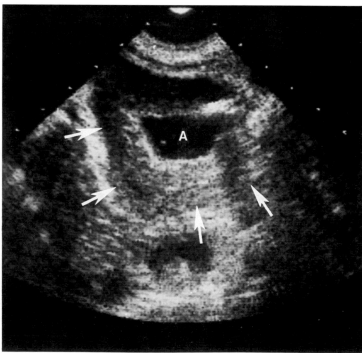

FIG. 9. Chronic granulomatous disease of children. **A:** Upper gastrointestinal series shows marked narrowing of the distal stomach. **B:** Longitudinal scan of the distal stomach in cross-section demonstrates a sonolucent fluid-containing antrum (*A*) surrounded by a hypoechoic thick wall (*arrows*). The stomach returned to normal after 1 month of conservative management.

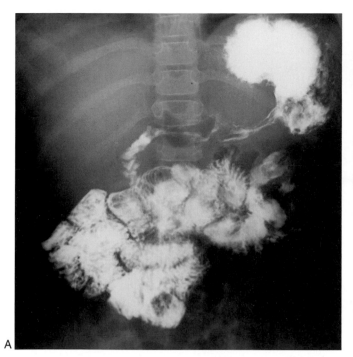

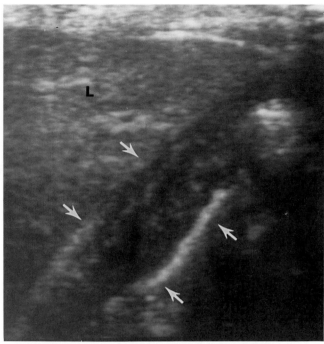

FIG. 10. Inflammatory pseudotumor. **A:** Upper gastrointestinal series shows marked narrowing of distal half of stomach. **B:** Longitudinal scan of involved area shows the gastric wall (*arrows*) to be hypoechoic and thickened. There is no fluid in the lumen of the stomach. *L,* liver.

owing, reflecting the presence of calcification. Intra- and extraluminal components typically are present (23).

Inflammatory Pseudotumor

Inflammatory pseudotumor, also known as plasma cell granuloma or fibroxanthoma, tends to occur along the greater curvature of the stomach and in the terminal ileum (71). The etiology is unknown, but it may represent an unusual variant of an inflammatory response. Clinically, patients present with fever, weight loss, abdominal mass, and anemia. On sonography, inflammatory pseudotumor may appear as a poorly defined lesion with mixed echogenicity due to hemorrhage and necrosis or as diffuse wall thickening (Fig. 10). Associated adenopathy may be noted. The tumor is aggressive and tends to recur if not completely resected.

Focal Foveolar Hyperplasia

Focal or polypoid foveolar hyperplasia is a type of gastric polyp. The normal gastric fovea are pits within the mucosa into which the deep gastric glands empty. Occasionally these pits become prominent and tortuous, possibly secondary to obstruction, and appear as one or more polypoid masses. Patients may present with symptoms of obstruction or with hematemesis. On sonography, focal foveolar hyperplasia appears as an echogenic polypoid mass that is superficial to muscle and therefore mucosal in origin (Fig. 11) (72). The localized extent of involvement is important in differentiating this condition from diffuse inflammatory disease.

Bezoars

Trichobezoars (hair) are more common than phytobezoars (vegetable matter) in childhood. Although sonography is not the imaging study of choice, it may be the initial examination because many of these patients present with an epigastric mass or tenderness and weight loss. Sonographic findings of a trichobezoar consist of a hyperechoic curvilinear band surrounding an echogenic intraluminal gastric mass that has marked acoustic shadowing and no through-transmission (70,73). Administration of oral fluid can be useful in confirming the intraluminal location of the

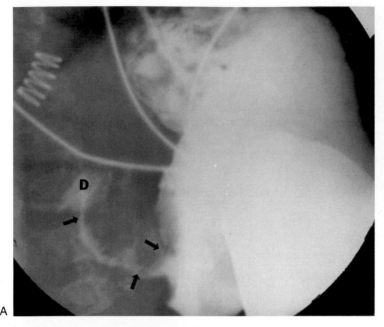

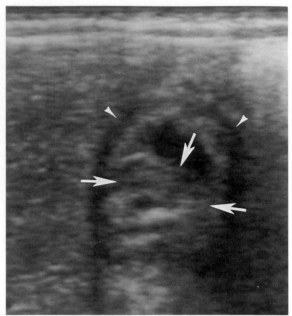

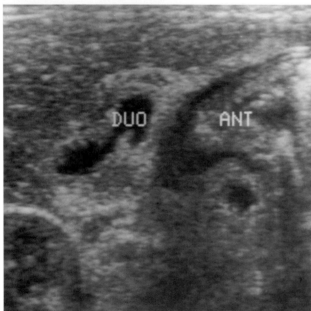

FIG. 11. Focal foveolar hyperplasia in a 6-week-old with vomiting. **A:** Upper gastrointestinal series shows a mass in the distal stomach with an irregular central channel (*arrows*), suggestive of pyloric stenosis. *D,* duodenal bulb. **B:** Scan along the long axis of the distal stomach and duodenum (*DUO*) shows the antral mucosa (*ANT*) to be thickened. **C:** Scan of the distal stomach in cross-section shows thickened echogenic polypoid mucosa (*arrows*) surrounded by normal hypoechoic muscle (*arrowheads*).

mass. Phytobezoars are generally seen in older patients and may be echogenic or complex. They do not have the marked shadowing seen with trichobezoars.

Miscellaneous

Although gastric neoplasms are rare, benign lesions such as leiomyoma, polyps (Fig. 12), and malignant tumors, including carcinoma and lymphoma, have been reported. These tumors are generally hypoechoic. There may be marked thickening of the gastric wall due to tumor infiltration, producing a target appearance. While the target appearance may be seen with tumor, it also may be observed secondary to inflammatory conditions. Differentiation requires tissue sampling (80,92).

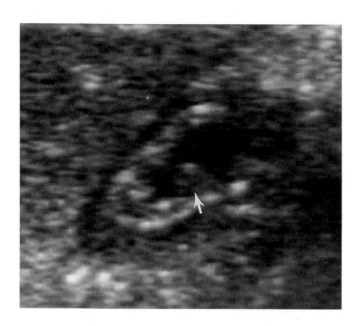

FIG. 12. Gastric polyp. Scan of the distal stomach in cross-section demonstrates a polyp (*arrow*), confirmed at endoscopy.

SMALL BOWEL

Normal Anatomy

Most of the small bowel, other than the duodenal bulb, is not visualized by sonography. When fluid-filled and with the patient in the right lateral decubitus position, the duodenal bulb can be seen as a discrete structure adjacent to the antrum (Fig. 13) (30). Fluid also can be noted to pass from the duodenal bulb into the descending and transverse portions of the duodenum. The fourth portion of the duodenum usually is not visualized by sonography.

Gas generally obscures visualization of the remainder of the small bowel. However, if there is adequate fluid within the bowel lumen, the small bowel can be

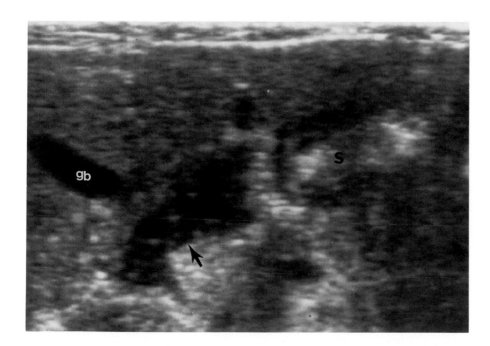

FIG. 13. Normal duodenum. Transverse scan of the abdomen shows the fluid-filled duodenal bulb (*arrow*) medial to the the gallbladder (*gb*). Small echodensities in the duodenum represent gas bubbles. *S*, stomach.

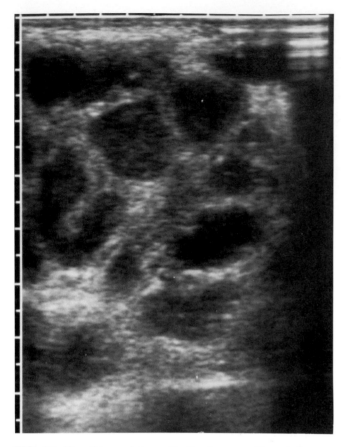

FIG. 14. Small bowel. Longitudinal scan of the abdomen shows multiple dilated small bowel loops without peristalsis in a patient with megacystis-microcolon-hypoperistalsis syndrome.

identified (Fig. 14) and the valvulae conniventes may be seen as separate linear echogenic structures 3 to 5 mm apart within the bowel lumen. Thickness measurements can be obtained if there is associated ascites. In adults, when the bowel is distended, the thickness of the wall, measured from the free edge of the fluid to the outer sonolucent muscle rim, should not exceed 3 mm. Wall thickness may range from 5 to 7 mm if the bowel is contracted. Strong echoes corresponding to gas bubbles or food particles may be seen in the fluid-filled bowel. On cross-section the small bowel, like all segments of the gastrointestinal tract, has a target appearance (43).

Obstruction

Small bowel obstruction in neonates may be due to duodenal atresia, malrotation, ileal or jejunal atresia, or meconium ileus; in older neonates and children, it is often due to intussusception, malrotation, or incarcerated hernia. Plain radiographs with contrast studies usually provide the correct diagnosis, but sonography may be helpful when there is complicated small bowel obstruction with perforation or a pseudocyst, when there is associated esophageal and small bowel atresia and air cannot enter the bowel lumen, or when conventional studies are equivocal (35,94). The sonographic appearance of small bowel obstruction is hyperactive, dilated, fluid-filled bowel, although this is a nonspecific appearance and can be seen with gastroenteritis.

Duodenal Atresia, Stenosis, and Diaphragms

Duodenal atresia and stenosis are common causes of neonatal bowel obstruction. The etiology is unknown, but most cases are believed to be the result of failure of recanalization of the fetal gut. Typically duodenal atresia and stenosis occur near the ampulla of Vater. Affected patients present within the first 24 hr of life with bilious vomiting. Associated anomalies are present in approximately one-half of patients. As many as 30% of patients with duodenal atresia have Down syndrome. Other anomalies include esophageal or small bowel atresia, malrotation, imperforate anus, congenital heart disease, and renal anomalies. Plain radiographs typically demonstrate dilatation of the stomach and duodenum with a characteristic double-bubble sign. With this appearance, additional imaging studies are unnecessary. However, when patients have been vomiting or when duodenal atresia is associated with esophageal atresia without an associated tracheoesophageal fistula, the diagnosis can be difficult to accomplish with conventional radiography since the abdomen is gasless (Fig. 15). Sonography is valuable in these situations because the distal esophagus, stomach, and duodenum are filled with fluid, providing an ideal window for sonography (Figs. 15,16) (94).

Duodenal diaphragms are thin webs that obstruct the second part of the duodenum at the level of the ampulla of Vater. Variable degrees of obstruction are present depending on the presence and size of an aperture in the diaphragm. If the diaphragm is complete, an obstruction similar to duodenal atresia is seen; if the aperture is substantial, obstruction can be incomplete or absent. On sonography, the diaphragm appears as an echogenic band in the dilated proximal duodenum (33).

Malrotation

Intestinal malrotation is a congenital anomaly of rotation involving the bowel segment that receives its blood supply from the superior mesenteric artery. Most patients are diagnosed in the first month of life

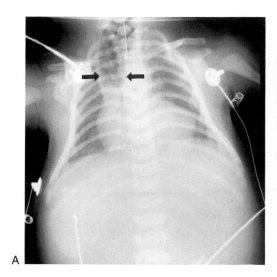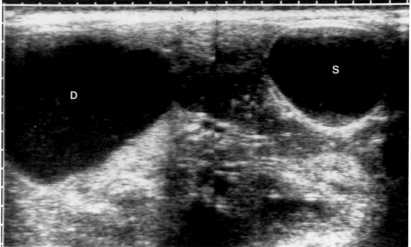

FIG. 15. Duodenal atresia with associated esophageal atresia. **A:** Chest and abdominal radiograph shows a dilated proximal esophageal pouch (*arrows*) with a distended gasless abdomen in a patient with Down syndrome. **B:** Transverse dual image scan of the upper abdomen demonstrates a dilated duodenal bulb (*D*) and stomach (*S*).

when they have sudden onset of bilious vomiting. Symptoms usually are due to volvulus or peritoneal bands. Normally the small bowel mesentery has a broad attachment extending from the ligament of Treitz to the ileocecal valve. The rotation anomalies are associated with a shortened base of the mesentery which predisposes to midgut volvulus. They also are accompanied by embryonic peritoneal bands that extend from the malpositioned colon to the posterolateral abdomen and porta hepatis. These bands may produce obstruction at the point where they cross the descending or transverse duodenum.

Plain radiographs of the abdomen in patients with malrotation may be normal or show evidence of high or low small-bowel obstruction. Upper gastrointestinal series can demonstrate the level of obstruction and the presence of an associated volvulus. Recently sonography has been used to demonstrate duodenal obstruction secondary to Ladd's bands or midgut volvulus. The duodenum proximal to the site of obstruction is dilated and hyperperistaltic with antegrade and retrograde peristalsis (51). Only the descending duodenum and the transverse portion of the duodenum to the right of the spine are visualized. These observations establish that the level of obstruction is at the third or transverse portion of the duodenum. Demonstration of an obstruction in the transverse duodenum in the neonate is strong presumptive evidence of malrotation with ob-

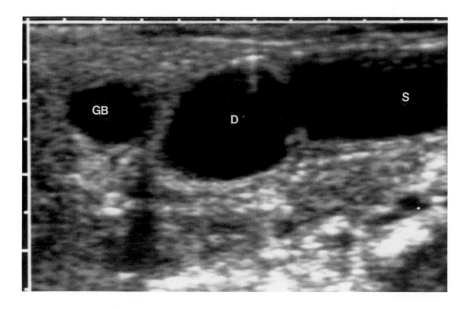

FIG. 16. Duodenal atresia. A 2-day-old infant with projectile vomiting and a gasless abdomen. Transverse scan of the upper abdomen shows the stomach (*S*), dilated pylorus, and blind-ending duodenal bulb (*D*) adjacent to the gallbladder (*GB*).

struction due either to duodenal bands or volvulus (Fig. 17). Other findings of malrotation include an abnormal relationship of the superior mesenteric artery and vein. The superior mesenteric vein normally is anterior and to the right of the superior mesenteric artery (Fig. 18). In malrotation, the superior mesenteric vein lies either directly anterior or to the left of the artery (66,78). It has not been established how frequently this anomalous relationship of the superior mesenteric artery and vein occurs in patients with malrotation, especially those without volvulus. Although sonography can determine that the duodenum is obstructed in pa-

tients with malrotation, it has not replaced the upper gastrointestinal series as the examination of choice for diagnosing malrotation. However, awareness of the findings of malrotation is important because it may be encountered incidentally in a child undergoing abdominal sonographic examination (1).

Jejunoileal Atresia and Meconium Ileus

Jejunoileal atresia is the result of an *in utero* vascular accident, whereas meconium ileus results from inspis-

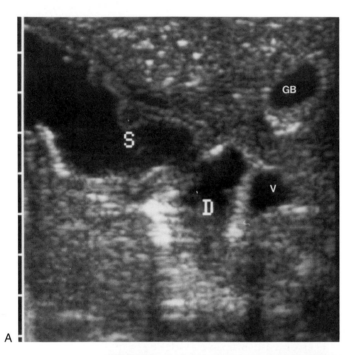

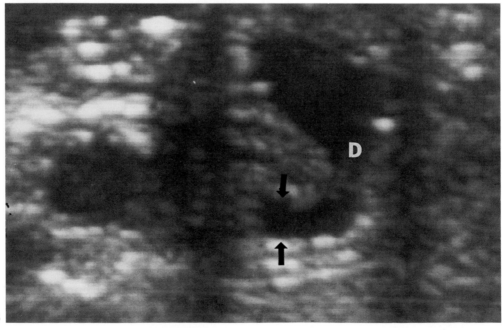

FIG. 17. Malrotation. **A:** Transverse abdominal scan in a patient with situs inversus and malrotation showing the stomach (*S*) and a slightly dilated duodenal bulb (*D*). Also noted are a preduodenal vein (*V*) and gallbladder (*GB*). **B:** A more caudal transverse scan shows obstruction of the descending duodenum (*D*) at the site of Ladd's band (*arrows*).

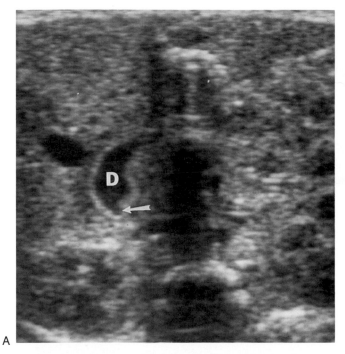

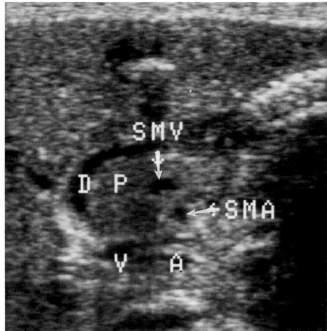

A

B

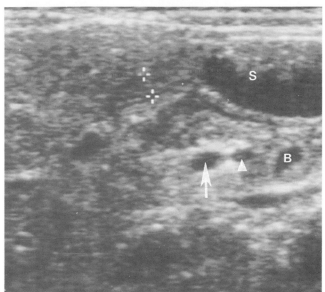

C

FIG. 18. Malrotation in a premature infant with bilious vomiting. **A:** Transverse scan of abdomen shows abrupt termination of the descending duodenum which has a tapering end (*arrow*). Hyperactive peristalsis was noted on real-time sonography. **B:** Anomalous relationship of the superior mesenteric artery (SMA) and superior mesenteric vein (*SMV*). The vein lies farther to the left than usual. Other structures in the image include the duodenum (*D*), pancreas (*P*), inferior vena cava (*V*), and aorta (*A*). **C:** Transverse abdominal scan showing the normal relationship of superior mesenteric vein (*arrow*) and artery (*arrowhead*) with vein at almost the same level as the artery. Stomach (*S*), hypertrophied muscle (*cursors*) of pyloric stenosis, and a bowel loop (*B*) are seen.

sation of abnormally thick and tenacious meconium in the distal small bowel. Both produce congenital bowel obstruction. The diagnosis of obstruction usually is evident on plain radiographs of the abdomen. If obstruction involves the jejunum, further radiographic evaluation usually is not required. If, however, distal bowel obstruction is suspected, a contrast enema may be useful for separating meconium ileus, ileal atresia, and other causes of obstruction. Sonography has no role in the evaluation of uncomplicated small bowel obstruction due to atresia or meconium ileus, but can be valuable in cases of complicated meconium ileus or ileal atresia. These complications include meconium peritonitis and pseudocysts.

Meconium peritonitis is a nonbacterial chemical peritonitis resulting from antenatal bowel perforation. Extrusion of sterile meconium produces an inflammatory reaction with subsequent dystrophic calcification. Calcifications may develop as soon as 12 hr after *in utero* perforation. When the calcified masses are sufficiently large, they can be visualized on sonography as foci of intense echogenicity with acoustic

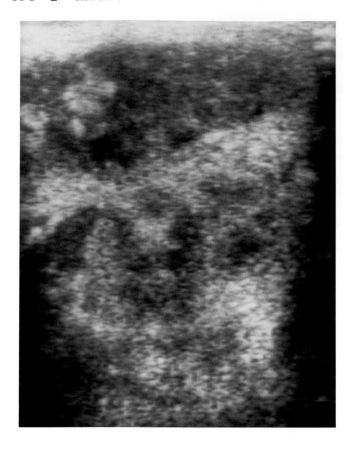

FIG. 19. Meconium peritonitis. Longitudinal scan of the abdomen demonstrates diffuse peritoneal echogenicity or "snowstorm" appearance. The patient had an ileal perforation proximal to an area of atresia.

shadowing. Occasionally the echogenicity is diffuse and referred to as a "snowstorm" appearance (Fig. 19). Calcifications also may extend into the scrotum through a patent process vaginalis.

In some cases of meconium peritonitis, the extruded meconium becomes walled off by fibrous adhesions, producing a cyst-like mass or pseudocyst (27). The cysts may contain only meconium or both meconium and encased bowel loops. Calcifications frequently develop in the cyst wall. On sonography, the cyst is usually well-defined and may be diffusely echogenic or heterogeneous, with areas of increased echogenicity that shadow (Fig. 20). The walls are usually well-defined, of variable thickness, and echogenic (22,28).

Rarely, sonography is performed on newborns with uncomplicated congenital bowel obstruction because the clinical findings are atypical, and perhaps suggest an abdominal mass. The usual appearance of uncomplicated ileal atresia and meconium ileus is multiple, dilated, fluid-filled bowel loops with active peristalsis. Occasionally in meconium ileus, the distal portion of the small bowel may appear echogenic with decreased peristalsis, reflecting obstruction by masses of thick, tenacious meconium (Fig. 21) (47). A small amount of ascites may be seen with either small bowel atresia or meconium ileus.

Intussusception

Intussusception is a frequent problem in childhood with peak incidence between the ages of 6 months and 2 yr. The disorder is more common in boys than girls (2 to 1 ratio). Peak seasonal incidence is during the time of year when respiratory and gastrointestinal infections occur. Signs and symptoms include pain, vomiting, rectal bleeding, and abdominal mass. Almost all pediatric intussusceptions are ileocolic; over 90% have no pathologic lead points and probably are due to hypertrophied Peyer's patches (40). Lead masses are more frequent in neonates and older children and tend to be duplications, polyps, Meckel's diverticulum, lymphoma, and hematomas (45,84). There is an increased incidence of intussusception in patients with cystic fibrosis (79) and following surgery (45).

Sonography is certainly not the primary radiologic means of diagnosing intussusception, but occasionally it has been requested for confusing abdominal symptoms and intussusception may then be noted. Several sonographic patterns of intussusception include the following: (a) a "donut" sign with a sonolucent outer rim surrounding a central echogenic area on cross-sectional images and a pseudokidney appearance on longitudinal scans; (b) multiple concentric circles with a

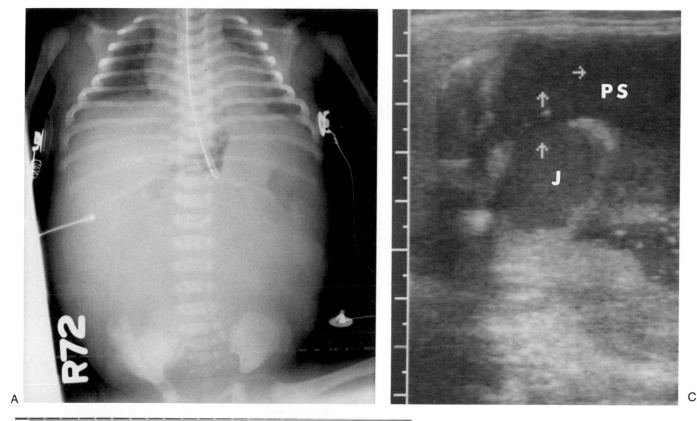

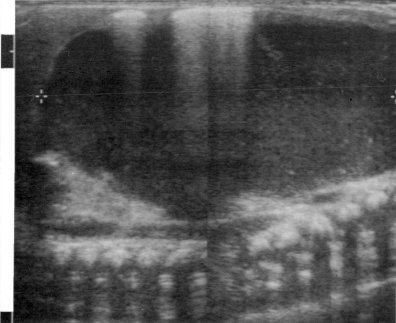

FIG. 20. Abdominal pseudocyst. **A:** Chest and abdomen radiograph demonstrates a small amount of bowel gas in a patient with a 6-hr distended abdomen. An abdominal mass was palpated. **B:** Longitudinal dual image scan of the abdomen demonstrates a huge, well-defined, fluid-filled mass (*cursors*) containing echogenic debris and a small amount of air anteriorly that produces distal shadowing. **C:** Longitudinal scan of the right upper quadrant shows a communication between the jejunum (*J*) and pseudocyst (*PS*) on real-time sonography; passage of fluid along the course designated by the *arrows* was seen.

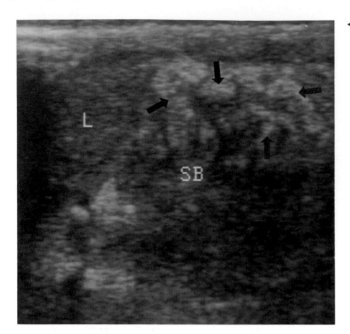

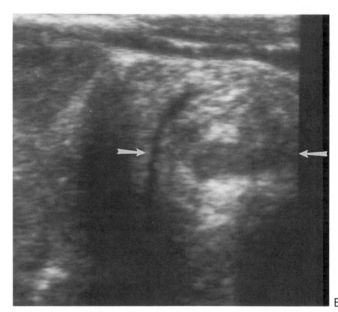

◀**FIG. 21.** Meconium ileus. Longitudinal scan of the abdomen shows small bowel (*SB*) filled with echogenic meconium (*arrows*). Echogenic meconium obscures visualization of small bowel posteriorly. *L*, liver.

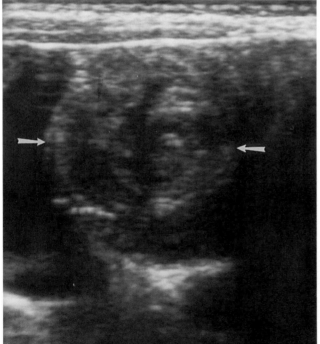

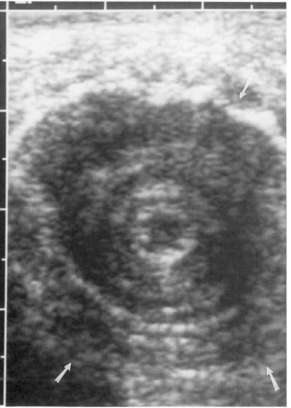

FIG. 22. Intussusception **A, B:** Longitudinal scans of the right upper quadrant in two patients and **C:** transverse scan in another patient show masses (*arrows*) with variable numbers of concentric rings. The layers have varying echogenicity, reflecting varying degrees of edema.

sonolucent center; and (c) a complex mass (24,26,103). The appearance varies with the degree of edema, and impaction of the mucosa and serosa of the various layers of the intussusception. With advanced edema only two layers are visible; with milder degrees of edema, there is less stretching and thinning of the serosa and mucosa, and multiple concentric rings can be identified (Fig. 22). When a lead mass is present, it may be directly imaged as a discrete soft tissue mass in the inner loop of bowel (3). Once intussusception has been diagnosed, hydrostatic reduction under sonographic control is possible (19).

Bowel Wall Thickening

Lymphangiectasia

Lymphangiectasia is a rare entity that produces dilated lacteals within intestinal villi. Presenting symptoms are generally peripheral edema or malabsorption with growth failure. Sonography demonstrates bowel wall thickening, separation of bowel loops by ascites,

and mesenteric edema (Fig. 23). At times dilated mesenteric lymphatics may be recognized (39). These can be distinguished from mesenteric blood vessels by Doppler studies, particularly color flow Doppler.

Crohn's Disease

Crohn's disease, or regional enteritis, is a chronic inflammatory bowel disease affecting children over 10 years of age. Patients typically present with chronic abdominal pain, diarrhea, weight loss, and fever, but occasionally the presentation is acute, suggesting appendicitis (4). The ileocecal area is involved in 35% to 60% of patients. In the remainder of patients, the disease involves the jejunum, proximal ileum, or colon alone.

Barium studies remain the primary method for demonstrating the mucosal extent of Crohn's disease. Sonography can be useful in detecting extramural complications, such as mesenteric abscesses and ureteral obstruction (99). On sonography, Crohn's disease appears as uniformly thickened bowel wall with a nar-

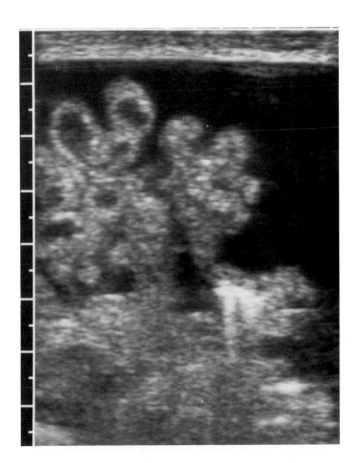

FIG. 23. Intestinal lymphangiectasia. Longitudinal scan of the right lower quadrant shows thickened small bowel loops projecting into chylous ascites.

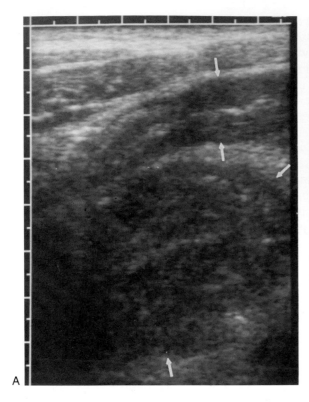

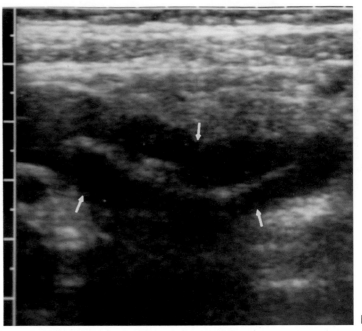

FIG. 24. Crohn's disease. **A, B:** Scans of the right lower quadrant in two patients. In each patient the ileum is abnormal, with markedly thickened hypoechoic bowel walls (*arrows*) surrounding echogenic mucosa centrally. The bowel lumen is collapsed.

rowed echogenic lumen (Fig. 24) (37). The abnormal bowel is contiguous with normal bowel lumen and is slightly compressible (Fig. 25). Enlarged lymph nodes also can be seen. An associated abscess appears as a poorly defined, irregular, hypoechoic, or complex mass, with or without echogenic densities representing air.

Acute Terminal Ileitis and Mesenteric Adenitis

Yersinia enterocolitis is one of the most common causes of acute terminal ileitis, usually presenting as mild gastroenteritis. In a few instances the enteritis may be severe, causing abdominal pain simulating appendicitis. The distal ileum is the most frequent site

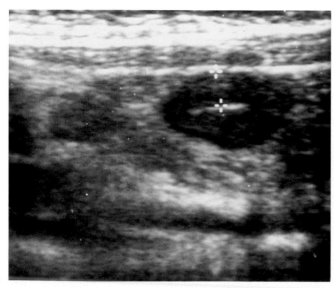

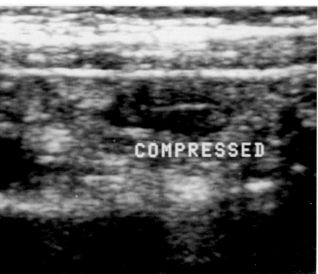

FIG. 25. Crohn's disease. **A:** Scan of the right lower quadrant shows a thickened loop of terminal ileum (*cursors*). **B:** Scan in same area shows the involved loop to be slightly compressible.

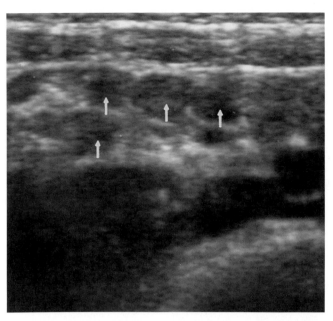

FIG. 26. *Yersinia enterocolitis.* Scan of the right lower quadrant demonstrates enlarged hypoechoic mesenteric lymph nodes (*arrows*).

of involvement, but changes in the colon can occur, especially later in the course of disease.

Sonographic examination can differentiate acute terminal ileitis from acute appendicitis. The sonographic findings of *Y. enterocolitis* include visualization of mural thickening of the terminal ileum with a target appearance on cross-section, slightly compressible bowel wall, and enlarged mesenteric lymph nodes (Fig. 26) (85). Bowel peristalsis is present, but usually diminished. Enlarged nodes are larger than 4 mm in diameter, are more numerous and sonolucent than normal nodes, and tend to be spherical in contrast to the disc-like shape of normal nodes. Mesenteric lymphadenopathy may be found in association with regional

enteritis, but generally the nodes are not as numerous or large as the nodes in patients with *Y. enterocolitis*. However, overlap does occur and a specific diagnosis will require fecal cultures, serologic studies for specific antibodies, or tissue sampling. In contrast to Crohn's disease, abscess is not a recognized feature of *Y. enterocolitis*. Complete resolution of lesions usually occurs spontaneously within a few weeks.

Other conditions that can cause a thick-walled terminal ileum include tuberculosis, histoplasmosis, *Campylobacter jejuni*, *Salmonella typhosa*, and Behçet's syndrome (85,87,99). Diagnosis requires stool culture or tissue sampling.

Masses

Small Bowel Tumors

Polyps and vascular neoplasms are the most common primary small bowel neoplasms; they may be isolated or associated with specific syndromes, such as Peutz-Jeghers, Cronkhite-Canada, Gardner's, or Sturge-Weber. The tumors can be seen sonographically if they are large enough, appearing as intraluminal oval structures or polyps.

Lymphoma is the most common small bowel malignancy. The peak age incidence in childhood is 5 to 8 years, with a male predominence. Clinical features include anemia, weight loss, anorexia, and a palpable abdominal mass. Abdominal pain may be present if there is an associated intussusception. Lymphoma may affect the small bowel primarily or as part of systemic involvement. The most frequent site of involvement is the ileocolic region. On sonography, the tumor may present as thickened bowel wall or as a complex mass with large anechoic areas due to necrosis (Fig. 27) (110). Small anechoic masses representing subse-

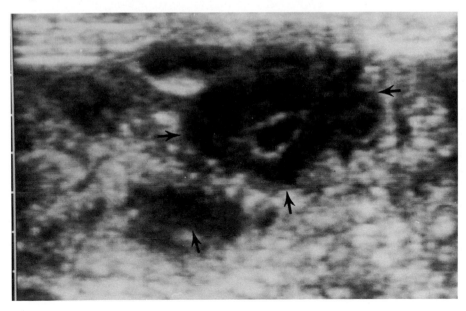

FIG. 27. Lymphoma. Transverse scan of the right mid abdomen demonstrates thickened bowel loops (*arrows*) with hypoechoic walls. (Courtesy of L. Magill, M.D., Memphis, TN.)

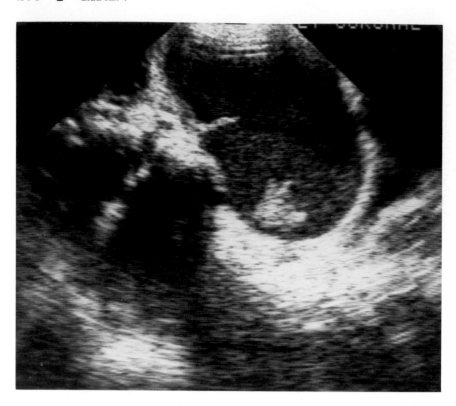

FIG. 28. Duplication in a 7-year-old with a palpable abdominal mass. Coronal scan of the mid abdomen shows a large cystic mass containing echogenic debris. Marked through-transmission is noted.

rosal or mesenteric nodal involvement also may be observed. Intussusception is an occasional finding. When present, splenomegaly and marked retroperitoneal adenopathy can help make the diagnosis of lymphoma.

Duplication

Small bowel duplications are believed to be the result of abnormal canalization, and are most common in the ileocecal area. The vast majority are diagnosed within the first year of life; clinical features include a palpable abdominal mass, abdominal distention, and vomiting. Bleeding may occur from ulceration of gastric mucosa within the duplication.

On sonography, the internal contents vary from anechoic or hypoechoic to echogenic, presumably because of thick contents, mucus, or blood (Figs. 28,29). Increased through-transmission is common. Occasionally an inner layer of echogenic mucosa is seen (Fig. 30), and when present can help separate duplications from mesenteric, ovarian, or choledochal cysts which do not have an echogenic lining (107). Often, however, the echogenic lining is not visualized and distinguishing between a duplication cyst and other abdominal cysts or chronically obstructed bowel loops may be difficult (Fig. 31).

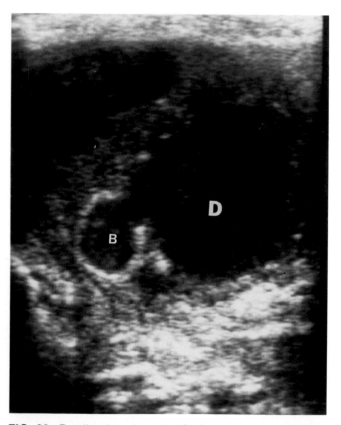

FIG. 29. Duplication. Longitudinal scan demonstrates a small bowel loop (*B*) communicating with a large hypoechoic duplication (*D*).

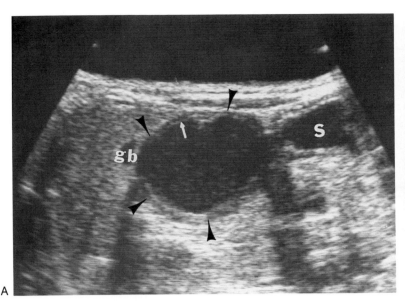 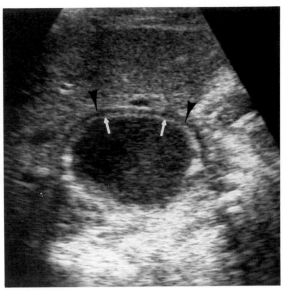

FIG. 30. Duodenal duplication. **A, B:** Transverse scans of upper abdomen show a hypoechoic duplication with echogenic mucosa (*arrows*) and hypoechoic muscle wall (*arrowheads*). *S,* stomach; *gb,* gallbladder. Echodensities within the duplication represent mucoid material.

Hematoma

Hematoma may result from accidental or nonaccidental trauma, Henoch-Schönlein purpura, bleeding diathesis, or leukemia (59,109). Since the duodenum is fixed in position, it is more often affected by trauma than is the rest of the gastrointestinal tract. Duodenal hematoma results from shearing of the duodenum between the superior mesenteric artery and spine, with extravasation of blood between the mucosa and serosa. Computerized tomography is the imaging procedure of choice to evaluate patients with severe, multiorgan, abdominal trauma (9). However, sonography may be used if there is localized injury (42,44,50,53,59,65). Hematoma may produce diffuse thickening of the bowel wall or a focal, eccentric mass

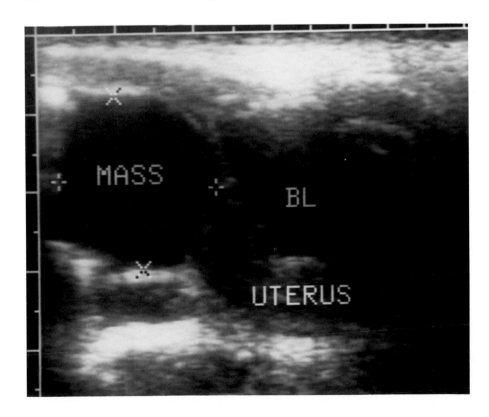

FIG. 31. Chronic obstructed bowel loop. Longitudinal scan of lower abdomen shows a cystic mass (*cursors*) superior to the bladder (*BL*) and uterus. At operation the mass was a loop of small bowel twisted around a peritoneal band.

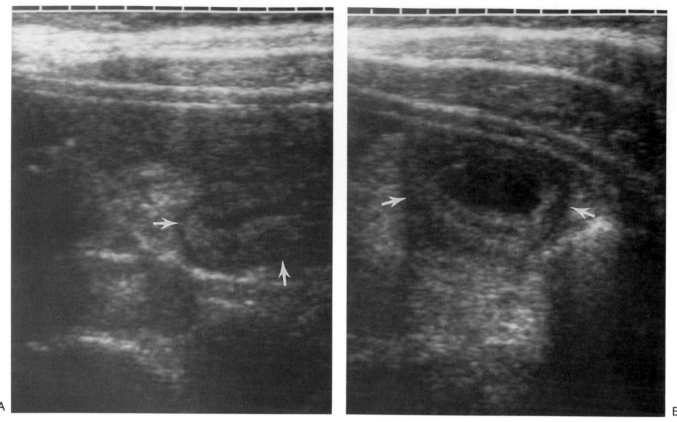

FIG. 32. Henoch-Schönlein's purpura. **A:** Longitudinal and **B:** transverse scans demonstrating thickening of the distal small bowel (*arrows*).

(Fig. 32). The echotexture is variable depending on the age of the hematoma. Initially, the hematoma is complex or mixed. With subsequent liquefaction it becomes more sonolucent. Later, it may become more echogenic as clot forms and retracts. Sonography also may detect associated injuries to the liver, spleen, or kidney.

APPENDIX

Appendicitis

Appendicitis is the most common cause of an acute surgical abdomen in childhood, usually occurring in patients between 6 and 12 years of age. The diagnosis generally is made on the basis of characteristic history and clinical findings. Radiologic evaluation is needed only if the clinical features are atypical. In the past, the primary method of investigation had been conventional abdominal radiographs and barium studies of the colon, but these provided only indirect evidence of acute appendicitis (90,91). Recently, sonography with a high-resolution linear array transducer and graded

compression has proven useful for making a diagnosis (36,56,58,74,86,88). In experienced hands, the sensitivity of sonography is about 90%, the specificity 95%, and the accuracy 93% (56).

At the start of the examination, the patient is asked to point to the site of maximal abdominal tenderness with a single finger. Scanning this area may result in rapid identification of the appendix, thereby shortening the examination time and decreasing associated patient discomfort. It is also helpful in identifying an aberrantly located appendix. Scanning is begun in the transverse plane just above the level of the umbilicus and continued caudally in the right lower quadrant, with moderate pressure on the transducer. On a transverse view, the right colon with its hypoechoic muscular wall and inner echogenic mucosa, iliopsoas muscle, and iliac vessels can be identified. The inflamed appendix usually is visualized at the base of the cecal tip. Longitudinal and oblique scans are then obtained of the lower quadrant, again with graded compression. In addition to scanning anteriorly over the right lower quadrant, it also may be useful to scan laterally in the right flank. Occasionally a retrocecal appendix can be visualized only by scanning through the lateral flank.

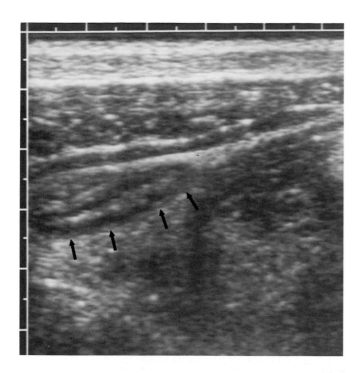

FIG. 33. Normal appendix. Right lower quadrant scan shows a tubular structure with a thin hypoechoic wall and echogenic mucosal center (*arrows*). At operation, the appendix was normal without evidence of inflammation.

Infrequently, a normal appendix can be seen sonographically (Fig. 33). When visualized, the normal appendix has a thin echogenic lining, hypoechoic wall, and tapered end, and may be slightly compressible. In adults, it measures 6 mm or less in maximal outer diameter.

A sonographic diagnosis of acute appendicitis is based on demonstration of a noncompressible appendix. The abnormal appendix appears as a blind-ending tubular structure on long axis view or as a target lesion on transverse scans (Fig. 34). The lumen of the obstructed appendix usually is fluid-filled, although in-

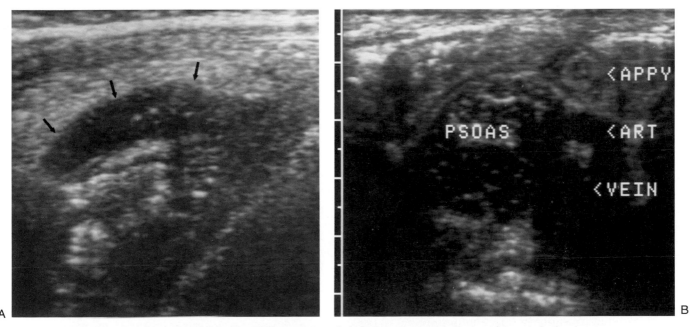

A   B

FIG. 34. Acute appendicitis. **A:** Oblique scan of right lower quadrant showing a tubular hypoechoic fluid-filled appendix (*arrows*). Several echogenic foci within lumen represent gas bubbles. **B:** Transverse scan of the right lower quadrant shows the abnormal appendix (*APPY*) with a target appearance. Also noted are the psoas muscle, and iliac artery (ART) and vein.

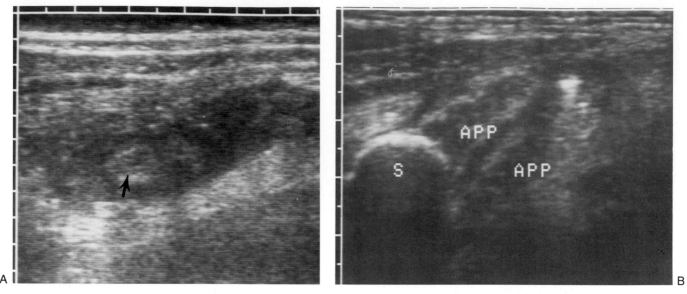

FIG. 35. Acute appendicitis with fecalith. **A:** Longitudinal right lower quadrant scan shows a fluid-filled tubular structure containing an echogenic area representing a fecalith (*arrow*). **B:** In another patient an oblique scan of the right lower quadrant demonstrates an appendiceal fecalith or stone (*S*), proximal to the fluid-filled appendix (*APP*) which is turned 180° on itself.

traluminal echogenic foci often are present and may be caused by gas or solid material, such as inspissated feces or appendicolith (Fig. 35). The fluid-filled lumen usually is surrounded by an inner echogenic layer representing mucosa and a peripheral hypoechoic mus-

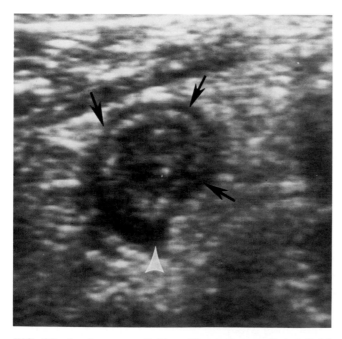

FIG. 36. Acute appendicitis with periappendiceal fluid. Cross-sectional view of the right lower quadrant shows a target lesion (*arrows*) corresponding to edematous, obstructed appendix. The various layers are a fluid-filled canal, adjacent echogenic mucosa, and a hypoechoic muscle wall. A small amount of fluid is seen around the appendix (*arrowhead*).

cular zone which has a thickness of 3 mm or more. Lack of sonographic visualization of the echogenic mucosal layer reflects submucosal ulceration and necrosis and indicates a greater likelihood of perforation (21). The diameter of the appendix is equal to or greater than 7 mm (56). A small amount of periappendiceal fluid also may be observed (Fig. 36).

A small percentage of patients will have false-negative studies and a few patients will have nondiagnostic studies due to inability to compress the right lower quadrant because of marked pain or obesity. Although sonography is quite sensitive for detecting appendicitis, most patients referred for sonographic evaluation of suspected appendicitis will not have appendicitis. In fact, approximately half of the patients will have no etiology for the pain, 25% will have appendicitis, and the other 25% will have a variety of genitourinary or gastrointestinal abnormalities (102). Thus, sonography of the upper abdomen and pelvis is indicated in children without sonographic evidence of acute appendicitis.

Following appendectomy, sonography can be used to detect fluid collections in the pelvis and abdomen (10). In cases of suspected abscess, sonography can guide percutaneous needle aspiration.

Perforated Appendicitis and Appendiceal Abscesses

Sonographic findings of a perforated appendix are a pericecal fluid collection, increased pericecal echogenicity, and nonvisualization of the echogenic mucosa of the appendix (21). Each finding alone is non-

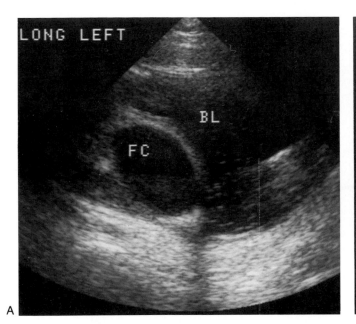
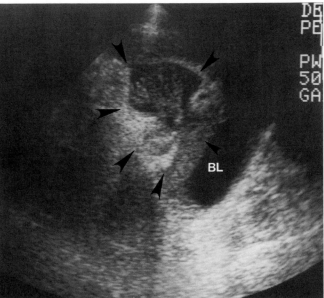

FIG. 37. Appendiceal abscess. **A:** Longitudinal scan in the left lower quadrant shows a nearly anechoic fluid collection (*FC*) posterior to the bladder (*BL*). **B:** In another patient, longitudinal scan of the pelvis demonstrates a complex mass (*arrowheads*) with a hypoechoic center displacing the bladder (*BL*) posteriorly.

specific and may be seen with a nonperforated appendix. With a combination of one or more findings, however, the sensitivity for the diagnosis of perforation is 86% and the specificity is 60% (21). Abscess formation secondary to perforation can be restricted to the right lower quadrant or may extend superiorly into the upper peritoneal cavity or inferiorly into the pelvis. On sonography, abscesses have a variable appearance and may be almost totally ano-, hypo-, or hyperechoic, or complex with both hypo- and hyperechoic areas (Fig. 37). The appendiceal stump may project into the abscess cavity (67).

It is important to recognize that a fluid collection in the right lower quadrant does not always indicate perforation, but may be a sympathetic response to inflammation. In addition, in girls it may be difficult to separate an appendiceal abscess from an ovarian process such as a tubo-ovarian abscess, ovarian torsion, or hemorrhagic ovarian cyst.

COLON

Sonography of the colon is usually limited to the evaluation of anorectal anomalies, necrotizing enterocolitis, and some colitides. Except for the right colon and rectum, most of the colon cannot be visualized as a discrete structure since it contains fecal material mixed with gas that produces intense echogenicity with acoustic shadowing (34).

Obstruction

Anorectal Anomalies

Anorectal malformation, also referred to as imperforate anus, is characterized by abnormal termination of the hindgut. The incidence is 1 in 5,000 births (13). Surgical management depends on the relationship of the most caudal portion of the hindgut to the levator sling. If the hindgut terminates above the sling, a high lesion is present and colostomy followed later by a pull-through operation is necessary. If the hindgut passes through the levator sling, the lesion is low and perineal surgery is performed. If the hindgut ends at the levator sling, the lesion is intermediate and a left-sided colostomy, followed later by either a pull-through procedure or perineal exploration, is indicated. Urinary tract anomalies, including crossed fused renal ectopia, unilateral renal agenesis, pelvic kidney, horseshoe kidney, and hydronephrosis, are present in 40% of infants with high anorectal malformations and in 25% of those with low lesions (14).

Traditionally, the radiologic evaluation begins with a plain lateral radiograph with the patient in an inverted or prone position. A lead marker is placed on the perineum at the site of the anal dimple and the distance between the rectal pouch and perineal marker is measured (13). This examination has limitations, however. A low lesion will mimic a high lesion if the distal pouch is plugged with meconium. Moreover, a high lesion will

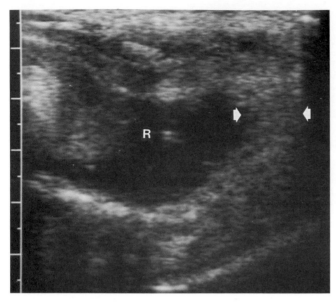

FIG. 38. Low imperforate anus. Longitudinal scan of the pelvis demonstrates the distance (*arrows*) between the perineum and the fluid-containing rectum (*R*) to be less than 1.5 cm.

The advantages of sonography are the ability to obtain measurements when the infant is quiet and to diagnose associated renal anomalies. Sagittal and transverse planes are obtained through the anterior abdominal wall with the infant supine. Longitudinal midline images also are performed through the perineum with the infant in a lithotomy position. After the examiner places a finger on the perineum at the site of the anal dimple, the relationship of the distal portion of the pouch to the perineum can be determined (Fig. 38). It has been suggested that a pouch-perineum distance of 1.0 cm or less indicates a low lesion, a distance of 1.0 to 1.5 cm represents an intermediate lesion, and a pouch-perineal distance of more than 1.5 cm implies a high lesion (38). Other signs of high lesions are gas within the bladder and intraluminal calcifications (7,77). Since sonography is time-consuming and there is some overlap between high and low lesions, it has not gained widespread acceptance for diagnosing imperforate anus.

mimic a low lesion if the lateral radiograph is taken when the infant is crying, since this displaces the pouch inferiorly. Other methods of evaluation include direct puncture of the rectal pouch (112), retrograde urethrography, and sonography (7,82,93).

Colon Atresia

Colon atresia is rare and probably the result of an *in utero* vascular accident. Plain radiography can show multiple dilated loops of bowel, but examination usually cannot be performed prior to 12 to 24 hr of age so that an adequate amount of gas can reach the site of obstruction. Sonography can determine the cause of

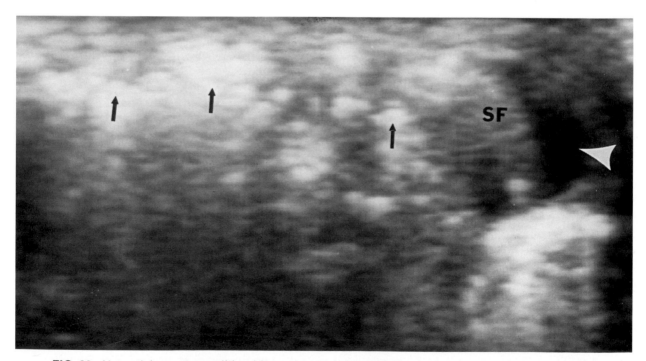

FIG. 39. Necrotizing enterocolitis with pneumatosis intestinalis and focal perforation. Transverse scan shows multiple echogenic areas consistent with gas (*arrows*) within the bowel wall and small fluid collection (*arrowhead*) adjacent to the splenic flexure (*SF*). A walled-off perforation at this site was proven surgically.

distention before gas is present in the distal bowel. The sonographic features of colon atresia are dilated distal small bowel and proximal colon, which often is markedly echogenic secondary to retained meconium (83).

Necrotizing Enterocolitis

Necrotizing enterocolitis is thought to be an ischemic bowel disease complicated by invasion of the bowel wall by enteric organisms. Approximately 80% of patients are premature infants; term or older infants often have underlying conditions such as heart disease, sepsis, and bowel obstruction. Affected patients have abdominal distention, feeding intolerance, and guaiac positive stools.

Early diagnosis of necrotizing enterocolitis is important, because if untreated the disease leads to sepsis, bowel perforation, and death. Plain abdominal radiography has been the method of confirming necrotizing enterocolitis, but sonography can be useful when plain radiographs are equivocal. On sonography

the abnormal bowel is thickened, demonstrating a target or bull's-eye appearance on transverse scans. Focal areas of intense echogenicity with acoustic shadowing may be noted in the wall, consistent with pneumatosis intestinalis (Fig. 39) (60). Peritoneal abscesses secondary to perforation and portal venous gas may be seen (95).

Recent reports have shown that Doppler imaging can be used to measure blood flow in the superior mesenteric artery (SMA) in full-term and premature infants. One study showed abnormal blood flow velocity in the SMA in neonates predisposed to necrotizing enterocolitis, such as small-for-gestational-age infants. These measurements of changes in SMA blood flow have important potential significance in the diagnosis and management of necrotizing enterocolitis (106,111).

Inflammatory Diseases of the Colon

A variety of inflammatory diseases affect the colon. Most arise in the mucosa or submucosa and produce

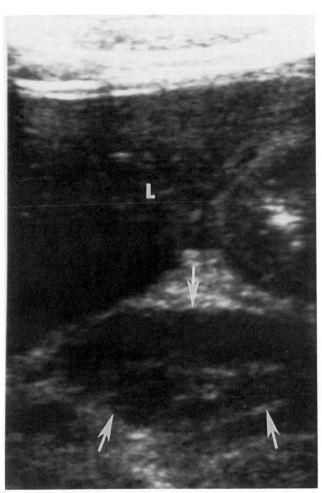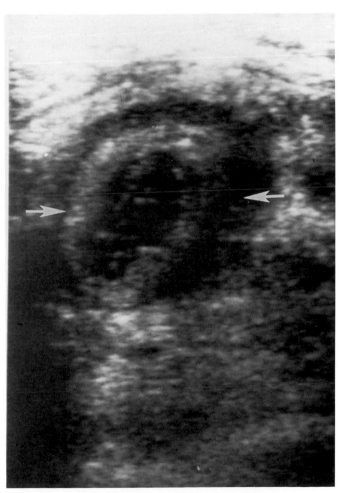

A   B

FIG. 40. Neutropenic colitis. **A:** Longitudinal, and **B:** transverse scans demonstrate a markedly thickened right colon (*arrows*). *L,* liver.

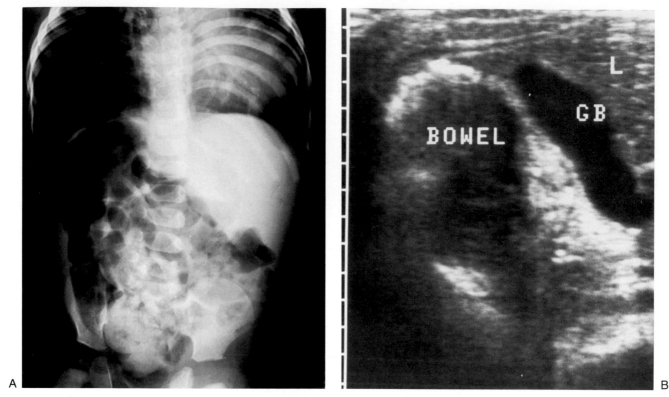

FIG. 41. Chilaiditi syndrome. **A:** Abdominal radiograph. There is cardiomegaly, and no normal hepatic outline is seen in the right upper quadrant. A sonogram was performed to rule out abdominal situs inversus. **B:** Transverse scan of the right upper quadrant demonstrates the colon (BOWEL) interposed between the right abdominal wall and right lobe of the liver (*L*) and gallbladder (*GB*). The spleen was in the normal position.

mucosal edema and ulceration early. Eventually wall thickening develops. Crohn's disease and ulcerative colitis are the most common diseases producing thickening of the wall of the bowel. Less frequently yersinia, salmonella or shigella colitis, hemolytic uremic syndrome; Behçet's syndrome (oral and genital ulceration with colitis); pseudomembranous colitis, and typhlitis are encountered (2,54,100). Typhlitis or inflammation of the right colon and cecum is associated with advanced leukemia or terminal aplastic anemia (99). The sonographic findings of colitis are a thickened bowel wall with echogenic mucosa (Fig. 40). Occasional findings include peritoneal fluid and a pericolonic abscess (6,20,46). The findings are nonspecific and may also be seen with ischemic bowel disease or vasculitis.

Ascariasis can be identified as multiple linear echolucencies in the bowel lumen.

Neoplasms

Polyps are the most frequent benign colonic lesion; malignant lesions are either lymphoma or carcinoma. Most tumors are evaluated by barium enema studies or sigmoidoscopy. Occasionally, however, the diagnosis is unsuspected and the patient is referred for son-

ography for evaluation of a palpable mass. Malignant tumors appear sonographically as target or bull's-eye lesions or as hypoechoic masses (32). Neoplasms need to be differentiated from fecalomas, which appear as highly echogenic masses with posterior acoustic shadowing (34).

Miscellaneous

Sonography can be used to diagnose Chilaiditi syndrome in patients suspected of having abdominal situs inversus on plain abdominal radiographs. Chilaiditi syndrome is characterized by interposition of the hepatic flexure between the liver and anterior abdominal wall (Fig. 41).

INTRAOPERATIVE AND ENDOSCOPIC SONOGRAPHY

Intraoperative sonography has been used to determine the extent of tumor prior to resection and to diagnose intraloop fluid collections (68). Endoscopic sonography has been used to stage tumors of the stomach and rectum in adults (28). Its role in pediatrics is currently limited.

REFERENCES

1. Abramson SJ, Berdon WE, Altman RP, Amodio JB, Levy J. Biliary atresia and noncardiac polysplenic syndrome: US and surgical considerations. *Radiology* 1987;163:377–379.
2. Abramson SJ, Berdon WE, Baker DH. Childhood typhlitis: Its increasing associations with acute myelogenous leukemia. *Radiology* 1983;146:61–64.
3. Adamsbaum C, Sellier N, Helardot P. Ileocolic intussusception with enterogenous cyst: Ultrasonic diagnosis. *Pediatr Radiol* 1989;19:325.
4. Agha FP, Ghahremani GG, Panella JS, Kaufman MW. Appendicitis as the initial manifestation of Crohn's disease: Radiologic features and prognosis. *AJR* 1987;149:515–518.
5. Aintablian NH, Slim MS, Antoun BW. Congenital microgastria. Case report and review of the literature. *Pediatr Surg Int* 1987;2:307–310.
6. Alexander JE, Williamson SL, Seibert JJ, Golladay ES, Jimenez JF. The ultrasonographic diagnosis of typhlitis (neutropenic colitis). *Pediatr Radiol* 1988;18:200–204.
7. Anderson S, Savader B, Barnes J, Savader S. Enterolithiasis with imperforate anus. Report of two cases with sonographic demonstration and occurrence in a female. *Pediatr Radiol* 1988;18:130–133.
8. Atwell JD, Levick P. Congenital hypertrophic pyloric stenosis and associated anomalies in the genitourinary tract. *J Pediatr Surg* 1981;16:1029–1035.
9. Babcock DS, Kaufman RA. Ultrasonography and computed tomography in the evaluation of the acutely ill pediatric patient. *Radiol Clin North Am* 1983;21:527–550.
10. Baker DE, Silver TM, Coran AG, McMillin KI. Postappendectomy fluid collections in children: Incidence, nature, and evolution evaluated using US. *Radiology* 1986;161:341–344.
11. Ball TI, Atkinson GO, Gay BB Jr. Ultrasound diagnosis of hypertrophic pyloric stenosis: Real-time application and the demonstration of a new sonographic sign. *Radiology* 1983;147:499–502.
12. Bar-Ziv J, Barki Y, Weizman Z, Urkin J. Transient protein-losing gastropathy (Ménétrier's disease) in childhood). *Pediatr Radiol* 1988;18:82–84.
13. Berdon WE, Baker DH, Santulli TV, et al. The radiologic evaluation of imperforate anus: An approach correlated with current surgical concepts. *Radiology* 1968;90:466–471.
14. Berdon WE, Hochberg D, Baker DH, et al. The association of lumbosacral spine and genitourinary anomalies with imperforate anus. *AJR* 1966;98:181–191.
15. Bisset RAL, Gupta SC. Hypertrophic pyloric stenosis, ultrasonic appearances in a small baby. *Pediatr Radiol* 1988;18:405.
16. Blumhagen JD. The role of ultrasonography in the evaluation of vomiting in infants. *Pediatr Radiol* 1986;16:267–270.
17. Blumhagen JD, Noble HGS. Muscle thickness in hypertrophic pyloric stenosis: Sonographic determination. *AJR* 1983;140:221–223.
18. Blumhagen JD, Weinberger E. Pediatric gastrointestinal ultrasonography. In: Sanders RC, Hill MC, eds. *Ultrasound annual*. New York: Raven Press, 1986;99–140.
19. Boli AA. Case report. Diagnosis and hydrostatic reduction of an intussusception under ultrasound guidance. *Clin Radiol* 1985;36:655–657.
20. Bolondi L, Ferrentino M, Trevisani F, Bernardi M, Gasbarrini G. Sonographic appearance of pseudomembranous colitis. *J Ultrasound Med* 1985;4:489–492.
21. Borushok KF, Jeffrey RB Jr, Laing FC, Townsend PR. Sonographic diagnosis of perforation in patients with acute appendicitis. *AJR* 1990;154:275–278.
22. Bowen A, Mazer J, Zarabi M, Fujioka M. Cystic meconium peritonitis: Ultrasonographic features. *Pediatr Radiol* 1984;14:18–22.
23. Bowen B, Ros PR, McCarthy MJ, Olmsted WW, Hjermstad BM. Gastrointestinal teratomas: CT and US appearance with pathologic correlation. *Radiology* 1987;162:431–433.
24. Bowerman RA, Silver TM, Jaffe MH. Real-time ultrasound diagnosis of intussusception in children. *Radiology* 1982;143:527–529.
25. Breaux CW Jr, Georgeson KE, Royal SA, Curnow AJ. Changing patterns in the diagnosis of hypertrophic pyloric stenosis. *Pediatrics* 1988;81:213–217.
26. Burke LF, Clark E. Ileal colic intussusception. A case report. *JCU* 1977;5:346–347.
27. Carroll BA, Moskowitz PS. Sonographic diagnosis of neonatal meconium cyst. *AJR* 1981;137:1262–1264.
28. Carroll BA. US of the gastrointestinal tract. *Radiology* 1989;172:605–608.
29. Claiborne AK, Blocker SH, Martin CM, McAlister WH. Prenatal and postnatal sonographic delineation of gastrointestinal abnormalities in a case of the VATER syndrome. *J Ultrasound Med* 1986;5:45–47.
30. Cohen HL, Haller JO, Mestel AL, Coren C, Schecter S, Eaton DH. Neonatal duodenum: Fluid-aided US examination. *Radiology* 1987;164:805–809.
31. Cohen HL, Schecter S, Mestel AL, Eaton DH, Haller JO. Ultrasonic "double track" sign in hypertrophic pyloric stenosis. *J Ultrasound Med* 1987;6:139–143.
32. Cremin BJ, Brown RA. Carcinoma of the colon: Diagnosis by ultrasound and enema. *Pediatr Radiol* 1987;17:319–320.
33. Cremin BJ, Solomon DJ. Ultrasonic diagnosis of duodenal diaphragm. *Pediatr Radiol* 1987;17:489–490.
34. Derchi LE, Musante F, Biggi E, Cicio GR, Oliva L. Sonographic appearance of fecal masses. *J Ultrasound Med* 1985;4:573–575.
35. Derchi LE, Ierace T, De Pra L, Solbiati L, Rizzatto G, Musante F. The sonographic appearance of duodenal lesions. *J Ultrasound Med* 1986;5:269–273.
36. Deutsch A, Leopold GR. Ultrasound demonstration of the inflamed appendix: Case report. *Radiology* 1981;140:163–164.
37. Dinkel E, Dittrich M, Peters H, Baumann W. Real-time ultrasound in Crohn's disease: Characteristic features and clinical implications. *Pediatr Radiol* 1986;16:8–12.
38. Donaldson JS, Black CT, Reynolds M, Sherman JO, Shkolnik A. Ultrasound of the distal pouch in infants with imperforate anus. *J Pediatr Surg* 1989;24:465–468.
39. Dorne HL, Jequier S. Sonography of intestinal lymphangiectasis. *J Ultrasound Med* 1986;5:13–16.
40. Ein SH. Leading points in childhood intussusception. *J Pediatr Surg* 1976;11:209–211.
41. Elam EA, Hunter TB, Hunt KR, Fajardo L, Boren W, Gaines J. The lack of sonographic image degradation after barium upper gastrointestinal examination. *AJR* 1989;153:993–994.
42. Filiatrault D, Longpre D, Patriquin H, Perreault G, Grignon A, Pronovost, Boisvert J. Investigation of childhood blunt abdominal trauma: A practical approach using ultrasound as the initial diagnostic modality. *Pediatr Radiol* 1987;17:373–379.
43. Fleischer AC, Muhletaler CA, James AE Jr. Sonographic patterns arising from normal and abnormal bowel. *Radiol Clin North Am* 1980;18:145–159.
44. Foley LC, Teele RL. Ultrasound of epigastric injuries after blunt trauma. *AJR* 1979;132:593–598.
45. Franken EA Jr, King H. Postoperative intussusception in children. *AJR* 1972;116:584–586.
46. Glass-Royal MC, Choyke PL, Gootenberg JE, Grant EG. Sonography in the diagnosis of neutropenic colitis. *J Ultrasound Med* 1987;6:671–673.
47. Goldstein RB, Filly RA, Callen PW. Sonographic diagnosis of meconium ileus *in utero*. *J Ultrasound Med* 1987;6:663–666.
48. Graif M, Itzchak Y, Avigad I, Strauss S, Ben-Ami T. The pylorus in infancy: Overall sonographic assessment. *Pediatr Radiol* 1984;14:14–17.
49. Haller JO, Cohen HL. Hypertrophic pyloric stenosis: Diagnosis using US. *Radiology* 1986;161:335–339.
50. Hayashi K, Futagawa S, Kozaki S, Hirao K, Hombo Z. Ultrasound and CT diagnosis of intramural duodenal hematoma. *Pediatr Radiol* 1988;18:167–168.
51. Hayden CK Jr, Boulden TF, Swischuk LE, Lobe TE. Sonographic demonstration of duodenal obstruction with midgut volvulus. *AJR* 1984;143:9–10.
52. Hayden CK Jr, Swischuk LE, Rytting JE. Gastric ulcer disease in infants: US findings. *Radiology* 1987;164:131–134.
53. Hernanz-Schulman M, Genieser NB, Abrosino M. Sono-

8

Adrenal Glands, Pancreas, and Other Retroperitoneal Structures

Gary D. Shackelford

The retroperitoneum is bounded anteriorly by the posterior parietal peritoneum, posteriorly by the transversalis fascia, superiorly by the diaphragm, and inferiorly by the pelvic brim (118). It contains the pancreas, the kidneys and ureters, the adrenal glands, the duodenal loop, the great vessels and branches, the ascending and descending colon, and miscellaneous structures such as lymph nodes, lymphatic channels, and nerves. Although they are technically contained within the retrofascial space posterior to the retroperitoneum, the psoas muscles and adjacent soft tissue structures such as the sympathetic trunks will be included in the discussion of miscellaneous retroperitoneal structures. The presacral soft tissue space will also be included, since many pathological conditions affecting this space also affect retroperitoneal structures. Diseases related to the kidney, duodenum, and colon are discussed in other chapters.

ADRENAL GLANDS

The adrenal glands are paired retroperitoneal structures within the confines of the perirenal fascia, anteromedial to the upper pole of each kidney. The right adrenal gland is situated in the small space between the diaphragmatic crus, right lobe of the liver, inferior vena cava, and upper pole of the right kidney. The left adrenal is located lateral to the aorta and left diaphragmatic crus, medial to the spleen, posterior to the stomach and pancreatic tail, and anteromedial to the upper pole of the left kidney. Both adrenals are only partly suprarenal, and the left gland frequently extends caudad as far as the level of the renal hilum (121).

Although they are closely associated anatomically with the kidneys, the adrenal glands and kidneys have unrelated embryologic origins. The adrenal has a dual origin: the medulla develops from neural crest tissue of neuroectodermal lineage; the cortex, which envelops the medulla in humans, arises from coelomic mesoderm. During fetal and early postnatal development, the adrenal cortex is thickened and is comprised of two layers. The thick inner fetal cortex predominates and is in turn surrounded by a thin outer zone which is destined to become the adult cortex. The large bulk of the fetal cortex is primarily responsible for the large size of the adrenal gland at birth (up to one-third the size of the kidney). Shortly after birth the fetal cortex begins to involute, primarily by a process of hemorrhagic necrosis, and it gradually shrinks and is almost completely replaced by connective tissue within 1 year (14). The glands lose about one-third of their weight in the first 2 to 3 weeks after birth, and they do not regain their birth weight until the end of the second year (123).

Technical Considerations

With modern real-time equipment the fetal adrenal glands can be identified early during the third trimester (109,148). After birth the adrenal gland can be visualized on the right in 97% to 100% of neonates and on the left in 83% to 96% (90,135). Corresponding reported figures for adults—and presumably older children—are 92% and 71%, respectively (112). Considerable technical skill is required to visualize the normal adrenal glands on a consistent basis beyond infancy, and the examination can at times be very time-consuming.

In neonates and young infants, the right adrenal gland can usually be easily visualized from either an anterolateral or right flank approach, using the relatively large right hepatic lobe as an acoustic window. Visualization of the left adrenal usually requires a left flank approach. In older patients, visualization of the right adrenal gland may require an intercostal approach using the liver as an acoustic window. Visualization of the left adrenal requires a more posterior approach using the spleen and left kidney as acoustic windows (188).

Shape

Each adrenal gland consists of an anteromedial ridge and two wings that open posterolaterally. On coronal and longitudinal sonographic scans, the adrenals as-

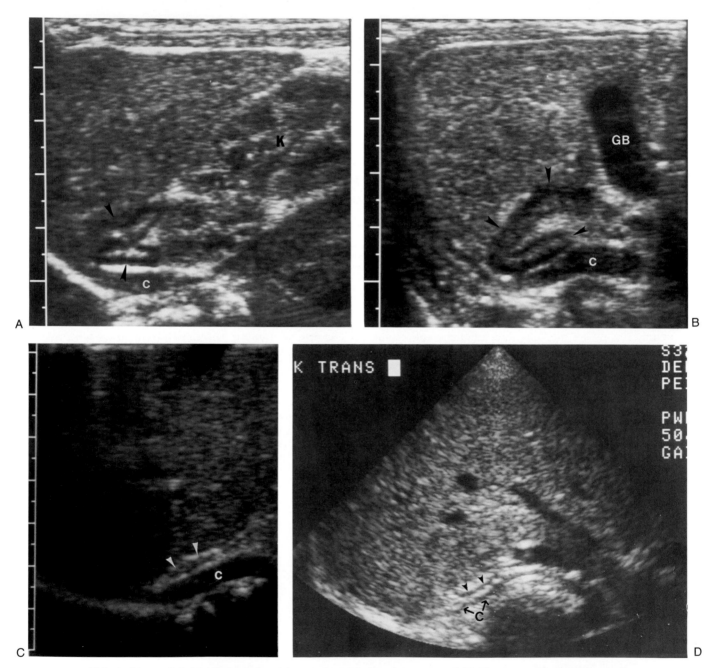

FIG. 1. Normal right adrenal gland (*arrowheads*) at various ages. **A,B:** Newborn. The hyperechoic medulla is surrounded by hypoechoic cortex. On the longitudinal scan (**A**) the adrenal has a "V" configuration; on the transverse scan (**B**) it conforms to the shape of a folded "L." **C:** Age 18 months; transverse scan. The adrenal is linear, nearly uniformly hypoechoic, and surrounded by hyperechoic fat. A faintly hyperechoic medulla is visible. **D:** Age 8 years; transverse scan. The adrenal is a thin, linear, hypoechoic structure without differentiation between cortex and medulla. On all scans the adrenal lies anterior to the diaphragmatic crus (*C*). *GB*, gallbladder; *K*, kidney.

TABLE 1. *Sonographic features of normal adrenal gland versus age*

Age	Shape and size	Echogenicity
Newborn	Cortex thick, with convex borders Medulla small	Cortex hypoechoic Medulla hyperechoic
1.5–2 months	Cortex smaller, with convex borders Medulla proportionately larger	Cortex hypoechoic Medulla hyperechoic
5–6 months	Gland smaller, with straight borders	Gland hyperechoic with indistinct corticomedullary differentiation
>1 year	Borders straight or concave, similar to adult gland	Gland hypoechoic

Adapted from Kangarloo et al., ref. 90.

sume the shape of a "V" or "Y" (135,188). On transverse scans, the shape differs depending on the scan plane, ranging from linear on more cranial scans to the shape of a "V," "Y," or "L" as one proceeds caudad (Fig. 1) (188).

Echo Texture

Each wing or limb of the neonatal adrenal is characterized by a thin hyperechoic core representing the medulla, surrounded by a thick hypoechoic rim which is the hypertrophied cortex. Correlative anatomic studies suggest that the decreased cortical echogenicity is due to two factors: (a) dilated, blood-filled cortical sinusoids due to cortical vascular congestion; and (b) orderly parallel orientation of the cuboidal cells that line the cortical columns (135). The increased medullary echogenicity is probably produced by random orientation of its cell population, producing multiple reflective interfaces (135).

The sonographic appearance of the normal adrenal gland varies with age (90) (Table 1). Early postnatally, the cortex remains hypoechoic relative to the medulla but becomes proportionately smaller due to involution of the fetal zone. As the fetal zone is progressively replaced by fibrous tissue, the gland increases in relative echogenicity, and by age 5 to 6 months there is poor or absent differentiation between the cortex and medulla. With subsequent disappearance of the fibrous tissue between 1 and 3 years of age, the gland returns to a hypoechoic appearance, with little qualitative change thereafter. On good quality scans in older children, the medulla can sometimes be seen as a thin, echogenic line. The prominent triangular or crescent-shaped hyperechoic suprarenal structure seen in older children represents perirenal fat, not the adrenal gland (Fig. 1) (188).

Size

Normal sonographic standards for adrenal size have been determined for neonates (135). The method used to measure the glands is illustrated in Fig. 2. The ad-

renal length ranges between 0.9 and 3.6 cm (mean, 1.5 cm), and the thickness ranges between 0.2 and 0.5 cm (mean, 0.3 cm). There is no statistically significant difference between the right and left glands. The generally accepted standards for adult adrenal glands are 4 to 6 cm in length, 0.2 to 0.6 cm in thickness, and 2 to 3 cm in width (188). In neonates and young children, age-related changes in the sonographic appearance and relative size of the cortex and medulla (Table 1) appear to be more diagnostically useful than actual sizes (90).

Congenital Anomalies

Absence

Absence of an adrenal gland is a rare anomaly. In an autopsy series of patients with renal agenesis and dysgenesis, the homolateral adrenal was found to be absent in 21 of 332 cases (6%) (10). Accessory adrenal tissue is a more common condition than agenesis. Only if cortical and medullary tissue are found together can the anomaly be termed an accessory adrenal gland (121).

Hypoplasia

The adrenal glands are hypoplastic in anencephalic infants due to failure of the pituitary gland to develop normally. The resulting inadequate production of adrenocorticotropic hormone (ACTH) leads to failure of normal development of the fetal adrenal cortex (123).

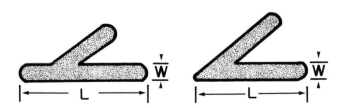

FIG. 2. Method used to measure the normal neonatal adrenal glands. *L*, length; *W*, width. (Adapted from ref. 135.)

In these patients, the weight of each adrenal gland is only about 8% of normal (166). Similar adrenal changes occur in infants with prenatal pituitary and central nervous system degenerative disorders, as well as in pregnancies with subnormal maternal urinary estriol levels or preeclampsia (166). There are also several forms of idiopathic hypoplasia in which the pituitary and hypothalamus are morphologically unremarkable. Other conditions associated with adrenal hypoplasia include neonatal adrenoleukodystrophy (104), Zellweger (cerebro-hepato-renal) syndrome (104), and infantile glycerol kinase deficiency (113). The adrenal glands of patients with these rare conditions have not been systematically evaluated with sonography.

Renal Agenesis

The ipsilateral adrenal gland is usually present in patients with renal agenesis or ectopia (10,141). A characteristic sonographic appearance of the adrenals has been noted in such infants (115,161). The adrenal retains its characteristic hyperechoic medulla and hypoechoic cortex, but elongates and increases in thickness, losing its "Y" or "V" shape on coronal and longitudinal scans, and assuming a discoid shape with slightly increased thickness centrally (Fig. 3) (115). In a small series of six neonates with renal agenesis or ectopia, the average length of the adrenal was 2.9 cm on the left and 3.4 cm on the right, compared with an average of 1.5 cm in the normal neonate. The adrenal was also increased slightly in thickness to 0.5 cm, compared with 0.3 cm in normals (115). The anomalous adrenal shape has been attributed to lack of pressure exerted by the kidney on the developing adrenal gland (141).

Since an elongated adrenal gland can occur with renal ectopia (115), careful search for renal tissue elsewhere in the abdomen or pelvis is always indicated. Although the ipsilateral adrenal has been described as "hypertrophied" in the presence of renal agenesis or ectopia (115), the adrenal is actually of normal weight and is normal in all other respects except for shape (141). Acquired atrophy of the kidney or nephrectomy results in retention of normal postnatal adrenal shape, at least in adults (94).

Metabolic Disease

Hyperplasia

Congenital adrenal hyperplasia (CAH) refers to a group of autosomal recessive disorders whose common denominator is an enzymatic deficiency in the adrenal cortex required for cortisol biosynthesis. In more than 90% of cases the defect involves the enzyme 21-hydroxylase, while deficiencies of 11β-hydroxylase and 3β-hydroxysteroid dehydrogenase account for most of the remaining cases. The clinical manifestations of 21-hydroxylase deficiency arise primarily from the overproduction and accumulation of steroidal precursors proximal to the site of enzymatic block, with subsequent diversion into the androgen biosynthesis pathway. This produces virilism in newborn females, premature masculinization in males, and advanced somatic development in both sexes. Chronic androgen excess may cause decreased fertility due to disruption of the hypothalamic-pituitary axis (130). Three-fourths of patients with 21-hydroxylase deficiency also have an inability to synthesize aldosterone, and these individuals are at risk for a potentially life-threatening

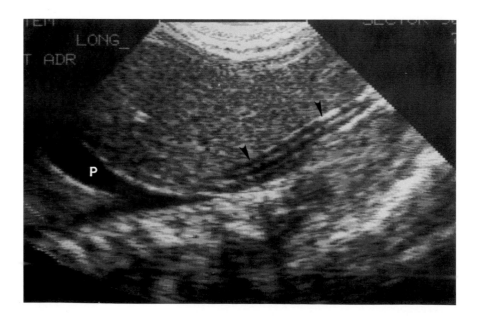

FIG. 3. Bilateral renal agenesis. The right adrenal gland is elongated and discoid-shaped, with slightly increased thickness centrally (*arrowheads*). Corticomedullary differentiation is preserved. Autopsy confirmation. *P,* pleural fluid.

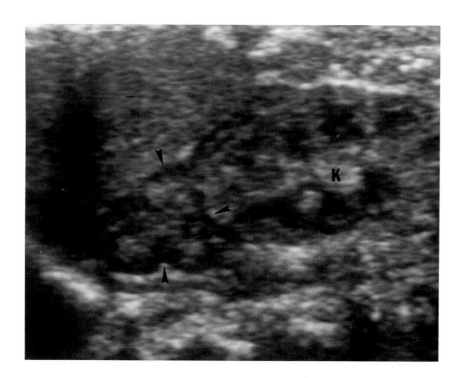

FIG. 4. Congenital adrenal hyperplasia due to 21-hydroxylase deficiency. Newborn female infant with ambiguous genitalia. Longitudinal scan through the right adrenal (*arrowheads*) and kidney (*K*). The adrenal is enlarged and triangular in shape. Although corticomedullary differentiation is present, it is less well-defined than normal.

crisis due to salt wasting in the neonatal period (130). Infants with 11β-hydroxylase deficiency are clinically similar to those with 21-hydroxylase deficiency. Deficiency of 3β-hydroxysteroid dehydrogenase causes ambiguous genitalia (usually severe hypospadias) in genotypic males; affected females are normal or only slightly virilized (130).

Congenital adrenal hyperplasia is the most common cause of female pseudohermaphroditism (29), and sonography can be useful in establishing the presence of a uterus and in demonstrating enlargement of the adrenals (29,66). The adrenals are usually either enlarged or at the upper limit of normal in size in CAH (29). The enlarged glands lose their flattened shape and appear triangular. The increased thickness involves the hypoechoic cortex. Although the medulla is uninvolved, corticomedullary differentiation is often indistinct (Fig. 4). Recognition of adrenal enlargement is important, since infants with ambiguous genitalia due to causes other than CAH have normal adrenals (29). Congenital adrenal hyperplasia is the most likely diagnosis in a newborn female infant with ambiguous external genitalia and bilateral adrenal enlargement, but normal adrenal size does not exclude the diagnosis.

Lipoid adrenal hyperplasia is a rare form of CAH due to cholesterol desmolase deficiency. There is failure of conversion of cholesterol to pregnenolone in the initial step of adrenal steroidogenesis, with impaired synthesis of all three classes of adrenal steroids: mineralocorticoids, glucocorticoids, and sex steroids. The adrenal glands are markedly enlarged due to massive accumulation of lipoid material consisting of cholesterol and cholesterol esters. Affected males have

markedly ambiguous external genitalia, suggesting that the enzyme defect is also present in the testes (130). To date there has been no report of the sonographic appearance of the adrenals in this condition, but a report of the CT features in an affected infant described massively enlarged adrenal glands with attenuation similar to that of fat (131).

Adrenocortical hyperplasia in older children may be primary; it may also be seen with ACTH administration or in conditions associated with excessive endogenous ACTH (Cushing's disease and ectopic ACTH-secretion syndrome). Primary hyperplasia most commonly results in Cushing's syndrome, and less commonly in primary aldosteronism. Although adrenal carcinoma is the most common cause of Cushing's syndrome in young children (143), after 10 years of age hyperplasia accounts for approximately 70% of cases (166). A rare cause of Cushing's syndrome is micronodular adrenal disease (microadenomatous hyperplasia, nodular adrenocortical dysplasia), a condition seen primarily in children and adolescents and characterized by multiple small (≤2 mm) autonomous cortisol-secreting adenomas in normal size glands (35,166). Primary aldosteronism in children less than 16 years of age is usually due to adrenal hyperplasia rather than adenoma (58). At the present time, the sensitivity of sonography in the detection of hyperplastic adrenal glands beyond infancy is unknown.

Wolman Disease

Wolman disease is a rare inborn error of lipid metabolism due to deficient activity of the lysosomal acid lipase, leading to massive accumulation of cholesterol esters and triglycerides in most tissues of the body (152). The disease occurs in infancy, with onset of symptoms in the first weeks of life, and death usually follows by the end of the first year. Hepatosplenomegaly, vomiting, diarrhea, steatorrhea, abdominal distention, and anemia are the major clinical signs and symptoms. One of the most striking findings is marked and symmetric enlargement of the adrenal glands, which almost invariably contain diffuse, punctate calcifications. The normal shape of the adrenals is retained. Pathologically, the inner zones of the cortex contain lipid-laden cells, with prominent areas of necrosis and calcification. The adrenal medulla is uninvolved.

Plain radiography demonstrates diffuse punctate calcifications distributed throughout normally shaped adrenals (142). Computerized tomography shows the enlarged adrenals with cortical distribution of the calcification (52,81). Sonography shows hyperechoic pyramidal adrenals with distal acoustic shadowing (52). Bilateral adrenal calcification can also be seen in adrenal hemorrhage and, apparently, in disseminated herpes simplex infection (124), but when seen in association with hepatosplenomegaly and gastrointestinal symptoms, Wolman disease is likely (152).

Adrenal Hemorrhage

Adrenal hemorrhage in the pediatric age group is primarily a neonatal condition. It is the most common cause of an adrenal mass in the neonate, but its frequency is unknown because many cases are believed to go undetected. In an autopsy series of perinatal deaths covering the period 1948 to 1970, adrenal hemorrhage occurred with a frequency of 1.7 per 1,000 live births (47). The lesion can also occur *in utero,* long enough before delivery to show faint radiographic calcifications at birth (128,140).

Conditions associated with neonatal adrenal hemorrhage include birth trauma, especially in infants of diabetic mothers or infants who are large for gestational age, perinatal stress, hypoxia, coagulation disorders, septicemia, and shock. Involvement may be either unilateral (usually right-sided) or bilateral. Hemorrhage is usually intracapsular, but if there is capsular rupture, it may extend into the retroperitoneal or intraperitoneal space (79,129,170). Involvement of the gland may be total or segmental, and segmental lesions range in size from single or multiple small areas to those involving almost the entire gland (47). In older children, adrenal hemorrhage can occur due to abdominal trauma, or as a complication of ACTH or anti-

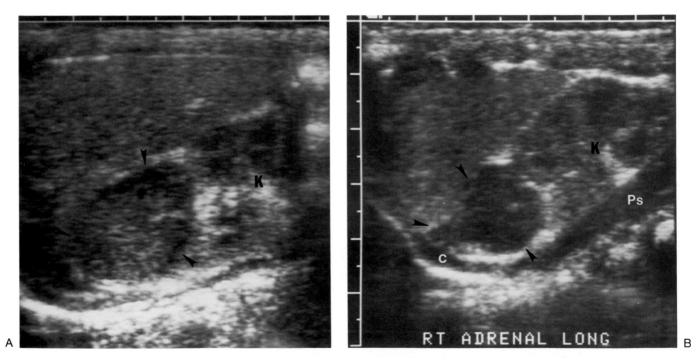

FIG. 5. Neonatal adrenal hemorrhage with echogenic gland seen initially. **A:** Longitudinal scan at 10 days of age shows a well-defined, uniformly echogenic right adrenal mass (*arrowheads*). **B:** At 18 days of age the mass is slightly smaller and is more hypoechoic. *c,* diaphragmatic crus; *K,* kidney; *Ps,* psoas muscle.

coagulant therapy, severe stress, or overwhelming sepsis, especially due to *Neisseria meningitidis* or *Haemophilus influenzae* (87).

The etiology of neonatal adrenal hemorrhage is unknown. One proposed cause is passive venous engorgement (16). The right adrenal vein drains directly into the inferior vena cava, without significant contribution from other veins. Increased pressure in the inferior vena cava, possibly due to prolonged abdominal compression during delivery, could produce severe venous engorgement in the right adrenal gland. The left adrenal vein, which drains into the left renal vein, is well supplied with alternative venous channels; in the event of a prolonged rise in inferior vena caval pressure, it would be less likely to undergo thrombosis. An alternative theory proposes that hypoxia or asphyxia, with reflex shunting of blood away from the splanchnic and visceral bed, produces hemorrhagic infarctions, ischemic in nature (47).

Clinical presentation of neonatal adrenal hemorrhage is usually due either to the presence of a mass, detected either by palpation or sonography, or to manifestation of complications, such as uncontrollable bleeding or jaundice. Other complications include in-

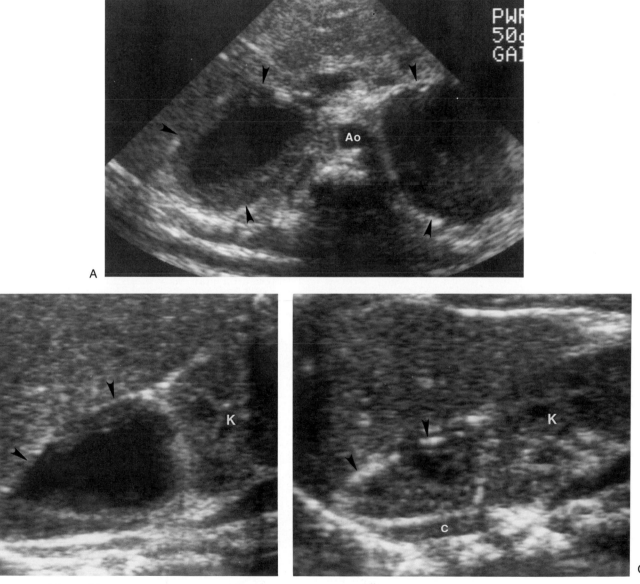

FIG. 6. Bilateral adrenal hemorrhage with cystic appearance on initial scan. Jaundiced infant with a history of traumatic delivery and hypoxia. **A,B:** Five days of age. Transverse scan (**A**) demonstrates large bilateral adrenal masses (*arrowheads*) with central cystic components containing internal debris. A peripheral rim of solid tissue is present in the right adrenal. **B:** Right adrenal, longitudinal scan. **C:** Five weeks of age; right adrenal, longitudinal scan. The central hematoma has nearly resolved. The adrenal is smaller and is now more uniformly echogenic. *Ao,* aorta; *c,* diaphragmatic crus; *K,* kidney.

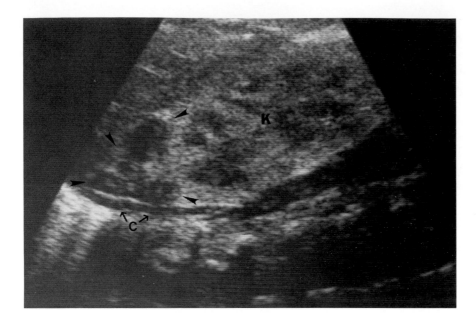

FIG. 7. Neonatal adrenal hemorrhage with retention of "V" configuration of gland. Two-day old infant with birth asphyxia. Longitudinal scan through the right adrenal (*arrowheads*) and kidney (*K*) showing mild adrenal enlargement, poor corticomedullary differentiation, and inhomogeneous echo texture. Autopsy confirmation. *C*, diaphragmatic crus.

testinal obstruction (107), hypertension (129,170), adrenal abscess (11), and impaired renal function (16,170). Renal vein thrombosis (almost exclusively left-sided) may be the most common lesion causing diminished ipsilateral renal function (23,26,98,105, 107,170). Adrenal insufficiency is very rare, even in bilateral cases, and when shock occurs, it is more likely related to blood loss than to adrenal insufficiency.

In the past, diagnosis of adrenal hemorrhage was confirmed with intravenous urography, which showed an avascular suprarenal mass—lucent during the phase of total-body opacification—with inferolateral displacement of the kidney (147). Follow-up plain radiographs often showed development of rim-like calcification, with more compact, flocculent calcifications observed months or years later.

Sonography is now the primary imaging study in the diagnosis of neonatal adrenal hemorrhage (37,79,119, 120,137,182). Large lesions affecting most of the gland' appear round, while smaller lesions are triangular or crescentic (Figs. 5–7). With focal lesions, the hemorrhagic area may be visualized adjacent to a normal portion of the gland (Fig. 8) (37). Hemorrhage cen-

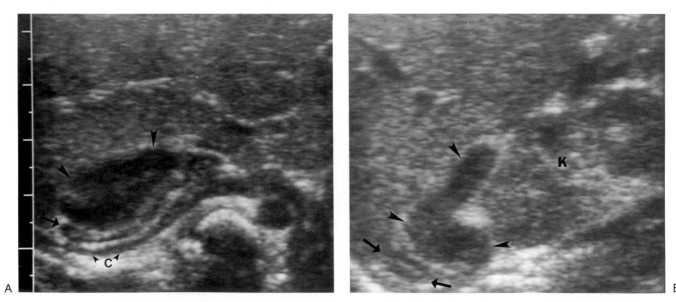

FIG. 8. Segmental adrenal hemorrhage in a 1-day-old infant with a history of traumatic delivery. Transverse (**A**) and longitudinal (**B**) scans of the right adrenal gland show a hypoechoic mass involving the anteromedial ridge and lateral wing (*arrowheads*). The medial wing (*arrows*) is uninvolved and is compressed against the diaphragmatic crus (*c*).

tered in the medulla may be associated with an intact cortex and a relatively normal adrenal configuration. On initial sonographic scanning, adrenal hemorrhage may appear as an echo-free, mixed, or echogenic suprarenal mass, depending on both the age of the lesion and the extent of hemorrhage. Most lesions exhibit mixed echogenicity early in their natural history and tend to develop an echo-free center over several days as the hematoma lyses and coalesces. During the next several weeks, the cystic mass regresses and eventually disappears, often leaving a residual focus of calcification in the adrenal (Fig. 9). The rate at which these changes occur varies from patient to patient.

It is important to appreciate that there are no pathognomonic sonographic features of neonatal adrenal hemorrhage. The most important condition in the differential diagnosis is neuroblastoma. In fact, neonatal neuroblastoma can be complicated by hemorrhage (see

Fig. 14) (54,127,165), and rim-like calcification on conventional radiographs, a finding generally considered to be characteristic of adrenal hemorrhage, can also occur when neuroblastoma coexists with hemorrhage (54). Serial sonographic examinations can help to differentiate between these lesions. A hematoma usually begins to lyse and decrease in size within 1 to 2 weeks, whereas neuroblastoma tends to retain its echogenicity and to remain stable or increase in size during the second week of life (54). Urinary catecholamine levels, which are elevated in approximately 85% to 90% of patients with neuroblastoma, should be obtained in all cases of presumed neonatal adrenal hemorrhage. Recent experience with magnetic resonance imaging suggests that it may increase diagnostic specificity early in the course of neonatal adrenal hemorrhage, when the diagnosis is uncertain (26,98,182).

The sonographic features of adrenal hemorrhage in

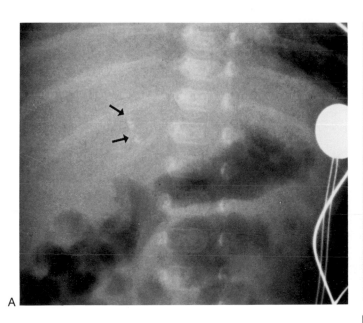

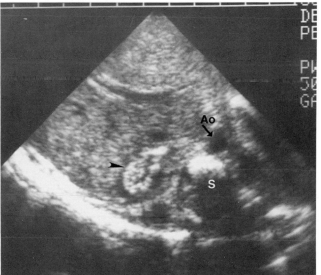

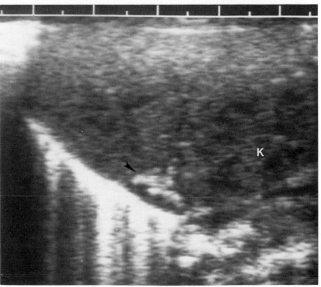

FIG. 9. Neonatal adrenal calcification, presumably secondary to antecedent hemorrhage. Premature infant with 740 g birth weight. **A:** Plain abdominal radiograph at 3 weeks of age shows a right upper quadrant calcification (*arrows*). Transverse (**B**) and longitudinal (**C**) sonograms through the right adrenal show irregular hyperechogenicity conforming roughly to the shape of the medulla (*arrowhead*), without distal acoustic shadowing. *Ao,* aorta; *K,* kidney; *S,* spine.

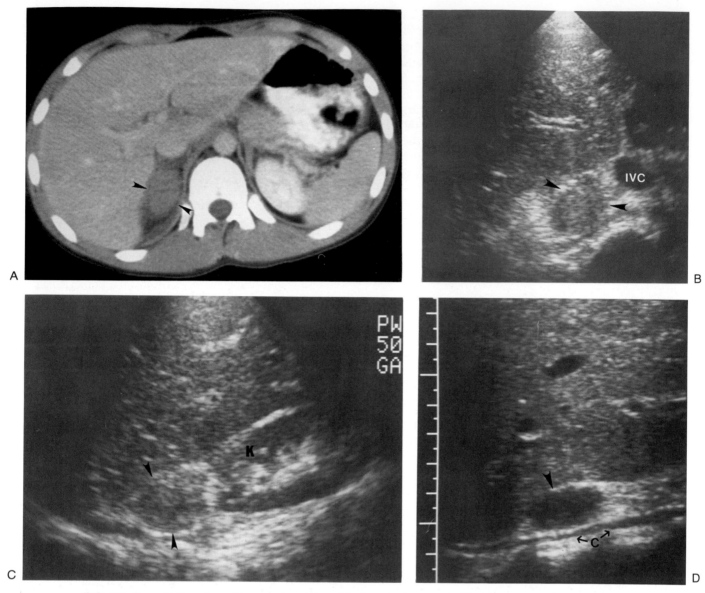

FIG. 10. Traumatic adrenal hemorrhage in a 14-year old boy who was thrown from an all-terrain vehicle. **A:** Contrast-enhanced CT scan through the upper abdomen shows a nonenhancing homogeneous right upper quadrant retroperitoneal mass (*arrowheads*) with increased attenuation of surrounding fat. More caudal scans showed a normal right kidney. Transverse (**B**) and longitudinal (**C**) sonograms were performed to establish a baseline for sonographic follow-up. There is a solid, homogeneously echogenic, round mass in the adrenal bed (*arrowheads*) with increased echogenicity of periadrenal fat. **D:** Oblique longitudinal scan 6 weeks later. The mass is smaller and is now hypoechoic. A later scan 6 months after the injury showed complete resolution. *C,* diaphragmatic crus; *IVC,* inferior vena cava; *K,* kidney.

older children are generally similar to those seen in the neonate. If performed early in the course, sonography shows an echogenic suprarenal mass (Figs. 10, 11). Serial studies show decrease in size of the mass and conversion to a cystic appearance, with eventual resolution (126,151,184).

Inflammatory Disease

Abscess

Adrenal abscess is a rare cause of suprarenal mass in the neonate. The majority of cases are believed to develop as a result of bacterial seeding of adrenal hem-

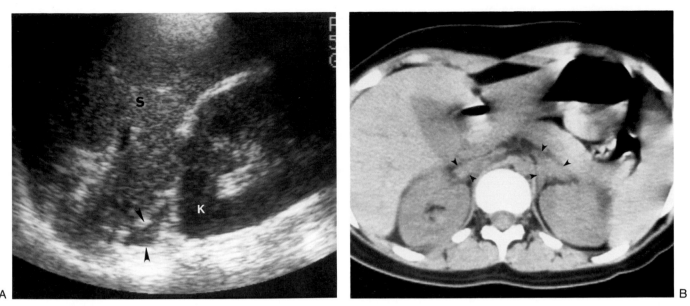

FIG. 11. Spontaneous bilateral adrenal hemorrhage with acute adrenal insufficiency in a 17-year-old girl with systemic lupus erythematosus. **A:** Coronal ultrasound scan through the left flank shows enlargement of the left adrenal gland (*arrowheads*), which is intermediate in echogenicity between that of the spleen (*S*) and left kidney (*K*). The right adrenal gland was similarly enlarged. **B:** Non–contrast-enhanced CT scan shows bilateral adrenal enlargement (*arrowheads*). Adrenal insufficiency was documented with laboratory studies, and the adrenal enlargement was resolved on follow-up CT scans.

orrhage. Hematogenous bacterial seeding of a normal gland is an alternative but less popular hypothesis. As with adrenal hemorrhage, most cases are unilateral, but bilateral cases have been documented (34,53,73). Maternal infection at the time of delivery occurs in approximately one-third of cases (11). Clinical signs are generally similar to those seen with adrenal hemorrhage, but fever and leukocytosis are also common. In a review of 14 cases of neonatal adrenal abscess,

offending organisms included *Escherichia coli,* Group B streptococci, *Staphylococcus aureus,* and *Bacteroides* species (11).

Sonography can easily identify the suprarenal origin of the abscess. It is usually hypoechoic, with echogenic debris that shifts and layers with change in position of the patient. Sometimes an abscess can appear as a solid mass (Fig. 12). Sonographic distinction between adrenal abscess and other lesions, such as adrenal hem-

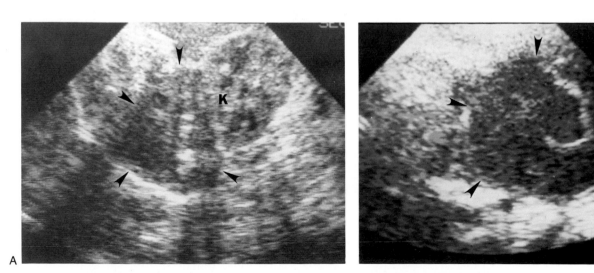

FIG. 12. Adrenal abscess in a 4-week old girl with a history of traumatic delivery. Coronal (**A**) and transverse (**B**) scans show a large left suprarenal mass (*arrowheads*). The mass at this stage appears predominantly solid, with focal high-amplitude echoes. Surgical confirmation. *K,* left kidney. (Courtesy of Dr. Harry J. Presberg, Norfolk, Virginia.)

orrhage and neuroblastoma with central hemorrhage and necrosis, can be difficult. Failure of a presumed adrenal hemorrhage to resolve or increase in size of the mass should raise the suspicion of abscess (11). Early diagnosis and treatment are necessary to prevent complications. Surgical excision or incision and drainage are usually necessary, and extension of the suppurative process to the adjacent kidney or spleen may require removal of these organs.

Other Lesions

Other infectious conditions may affect the adrenals, including tuberculosis and fungal infections such as histoplasmosis. Chronic disseminated histoplasmosis is known to affect the adrenals; the sonographic features have been described in adults (185), but not in children. The most common sonographic observation is bilateral and symmetrical adrenal gland enlargement.

Bilateral adrenal calcification in a 7-week old infant with documented herpes simplex type I infection at 2 weeks of age has been reported (124). This infant displayed diffuse punctate hepatic calcifications and bilateral calcifications in normal size or slightly small adrenals. The child later developed an addisonian crisis.

Tumors

Neuroblastoma

Neuroblastoma is the most common solid tumor of extracranial origin in children, and during infancy it ranks as the most common malignant tumor. At the time of presentation, more than 50% of patients are less than 2 years of age, and 75% are under 4 years (57). Both sexes are affected with equal frequency. Arising from neural crest tissue, neuroblastoma can originate anywhere along the sympathetic chain. The primary site in approximately two-thirds of cases is the abdomen, and approximately two-thirds of abdominal tumors arise from the adrenal medulla. Most remaining abdominal and pelvic tumors originate in the paravertebral sympathetic chain or the presacral soft tissue region, and a small percentage arise from the paraaortic bodies.

Neuroblastoma belongs to the neuroblastoma-ganglioneuroblastoma-ganglioneuroma complex. These three neural crest tumors are distinguished by their degree of maturation and cellular differentiation. Neuroblastoma is the most common and most primitive tumor in this complex. Ganglioneuroma is a benign tumor at the completely differentiated end of the spectrum, and ganglioneuroblastoma represents a pathologically intermediate lesion (78).

Pathologically, neuroblastoma is grossly or finely nodular with a peripheral rim of cortex. Necrosis, hemorrhage, cystic degeneration, and calcification are common. Microscopically the tumor is composed of small, darkly staining, round cells that are characteristically arranged in rosettes (166). To confirm the diagnosis, some histologic evidence of neural origin or differentiation is required. This can be accomplished by light microscopy, electron microscopy, or immunohistology (28). Foci of immature or mature neurons and nerve fibers, with recognizable ganglion cells, characterize ganglioneuroblastoma. Benign ganglioneuroma is composed of mature ganglion cells, Schwann cells, and nerve bundles (166).

Children with abdominal neuroblastoma most commonly present with a palpable mass. Less commonly, presenting signs or symptoms are due to metastases. Rarely, there may be manifestations of a paraneoplastic syndrome, such as myoclonic encephalopathy, or intractable diarrhea and hypokalemia secondary to tumor secretion of vasoactive intestinal peptide (VIP). Pelvic tumors may cause urinary or gastrointestinal symptoms such as oliguria or constipation, respectively, secondary either to local mechanical compression or neural involvement (22). Systemic signs and symptoms such as fever, weight loss, abdominal distention, irritability, hypertension, and anemia may be present. Urinary levels of catecholamine metabolites, particularly vanillymandelic acid (VMA) and homovanillic acid (HVA), are increased in 85% to 90% of patients with neuroblastoma (78).

TABLE 2. *International staging system for neuroblastoma*

Stage 1	Localized tumor confined to the area of origin; complete gross excision, with or without microscopic residual disease; identifiable ipsilateral and contralateral lymph nodes negative microscopically.
Stage 2A	Unilateral tumor with incomplete gross excision; identifiable ipsilateral and contralateral lymph nodes negative microscopically.
Stage 2B	Unilateral tumor with complete or incomplete gross excision; with positive ipsilateral regional lymph nodes; identifiable contralateral lymph nodes negative microscopically.
Stage 3	Tumor infiltrating across the midline with or without regional lymph node involvement; or, unilateral tumor with contralateral regional lymph node involvement; or, midline tumor with bilateral regional lymph node involvement.
Stage 4	Dissemination of tumor to distant lymph nodes, bone, bone marrow, liver, and/or other organs (except as defined in stage 4S).
Stage 4S	Localized primary tumor as defined for stage 1 or 2 with dissemination limited to liver, skin, and/or bone marrow.

From Brodeur et al., ref. 28, with permission.

Neuroblastoma tends to metastasize early, and over one-half of patients have metastases when initially diagnosed. Common sites of metastases are lymph nodes, liver, skeleton, bone marrow, and skin. The pattern of metastases varies with age. Skin lesions are common in infants but rare in older children, and skeletal metastases are very common in older infants and children but rare in neonates (22,57,153). Liver metastases may occur at any age, but extensive hepatic involvement tends to occur in young infants. Extraadrenal abdominal tumors arising from the paravertebral sympathetic chain have a particular predilection for direct extradural intraspinal extension.

The most important factors that affect prognosis are age at diagnosis, site of origin of the primary tumor, and stage of disease at diagnosis. Tumors occurring in the younger age group and arising in extraabdominal sites have a more favorable prognosis. There are several major staging systems used for neuroblastoma. The system of Evans et al., which is based on the clinical extent of tumor, is the one most widely used by radiologists in the United States during preoperative imaging evaluation (55). In an attempt to reconcile differences between the various staging systems, a new staging system that takes into account the most important elements of current but incompatible systems has been proposed (Table 2) (28). The proposed new system is based on clinical, radiographic, and surgical findings. It is incumbent on the radiologist to understand the staging classification utilized at his or her

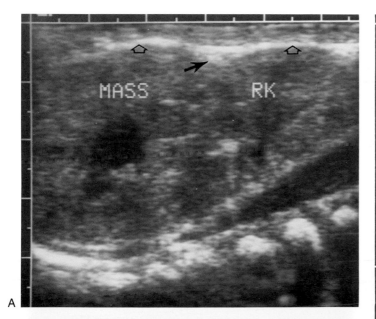

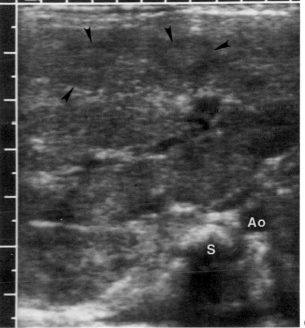

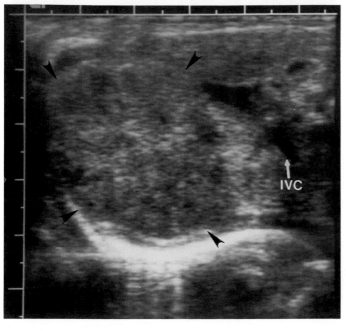

FIG. 13. Neuroblastoma stage 4S in a newborn infant with a right abdominal mass. **A:** Longitudinal scan shows a predominantly solid right suprarenal mass (*mass*) with a central hypoechoic zone. Anterior displacement of retroperitoneal fat (*open arrows*) indicates that the mass is retroperitoneal in origin. Although the mass cannot be separated from the right kidney (*RK*), wedging of a portion of the retroperitoneal fat into a triangular shape (*arrow*) confirms that it arises from the adrenal. **B:** Transverse scan. The adrenal mass (*arrowheads*) is slightly inhomogeneous. The inferior vena cava (*IVC*) is compressed and displaced to the left. At operation, the mass could be separated from the kidney. **C:** Transverse scan through the liver shows diffuse inhomogeneity of hepatic parenchyma and several discrete, slightly hyperechoic metastases (*arrowheads*) with surrounding hypoechoic zones. *Ao*, aorta; *S*, spine.

institution and to direct the imaging evaluation to determine the margins of the primary tumor and the extent of metastatic disease (181).

Pretreatment evaluation of patients with neuroblastoma can be provided by sonography, CT, plain radiography, intravenous urography, scintigraphy, and, more recently, magnetic resonance imaging. In patients presenting with a palpable abdominal mass, either plain radiography or sonography is usually the initial study. Plain radiography can be very helpful in confirming the presence and general location of a mass, as well as in determining the presence or absence of calcifications. Calcifications can be seen in approximately 50% of primary abdominal tumors, and if thoracic paravertebral lymph node metastases are also present, neuroblastoma is the most likely diagnosis. Once a mass has been detected clinically or radiographically, other imaging studies are necessary. Intravenous urography is now rarely utilized in the workup of a pediatric abdominal mass. When performed, it classically shows an extrarenal mass displacing the kidney without intrinsic distortion of the collecting system. Most authors consider CT to be superior to sonography in the evaluation of patients with neuroblastoma, especially beyond early infancy (9,22,42,159,171). Computerized tomography better delineates the extent of primary tumor and its relationship to surrounding structures, i.e., the clinical stage of disease. However, in some cases, the multi-planar imaging capabilities of sonography may offer an advantage over CT in determining whether the tumor mass is intrinsic or extrinsic to the kidney. Magnetic resonance imaging appears to be comparable to CT in detection and preoperative staging of neuroblastoma, including prediction of resectability (48).

Classic adrenal neuroblastoma appears sonographically as a suprarenal mass extrinsic to the kidney, displacing it caudad (Figs. 13, 14). The features of a primary extraadrenal tumor depend on its site of origin (Fig. 15). The range of sonographic textures varies, but the tumor is usually predominantly solid. It may be either hyperechoic or hypoechoic with respect to hepatic parenchyma (181). Reflecting the absence of a well-defined capsule, the tumor margins are usually poorly defined. Inhomogeneity of the mass is common, with hyperechoic areas intermixed with less echogenic areas (Fig. 13) (76). High-amplitude echoes with distal acoustic shadowing are usually secondary to calcification. Echo-free areas may be seen and may even predominate (13,80,122), and are secondary to hemorrhage, necrosis, cystic change, or some combination thereof. In one small series of patients, a distinctive sonographic pattern which the authors believe may be specific for neuroblastoma was described (5). In 40% of patients with neuroblastoma a round, smoothly marginated, uniformly hyperechoic lobule that occupied a part of the larger tumor mass was found. Histologically, the lobule represented uniform aggregates of

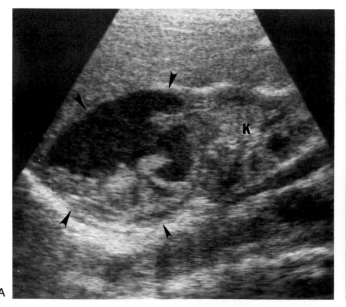 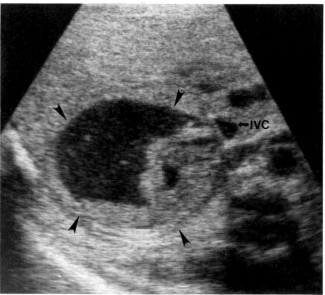

FIG. 14. Hemorrhagic neuroblastoma in a 2-week old infant. Longitudinal (**A**) and transverse (**B**) scans show a complex right suprarenal mass with a large cystic component containing debris (*arrowheads*). Eccentric solid tissue within the mass has irregular margins. At operation, the adrenal mass could be separated from the right kidney. Pathologically, most of the tumor was cystic and contained necrotic debris and old blood. *IVC,* inferior vena cava; *K,* right kidney.

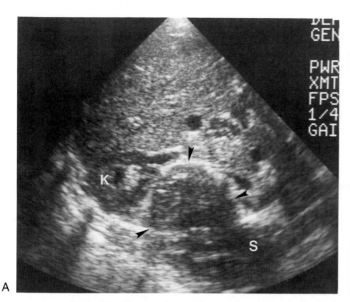

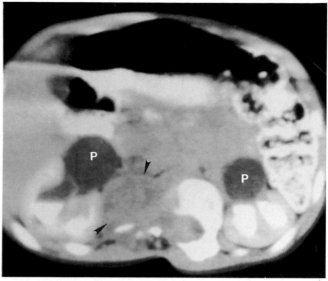

FIG. 15. Extraadrenal neuroblastoma maturing into a benign ganglioneuroma. Seven-year-old girl with congenital paraplegia secondary to neuroblastoma with intraspinal extension. A posterior laminectomy without resection of the tumor was done during infancy, and she was treated with chemotherapy and radiation. **A:** Transverse ultrasound scan from the right anterolateral approach shows a solid right paraspinal mass (*arrowheads*) medial to the right kidney (*K*). S, spine. **B:** Contrast-enhanced CT scan shows slight inhomogeneity of the mass (*arrowheads*), which invades the spinal canal. Contrast medium pools in dilated calyces, and dilated renal pelves (*P*) are not yet opacified. The abdominal portion of the tumor was resected and found to be a benign ganglioneuroma.

neuroblastoma cells with scant stroma and few blood vessels. This sonographic pattern was not seen in any other pediatric abdominal and pelvic tumors, including Wilms' tumor.

Neuroblastoma and Wilms' tumor represent the two most common solid abdominal malignancies of childhood, and sonographic distinction between these tumors is important. Differentiation is usually possible by determining whether the mass is intrarenal or extrarenal. The pattern of displacement of anterior retroperitoneal fat on parasagittal scans can be helpful in determining the origin of a mass in the right upper quadrant (70). Hepatic or intraperitoneal subhepatic masses displace the hyperechoic fat posteriorly, while retroperitoneal masses displace it anteriorly. When wedged into a triangular shape, an anteriorly displaced retroperitoneal fat echo further indicates an adrenal mass rather than an upper pole renal mass (Figs. 13, 16). However, because of a paucity of retroperitoneal fat in many children, this sign is unfortunately not consistently useful. In cases where it is impossible to determine whether a mass arises from the kidney or adrenal, analysis of its sonographic textural features may be helpful to differentiate neuroblastoma from Wilms' tumor. Neuroblastoma is typically markedly heterogeneous, whereas Wilms' tumor is usually evenly echogenic or relatively evenly echogenic, except for scat-

tered discrete holes corresponding to areas of cystic necrosis (76).

Although neuroblastoma in the neonatal period is much less common than adrenal hemorrhage, it should always be considered in the differential diagnosis of a neonatal suprarenal mass. Adrenal neuroblastoma has even been sonographically detected *in utero* (13,57). Although adrenal hemorrhage can occur *in utero* (128,140), an adrenal mass in a fetus more likely represents neuroblastoma than hemorrhage (68). As discussed in the section on adrenal hemorrhage, sonographic differentiation between neonatal neuroblastoma and adrenal hemorrhage may be difficult or impossible. Neonatal neuroblastoma can be complicated by hemorrhage (54,127,165). The most important feature in the sonographic distinction between these two conditions is the tendency of adrenal hemorrhage to change over the course of a few weeks, becoming more cystic and decreasing in size. Neuroblastoma, by contrast, tends to remain static in echo texture over the first 2 weeks of life and to retain the same size or enlarge slightly (32,54). Urinary catecholamines, which are elevated in 85% to 90% of patients with neuroblastoma, should be measured in all neonates with a suprarenal mass, and the sonographic evaluation should include the search for retroperitoneal or hepatic metastases.

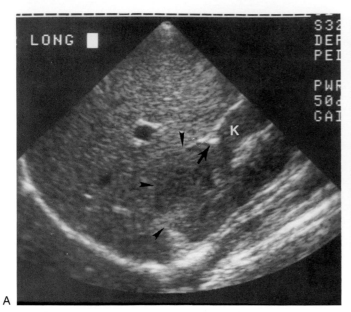
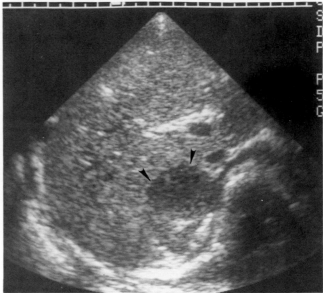

FIG. 16. Lymphoma involving the right adrenal gland. Three-year-old boy with newly diagnosed B-cell lymphoma presenting as a supraorbital scalp mass with bone destruction. During preoperative workup, sonography revealed a slightly inhomogeneous, solid right suprarenal mass (*arrowheads*). **A:** Longitudinal scan. The triangular wedge of echogenic retroperitoneal fat (*arrow*) between the kidney (*K*) and the mass indicates that the mass arises from the adrenal. **B:** Transverse scan. The preoperative diagnosis was neuroblastoma, but biopsy of the scalp lesion revealed B-cell lymphoma. The adrenal mass was not biopsied, but it rapidly resolved after institution of chemotherapy.

In evaluating the intraabdominal extent of tumor, sonography may be very helpful in detecting encasement of the inferior vena cava, aorta, or its major branches, a common feature of neuroblastoma and a finding that excludes complete resectability (20). Sonography may also be valuable in identifying metastatic involvement of retroperitoneal and retrocrural lymph nodes, but it is generally considered to be less reliable in this regard than CT (22). Except in small infants, sonography is usually unable to detect extradural extension into the spinal canal. Hepatic metastases have a variable sonographic appearance. Discrete lesions may be hyperechoic, hypoechoic, or rarely cystic (13,181), and diffuse metastatic infiltration may be manifested by either inhomogeneity of hepatic parenchyma or normal hepatic echo texture with hepatomegaly (see Fig. 13C).

Adrenocortical Tumors

Adrenocortical tumors are rare lesions, accounting for <1% of all neoplasms in children. They are far less common than neuroblastoma but slightly outnumber pheochromoctyoma (42). Carcinoma is the more common adrenocortical tumor, outnumbering adenoma by a ratio of approximately 3 to 1 (43). In children these neoplasms tend to be hormonally active, most commonly producing virilism in females and pseudoprecocious puberty in males (42). Cushing's syndrome, feminization, and hyperaldosteronism are much less common manifestations. In infancy the adrenogenital syndrome is usually caused by congenital adrenal hyperplasia, whereas onset of virilism in females after birth but before puberty is most commonly the consequence of adrenal carcinoma (143). Whereas Cushing's syndrome is usually caused by adrenal hyperplasia in adults, in young children adrenal carcinoma is the most common cause (143). Carcinoma and, less commonly, adenoma and cortical macrocysts are known to occur in association with the Beckwith-Wiedemann syndrome, including its incomplete form, the so-called congenital asymmetry-intraabdominal malignancy syndrome (114,168,169). Cortical macrocysts may be complicated by hemorrhage (114). Pediatric adrenocortical tumors have been reported more frequently in females than males (43), but it is unclear whether this reflects a true female preponderance or merely a selection bias because of the noticeable tumor-induced virilism (143). In a series of 17 pediatric adrenocortical neoplasms (13 carcinomas, four adenomas), the mean ages of presentation for adrenal carcinoma and adenoma were 6 years and 3 years, respectively (43). Carcinoma during the neonatal period has been reported (32).

Adrenal carcinomas tend to be highly malignant neoplasms, undergoing local invasion early and metastasizing widely. In the abdomen, hepatic, nodal, and intravascular spread can be seen. Since the only curative therapy is complete surgical removal, preoperative determination of the tumor extent is very important. Although there is no large pediatric series that critically compares CT with sonography, the general impression is that CT is superior to sonography in determining extent of tumor, but sonography may be particularly useful to determine vascular invasion and to confirm extrarenal and extrahepatic location of tumor (46). Experience with magnetic resonance imaging has thus far been insufficient to determine its ultimate role in the evaluation of pediatric adrenocortical tumors.

Because of the high frequency of hormonal activity of pediatric adrenocortical tumors, most present early and are <6 cm in greatest dimension at the time of initial presentation. Sonographically, these relatively small tumors are usually homogeneous, moderately echogenic, well-defined masses, often with a capsule-like rim. Larger lesions are commonly heterogeneous, with scattered hypoechoic or hyperechoic zones representing necrosis, hemorrhage, or calcification (75); these features are seen more commonly in carcinoma than adenoma but are not specific for malignancy (42,75,166). In the absence of metastatic spread, the differentiation between adenoma and carcinoma is usually impossible with imaging studies. Pheochromocytoma may be sonographically indistinguishable from adrenocortical tumors, but biochemical studies will usually allow differentiation. Sonographic features of adrenal carcinoma that may be helpful in the differentiation from neuroblastoma include absence of vascular encasement (common in neuroblastoma) and presence of intravascular extension (rare in neuroblastoma) (46).

Pheochromocytoma

Pheochromocytoma is a rare catecholamine-secreting tumor arising from chromaffin cells of the sympathetic nervous system. Fewer than 5% of all cases occur in children (42). Primary adrenal pheochromocytomas arise from the medulla; extraadrenal tumors arise from the paravertebral sympathetic chain, paraaortic bodies, or bladder wall. In contrast to adults, children have fewer malignant tumors (<10%), more extraadrenal tumors (20–30%), and a higher frequency of bilaterality and multiple tumors (30%) (35,42,92). Most pediatric malignant pheochromocytomas arise from extraadrenal sites (138). It may be difficult or impossible to differentiate benign from malignant tumors on histologic grounds (166), and determination of malignancy often depends on detection of metastases.

Although most tumors are sporadic, pheochromocytoma can be heritable, either as an isolated lesion or, more commonly, associated with other disorders such as multiple endocrine neoplasia types II$_a$ and II$_b$ (MEN II$_a$ and MEN II$_b$) and phakomatoses (neurofibromatosis, tuberous sclerosis, von Hippel-Lindau disease and Sturge-Weber syndrome) (35). Bilateral tumors occur more often in familial cases (166).

Most patients with pheochromocytoma come to medical attention during evaluation for hypertension. Hypertension is usually sustained in children and is associated with increased levels of plasma and 24-hr urinary catecholamines and their metabolites (35). Less common presenting manifestations include a palpable mass or a history of a familial condition associated with pheochromocytoma.

Because of the relatively high frequency of bilaterality, multiplicity, and extraadrenal site of origin, CT is the preferred imaging procedure in pediatric patients with biochemical evidence of pheochromocytoma, since it allows more effective evaluation of the entire retroperitoneum and pelvis than does sonography. Scintigraphic localization of pheochromocytoma can be accomplished with [123]I- or [131]I-*meta*-iodobenzylguanidine (MIBG), which is taken up by cytoplasmic catecholamine-containing neurosecretory granules in the same manner as norepinephrine (21,162).

There is a paucity of information in the literature on the sonographic appearance of adrenal pheochromocytoma, and most descriptions refer to adults (24). A spectrum of sonographic findings has been described, but most tumors are relatively large, sharply marginated lesions that are entirely or predominantly solid. Solid lesions may be either homogeneous or heterogeneous. Correlative pathologic studies have shown hypoechoic or anechoic areas to represent necrosis or old blood, and hyperechoic zones to represent recent hemorrhage (24). Calcification can be seen occasionally. The sonographic appearance of pheochromocytoma is not distinctive, and differentiation from other adrenal tumors, particularly adrenocortical neoplasms, requires biochemical studies. Sonographic detection of extension of an adrenal pheochromocytoma into the inferior vena cava, apparently through a venous channel, has been described (83).

Metastases

Adrenal metastases occur commonly in a variety of adult malignancies, but they are rare in children. Lymphomatous involvement of the adrenal can occur; tumor deposits produce solid, homogeneous masses that cannot be sonographically differentiated from other neoplasms (Fig. 16).

PANCREAS

The pancreas is located in the anterior pararenal space of the retroperitoneum. The pancreatic head is nestled in the curve of the descending duodenum, and the tail extends into the splenic hilum, where, ensheathed within the splenorenal ligament, it becomes intraperitoneal for a short distance (118). Several important vascular relationships serve to define pancreatic anatomy and provide useful landmarks during sonographic scanning. The inferior vena cava lies posterior to the pancreatic head. The uncinate process, a caudal extension of the head, is located posterior to the superior mesenteric artery and vein. The pancreatic neck joins the head and body and is situated anterior to the portal vein at its point of origin at the confluence of the superior mesenteric vein and splenic vein. The body and tail lie immediately ventral to the splenic vein, caudal to the splenic artery. The duodenojejunal junction demarcates the junction between the body and tail (118). Immediately anterior to the pancreas lies the lesser peritoneal sac, a potential space between the stomach and pancreas.

The pancreas develops from dorsal and ventral buds that arise from the caudal part of the developing foregut. During the process of duodenal rotation, the ventral pancreatic bud is carried dorsally with the bile duct and fuses with the larger dorsal pancreatic bud. As the buds fuse, their ducts anastomose. The main pancreatic duct (Wirsung) forms from the ventral pancreatic duct and the distal portion of the duct of the dorsal bud. The proximal portion of the dorsal duct frequently persists and forms an accessory pancreatic duct (Santorini) superior to the main duct. Rarely, the ductal systems do not fuse, resulting in two separate ducts that drain their respective anlage, a condition know as pancreas divisum. Autopsy studies have shown pancreas divisum to occur in 4% to 11% of glands, making it the most common congenital anomaly of the pancreas (144). Annular pancreas may cause duodenal obstruction shortly after birth. This anomaly most likely results from development of a bifid ventral pancreatic bud, with encirclement of the duodenum by the separate buds as they move in opposite directions to fuse with the dorsal bud (123).

Technical Considerations

The pancreas can be visualized with sonography in a high percentage of pediatric patients. In one study using real-time and static equipment, the pancreas was successfully visualized in 86% of 110 children (38). In another study using only modern real-time equipment, satisfactory examinations were obtained in 94% of 300 consecutive pediatric patients (158). Thin body habitus with generally low body fat content and a relatively large left hepatic lobe are largely responsible for a higher frequency of satisfactory examinations in children than in adults.

Patients should be examined in a fasting state to prevent image degradation by gas and food in the stomach and adjacent bowel loops. The highest frequency transducer possible should be used. Linear array transducers, which have excellent near-field resolution, can frequently be employed with success to visualize the

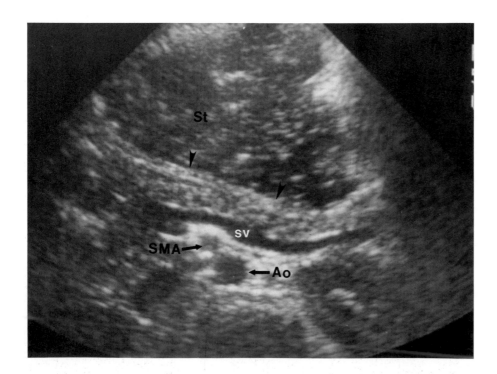

FIG. 17. Normal pancreas visualized through a water-filled stomach (*St*). Six-year-old child. Transverse view shows the pancreatic body and tail (*arrowheads*) anterior to the splenic vein (*sv*). *Ao*, aorta; *SMA*, superior mesenteric artery.

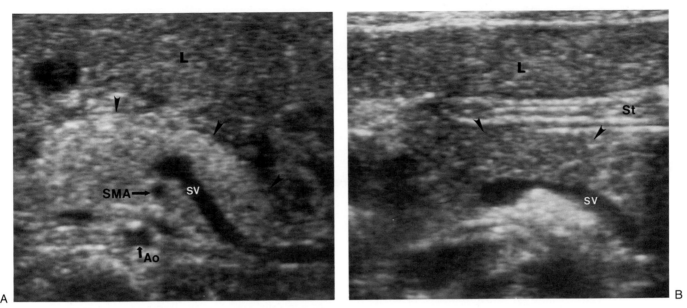

FIG. 18. Transverse scans of the normal pancreas in two children showing variability of pancreatic echogenicity. **A:** Age 3 months. **B:** Age 3 years. In (**A**) the pancreas (*arrowheads*) is hyperechoic with respect to liver (*L*), and in (**B**) the pancreas and liver are isoechoic. *Ao*, aorta; *St*, Stomach (compressed); *SMA*, superior mesenteric artery; *sv*, splenic vein.

pancreatic head and body. As with any sonographic examination, the key to success is finding a suitable acoustic window to visualize the region of interest. Scanning through the left hepatic lobe from an anterior approach usually produces satisfactory images of the head and body. If the left lobe is small or if gas overlies the pancreas, distending the stomach with water can provide an acoustic window (Fig. 17). The most problematic area of the pancreas to visualize is the tail. If routine anterior views are not successful, coronal scanning through the spleen may be employed with success.

The normal pediatric pancreas is homogeneous, with echogenicity equal to or slightly greater than that of adjacent liver (Fig. 18) (40,158). A hypoechoic pancreas relative to adjacent liver can be seen in up to 10% of cases (158). The overall echogenicity of the pancreas is generally less than in adults, probably due to the lower fat content of pancreatic lobules in children (59). Both age and body fat deposition appear to be determinants of increasing pancreatic echogenicity, and these factors have been demonstrated to function independently (187). It has also been shown that adult patients on oral prednisone for a period exceeding 6 months have higher pancreatic echogenicity than controls, when the effects of body fat have been accounted for (74).

The pancreatic head and tail are similar in size and are separated by thinner neck and proximal body seg-

ments (38,158). The method used to measure the maximum anteroposterior dimensions of the head, body, and tail is illustrated in Fig. 19. The pancreas grows

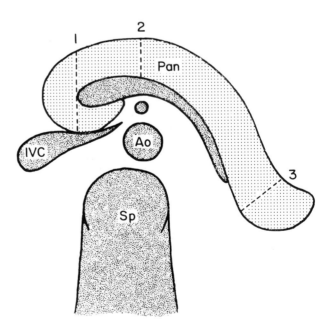

FIG. 19. Diagram of the normal pediatric pancreas (*Pan*) illustrating the points for measurement of the maximum anteroposterior dimensions. *1*, head; *2*, body; *3*, tail; *Ao*, aorta; *IVC*, inferior vena cava; *Sp*, spine. (Adapted from ref. 158.)

TABLE 3. *Normal dimensions of the pancreas as a function of age*

Patient age	Maximum anteroposterior dimensions of pancreas (cm ± 1 standard deviation)		
	Head	Body	Tail
<1 month	1.0 ± 0.4	0.6 ± 0.2	1.0 ± 0.4
1 month–1 year	1.5 ± 0.5	0.8 ± 0.3	1.2 ± 0.4
1–5 years	1.7 ± 0.3	1.0 ± 0.2	1.8 ± 0.4
5–10 years	1.6 ± 0.4	1.0 ± 0.3	1.8 ± 0.4
10–19 years	2.0 ± 0.5	1.1 ± 0.3	2.0 ± 0.4

From Siegel et al., ref. 158, with permission.

substantially in the first year of life, with much slower growth between 1 and 18 years of age (Table 3) (158).

Using high-resolution, real-time equipment, the pancreatic duct can frequently be visualized, either as a single echogenic line in the body of the gland or, less commonly, as a smooth tubular structure with hyperechoic walls and an echo-free lumen (Fig. 20). The normal ductal diameter should be no greater than 1 to 2 mm.

Pancreatitis

Acute Pancreatitis

The prevalence of childhood pancreatitis is unknown, but it is undoubtedly an underdiagnosed condition. There are no clinical or laboratory features that unequivocally establish the diagnosis of acute pancreatitis, and in the majority of cases the diagnosis is inferred from a combination of clinical and imaging findings and an elevation of serum amylase activity greater

than three times normal (40). The frequency of proven causes in published series is influenced strongly by the source of the report, with abdominal trauma and anatomic abnormalities predominating in studies from surgical centers. Drug toxicity assumes an increasingly prominent role in tertiary care centers. Local factors, including the presence of a pediatric oncology unit, a renal transplant service, the autopsy rate, interest in the entity, and the prevalence of conditions such as sickle cell anemia, cystic fibrosis, and ascariasis, also skew the relative frequencies of the various etiologies (149).

Sonography is useful in acute pancreatitis to help substantiate the diagnosis in uncertain cases, to evaluate for biliary tract disorders or other surgically correctable abnormalities that may be associated with the disease, and to detect possible complications (Fig. 21). In most series, the most commonly described intrapancreatic sonographic findings in both children and adults are diffuse or focal enlargement of the gland, and hypoechoic parenchyma that is less echogenic than adjacent liver, assuming the liver to be normal (50,61,88,103). However, in a pediatric study using modern real-time equipment, pancreatic enlargement (46%) and dilatation of the pancreatic duct (46%) were found to be the most common indicators of pancreatitis (Fig. 21); decreased pancreatic echogenicity was not a reliable sign (158). Pancreatic echogenicity and dimensions vary widely throughout childhood, overlapping with those of acute pancreatitis; the limitations of sonography as a screening test for pediatric pancreatitis must be recognized (158).

In addition to intrapancreatic changes in size, echogenicity, and ductal dilatation, focal intrapancreatic masses representing acute fluid collection, phlegmon (a solid mass of indurated pancreas and adjacent re-

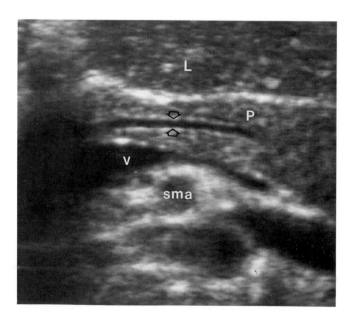

FIG. 20. Normal pancreas with visualization of pancreatic duct. Transverse scan of the pancreas (*P*) in a 17-year-old boy using a 5 MHz linear array transducer. The pancreatic duct (*open arrows*) is visualized as an anechoic tubular structure with hyperechoic walls and a diameter of 1.9 mm. *L*, liver; *sma*, superior mesenteric artery; *V*, portal venous confluence.

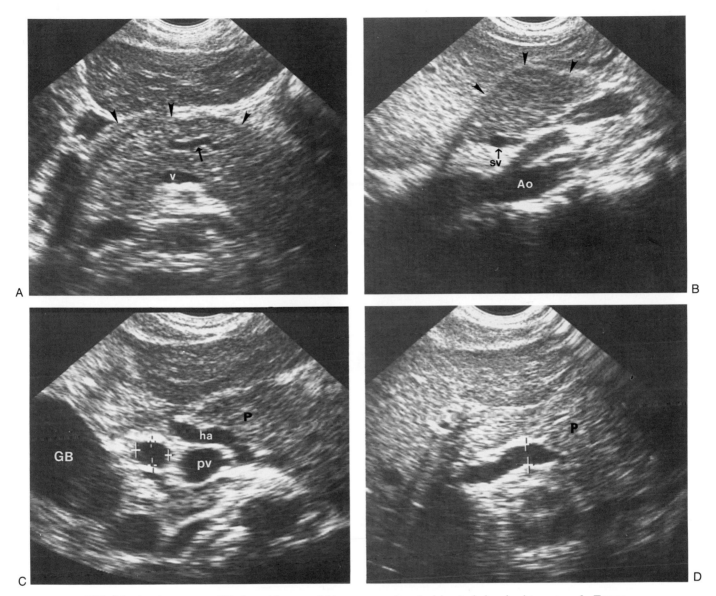

FIG. 21. Acute pancreatitis in a 13-year-old boy secondary to blunt abdominal trauma. **A:** Transverse scan showing a diffusely enlarged pancreas (*arrowheads*) with echogenicity equal to that of adjacent liver. The pancreatic duct (*arrow*) is dilated (4 mm diameter). **B:** Longitudinal scan through the body of the swollen pancreas. **C,D:** Repeat examination 2 weeks later at the time of recurrence of symptoms and elevation of serum bilirubin. On transverse scan (**C**) superior to the pancreatic head a dilated bile duct (7 mm diameter) is seen (*cursors*). The gallbladder (*GB*) is also dilated. On longitudinal scan (**D**) the dilated bile duct tapers as it enters the swollen pancreatic head (*P*). *Ao*, aorta; *ha*, hepatic artery; *pv*, portal vein; *v*, portal venous confluence; *sv*, splenic vein.

troperitoneal tissues), or hemorrhage may also occur. Acute fluid collections may extend outside the confines of the gland, most commonly into the lesser sac or anterior pararenal space. Extension into the anterior pararenal space usually appears in adults as a hypoechoic abnormality tracking along the perirenal (Gerota) fascia (88). Hyperechogenicity of the anterior pararenal space in a child has been described (173), a finding that has not been reported in adults. A small amount of ascitic fluid is commonly seen in acute pancreatitis,

but this does not represent so-called pancreatic ascites—which occurs when there is a communication between the pancreatic duct and the peritoneal cavity—unless the fluid has an abnormally elevated amylase level and a protein level greater than 2.5 g/dl (179).

Sonography is an ideal technique to follow pancreatic or extrapancreatic fluid collections once found, but, at least in adults, it is not as effective as CT in revealing the full extent of peripancreatic abnormalities (36,50,103). A fluid collection in acute pancreatitis may eventually lead to the development of a pseudocyst, defined as a chronic fluid collection limited by a fibrous capsule and devoid of an epithelial lining (103,160). Sonographically, pseudocysts are usually well-defined, ovoid or round in shape, and have a discrete wall. They may be unilocular or multilocular, and, depending on their age, may either be anechoic or contain internal echoes due to necrotic debris or hemorrhage (Figs. 22, 23) (103). When it occurs, spontaneous resolution usually takes place within the first 6 weeks after development (25). Spontaneous resolution of pseudocysts in children has been documented with sonography (17,164), but these may in fact have represented acute pancreatic fluid collections rather than bona fide pseudocysts. Complications of pseudocysts include massive intraperitoneal rupture, rupture into a contiguous part of the gastrointestinal tract, slow intraperitoneal leakage resulting in chronic pancreatic ascites, hemorrhage, infection and abscess, biliary ductal obstruction, and bowel obstruction (25). Hemorrhagic pseudocyst can be suspected when there is sudden increase in abdominal pain, a fall in hematocrit, increased cyst size, and development of extensive internal echoes (Fig. 23) (103). It is usually not possible to distinguish between infected and uninfected pseudocysts using sonographic criteria. Infected pseudocysts tend to have more extensive internal echoes, but are otherwise similar to uninfected ones (106).

A rare complication of pancreatitis is pseudoaneurysm. The splenic artery is most frequently affected, but any vessel contiguous with a fluid collection of pancreatic origin can be involved (30). If available, duplex and/or color flow Doppler should be utilized when a pancreatic fluid collection, focal mass, or suspected pseudocyst is encountered in order to look for turbulent arterial flow within it, which would be indicative of a pseudoaneurysm (56).

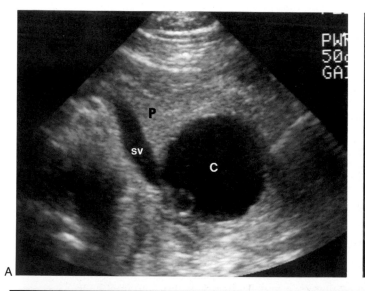

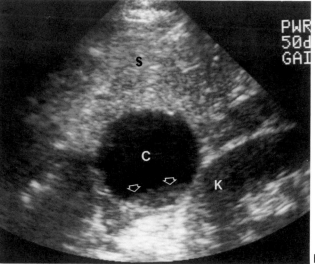

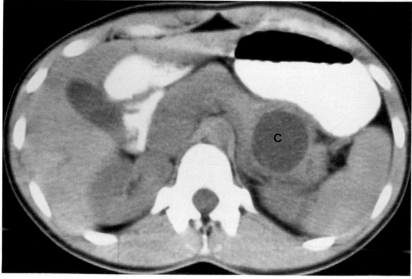

FIG. 22. Pancreatic pseudocyst complicating acute pancreatitis in a 16-year-old girl. **A:** Transverse sonogram shows a well-defined pseudocyst (*C*) adjacent to the splenic vein (*sv*) and pancreatic tail (*P*). **B:** Coronal scan through the spleen (*S*) shows a fluid-debris level in the pseudocyst (*arrows*). **C:** Non–contrast-enhanced CT scan shows the pseudocyst in the pancreatic tail. *K,* left kidney.

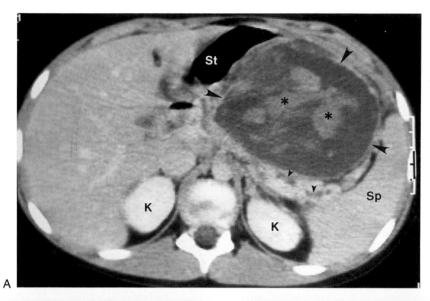

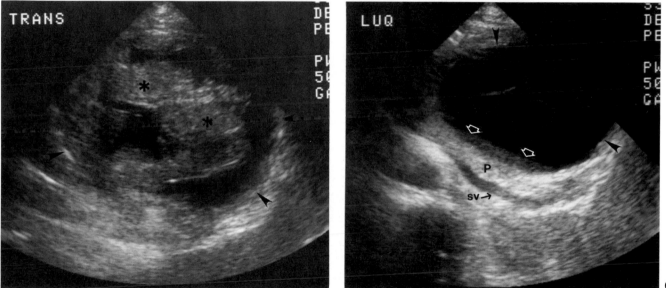

FIG. 23. Pseudocyst with hemorrhage in chronic (hereditary) pancreatitis. A 10-year-old boy with a known lesser sac pseudocyst who presented with sudden onset of severe abdominal pain. **A:** Contrast-enhanced CT scan shows the pseudocyst (*large arrowheads*) in the lesser sac, displacing the stomach (*St*) anteriorly and to the right. Foci of increased attenuation (*asterisks*) presumably represent clotted blood. The pancreas is atrophic, and the pancreatic duct (*small arrowheads*) is dilated. **B:** Transverse sonogram through the pseudocyst (*arrowheads*) on the same day as the CT scan, obtained as a baseline for sonographic follow-up. The solid echogenic material presumed to represent clotted blood (*asterisks*) is well-demonstrated. **C:** Transverse sonogram 2 weeks later. The pseudocyst (*arrowheads*) is slightly smaller, and there has been considerable clearing of the internal echoes. A fluid-debris level (*open arrows*) is seen. *K,* kidney; *P,* pancreas; *Sp,* spleen; *sv,* splenic vein.

Traumatic pancreatic injuries include acute pancreatitis with contusion and edema, peripancreatic fluid collections, hemorrhage, and frank laceration. Comparative studies of sonography and CT in patients with blunt abdominal trauma and surgically proven pancreatic fractures have shown that CT is superior to sonography in demonstrating changes of acute traumatic pancreatitis (89). Because of its ease of performance, sensitivity, and ability to give an accurate representation of the entire abdominal contents, CT is the preferred imaging examination for serious blunt abdominal trauma at our institution, particularly when there is a high likelihood of pancreatic injury. Published reports on the reliability of sonography in acute pancreatic trauma have shown conflicting results, probably due to differences in the time interval between the injury and the sonogram, the relatively small number of patients reported in each series, and the type of sonographic equipment used (63,71,89,178). The earliest sonographic signs of traumatic pancreatitis are enlargement of the gland and/or a peripancreatic collection of fluid, indistinguishable from nontraumatic pancreatitis (71). A condition in children referred to as "obstructive pancreatitis" has been reported in conjunction with traumatic duodenal hematoma. On sonography, there is diffuse pancreatic enlargement, dilatation of the pancreatic and extrahepatic bile ducts, and hematoma of the second part of the duodenum. Elevation of serum amylase and serum bilirubin may be delayed for several days after the injury.

Chronic Pancreatitis

Hereditary pancreatitis, an autosomal dominant disorder with incomplete penetrance, may be the most common cause of chronic pancreatitis in children (67,149). This entity is clinically and pathologically indistinguishable from idiopathic nonfamilial chronic pancreatitis, and the diagnosis can only be established with certainty if the family history is positive. Other causes of chronic pancreatitis include malnutrition, hyperparathyroidism, cystic fibrosis, benign or malignant obstruction of the main pancreatic duct, and possibly pancreas divisum (67,111,144). Studies reporting the experience with endoscopic retrograde cholangiopancreatography (ERCP) in patients with chronic pancreatitis have shown a statistically significant association with pancreas divisum (144). It has been suggested that in pancreas divisum, the accessory pancreatic duct (Santorini) and the accessory ampulla are too small in some patients to transmit the volume of pancreatic secretions that must pass through them. This condition results in a relative stenosis at the accessory ampulla (144). Pancreas divisum cannot be diagnosed with sonography.

The sonographic manifestations of chronic pancreatitis have been described mainly in adults, and include increased echogenicity secondary to fibrosis and/or fatty replacement, calcifications, ductal dilatation (often saccular), atrophy, focal or diffuse enlargement, and an irregular pancreatic outline (36,50). There is apparently a high frequency of both false-negative and false-positive examinations (111). Extrahepatic biliary tract dilatation has been reported in 19% of adults with chronic pancreatitis (2). Published experience and our own personal experience suggest that the sonographic findings of chronic pancreatitis in children are similar to those seen in adults (Fig. 24) (12).

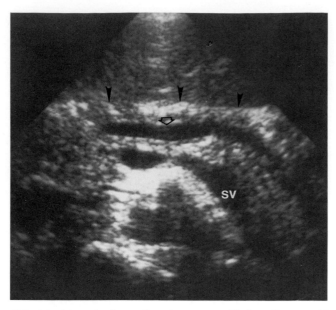

FIG. 24. Chronic (hereditary) pancreatitis in a 5-year-old girl (the sister of the patient illustrated in Fig. 23). The pancreas (*arrowheads*) is inhomogeneously hyperechoic, and the pancreatic duct (*open arrow*) is dilated (3 mm diameter). *sv,* splenic vein.

The complications of chronic pancreatitis are similar to those of acute pancreatitis and are readily demonstrated on sonography and CT. The importance of ERCP in the diagnosis and management of chronic pancreatitis should be emphasized. Endoscopic retrograde cholangiopancreatography is frequently the only test that can demonstrate the precise location and nature of ductal obstructive lesions, and it can aid in preoperative surgical planning for relief of that obstruction (67).

Cystic Fibrosis

The pancreas is abnormal in almost all cases of cystic fibrosis. Obstruction of ducts by inspissated secretions leads to ductal and acinar dilatation, with subsequent tissue destruction, atrophy, and replacement by fibrous tissue and fat. Intraluminal calcifications are common pathologically and are occasionally macroscopic. Small cysts occur frequently and primarily represent dilated ducts. Inflammatory changes are not prominent (136).

With the use of high-frequency, real-time equipment, the pancreas can usually be visualized in patients with cystic fibrosis (174). Bowel gas can be more of a problem than usual (116,186), but it can be minimized by examining the patient after a prolonged fast. The most common sonographic abnormality is moderate to marked increase in pancreatic echogenicity compared with liver at the same depth (Fig. 25).

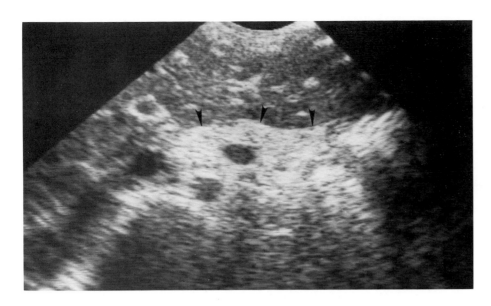

FIG. 25. Cystic fibrosis in an 18-year-old woman. The pancreas (*arrowheads*) is markedly hyperechoic. The patient died 1 month after this examination; autopsy disclosed replacement of virtually all exocrine pancreatic tissue by fibrous tissue and fat.

Echogenicity increases with age and is attributable to fatty replacement and/or fibrosis (44,49,72,139,174, 183,186). There may be a bias toward underestimation of the hyperechoic character of the pancreas since liver disease, especially fatty infiltration, may produce increased hepatic echogenicity. Other pancreatic abnormalities include atrophy, irregular and indistinct margins, calcifications, and small cysts. Pancreatic ductal dilatation is seen infrequently. There is no correlation between pancreatic morphology in cystic fibrosis, especially pancreatic ductal dilatation, and pancreatic exocrine function (174).

Pancreatitis is thought to occur in less than 1% of adolescents and adults with cystic fibrosis (19). When it occurs, it is usually found in those who have not lost all exocrine pancreatic function, and it is presumably secondary to ductal obstruction and leakage of pancreatic enzymes. Hypoechoic enlargement of the pancreas may occur in some patients with clinical signs of pancreatitis (183), but in most patients the appearance of the pancreas is indistinguishable from that seen in uncomplicated cystic fibrosis (139).

Tumors

Pancreatic tumors are rare pediatric neoplasms. They may be classified into nonfunctioning (usually exocrine) and functioning (islet cell) tumors. Symptoms vary according to the functional status of the tumor and the site of origin. Most nonfunctioning tumors are adenocarcinomas and are aggressive malignancies that frequently arise in the pancreatic head and commonly have local extension or metastases at the time of diagnosis (125,175). In contrast to pancreatic carcinoma in adults which shows a male predominance, distribution between the sexes is equal in chil-

dren. Pancreatoblastoma is an infantile type of pancreatic carcinoma with a distinctive histopathologic appearance resembling a fetal pancreas at the eighth week of development. It has a favorable outcome and requires differentiation from more aggressive neoplasms (3,85,86). This tumor is well encapsulated and almost always arises in the pancreatic head. Other nonfunctioning pediatric pancreatic tumors include lymphangioma, hamartoma (31), sarcoma, lymphoma, and hemangioendothelioma.

Islet cell tumors of the pancreas are functioning neoplasms whose presenting manifestations are usually related to their hormonal activity. They are believed to arise from neural crest tissue that gives rise to the cells of the islets of Langerhans. Islet cell tumors may elaborate more than one hormone, but they are usually named after the hormone most responsible for their clinical manifestations. The most common type is the insulinoma, with gastrinoma, VIPoma (which secretes vasoactive intestinal peptide), glucagonoma, and somatostatinoma occurring less frequently (35). Islet cell tumors are typically small lesions less than 2 cm in diameter. A small subset of tumors is hormonally inactive, and these neoplasms are usually clinically silent until they cause symptoms due to their size or to metastatic disease. Consequently, they are typically larger than functioning tumors at the time of diagnosis. Some of the cases that have been reported as nonfunctioning islet cell tumors are now thought to represent pancreatoblastomas (85). Approximately 50% of islet cell tumors are malignant at the time of discovery (35). Histologic criteria for malignancy are unreliable, and malignancy is usually based on demonstration of locally invasive growth or metastases (156). With the exception of somatostatinoma, each of the other functioning islet cell tumors has been seen in the context of multiple endocrine neoplasia type I (MEN I)

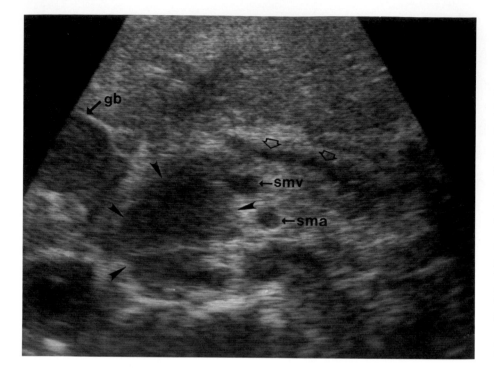

FIG. 26. Pancreatic hemangioendothelioma causing obstruction of the pancreatic duct and chronic pancreatitis. Three-year-old girl presenting with jaundice but no history of abdominal pain. Transverse scan through the pancreas shows a hypoechoic mass (*arrowheads*) in the pancreatic head. The body of the pancreas is poorly defined, and the pancreatic duct (*open arrows*) is dilated. The gallbladder (*gb*) is filled with echogenic bile. Other scans showed biliary ductal dilatation caused by the mass. At operation, the entire pancreas was found to be rock-hard, with considerable surrounding inflammatory reaction. sma, superior mesenteric artery; *smv,* superior mesenteric vein.

(35,156). About three-fourths of islet cell tumors in MEN I are gastrinomas, and most of the remaining ones are insulinomas (35).

The reported sonographic experience with pediatric pancreatic neoplasms is meager, especially utilizing high-resolution, real-time equipment. An inhomogeneously hyperechoic mass with scattered echo-free areas has been described in a neonate with pancreatic carcinoma (146), and a hypoechoic mass associated with chronic pancreatitis secondary to pancreatic ductal obstruction has been seen with pancreatic hemangioendothelioma (Fig. 26). In a series of adult patients with islet cell tumors, most of the tumors were homogeneous solid masses that contained low-level echoes (156). Tumor calcification and cystic spaces were occasionally encountered and were always in malignant lesions.

Sonographic examination of a child with a pancreatic mass should include a careful evaluation of the liver, porta hepatis, and adjacent retroperitoneum to search for metastases or evidence of local spread of tumor beyond the confines of the gland. Liver and regional lymph nodes are the most common metastatic sites for both exocrine adenocarcinoma and malignant islet cell tumors (125,156). Hepatic metastases from islet cell tumors are usually hyperechoic (156).

VASCULAR ABNORMALITIES

Sonography is a nearly ideal technique to evaluate the major retroperitoneal vessels in infants and children. When combined with duplex Doppler and/or color flow Doppler studies, sonography can be used to obtain not only morphologic details, but also information on vascular patency, flow direction, and both physiologic and pathologic changes in impedance (Fig. 27) (93).

Technical Considerations

The relatively large liver in infants and small children provides an excellent acoustic window for visualizing the superior portions of the inferior vena cava and abdominal aorta through the anterior abdominal wall. This approach frequently allows visualization of the aorta as far inferiorly as the level of origin of the superior mesenteric artery. Coronal scans through both flanks can provide excellent demonstration of the aorta and inferior vena cava in infants and older children (Fig. 28) (110,172). Advantages of coronal sonography in the evaluation of the neonatal retroperitoneum include limited manipulation of the infant, less

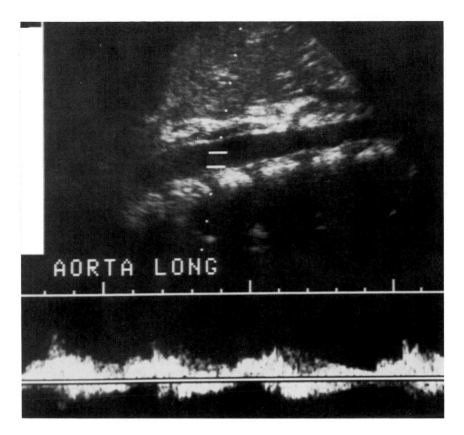

FIG. 27. Coarctation of thoracic aorta in a 5-year-old patient, with abnormal Doppler time-velocity profile in abdominal aorta. The real-time image of the abdominal aorta is normal, but Doppler interrogation superior to the origin of the celiac axis and superior mesenteric artery reveals diminished peak systolic shift, spectral broadening, and bidirectional flow during diastole, reflecting hemodynamic alterations secondary to the coarctation upstream.

hindrance from monitoring devices or tubes when positioning the transducer, and improved visualization of structures due to less interference by bowel gas (110). The highest frequency scanning probe possible should be used. A 5.0 MHz or higher-frequency linear array transducer provides the best images in very small infants.

Aorta

Umbilical Arterial Catheter Localization

Sonography can reliably localize the position of umbilical arterial catheters (64,110,132,134). The aorta normally is pulsatile, with an anechoic lumen. The

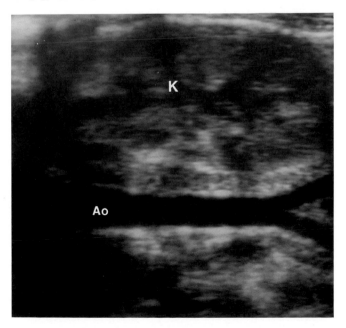

FIG. 28. Normal aorta in a neonate. Coronal scan via the left flank shows the aorta (*Ao*) and both common iliac arteries. *K*, left kidney.

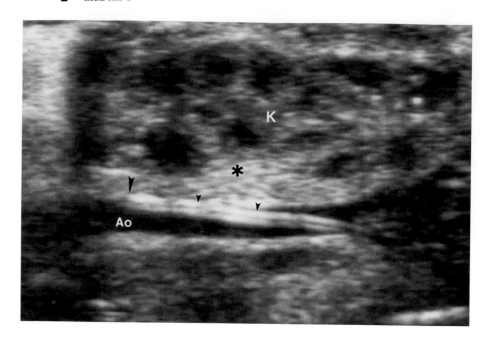

FIG. 29. Umbilical arterial catheter localization. Coronal scan through the left kidney (*K*) demonstrates the echogenic catheter (*arrowheads*) in the aortic lumen (*Ao*). The catheter tip (*large arrowhead*) lies superior to the renal hilum (*asterisk*).

catheter appears either as a brightly echogenic linear or parallel-walled structure within the lumen (Fig. 29). Unlike plain radiography, in which the position of the catheter tip with respect to important vascular structures such as the renal arteries is inferred from its relationship to the vertebral column, sonography allows direct visualization of the vessels and other important structures. Most neonatologists consider the optimal position of the catheter tip to be inferior to the renal arteries and superior to the aortic bifurcation. With coronal scanning, the origin of one or both renal arteries can be identified in approximately 50% of neonates (110). Color flow Doppler should allow an even higher frequency of success. Even without direct visualization, the position of the renal arteries can be reliably inferred by ascertaining the levels of the renal hila.

Thrombus

Thrombus formation can be readily identified with sonography (110,133,150,155). Most thrombi occur in neonates following catheterization of the umbilical artery, but rarely they may be secondary to clotting disorders or embolization from thrombi originating in other cardiovascular malformations (97). With sonography, the reported frequency of aortic thrombi in infants following umbilical arterial catheterization ranges from 17% to 26% (133,155). Significant risk factors associated with aortic thrombosis include (a) calcium in the catheter infusate, (b) placement of the catheter superior to the renal arteries, and (c) low birth weight (<1,500 g) (155). Clinical signs of vascular com-

promise or catheter malfunction are highly predictive of the presence of thrombus, but many thrombi are asymptomatic. The clinical significance of aortic thrombi in asymptomatic infants is at present unknown. Symptomatic infants may be candidates for surgical treatment with clot removal or medical treatment with fibrinolytic therapy.

Sonograms of infants with suspected clots should include scans of the entire abdominal aorta in both transverse and longitudinal planes, as localized mural thrombi may be missed on longitudinal scans if the scan plane does not pass through the clot. The proximal iliac arteries can usually be visualized on coronal scans. Evaluation of the kidneys should be included in the examination. Localized thrombi appear as echogenic foci resembling plaques or polyps attached to the vessel wall or catheter or, when larger, as echogenic material filling the vascular lumen (Fig. 30). Rarely, a thin, linear, mobile, flap-like structure may be identified within the aortic lumen, possibly representing either a floating thrombus or a piece of torn intima (Fig. 31) (133). Thrombi can resolve within a few days, but may last for several weeks. Arterial insufficiency of the lower extremities caused by a distended bladder can mimic thrombotic aortoiliac occlusion in small infants, and sonography can differentiate between these two conditions (101).

Aneurysm

Aortic aneurysm in infants is most commonly seen as a complication of umbilical arterial catheterization. Aortoiliac aneurysms in older children may be seen in

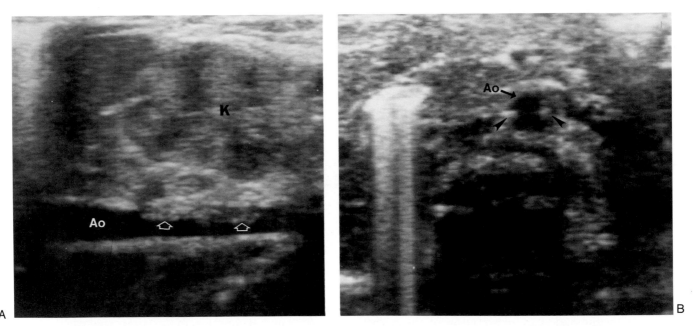

FIG. 30. Aortic thrombus. **A,B:** One-month-old infant with hypertension and a past history of umbilical arterial catheterization. A: Left coronal scan shows echogenic thrombus (*open arrows*) attached to the aortic wall at the level of the left kidney (*K*). B: Transverse scan shows thrombi (*arrowheads*) attached to both lateral aortic walls. *Ao,* aorta. **C** (see Colorplate 8): Aortic thrombus in another neonate with a history of umbilical arterial catheterization. Color Doppler image shows extensive thrombus in the abdominal aorta (*arrowheads*), with complete occlusion caudally. *S,* spine.

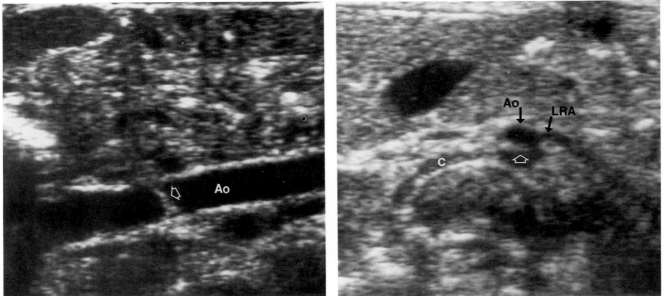

FIG. 31. Band-like defect in the aorta, presumed to represent a remnant of a prior larger thrombus. Three-week-old infant with a past history of umbilical arterial catheterization. Longitudinal (**A**) and transverse (**B**) scans show a well-defined echogenic linear structure (*open arrow*) in the aorta (*Ao*) at the level of the left renal artery (*LRA*); *c,* diaphragmatic crus.

the mucocutaneous lymph node syndrome (Kawasaki syndrome) (39), polyarteritis nodosa, and Takayasu arteritis (69). Most aneurysms associated with arterial catheters are of presumed mycotic origin, with localized trauma from the catheter playing a contributing role. The aneurysm typically develops at the site of the catheter tip (27). Sonography can identify the size, location, and number of aneurysms. In addition, it can be helpful in defining the relationship of the aneurysm to the major abdominal arteries and in detecting superimposed complications such as thrombosis and hemorrhage (27,96).

Inferior Vena Cava

The caliber of the inferior vena cava is highly variable. It normally decreases with inspiration; in cooperative patients Valsalva's maneuver can be used to distend it and render it more visible. Abnormal dilatation, with diminution or obliteration of the normal inspiratory decrease in caliber, occurs with right-sided heart failure, tricuspid insufficiency, and pericardial tamponade.

Congenital Anomalies

The inferior vena cava and azygos/hemiazygos systems are formed by the successive development and regression of three paired cardinal veins (Fig. 32). Infrahepatic interruption of the inferior vena cava with azygos (hemiazygos) continuation is an anomaly due to interruption or failure of fusion of the hepatic and prerenal (subcardinal) veins. This defect occurs in association with persistence of the mid-portion of either the right (azygos) or left (hemiazygos) supracardinal vein (6). The hepatic veins drain directly into the right atrium at the usual site of the caval orifice. The anomaly occurs with increased frequency in patients with congenital heart disease or other visceral abnormalities such as the asplenia and polysplenia syndromes, but it may also be seen as an isolated defect.

Sonography can readily demonstrate the pathognomonic features of inferior vena caval interruption, which include absence of the suprarenal caval segment at the level of the liver, independent drainage of the confluence of hepatic veins into the right atrium, and direct visualization of an enlarged posterior right-sided

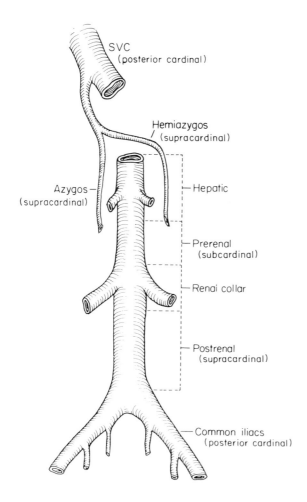

FIG. 32. Embryologic segments contributing to formation of the inferior vena cava, azygos, and hemiazygos veins. In infrahepatic interruption of the inferior vena cava, the hepatic and prerenal segments fail to unite. Persistence of the midportion of the right (azygos) or left (hemiazygos) supracardinal vein leads to azygos or hemiazygos continuation, respectively. (Adapted from ref. 65.)

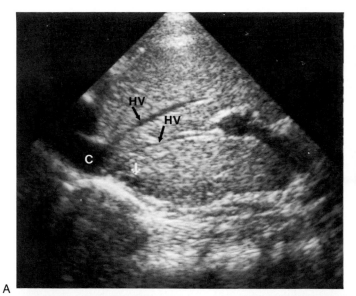

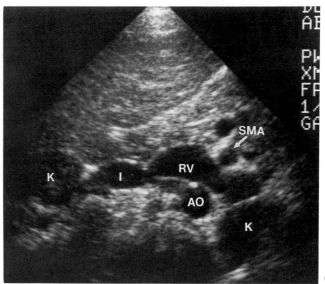

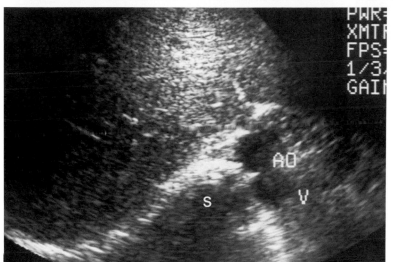

FIG. 33. Infrahepatic interruption of the inferior vena cava with hemiazygos continuation in a 12-year-old girl. **A:** Longitudinal scan shows absence of the inferior vena caval segment at the level of the liver (*cursor arrow*). The hepatic veins (*HV*) drain into a venous confluence (*C*). **B:** Transverse scan at the level of the liver. The enlarged hemiazygos vein (V) lies posterior to the aorta (*AO*). **C:** Transverse scan at the level of the kidneys (*K*). The inferior vena cava (*I*) is present at this level, and it drains into the left renal vein (*RV*), which is dilated because of increased flow. *S*, spine; *SMA*, superior mesenteric artery.

azygos or left-sided hemiazygos venous channel (Fig. 33) (65,145). Doppler studies can aid in confirming that the prominent channel is a central systemic vein (145). With hemiazygos continuation, flow is increased and reversed in an enlarged left renal vein, which is in continuity with the hemiazygos system.

Other anomalies affecting the inferior vena cava include retroaortic left renal vein, circumaortic left renal vein, transposition of the inferior vena cava, duplication of the inferior vena cava, and connection with an anomalous infradiaphragmatic pulmonary vein. There is a paucity of reported sonographic experience with these conditions, and most reports refer to adults (95,176).

Thrombus

Thrombosis of the inferior vena cava occurs in a variety of conditions, both neoplastic and non-neoplastic. Among the non-neoplastic causes are long-term indwelling catheters (62), clotting disorders, dehydration, sepsis, nephrotic syndrome, homocystinuria, phlebitis or periphlebitis (167), and extension from pelvic venous thrombosis. Neoplastic involvement of the venous lumen may occur with renal tumors (Wilms tumor, renal cell carcinoma, angiomyolipoma), hepatocellular carcinoma, adrenocortical carcinoma, pheochromocytoma, and retroperitoneal sarcomas (7,51,83,102,163). Thrombotic involvement by neo-

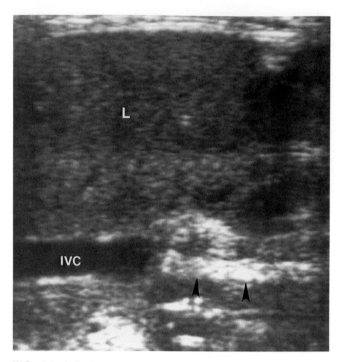

FIG. 34. Inferior vena caval thrombus in a 3-month-old infant with an indwelling venous hyperalimentation catheter. Longitudinal scan shows echogenic thrombus (*arrowheads*) filling the lumen of the inferior vena cava (*IVC*) caudal to the liver (*L*). Further craniad the vena cava is patent.

plasm may be the result of either direct invasion or retrograde extension through venous channels draining the primary tumor. The latter pattern appears to be the more common mechanism in most pediatric tumors.

Sonography can readily demonstrate the intraluminal thrombus, and in most cases of neoplastic disease it can distinguish between tumor extension and extrinsic compression (Figs. 34, 35). Most thrombi appear as echogenic defects filling the lumen, but following partial recanalization the thrombus they may resemble a plaque attached to the vessel wall.

An entity that appears to be unique to the pediatric age group is calcified thrombus in the inferior vena cava. The thrombus is characteristically located at the thoracolumbar junction and appears on plain radiography as a sharply marginated elliptical or bullet-shaped calcification located slightly to the right of the midline, with its long axis oriented vertically (Fig. 36A) (91). The etiology of this condition and the reason for the predilection for this site are unknown. It has been diagnosed in a newborn infant (91). Most thrombi are asymptomatic and are discovered incidentally during workup for an unrelated illness. Because of the abundance of retroperitoneal collaterals, there is no sign of venous obstruction, even in cases of complete occlusion of the lumen. The diagnosis can be readily con-

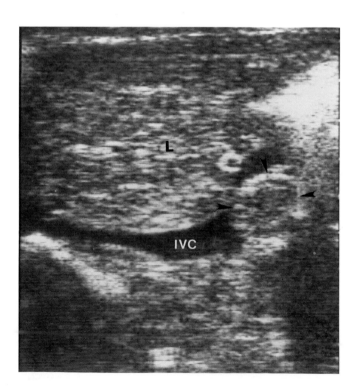

FIG. 35. Wilms' tumor thrombus extending into inferior vena cava in a 2-year-old girl. Longitudinal scan shows inhomogeneously echogenic thrombus (*arrowheads*) filling the lumen of the inferior vena cava (*IVC*). There was surgical confirmation. *L*, liver.

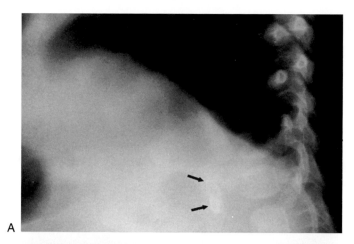

FIG. 36. Calcified thrombus in the inferior vena cava in a 2-month-old infant. **A:** Smooth, vertically elongated calcification (*arrows*) anterior to the twelfth thoracic vertebra noted as an incidental finding on a lateral chest radiograph. Longitudinal (**B**) and transverse (**C**) sonograms show an elongated hyperechoic structure (*arrowheads*) adherent to the posterior wall of the inferior vena cava (*IVC*). *K*, right kidney; *L*, liver; *RV*, right renal vein.

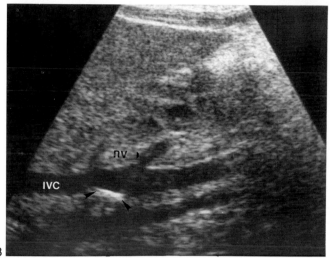

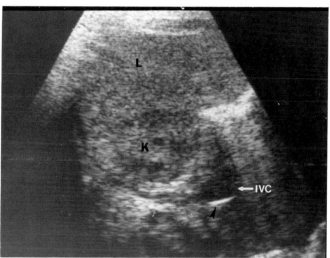

firmed with sonography (Fig. 36) (41,177), and the addition of duplex or color flow Doppler studies can aid in assessing vascular patency. The calcified thrombus appears as an elongated, hyperechoic mass with distal acoustic shadowing, partially or completely filling the lumen. Rarely, noncalcified thrombus may be seen inferior to the calcification (91).

The differential diagnosis of a membranous filling defect in the inferior vena cava at its junction with the right atrium includes a prolapsing Chiari malformation. A Chiari malformation results from excessive fenestration of the valve of the inferior vena cava and the valve of the coronary sinus, producing a network of fine filaments in the right atrium. It occurs with a frequency of 2% to 3%, and with two-dimensional echocardiography it is seen in approximately 1.5% of the normal population (108). When present, it normally appears echocardiographically as an oscillating echogenic membrane within the right atrium that moves toward the tricuspid valve during atrial systole, and away from it during atrial diastole. With tricuspid insufficiency, increased mobility may result in prolapse into the inferior vena cava during atrial diastole, pro-

ducing a flap-like intraluminal structure that should not be confused with thrombus. Pathologic prolapse has only been reported in adults (108), but since a Chiari malformation can also be demonstrated during pediatric echocardiography, prolapse into the inferior vena cava could theoretically be seen in children as well.

MISCELLANEOUS RETROPERITONEAL STRUCTURES

Normal Anatomy

The diaphragmatic crura are attached to the anterolateral surfaces of the upper lumbar vertebral bodies. The two crura are closely applied to the anterior surface of the aorta and enclose the retrocrural space, which contains fat, the thoracic duct, lymph nodes, and the azygos and hemiazygos veins. The right crus is larger and is readily visible on abdominal sonography of most infants and small children, appearing as a well-defined hypoechoic structure anterolateral to the upper lumbar spine and posteromedial to the caudate lobe of the liver, inferior vena cava, and right adrenal gland (Fig. 37). Care should be taken not to mistake the cephalic portion of the crus of the right hemidiaphragm for the right adrenal gland on transverse scans of small infants. A prominent inferior right crus can be mistaken for retroperitoneal adenopathy. If there is confusion, longitudinal scans, which demonstrate the crus as a linear structure, should resolve the issue (33).

The major muscles of the retrofascial space posterior to the retroperitoneum all appear as relatively homogeneous hypoechoic structures with occasional stria-

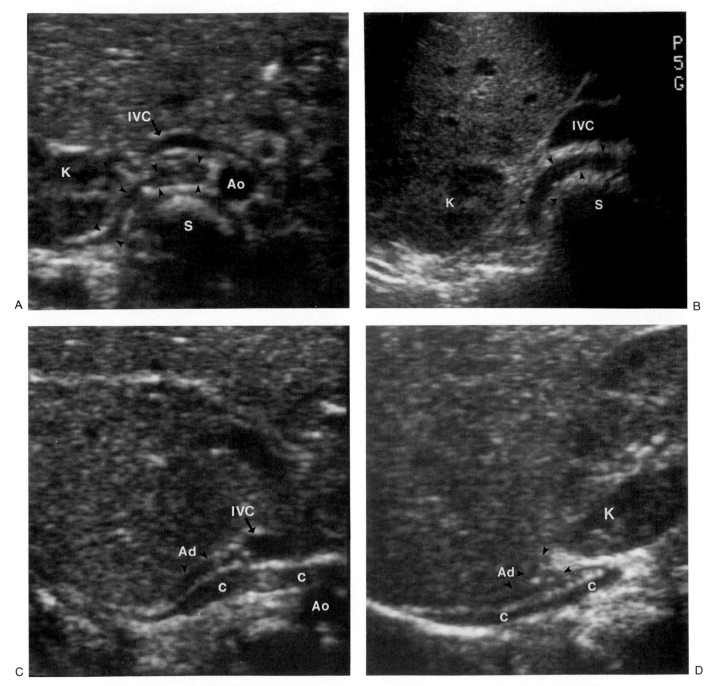

FIG. 37. Normal diaphragmatic crus. **A:** Age 5 weeks; transverse scan at the level of the left renal vein. The right crus (*arrowheads*) is thicker medially adjacent to the aorta (*Ao*). It lies posterior to the inferior vena cava (*IVC*) and extends posterolaterally adjacent to the spine (*S*). **B:** Seventeen years old; transverse scan at the level of the upper pole of the right kidney (*K*). The crus is a well-defined hypoechoic structure that is outlined by hyperechoic fat. **C,D:** Age 8 weeks. The adrenal gland (*Ad, arrowheads*) appears as a hypoechoic structure anterior to the crus (*c*). On the longitudinal scan (**D**) the crus is long and linear, extending superior to the adrenal.

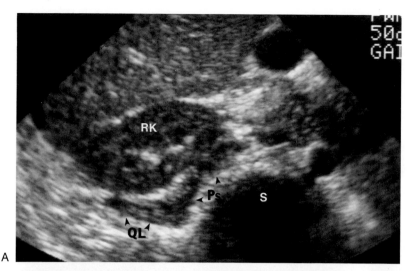

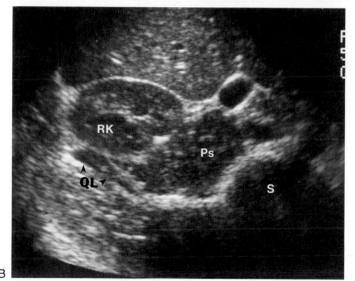

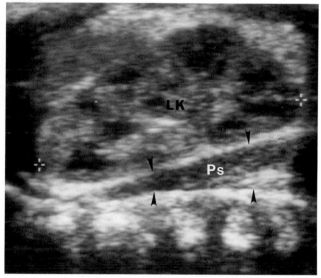

FIG. 38. Normal retroperitoneal muscles. Transverse scans at the level of the right kidney (*RK*) in a 5-year-old girl (**A**) and a muscular 15-year-old boy (**B**). The psoas muscle (*Ps, arrowheads*) lies between the kidney and the spine (*S*). In **B** it is larger and more rounded in shape. The quadratus lumborum muscle (*QL, arrowheads*) lies posterior to the kidney and is a relatively flat structure. **C:** Coronal scan via the left flank in a neonate shows the left psoas muscle tapering cephalad (*arrowheads*) in its position medial to the left kidney (*LK*).

tions. The psoas is the most consistently visualized muscle. It descends in a paravertebral location from the thoracolumbar junction into the iliac fossa, where it merges with the iliacus as the two muscles course into the true pelvis to become the iliopsoas. In the upper retroperitoneum, the psoas muscle lies posteromedial to the kidney and lateral to the spine. Depending on age, body habitus, and scan level, its shape varies on transverse scans, ranging from oval to round (Fig. 38). Contraction of the psoas causes the muscle to assume a more rounded shape. On coronal scans, the psoas tapers cephalad, disappearing near the upper pole of the kidney. Care should be exercised not to mistake the hypoechoic psoas muscle on coronal scans for a dilated ureter. The quadratus lumborum lies posterior to the kidney and appears as a relatively flat structure on both transverse and longitudinal scans (Fig. 38).

Inflammatory Disease

Retroperitoneal infection may involve the iliopsoas muscle. It may be secondary to bacteremia or to spread from adjacent inflammatory disease, such as a posteriorly perforated appendix or colon, Crohn's disease, suppurative iliac or pelvic lymphadenitis, or infections of the kidney, spine, or other retroperitoneal structures (60). Most psoas abscesses are now pyogenic rather than tuberculous. Identification of the causative organism(s) can often provide a clue to the etiology. Those that result from primary bacteremia, discitis, or vertebral osteomyelitis are usually caused by *Staphylococcus aureus,* whereas abscesses secondary to perforation of the appendix or colon are due to bowel flora. Suppurative iliac lymphadenitis in children is usually caused by streptococcal infection of the lower extremity (60). Bacteremic seeding of a primary psoas hematoma also can lead to development of an abscess.

Abscess of the psoas muscle or other retroperitoneal structures can be diagnosed with either sonography or CT (8,82,100,154). On sonography, early involvement is manifested as enlargement of the involved psoas muscle, followed by development of a hypoechoic or anechoic mass, often with either internal debris or septations (Fig. 39). Differentiation from other fluid-filled retroperitoneal masses such as hematoma or necrotic tumor may be difficult or impossible solely on sonographic grounds. Hematoma is usually seen in asso-

ciation with a bleeding disorder or major trauma, but abscess formation in a primary hematoma should be kept in mind in the appropriate clinical setting.

Retroperitoneal Lymph Nodes

Sonography can accurately detect retroperitoneal lymph node enlargement, especially in the upper retroperitoneum where bowel gas is less of a problem. Computerized tomography, however, is considered to be more accurate than sonography, even in children,

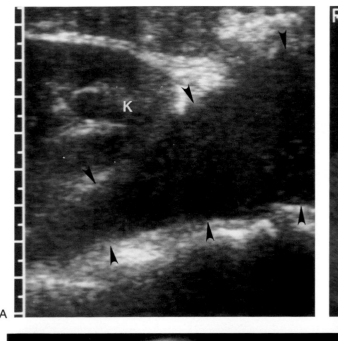

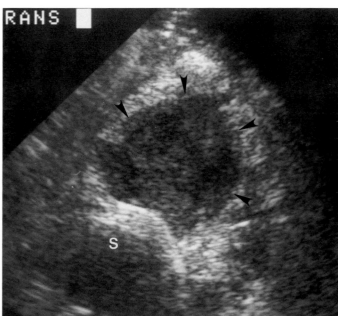

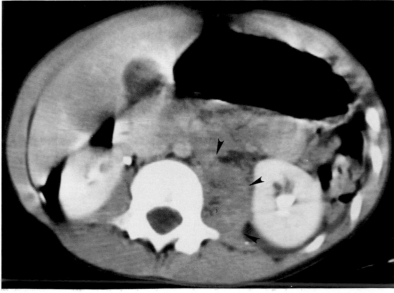

FIG. 39. Psoas abscess. Nine-year-old boy with a history of blunt trauma to the left flank and back 1 week earlier, with subsequent development of flank pain and fever. Left coronal (**A**) and transverse (**B**) sonograms show an enlarged psoas muscle (*arrowheads*). The psoas is relatively hypoechoic, with inhomogeneous echogenicity. **C:** Contrast-enhanced CT scan shows the left psoas enlargement, with inhomogeneous enhancement (*arrowheads*). At operation, a large psoas abscess containing thick purulent material was found, with edema of the psoas superior and inferior to the abscess. *K*, left kidney; *S*, spine.

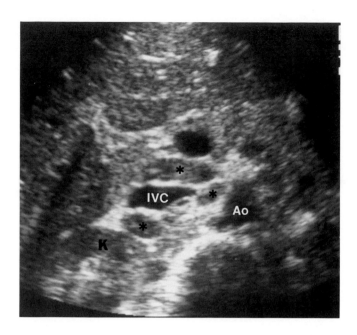

FIG. 40. Retroperitoneal lymphadenopathy in a 16-year-old boy with lymphoma. Transverse scan at the level of the right kidney (*K*) shows enlargement of paracaval and interaorto-caval lymph nodes (*asterisks*), which appear as discrete, rounded, hypoechoic structures. *Ao,* aorta; *IVC,* inferior vena cava.

who have less abdominal fat than adults, primarily because CT affords a better view of the entire abdomen and is not degraded by bowel gas.

Detection of nodal enlargement is important in the preoperative staging evaluation of abdominal neoplasms such as neuroblastoma and primary renal tumors. There are two basic sonographic patterns of lymphadenopathy: rounded focal lesions ranging from 1 to 3 cm in diameter; and larger confluent masses resulting from coalescence of multiple smaller nodes (99). The former are usually easy to differentiate from adjacent organs, but the latter may appear inseparable from contiguous structures. Enlarged nodes are usually relatively hypoechoic, with a homogeneous internal structure (Figs. 40, 41). Although sonography can detect nodal enlargement, it cannot distinguish between enlargement due to inflammatory conditions and enlargement due to neoplastic involvement.

Tumors and Cysts

Wilms tumor and neuroblastoma account for over 85% of primary retroperitoneal neoplasms (77). Excluding these tumors, primary retroperitoneal neoplasms are rare. Sonography can accurately distinguish cystic from solid retroperitoneal masses and can provide excellent definition of the internal features and wall structure of predominantly cystic masses. Sonography can also be very useful in determining the location of a retroperitoneal mass, but some masses may

be so large as to make determination of the organ of origin difficult or impossible. Contrast-enhanced CT and magnetic resonance imaging are more accurate for this purpose.

Most of the predominantly solid primary retroperitoneal tumors do not have specific sonographic characteristics. Rhabdomyosarcoma, the most common soft tissue sarcoma, appears as a solid mass of variable echogenicity, often with hypoechoic or anechoic areas that are probably secondary to necrosis or hemorrhage (117). Lipomas, lipoblastomas, liposarcomas, and fat-containing components of teratomas are all hyperechoic, but reliable sonographic differentiation of fat from other soft-tissue components is usually impossible. Calcifications can be identified in teratomas and other retroperitoneal sarcomas because of acoustic shadowing distal to the hyperechoic foci (45). Primary lymphangiomas arising in the retroperitoneum and elsewhere typically contain anechoic fluid in one or more contiguous cystic loculations separated by thin soft-tissue septa. The fluid may contain fine dependent or diffuse echoes. Hemorrhage or infection may produce fluid with a coarsely echogenic pattern or mobile solid structures (18).

Retroperitoneal Fibrosis

Retroperitoneal fibrosis is a disease in which a plaque-like fibrotic mass centered at or near the sacral promontory envelops the distal prevertebral vessels

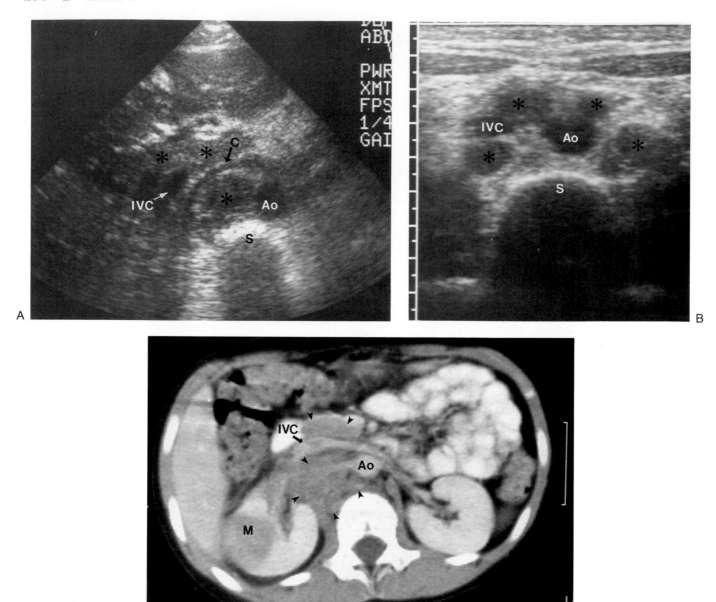

FIG. 41. Retroperitoneal lymphadenopathy in a 10-year-old boy with adenocarcinoma of the right kidney. **A:** Transverse sonogram through the upper abdomen shows retrocrural, paracaval, and interaorto-caval lymphadenopathy (*asterisks*), which is represented by confluent masses of coalesced nodes. **B:** Transverse sonogram caudal to the kidneys shows paraaortic and paracaval lymphadenopathy (*asterisks*). The lymph nodes at this level are more discrete than in **A**. **C:** Contrast-enhanced CT scan at a level slightly caudal to **A** shows the primary tumor mass (*M*) in the right kidney and extensive retrocrural, paracaval, and interaorto-caval lymphadenopathy (*arrowheads*). *Ao,* aorta; *C,* diaphragmatic crus; *IVC,* inferior vena cava; *S,* spine.

and/or one or both ureters. Although it is most commonly seen in middle-aged adults, rare cases have been reported in children (15,157). Retroperitoneal fibrosis is usually idiopathic, but the disease has been seen in association with several drugs, hemorrhage, infection, and a variety of systemic illnesses. There may be an

association with occult malignancy in adults, but apparently not in children (15,157).

The classic radiologic finding in both children and adults is hydronephrosis with medial deviation of the ureter(s) at the site of the fibrotic mass (15). Sonography shows a smooth-walled hypoechoic mass anterior to the sacral promontory. There is a tendency to envelop but not displace the aorta and inferior vena cava, in contrast to lymphoma and neuroblastoma which commonly encase and displace vascular structures. Since the disease is so rare in children, biopsy is usually necessary to establish the diagnosis.

Presacral Soft Tissues

Many of the conditions that affect the retroperitoneum also involve the presacral soft tissues. Approximately 40% of tumors of germ cell origin occur in the sacrococcygeal region, making this the most common site of these tumors in childhood (1). Most of these are teratomas, and they have been classified according to clinical presentation as follows: type I (47%), predominantly external with minimal presacral component; type II (34%), external with a significant intrapelvic component; type III (9%), predominantly internal, both pelvic and intraabdominal, with a smaller external component; and type IV (10%), entirely presacral, without an external component or significant intraabdominal extension (Fig. 42) (4). Early diagnosis and treatment, consisting of removal of the tumor in con-

tinuity with the coccyx, are of the utmost importance because of the tendency for malignant conversion. The prevalence of malignancy when the diagnosis is made at less than 2 months of age is approximately 10%, whereas after 2 months of age two-thirds of boys and nearly one-half of girls have malignant tumors (4).

The diagnosis is usually obvious when sacrococcygeal teratoma presents as a large mass with a significant external component. There may be a history of prenatal sonographic detection of a mass contiguous with the fetal sacrum (84). Calcifications and fat on plain radiographs provide strong confirmatory evidence. Sonography can provide useful information on the extent and internal tissue characteristics of teratomas (Fig. 43). Since compression or invasion of the bladder or ureters may occur, the kidneys should also be evaluated for evidence of hydronephrosis. Benign tumors are predominantly cystic, with solid components often projecting into one or more large cysts; malignant teratomas are predominantly solid but may contain finely polycystic areas (3).

Some of the other masses that may occur in the presacral region of children include neuroblastoma and other neurogenic tumors, soft tissue sarcoma, lymphoma, lipoma, lymphangioma, anterior meningocele,

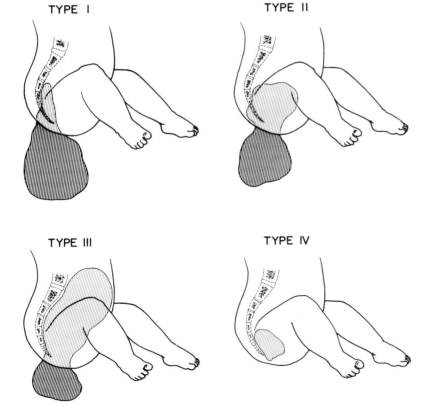

FIG. 42. Classification of sacrococcygeal teratomas. Type I: predominantly external with a small presacral component. Type II: external with a significant intrapelvic component. Type III: predominantly internal, both pelvic and intraabdominal, with a smaller external component. Type IV: entirely presacral, without an external component or significant intraabdominal extension. (Adapted from ref. 4.)

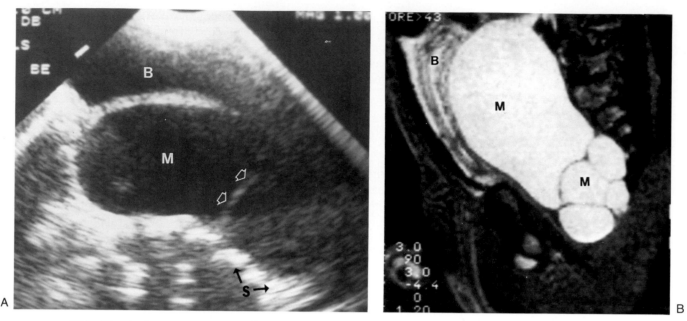

A

B

FIG. 43. Benign sacrococcygeal teratoma in a 3-month-old boy with a history of constipation. **A:** Longitudinal sonogram shows a predominantly cystic mass (*M*) posterior to the bladder (*B*), displacing it anteriorly and superiorly. The mass has internal septations in its caudal portion (*open arrows*). **B:** Midsagittal magnetic resonance image through the mass (TR = 3,000 msec, TE = 90 msec). The septations are better demonstrated than on the sonogram. This is a type III lesion, with a large pelvic and abdominal component and no significant external mass. *S,* spine. (Courtesy of Dr. Lakshmana Das Narla, Richmond, Virginia.)

neurenteric cyst, rectal duplication, chordoma, sacral bone tumors, and abscess (180). Although sonography can be helpful in characterizing the internal tissue characteristics of a mass and in defining its extent (Fig. 44),

the diagnosis is seldom determined without tissue sampling. In many cases, either CT or magnetic resonance imaging may provide more accurate and more complete presurgical evaluation.

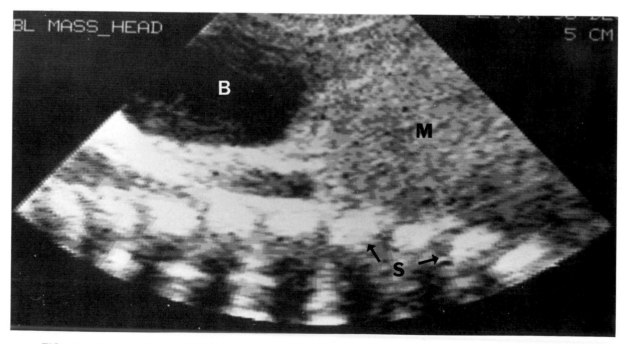

FIG. 44. Presacral neuroblastoma in a newborn infant. Longitudinal scan shows a solid, homogeneous mass (*M*) caudal to the bladder (*B*) and anterior to the sacrum (*S*).

REFERENCES

1. Ablin A, Isaacs H Jr. Germ cell tumors. In: Pizzo PA, Poplack DG, eds. *Principles and Practice of Pediatric Oncology*. Philadelphia: JB Lippincott, 1989;713–731.
2. Alpern MB, Sandler MA, Kellman GM, Madrazo BL. Chronic pancreatitis: Ultrasonic features. *Radiology* 1985;155:215–219.
3. Altman AJ, Schwartz AD. *Malignant Diseases of Infancy, Childhood and Adolescence,* 2nd ed. Philadelphia: Saunders, 1983.
4. Altman RP, Randolph JG, Lilly JR. Sacrococcygeal teratoma: American Academy of Pediatrics Surgical Section Survey—1973. *J Pediatr Surg* 1974;9:389–398.
5. Amundson GM, Trevenen CL, Mueller DL, Rubin SZ, Wesenberg RL. Neuroblastoma: A specific sonographic tissue pattern. *AJR* 1987;148:943–945.
6. Anderson RC, Adams P Jr, Burke B. Anomalous inferior vena cava with azygos continuation (infrahepatic interruption of the inferior vena cava). *J Pediatr* 1961;59:370–383.
7. Arenson AM, Graham RT, Shaw P, Srigley J, Herschorn S. Angiomyolipoma of the kidney extending into the inferior vena cava: Sonographic and CT findings. *AJR* 1988;151:1159–1161.
8. Arenson AM, Wilson SR, McKee JD. Psoas disease causing a characteristic change in the ultrasonographic appearance of the psoas compartment. *J Can Assoc Radiol* 1984;35:276–278.
9. Armstrong EA, Harwood-Nash DCF, Fitz CR, Chuang SH, Pettersson H, Martin DJ. CT of neuroblastomas and ganglioneuromas in children. *AJR* 1982;139:571–576.
10. Ashley DJB, Mostofi FK. Renal agenesis and dysgenesis. *J Urol* 1960;83:211–230.
11. Atkinson GO Jr, Kodroff MB, Gay BB Jr., Ricketts RR. Adrenal abscess in the neonate. *Radiology* 1985;155:101–104.
12. Atkinson GO Jr, Wyly JB, Gay BB Jr, Ball TI, Winn KJ. Idiopathic fibrosing pancreatitis: A cause of obstructive jaundice in childhood. *Pediatr Radiol* 1988;18:28–31.
13. Atkinson GO Jr, Zaatari GS, Lorenzo RL, Gay BB Jr, Garvin AJ. Cystic neuroblastoma in infants: Radiographic and pathologic features. *AJR* 1986;146:113–117.
14. Bech K, Tygstrup I, Nerup J. The involution of the foetal adrenal cortex: A light microscopic study. *Acta Path Microbiol Scand* 1969;76:391–400.
15. Birnberg FA, Vinstein AL, Gorlick G, Lee FA, Hales MS. Retroperitoneal fibrosis in children. *Radiology* 1982;145:59–61.
16. Black J, Williams DI. Natural history of adrenal haemorrhage in the newborn. *Arch Dis Child* 1973;48:183–190.
17. Bloom RA, Abu-Dalu K, Pollak D. Spontaneous resolution of a large pancreatic pseudocyst in a child. *J Clin Ultrasound* 1983;11:37–39.
18. Blumhagen JD, Wood BJ, Rosenbaum DM. Sonographic evaluation of abdominal lymphangiomas in children. *J Ultrasound Med* 1987;6:487–495.
19. Boat TF, Welsh MJ, Beaudet AL. Cystic fibrosis. In: Scriver CR, Beaudet AL, Sly WS, Valle D, eds. *The Metabolic Basis of Inherited Disease,* 6th ed. New York: McGraw-Hill, 1989;2649–2680.
20. Boechat MI, Ortega J, Hoffman AD, Cleveland RH, Kangarloo H, Gilsanz V. Computed tomography in Stage III neuroblastoma. *AJR* 1985;145:1283–1287.
21. Bomanji J, Levison DA, Flatman WD, Horne T, Bouloux PM-G, Ross G, et al. Uptake of iodine-123 MIBG by pheochromocytomas, paragangliomas, and neuroblastomas: A histopathological comparison. *J Nucl Med* 1987;28:973–978.
22. Bousvaros A, Kirks DR, Grossman H. Imaging of neuroblastoma: An overview. *Pediatr Radiol* 1986;16:89–106.
23. Bowen A, Smazal SF Jr. Ultrasound of coexisting right renal vein thrombosis and adrenal hemorrhage in a newborn. *J Clin Ultrasound* 1981;9:511–513.
24. Bowerman RA, Silver TM, Jaffe MH, Stuck KJ, Hinerman DL. Sonography of adrenal pheochromocytomas. *AJR* 1981;137:1227–1231.
25. Bradley EL III, Clements JL Jr, Gonzalez AC. The natural history of pancreatic pseudocysts: A unified concept of management. *Am J Surg* 1979;137:135–141.
26. Brill PW, Jagannath A, Winchester P, Markisz JA, Zirinsky K. Adrenal hemorrhage and renal vein thrombosis in the newborn: MR imaging. *Radiology* 1989;170:95–98.
27. Brill PW, Winchester P, Levin AR, Griffith AY, Kazam E, Zirinsky K. Aortic aneurysm secondary to umbilical artery catheterization. *Pediatr Radiol* 1985;15:199–201.
28. Brodeur GM, Seeger RC, Barrett A, Berthold F, Castleberry RP, D'Angio G, et al. International criteria for diagnosis, staging, and response to treatment in patients with neuroblastoma. *J Clin Oncol* 1988;6:1874–1881.
29. Bryan PJ, Caldamone AA, Morrison SC, Yulish BS, Owens R. Ultrasound findings in the adreno-genital syndrome (congenital adrenal hyperplasia). *J Ultrasound Med* 1988;7:675–679.
30. Burke JW, Erickson SJ, Kellum CD, Tegtmeyer CJ, Williamson BRJ, Hansen MF. Pseudoaneurysms complicating pancreatitis: Detection by CT. *Radiology* 1986;161:447–450.
31. Burt TB, Condon VR, Matlak ME. Fetal pancreatic hamartoma. *Pediatr Radiol* 1983;13:287–289.
32. Butler H, Bick R, Morrison S. Unsuspected adrenal masses in the neonate: Adrenal cortical carcinoma and neuroblastoma. *Pediatr Radiol* 1988;18:237–239.
33. Callen PW, Filly RA, Sarti DA, Sample WF. Ultrasonography of the diaphragmatic crura. *Radiology* 1979;130:721–724.
34. Carty A, Stanley P. Bilateral adrenal abscesses in a neonate. *Pediatr Radiol* 1973;1:63–64.
35. Chrousos GP. Endocrine tumors. In: Pizzo PA, Poplack DG, eds. *Principles and Practice of Pediatric Oncology*. Philadelphia: JB Lippincott, 1989;733–757.
36. Clark LR, Jaffe MH, Choyke PL, Grant EG, Zeman RK. Pancreatic imaging. *Radiol Clin North Am* 1985;23:489–501.
37. Cohen EK, Daneman A, Stringer DA, Soto G, Thorner P. Focal adrenal hemorrhage: A new US appearance. *Radiology* 1986;161:631–633.
38. Coleman BG, Arger PH, Rosenberg HK, Mulhern CB, Ortega W, Stauffer D. Gray-scale sonographic assessment of pancreatitis in children. *Radiology* 1983;146:145–150.
39. Cook A, L'Heureux P. Radiographic findings in the mucocutaneous lymph node syndrome. *AJR* 1979;132:107–109.
40. Cox KL, Ament ME, Sample WF, Sarti DA, O'Donnell M, Byrne WJ. The ultrasonic and biochemical diagnosis of pancreatitis in children. *J Pediatr* 1980;96:407–411.
41. Cunat JS, Morrison SC, Fletcher BD. Sonographic diagnosis of calcified thrombus of the inferior vena cava. *Br J Radiol* 1982;55:160–162.
42. Daneman A. Adrenal neoplasms in children. *Semin Roentgenol* 1988;23:205–215.
43. Daneman A, Chan HSL, Martin J. Adrenal carcinoma and adenoma in children: A review of 17 patients. *Pediatr Radiol* 1983;13:11–18.
44. Daneman A, Gaskin K, Martin DJ, Cutz E. Pancreatic changes in cystic fibrosis: CT and sonographic appearances. *AJR* 1983;141:653–655.
45. Davidson AJ, Hartman DS, Goldman SM. Mature teratoma of the retroperitoneum: Radiologic, pathologic, and clinical correlation. *Radiology* 1989;172:421–425.
46. Davies RP, Lam AH. Adrenocortical neoplasm in children: Ultrasound appearance. *J Ultrasound Med* 1987;6:325–328.
47. deSa DJ, Nicholls S. Haemorrhagic necrosis of the adrenal gland in perinatal infants: A clinico-pathological study. *J Pathol* 1972;106:133–149.
48. Dietrich RB, Kangarloo H, Lenarsky C, Feig SA. Neuroblastoma: The role of MR imaging. *AJR* 1987;148:937–942.
49. Dobson RL, Johnson MA, Hennig RC, Brown NE. Sonography of the gallbladder, biliary tree, and pancreas in adults with cystic fibrosis. *J Can Assoc Radiol* 1988;39:257–259.
50. Donovan PJ, Sanders RC, Siegelman SS. Collections of fluid after pancreatitis: Evaluation by computed tomography and ultrasonography. *Radiol Clin North Am* 1982;20:653–665.
51. Dunnick NR, Doppman JL, Geelhoed GW. Intravenous extension of endocrine tumors. *AJR* 1980;135:471–476.
52. Dutton RV. Wolman's disease: Ultrasound and CT diagnosis. *Pediatr Radiol* 1985;15:144–146.
53. Eklöf O, Grotte G, Jorulf H, Löhr G, Ringertz H. Perinatal haemorrhagic necrosis of the adrenal gland: A clinical and ra-

diological evaluation of 24 consecutive cases. *Pediatr Radiol* 1975;4:31–36.

54. Eklöf O, Mortensson W, Sandstedt B. Suprarenal haematoma versus neuroblastoma complicated by haemorrhage: A diagnostic dilemma in the newborn. *Acta Radiol* 1986;27:3–10.

55. Evans AE, D'Angio GJ, Randolph J. A proposed staging for children with neuroblastoma: Children's Cancer Study Group A. *Cancer* 1971;27:374–378.

56. Falkoff GE, Taylor KJW, Morse S. Hepatic artery pseudoaneurysm: Diagnosis with real-time and pulsed Doppler US. *Radiology* 1986;158:55–56.

57. Ferraro EM, Fakhry J, Aruny JE, Bracero LA. Prenatal adrenal neuroblastoma: Case report with review of the literature. *J Ultrasound Med* 1988;7:275–278.

58. Filiatrault D, Perreault G, Laberge JM, Ducharme JC. CT localization of an aldosteronoma in a 10-year-old boy. *Pediatr Radiol* 1986;16:85–86.

59. Filly RA, London SS. The normal pancreas: Acoustic characteristics and frequency of imaging. *J Clin Ultrasound* 1979;7:121–124.

60. Finegold SM. Retroperitoneal infection. In: Feigin RD, Cherry JD, eds. *Textbook of Pediatric Infectious Diseases,* 2nd ed. Philadelphia: Saunders, 1987;757–758.

61. Fleischer AC, Parker P, Kirchner SG, James AE Jr. Sonographic findings of pancreatitis in children. *Radiology* 1983;146:151–155.

62. Fliegel CP, Signer E, Stahl M, Lo S. Thrombotic complications of long term intravenous alimentation in infants. *Ann Radiol* 1976;19:15–22.

63. Foley LC, Teele RL. Ultrasound of epigastric injuries after blunt trauma. *AJR* 1979;132:593–598.

64. Garg AK, Houston AB, Laing JM, Mackenzie JR. Positioning of umbilical arterial catheters with ultrasound. *Arch Dis Child* 1983;58:1017–1018.

65. Garris JB, Kangarloo H, Sample WF. Ultrasonic diagnosis of infrahepatic interruption of the inferior vena cava with azygos (hemiazygos) continuation. *Radiology* 1980;134:179–183.

66. Ghiacy S, Dubbins PA, Baumer H. Ultrasound demonstration of congenital adrenal hyperplasia. *J Clin Ultrasound* 1985;13:419–420.

67. Ghishan FK, Greene HL, Avant G, O'Neill J, Neblett W. Chronic relapsing pancreatitis in childhood. *J Pediatr* 1983;120:514–518.

68. Giulian BB, Chang CCN, Yoss BS. Prenatal ultrasonographic diagnosis of fetal adrenal neuroblastoma. *J Clin Ultrasound* 1986;14:225–227.

69. Golding RL, Perri G, Cremin BJ. The arteriographic manifestations of Takayasu's arteritis in children. *Pediatr Radiol* 1977;5:224–230.

70. Gore RM, Callen PW, Filly RA. Displaced retroperitoneal fat: Sonographic guide to right upper quadrant mass localization. *Radiology* 1982;142:701–705.

71. Gorenstein A, O'Halpin D, Wesson DE, Daneman A, Filler RM. Blunt injury to the pancreas in children: Selective management based on ultrasound. *J Pediatr Surg* 1987;22:1110–1116.

72. Graham N, Manhire AR, Stead RJ, Lees WR, Hodson ME, Batten JC. Cystic fibrosis: Ultrasonographic findings in the pancreas and hepatobiliary system correlated with clinical data and pathology. *Clin Radiol* 1985;36:199–203.

73. Gross M, Kottmeier PK, Waterhouse K. Diagnosis and treatment of neonatal adrenal hemorrhage. *J Pediatr Surg* 1967;2:308–312.

74. Gupta AK, Arenson AM, McKee JD. Effect of steroid ingestion on pancreatic echogenicity. *J Clin Ultrasound* 1987;15:171–174.

75. Hamper UM, Fishman EK, Hartman DS, Roberts JL, Sanders RC. Primary adrenocortical carcinoma: Sonographic evaluation with clinical and pathologic correlation in 26 patients. *AJR* 1987;148:915–919.

76. Hartman DS, Sanders RC. Wilms' tumor versus neuroblastoma: Usefulness of ultrasound in differentiation. *J Ultrasound Med* 1982;1:117–122.

77. Hastings N, Pollock WF, Snyder W Jr. Retroperitoneal tumors in infants and children. *Arch Surg* 1961;82:950–974.

78. Hayes FA, Smith EI. Neuroblastoma. In: Pizzo PA, Poplack DG, eds. *Principles and Practice of Pediatric Oncology.* Philadelphia: JB Lippincott, 1989;607–622.

79. Heij HA, Taets van Amerongen AHM, Ekkelkamp S, Vos A. Diagnosis and management of neonatal adrenal haemorrhage. *Pediatr Radiol* 1989;19:391–394.

80. Hendry GMA. Cystic neuroblastoma of the adrenal gland—A potential source of error in ultrasonic diagnosis. *Pediatr Radiol* 1982;12:204–206.

81. Hill SC, Hoeg JM, Dwyer AJ, Vucich JJ, Doppman JL. CT findings in acid lipase deficiency: Wolman disease and cholesteryl ester storage disease. *J Comput Assist Tomogr* 1983;7:815–818.

82. Hoffer FA, Shamberger RC, Teele RL. Ilio-psoas abscess: Diagnosis and management. *Pediatr Radiol* 1987;17:23–27.

83. Hoffman JC, Weiner SN, Koenigsberg M, Morehouse HT, Smith T. Pheochromocytoma invasion of the inferior vena cava: Sonographic evaluation. *Radiology* 1983;149:793–795.

84. Hogge WA, Thiagarajah S, Barber VG, Rodgers BM, Newman BM. Cystic sacrococcygeal teratoma: Ultrasound diagnosis and perinatal management. *J Ultrasound Med* 1987;6:707–710.

85. Horie A, Yano Y, Kotoo Y, Miwa A. Morphogenesis of pancreatoblastoma, infantile carcinoma of the pancreas: Report of two cases. *Cancer* 1977;39:247–254.

86. Iseki M, Suzuki T, Koizumi Y, Hirose M, Laskin WB, Nakazawa S, et al. Alpha-fetoprotein-producing pancreatoblastoma: A case report. *Cancer* 1986;57:1833–1835.

87. Jacobs RF, Hsi S, Wilson CB, Benjamin D, Smith AL, Morrow R. Apparent meningococcemia: Clinical features of disease due to *Haemophilus influenzae* and *Neisseria meningitidis. Pediatrics* 1983;72:469–472.

88. Jeffrey RB Jr. Sonography in acute pancreatitis. *Radiol Clin North Am* 1989;27:5–17.

89. Jeffrey RB, Laing FC, Wing VW. Ultrasound in acute pancreatic trauma. *Gastrointest Radiol* 1986;11:44–46.

90. Kangarloo H, Diament MJ, Gold RH, Barrett C, Lippe B, Geffner M, et al. Sonography of adrenal glands in neonates and children: Changes in appearance with age. *J Clin Ultrasound* 1986;14:43–47.

91. Kassner EG, Baumstark A, Kinkhabwala MN, Ablow RC, Haller JO. Calcified thrombus in the inferior vena cava in infants and children. *Pediatr Radiol* 1976;4:167–171.

92. Kaufman BH, Telander RL, van Heerden JA, Zimmerman D, Sheps SG, Dawson B. Pheochromocytoma in the pediatric age group: Current status. *J Pediatr Surg* 1983;18:879–884.

93. Keller MS, Taylor KJW, Riely CA. Pseudoportal Doppler signal in the partially obstructed inferior vena cava. *Radiology* 1989;170:475–477.

94. Kenney PJ, Robbins GL, Ellis DA, Spirt BA. Adrenal glands in patients with congenital renal anomalies: CT appearance. *Radiology* 1985;155:181–182.

95. Kinard RE, Orrison WW. Ultrasound demonstration of the retroaortic left renal vein. *J Clin Ultrasound* 1986;14:151–152.

96. Kirpekar M, Augenstein H, Abiri M. Sequential development of multiple aortic aneurysms in a neonate post umbilical arterial catheter insertion. *Pediatr Radiol* 1989;19:452–453.

97. Knowlson GT, Marsden HB. Aortic thrombosis in the newborn period. *Arch Dis Child* 1978;53:164–166.

98. Koch KJ, Cory DA. Simultaneous renal vein thrombosis and bilateral adrenal hemorrhage: MR demonstration. *J Comput Assist Tomogr* 1986;10:681–683.

99. Koenigsberg M, Hoffman JC, Schnur MJ. Sonographic evaluation of the retroperitoneum. *Semin Ultrasound* 1982;3:79–96.

100. Kumari S, Pillari G, Phillips G, Pochaczevsky R. Fluid collections of the psoas in children. *Semin Ultrasound* 1982;3:139–155.

101. Kushner DC, Chin JK, Cleveland RH, Herman TE, Fugate JH. Neonatal aortoiliac compression caused by a distended bladder. *AJR* 1986;146:1273–1275.

102. Kutcher R, Rosenblatt R, Mitsudo SM, Goldman M, Kogan S.

Renal angiomyolipoma with sonographic demonstration of extension into the inferior vena cava. *Radiology* 1982;143:755–756.

103. Lawson TL. Acute pancreatitis and its complications: Computed tomography and sonography. *Radiol Clin North Am* 1983;21:495–513.

104. Lazarow PB, Moser HW. Disorders of peroxisome biogenesis. In: Scriver CR, Beaudet AL, Sly WS, Valle D, eds. *The Metabolic Basis of Inherited Disease*, 6th ed. New York: McGraw-Hill, 1989;1479–1509.

105. Lebowitz JM, Belman AB. Simultaneous idiopathic adrenal hemorrhage and renal vein thrombosis in the newborn. *J Urol* 1983;129:574–576.

106. Lee CM, Chang-Chien CS, Lin DY, Yang CY, Sheen IS, Chen WJ. The real-time ultrasonography of pancreatic pseudocyst: Comparison of infected and noninfected pseudocysts. *J Clin Ultrasound* 1988;16:393–398.

107. Levine C. Intestinal obstruction in a neonate with adrenal hemorrhage and renal vein thrombosis. *Pediatr Radiol* 1989;19:477–478.

108. Lewandowski B, Challender J, Dery R. Prolapsing Chiari malformation in tricuspid regurgitation: A moving filling defect in the inferior vena cava. *J Ultrasound Med* 1985;4:655–658.

109. Lewis E, Kurtz AB, Dubbins PA, Wapner RJ, Goldberg BB. Real-time ultrasonographic evaluation of normal fetal adrenal glands. *J Ultrasound Med* 1982;1:265–270.

110. Magill HL, Tonkin ILD, Bada H, Riggs W Jr. Advantages of coronal ultrasonography in evaluating the neonatal retroperitoneum. *J Ultrasound Med* 1983;2:289–295.

111. Malfertheiner P, Büchler M. Correlation of imaging and function in chronic pancreatitis. *Radiol Clin North Am* 1989;27:51–64.

112. Marchal G, Gelin J, Verbeken E, Baert A, Lauwerijns J. High-resolution real-time sonography of the adrenal glands: A routine examination? *J Ultrasound Med* 1986;5:65–68.

113. McCabe ERB. Disorders of glycerol metabolism. In: Scriver CR, Beaudet AL, Sly WS, Valle D, eds. *The Metabolic Basis of Inherited Disease*, 6th ed. New York: McGraw-Hill, 1989; 945–961.

114. McCauley RGK, Beckwith JB, Faerber EN, Berdon WE. Benign adrenal cortical macrocysts in the Beckwith-Wiedemann syndrome (BWS). Presented at the Annual Meeting of The Society for Pediatric Radiology, Cincinnati, OH, April 19–22, 1990.

115. McGahan JP, Myracle MR. Adrenal hypertrophy: Possible pitfall in the sonographic diagnosis of renal agenesis. *J Ultrasound Med* 1986;5:265–268.

116. McHugo JM, McKeown C, Brown MT, Weller P, Shah KJ. Ultrasound findings in children with cystic fibrosis. *Br J Radiol* 1987;60:137–141.

117. McLeod AJ, Lewis E. Sonographic evaluation of pediatric rhabdomyosarcomas. *J Ultrasound Med* 1984;3:69–73.

118. Meyers MA. *Dynamic Radiology of the Abdomen: Normal and Pathologic Anatomy*, 3rd ed. New York: Springer-Verlag, 1988.

119. Mineau DE, Koehler PR. Ultrasound diagnosis of neonatal adrenal hemorrhage. *AJR* 1979;132:443–444.

120. Mittelstaedt CA, Volberg FM, Merten DF, Brill PW. The sonographic diagnosis of neonatal adrenal hemorrhage. *Radiology* 1979;131:453–457.

121. Mitty HA. Embryology, anatomy, and anomalies of the adrenal gland. *Semin Roentgenol* 1988;23:271–279.

122. Mohd TbH, Yip CH. Cystic neuroblastoma with colonic fistula. *Pediatr Radiol* 1988;18:406.

123. Moore KL. *The Developing Human: Clinically Oriented Embryology*, 4th ed. Philadelphia: Saunders, 1988.

124. Morrison SC, Comisky E, Fletcher BD. Calcification in the adrenal glands associated with disseminated herpes simplex infection. *Pediatr Radiol* 1988;18:240–241.

125. Moynan RW, Neerhout RC, Johnson TS. Pancreatic carcinoma in childhood: Case report and review. *J Pediatr* 1964;65:711–720.

126. Murphy BJ, Casillas J, Yrizarry JM. Traumatic adrenal hemorrhage: Radiologic findings. *Radiology* 1988;169:701–703.

127. Murthy TVM, Irving IM, Lister J. Massive adrenal hemorrhage in neonatal neuroblastoma. *J Pediatr Surg* 1978;13:31–34.

128. Naidech HJ, Chawla HS. Bilateral adrenal calcifications at birth in a neonate. *AJR* 1983;140:105–106.

129. Neuenschwander S, Montagne J Ph, Lavollay B, Gruner M. Une cause rare d'hypertension néonatale. *Ann Radiol* 1982;25:142–145.

130. New MI, White PC, Pang S, Dupont B, Speiser PW. The adrenal hyperplasias. In: Scriver CR, Beaudet AL, Sly WS, Valle D, eds. *The Metabolic Basis of Inherited Disease*, 6th ed. New York: McGraw-Hill, 1989;1881–1917.

131. Ogata T, Ishikawa K, Kohda E, Matsuo N. Computed tomography in the early detection of congenital lipoid adrenal hyperplasia. *Pediatr Radiol* 1988;18:360–361.

132. Oppenheimer DA, Carroll BA. Ultrasonic localization of neonatal umbilical catheters. *Radiology* 1982;142:781–782.

133. Oppenheimer DA, Carroll BA, Garth KE. Ultrasonic detection of complications following umbilical arterial catheterization in the neonate. *Radiology* 1982;145:667–672.

134. Oppenheimer DA, Carroll BA, Garth KE, Parker BR. Sonographic localization of neonatal umbilical catheters. *AJR* 1982;138:1025–1032.

135. Oppenheimer DA, Carroll BA, Yousem S. Sonography of the normal neonatal adrenal gland. *Radiology* 1983;146:157–160.

136. Oppenheimer EH, Esterly JR. Pathology of cystic fibrosis: Review of the literature and comparison with 146 autopsied cases. *Perspect Pediatr Pathol* 1975;2:241–278.

137. Pery M, Kaftori JK, Bar-Maor JA. Sonography for diagnosis and follow-up of neonatal adrenal hemorrhage. *J Clin Ultrasound* 1981;9:397–401.

138. Phillips AF, McMurtry RJ, Taubman J. Malignant pheochromocytoma in childhood. *Am J Dis Child* 1976;130:1252–1255.

139. Phillips HE, Cox KL, Reid MH, McGahan JP. Pancreatic sonography in cystic fibrosis. *AJR* 1981;137:69–72.

140. Pinck RL, Constantacopoulos CG, Felice A, Ippolito J, Rubin B, Haller JO. Adrenal hemorrhage in the newborn with evidence of bleeding while in utero. *J Urol* 1979;122:813–814.

141. Potter EL. Bilateral absence of ureters and kidneys: A report of 50 cases. *Obstet Gynecol* 1965;25:3–12.

142. Queloz JM, Capitanio MA, Kirkpatrick JA. Wolman's disease: Roentgen observations in 3 siblings. *Radiology* 1972;104:357–359.

143. Richie JP, Gittes RF. Carcinoma of the adrenal cortex. *Cancer* 1980;45:1957–1964.

144. Richter JM, Schapiro RH, Mulley AG, Warshaw AL. Association of pancreas divisum and pancreatitis, and its treatment by sphincteroplasty of the accessory ampulla. *Gastroenterology* 1981;81:1104–1110.

145. Ritter SB, Bierman FZ. Noninvasive diagnosis of interrupted inferior vena cava: Gated pulsed Doppler application. *Am J Cardiol* 1983;51:1796–1798.

146. Robey G, Daneman A, Martin DJ. Pancreatic carcinoma in a neonate. *Pediatr Radiol* 1983;13:284–286.

147. Rose J, Berdon WE, Sullivan T, Baker DH. Prolonged jaundice as presenting sign of massive adrenal hemorrhage in newborn: Radiographic diagnosis by IVP with total-body opacification. *Radiology* 1971;98:263–272.

148. Rosenberg ER, Bowie JD, Andreotti RF, Fields SI. Sonographic evaluation of fetal adrenal glands. *AJR* 1982;139:1145–1147.

149. Rosenblum JL. Pancreatitis. In: Feigin RD, Cherry JD, eds. *Textbook of Pediatric Infectious Diseases*, 2nd ed. Philadelphia: Saunders, 1987;750–753.

150. Rudas G, Bors S. Aortic thrombosis diagnosed by ultrasound. *Pediatr Radiol* 1988;18:77–78.

151. Sarnaik AP, Sanfilippo DJ, Slovis TL. Ultrasound diagnosis of adrenal hemorrhage in meningococcemia. *Pediatr Radiol* 1988;18:427–428.

152. Schmitz G, Assmann G. Acid lipase deficiency: Wolman disease and Cholesteryl ester storage disease. In: Scriver CR, Beaudet AL, Sly WS, Valle D, eds. *The Metabolic Basis of*

Inherited Disease, 6th ed. New York: McGraw-Hill, 1989; 1623–1644.

153. Schneider KM, Becker JM, Krasna IH. Neonatal neuroblastoma. *Pediatrics* 1965;36:359–366.

154. Schut JM, Meradji M, Oranje AP, Bergmeijer JH, Schuller JL. Double-sided psoas abscess in a young infant: Sonographic and radiographic findings. *Pediatr Radiol* 1988;18:176–177.

155. Seibert JJ, Taylor BJ, Williamson SL, Williams BJ, Szabo JS, Corbitt SL. Sonographic detection of neonatal umbilical-artery thrombosis: Clinical correlation. *AJR* 1987;148:965–968.

156. Shawker TH, Doppman JL, Dunnick NR, McCarthy DM. Ultrasonic investigation of pancreatic islet cell tumors. *J Ultrasound Med* 1982;1:193–200.

157. Sherman C, Winchester P, Brill PW, Mininberg D. Childhood retroperitoneal fibrosis. *Pediatr Radiol* 1988;18:245–247.

158. Siegel MJ, Martin KW, Worthington JL. Normal and abnormal pancreas in children: US studies. *Radiology* 1987;165:15–18.

159. Siegel MJ, Sagel SS. Computed tomography as a supplement to urography in the evaluation of suspected neuroblastoma. *Radiology* 1982;142:435–438.

160. Siegelman SS, Copeland BE, Saba GP, Cameron JL, Sanders RC, Zerhouni EA. CT of fluid collections associated with pancreatitis. *AJR* 1980;134:1121–1132.

161. Silverman PM, Carroll BA, Moskowitz PS. Adrenal sonography in renal agenesis and dysplasia. *AJR* 1980;134:600–602.

162. Sisson JC, Frager MS, Valk TW, Gross MD, Swanson DP, Wieland DM, et al. Scintigraphic localization of pheochromocytoma. *N Engl J Med* 1981;305:12–17.

163. Slovis TL, Philippart AI, Cushing B, Das L, Perlmutter AD, Reed JO, et al. Evaluation of the inferior vena cava by sonography and venography in children with renal and hepatic tumors. *Radiology* 1981;140:767–772.

164. Slovis TL, VonBerg VJ, Mikelic V. Sonography in the diagnosis and management of pancreatic pseudocysts and effusions in childhood. *Radiology* 1980;135:153–155.

165. Sober I, Hirsch M. Unilateral massive adrenal hemorrhage in newborn infant. *J Urol* 1965;93:430–434.

166. Sommers SC. Adrenal glands. In: Kissane JM, ed. *Anderson's Pathology,* 8th ed. St. Louis: Mosby, 1985;1429–1450.

167. Sonnenfeld M, Finberg HJ. Ultrasonographic diagnosis of incomplete inferior vena caval thrombosis secondary to periphlebitis: The importance of a complete survey examination. *Radiology* 1980;137:743–744.

168. Sotelo-Avila C, Gonzalez-Crussi F, Fowler JW. Complete and incomplete forms of Beckwith-Wiedemann syndrome: Their oncogenic potential. *J Pediatr* 1980;96:47–50.

169. Sotelo-Avila C, Gooch WM III. Neoplasms associated with the Beckwith-Wiedemann syndrome. *Perspect Pediatr Pathol* 1976;3:255–272.

170. Starinsky R, Manor A, Segal M. Non-functioning kidney associated with neonatal adrenal hemorrhage. *Pediatr Radiol* 1986;16:427–429.

171. Stark DD, Moss AA, Brasch RC, deLorimier AA, Albin AR, London DA, et al. Neuroblastoma: Diagnostic imaging and staging. *Radiology* 1983;148:101–105.

172. Steiner E, Rubens D, Weiss SL, Lerner R, Asztely M. Sonographic examination of the abdominal aorta through the left flank: A prospective study. *J Ultrasound Med* 1986;5:499–502.

173. Swischuk LE, Hayden CK Jr. Pararenal space hyperechogenicity in childhood pancreatitis. *AJR* 1985;145:1085–1086.

174. Swobodnik W, Wolf A, Wechsler JG, Kleihauer E, Ditschuneit H. Ultrasound characteristics of the pancreas in children with cystic fibrosis. *J Clin Ultrasound* 1985;13:469–474.

175. Taxy JB. Adenocarcinoma of the pancreas in childhood: Report of a case and a review of the English language literature. *Cancer* 1976;37:1508–1518.

176. Trigaux JP, Marchandise B, Schoevaerdts JC, Kremer R, Chalant CH. Partial abnormal infradiaphragmatic pulmonary venous connection visualized by two-dimensional abdominal ultrasonography. *J Clin Ultrasound* 1984;12:425–428.

177. Uglietta JP, Woodruff WW, Effmann EL, Carroll BA. Duplex Doppler ultrasound evaluation of calcified inferior vena cava thrombosis. *Pediatr Radiol* 1989;19:250–252.

178. Van Steenbergen W, Samain H, Pouillon M, Van Roost W, Marchal G, Baert A, et al. Transection of the pancreas demonstrated by ultrasound and computed tomography. *Gastrointest Radiol* 1987;12:128–130.

179. Weaver DW, Walt AJ, Sugawa C, Bouwman DL. A continuing appraisal of pancreatic ascites. *Surg Gynecol Obstet* 1982; 154:845–848.

180. Werner JL, Taybi H. Presacral masses in childhood. *AJR* 1970;109:403–410.

181. White SJ, Stuck KJ, Blane CE, Silver TM. Sonography of neuroblastoma. *AJR* 1983;141:465–468.

182. Willemse APP, Coppes MJ, Feldberg MAM, Kramer PPG, Witkamp ThD. Magnetic resonance appearance of adrenal hemorrhage in a neonate. *Pediatr Radiol* 1989;19:210–211.

183. Willi UV, Reddish JM, Teele RL. Cystic fibrosis: Its characteristic appearance on abdominal sonography. *AJR* 1980; 134:1005–1010.

184. Wilms G, Marchal G, Baert A, Adisoejoso B, Mangkuwerdojo S. CT and ultrasound features of post-traumatic adrenal hemorrhage. *J Comput Assist Tomogr* 1987;11:112–115.

185. Wilson DA, Nguyen DL, Tytle TL, Swaney CM, Muchmore HG. Sonography of the adrenal glands in chronic disseminated histoplasmosis. *J Ultrasound Med* 1986;5:69–73.

186. Wilson-Sharp RC, Irving HC, Brown RC, Chalmers DM, Littlewood JM. Ultrasonography of the pancreas, liver, and biliary system in cystic fibrosis. *Arch Dis Child* 1984;59:923–926.

187. Worthen NJ, Beabeau D. Normal pancreatic echogenicity: Relation to age and body fat. *AJR* 1982;139:1095–1098.

188. Yeh HC. Adrenal gland and nonrenal retroperitoneum. *Urol Radiol* 1987;9:127–140.

9

Urinary Tract

Marilyn J. Siegel

Sonography has become increasingly important in the evaluation of urinary tract disease because it can be performed easily and it is noninvasive, with no risk to the patient or operator. Both the normal and abnormal kidneys can be accurately depicted with sonography, and with the advent of Doppler sonography, renal blood flow abnormalities also can be recognized.

The most common indications for renal sonography are the determination of the existence and character of a renal mass, determination of the cause of renal failure, detection of complications of urinary tract infection, and evaluation of renal allografts. Less frequent indications for sonography include diagnosis of perirenal or pararenal disease; detection of calculi; evaluation of renal vein thrombosis, renal ischemia, or infarction; and the assessment of bladder and perivesical abnormalities.

TECHNIQUE

The kidneys are traditionally examined by transverse and longitudinal scans with the patient in the supine position. In this position, the liver serves as an acoustic window for imaging the right kidney. For the left kidney, the supine approach is often inadequate because of interposed bowel gas, and scans with the patient in the decubitus position often are required. Occasionally the prone position is needed if abundant bowel gas prevents optimal visualization of the kidneys when the patient is in the supine or decubitus positions.

Real-time scanning, particularly with sector scanners, is advantageous for identification of renal anatomy because it can image between ribs. A high-frequency transducer also is needed to maximize resolution. In most children and thin adolescents, a 5 MHz transducer is routinely used; a 3.5 MHz transducer usually is required for larger adolescents, and a 7.0 or 7.5 MHz transducer may be used in small infants. Duplex Doppler and color Doppler flow imaging are useful to evaluate the integrity of the renal vessels.

NORMAL ANATOMY

Normal sonographic standards for kidney length in premature and term infants as well as in children have been established and have facilitated evaluation of abnormal kidneys (12,36,143,149). Variations in normal morphology with age also have been reported (60,61,69,76,173). Knowledge of these various appearances is essential for proper sonographic interpretation.

Normal neonatal and infant kidneys have three unique features that differentiate them from the kidneys of older children and adults (Fig. 1). First, the echogenicity of the renal cortex usually is equal to that of the liver or spleen, rather than hypoechoic relative to those structures. The glomeruli in the neonate occupy about 20% of the cortical volume as compared with about 9% in the adult. Moreover, the cellular component occupies a proportionally greater volume of the glomerular tuft (60,61,69). The increased number of anatomical structures and, thus, of interfaces presumably accounts for the increased echogenicity. The renal cortex of the right kidney and adjacent liver are equally echogenic in 65% of neonates, while the cortex of the left kidney and spleen are equally echogenic in 50% of neonates (61). In the remaining patients, the cortex is slightly less echogenic. Second, the medullary pyramids are hypoechoic and prominent, the result of a larger medullary and smaller cortical volume relative to that of older children and adults (61,76). Finally, the renal sinus in neonates and young infants is not as echogenic as it is in older patients because of the paucity of renal sinus fat (Fig. 2). The renal cortex becomes less echogenic than liver or spleen and the renal pyramids become less prominent in the majority of patients by 2 or 3 months, and by 6 months almost 100% of infants demonstrate an adult echopattern. The intensity of the central sinus gradually increases with age and the adult pattern is attained by adolescence (61).

Other normal anatomic structures are the junctional parenchymal defect and the interrenicular septum (74).

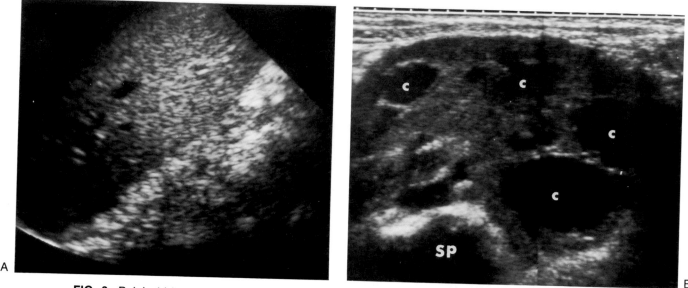

FIG. 3. Pelvic kidney. **A:** The right kidney cannot be identified on a coronal scan of the right upper quadrant. **B:** Transverse scan of the pelvis shows a dysplastic kidney with dilated calyces (*c*). *Sp*, spine.

morphic with bizarre shapes, tilted axes, and unusual calyces (Fig. 3).

Cross ectopia is a form of renal ectopia in which the ectopic kidney lies on the opposite side of the retroperitoneum with its ureter occupying a normal position in the bladder. Ninety percent of crossed ectopic kidneys are fused to the normal ipsilateral kidney, usually side by side longitudinally. The resultant renal mass appears dysmorphic with a sigmoid or S-shape. Patients with ectopic kidneys are at increased risk for developing complications such as hydronephrosis, infection, and calculus formation. Multicystic dysplasia of the crossed unit has also been described (105,127). The sonographic findings of simple crossed fused ectopia include a mass with a reniform contour and two renal sinuses and absence of the kidney in the contra-

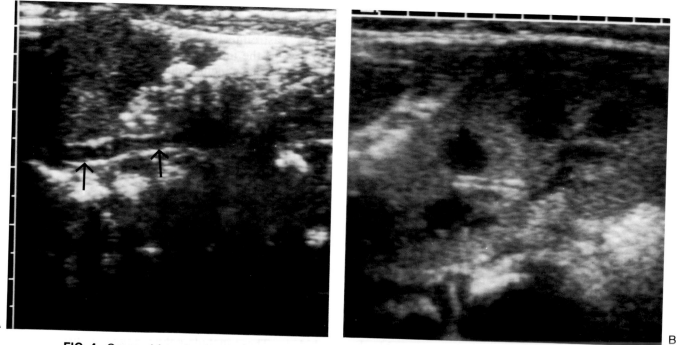

FIG. 4. Crossed fused ectopia with dysplastic kidney in a neonate. **A:** Scan through the left flank shows an elongated adrenal gland (*arrows*) and no demonstrable kidney. **B:** Longitudinal sonogram of the right lower quadrant demonstrates a normal left kidney with prominent pyramids.

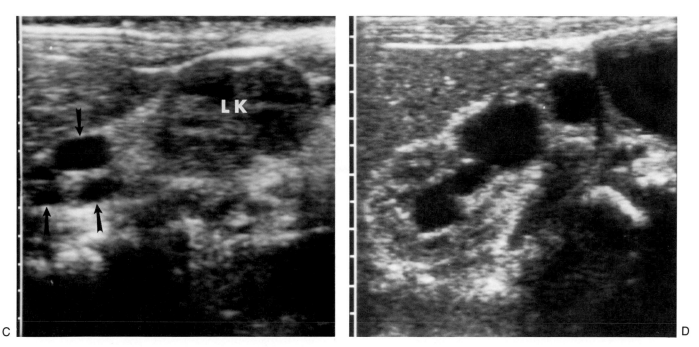

FIG. 4 *Continued.* **C:** Oblique scan slightly further to the right reveals the lower pole of the right kidney with several cysts (*arrows*), lying adjacent to the left kidney (*LK*). **D:** Longitudinal scan of the upper right abdomen reveals a cystic dysplastic right kidney.

lateral renal fossa (54). The fused lower pole unit is positioned medially, extending anteriorly to the spine. In cases with multicystic dysplasia, a multicystic mass of variable size is contiguous with the lower pole of the upper kidney (Fig. 4).

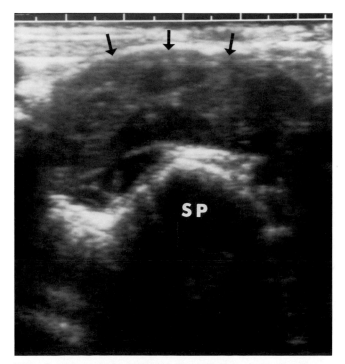

FIG. 5. Horseshoe kidney. Transverse scan shows an isthmus of tissue (*arrows*) anterior to the spine (*SP*) connecting the lower poles of the kidneys.

Horseshoe Kidney

Horseshoe kidney is the most common renal fusion anomaly, with an incidence of 1 in 400 births. In this condition there is fusion of the lower poles of the kidneys, producing a parenchymal or fibrous isthmus across the midline. The ureters typically cross in front of the isthmus, descending from anteriorly positioned renal pelves. The arterial supply is variable, arising from either the lower aorta or from common iliac arteries. Associated anomalies of the genitourinary, cardiovascular, or skeletal systems as well as the gastrointestinal tract occur in about one-third of patients. As in ectopia, there is an increased risk of hydronephrosis, infection, and stones. Rare complications of horseshoe kidneys include Wilms' tumor and renal cell carcinoma. The sonographic findings of horseshoe kidney include a normal retroperitoneal position of the kidneys, medially oriented inferior poles, and an isthmus of tissue crossing the midline (Fig. 5).

HYDRONEPHROSIS

Ureteropelvic junction obstruction; obstruction of the distal ureter, usually primary megaureter; upper pole hydronephrosis due to duplex anomalies; and posterior urethral valves are the most common causes of neonatal hydronephrosis, accounting for 87% of cases (20). Less frequently, reflux and prune-belly syndrome are responsible for neonatal hydronephrosis. Many cases are detected *in utero;* after delivery, patients with hydronephrosis are almost always discovered because of signs of an abdominal mass or urinary tract infection. When intrauterine hydronephrosis is diagnosed, a postpartum examination is indicated to confirm the diagnosis. It is recommended that the initial postpartum sonogram be performed several days after delivery. A renal sonogram performed earlier may be falsely negative or may underestimate the severity of hydronephrosis, probably due to a relative state of dehydration and decreased glomerular filtration rate immediately after delivery. With patient rehydration in the first few days of life and improvement in the glomerular filtration rate, obstructing lesions become more apparent (Fig. 6) (98).

Ureteropelvic Junction Obstruction

Ureteropelvic junction obstruction is the most frequent type of upper urinary tract obstruction in childhood. The etiology is controversial but believed to be congenital in origin and caused by intrinsic stenosis or extrinsic compression from a band, adhesion, or aberrant vessel. Occasionally the obstruction may be functional due to abnormal development of the muscle fibers at the ureteropelvic junction. Approximately 55% of children with this condition are diagnosed before the age of 5 years and 25% are diagnosed during the first year of life (161).

A palpable mass is the usual finding in infants with ureteropelvic junction obstructions; abdominal pain, hematuria, or urinary tract infection are more common in older children. Recurrent flank pain associated with increased fluid intake is another presenting symptom. The characteristic sonographic findings include multiple cystic structures of uniform size; communication between the cysts; a moderate or large renal pelvis; visible renal parenchyma; and lack of visualization of a distal ureter (Fig. 7) (146). The renal parenchyma may have increased echogenicity or contain cysts corresponding to histologic areas of renal dysplasia (94,146). With severe obstruction, the renal collecting system may rupture and cause urine to collect in the perirenal space. Rarely, ipsilateral ureteral dilatation is present secondary to coexisting vesicoureteral reflux or distal ureteral obstruction. Although the diagnosis of obstruction at the ureteropelvic junction can be established with a high degree of certainty by sonography, a urogram or scintigram is necessary to determine function. Demonstration of a well-perfused kidney with progressive increase in radionuclide ac-

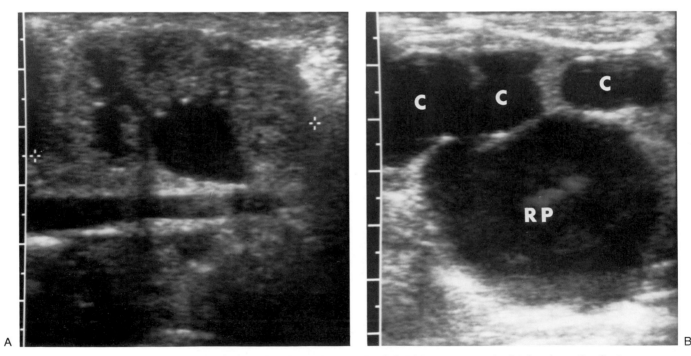

FIG. 6. Hydronephrosis. **A:** Longitudinal scan of the left kidney (*cursors*) obtained on the first day of life shows mild hydronephrosis. **B:** Scan on the fourth day of life reveals marked dilatation of the renal pelvis (*RP*) and calyces (*C*).

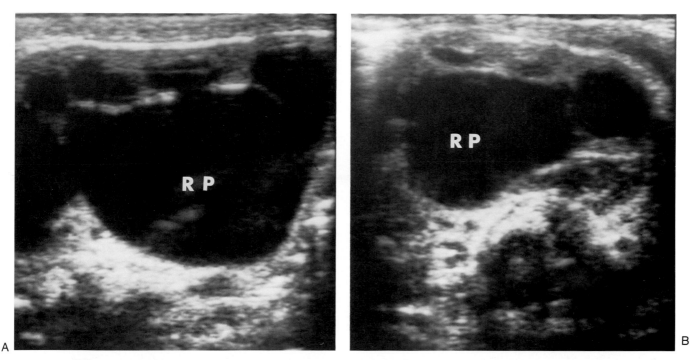

FIG. 7. Ureteropelvic junction obstruction. **A:** Longitudinal and **B:** transverse scans of the left kidney demonstrate moderately dilated calyces communicating with a markedly dilated renal pelvis (*RP*). A thin rim of normal parenchyma surrounds the dilated collecting system. No dilated ureter is identified.

tivity within the collecting system supports the diagnosis of obstructive hydronephrosis. If there is ipsilateral ureteral enlargement, the presence or absence of reflux should be evaluated by cystourethrography.

Ureteral Duplication

Ureteral duplication is the most frequent renal anomaly, occurring in 1 in 125 patients or 0.8% of the population. The right and left kidneys are affected equally and bilateral duplication is present in 40% of patients. Duplications range from partial to complete separation of the collecting system.

In incomplete ureteral duplication, a common distal ureter enters the bladder. The spectrum of incomplete duplication ranges from a bifid renal pelvis to Y-shaped ureters with the two ureters fusing somewhere along their course, producing a single common ureter distally. On sonography, the simple nonobstructed duplicated kidney is larger than the normal single system kidney; frequently a cleft in the central echo complex representing the duplication anomaly is observed (148).

With complete ureteral duplication, the kidney has two pelvocalyceal systems and two ureters with sep-

arate insertions. The ureteral orifice of the upper pole moiety will lie medial and inferior to the orifice of the ureter draining the lower pole segment (Weigert-Meyer rule). The end result is that the upper pole system terminates ectopically. Ectopic ureters may insert into the vestibule, vagina, uterus, or urethra in girls and into the posterior urethra, epididymis, seminal vesicle, or vas deferens in boys. In both sexes, the ectopic ureters may end in the bladder neck or in the trigone inferomedial to the normal location. When the ectopic ureter drains above the external sphincter, the symptoms are those of infection; when the orifice inserts below the external sphincter, urinary incontinence is a frequent complaint. The distal portion of the ectopic ureter may be stenotic or associated with a ureterocele; both of these anomalies can obstruct the ureter of the upper pole moiety. The ureter draining the lower pole moiety inserts slightly superior and lateral to its normal trigonal position, predisposing it to vesicoureteral reflux.

Typical sonographic features of a duplicated system with an ectopic ureter are a dilated upper pole collecting system, with a thin rim of parenchyma of normal echogenicity. The draining ureter is tortuous and dilated; the distal portion of the ectopic ureter either enters into an intravesical cyst, the ureterocele,

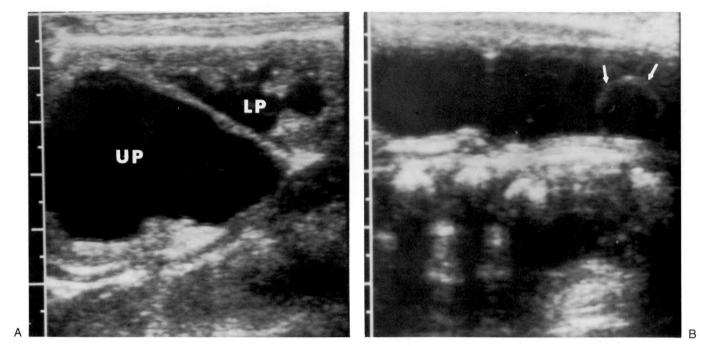

FIG. 8. Ureteral duplication with a ureterocele. **A:** Longitudinal sonogram of the left kidney demonstrates marked dilated upper pole (*UP*) and mildly dilated lower pole (*LP*) renal pelves. **B:** Longitudinal sonogram of the bladder shows a cyst with an echogenic wall (*arrows*), representing the ureterocele, at the base of the bladder.

or terminates outside the bladder (Figs. 8,9) (4,45, 62,126). Occasionally the upper pole moiety may appear highly echogenic with small cysts due to dysplasia, or it may be hypoplastic, rather than dilated, and have a diminutive ureter (151). The lower pole ureter may be dilated secondary to reflux. In severe cases, the ectopic ureterocele obstructs the lower pole ureter on the ipsilateral side and may even obstruct the ureter on the contralateral side.

Simple Ureterocele

In its simple form, the ureterocele arises from a normally positioned ureteral orifice near the corner of the

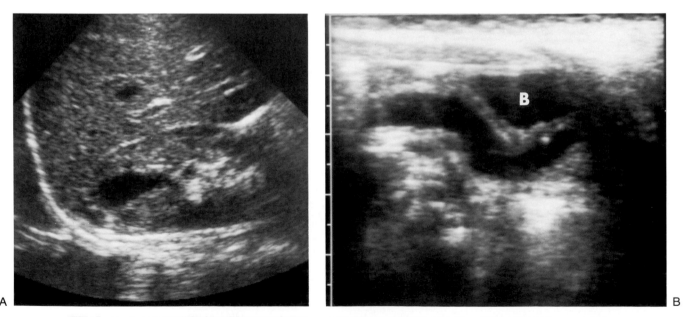

FIG. 9. Ureteral duplication with an ectopic ureter. **A:** Longitudinal view of the left kidney reveals a dilated upper pole collecting system. **B:** Longitudinal sonogram through the lower pelvis shows a dilated ureter extending below the bladder (*B*) base.

trigone. Simple ureteroceles are more commonly discovered in adults than in children and usually are small, with little or no evidence of obstruction. In children, however, they more often are associated with hydronephrosis. Symptoms typically are those of urinary tract infection. On sonography, the ureterocele appears as an intravesical sonolucent mass with a thin echogenic wall near the lateral margin of the trigone.

Megaureter

Megaureter may be due to obstruction or reflux, or it may be idiopathic. Each of these major groups may be further subdivided into primary and secondary causes.

Primary obstructed megaureter occurs just at or above the ureterovesical junction. Possible etiologies include ureteral stenosis, valves or stricture, or an adynamic distal ureteral segment. In the latter instance, the terminal 0.5 to 4 cm of ureter is unable to conduct a peristaltic wave, producing a functional rather than anatomical obstruction. In secondary obstructive megaureter, the ureterectasis occurs as a result of ureteral obstruction, neurogenic bladder, ureterocele, or calculi.

Primary refluxing megaureter is due to a short or absent intravesical ureter. In secondary refluxing megaureter, the reflux is due to a neurogenic bladder or

infravesical obstruction, such as posterior valves or ureteroceles.

In primary nonobstructive, nonrefluxing megaureter, there is no juxtavesical obstruction, reflux, or outlet obstruction. The dilatation may involve the entire ureter or be segmental. Upper tract drainage usually is not significantly abnormal. The diagnosis of nonrefluxing, nonobstructing megaureter is one of exclusion. Secondary nonrefluxing, nonobstructing megaureter may by due to urinary tract infection or to high urine flow and volume, such as that occurring in diabetes insipidus. Most children with megaureter, regardless of type, present with urinary tract infection.

The sonographic findings of megaloureter are dilatation of the ureter which may terminate in a narrow distal segment; hyperperistalsis of the lower ureter, ending in an adynamic narrowed segment; and disproportionate dilatation of the lower ureter with respect to the upper ureter and renal pelvis (Fig. 10) (178).

Differentiation of the obstructed from the nonobstructed dilated renal collecting system, usually due to reflux, is a difficult problem. When a dilated collecting system is imaged, additional evaluation with duplex Doppler has been shown to be helpful in adults for detecting the presence or absence of true obstruction. The presence of a resistive index (peak systolic frequency shift minus end diastolic frequency shift divided by peak systolic frequency shift) of 0.70 or greater is suspicious for obstruction; conversely, a

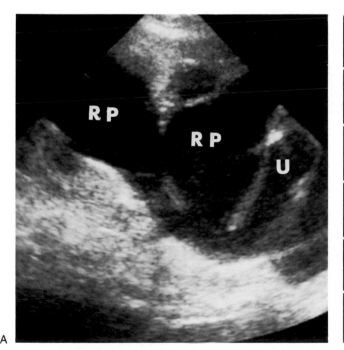
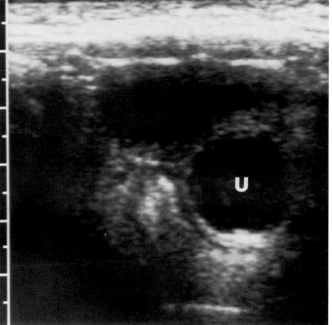

FIG. 10. Megaureter. **A:** Longitudinal scan of the left flank reveals a dilated bifid renal pelvis (*RP*) with a dilated tortuous ureter (*U*). **B:** Transverse image through the lower pelvis shows a markedly dilated distal ureter (*U*) posterior to the bladder. At surgery, there was a stricture at the ureterovesical junction.

nonobstructed kidney has a resistive index below 0.70 (134).

Posterior Urethral Valves

Posterior urethral valves are the most common cause of urethral obstruction in boys. They are generally classified into 3 types, but the existence of type 2 and type 3 valves is controversial and only type 1 valves will be discussed. Type 1 valves are folds which extend distally from either side of the verumontanum to attach to the anterior lateral wall of the urethra. The clinical presentation is variable. Approximately half of the patients present in the neonatal period with bilateral flank masses and a distended bladder secondary to significant urethral obstruction. Urinary ascites is a common associated finding. With lesser degrees of obstruction, the patients may present later in childhood with urinary tract infection, voiding abnormalities, or chronic retention with failure to thrive.

Sonography demonstrates bilateral hydroureteronephrosis with parenchymal thinning, a thick-walled bladder, and a dilated prostatic urethra (30,106). Occasionally parenchymal cysts or increased echogenicity of the kidneys is noted secondary to associated cystic renal dysplasia (Fig. 11) (147). Other findings include urinary ascites and subcapsular or perirenal urinomas, resulting from urine extravasation, either through rupture of a caliceal fornix or a tear in the renal parenchyma. Urinomas may be either anechoic or septated fluid collections (38,110,111).

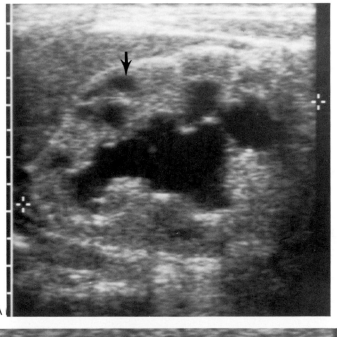

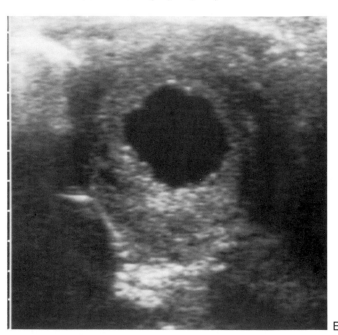

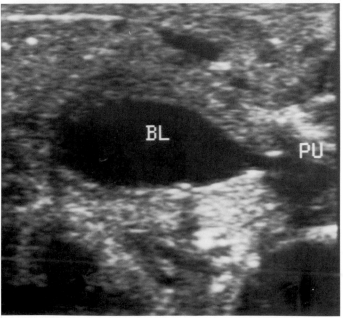

FIG. 11. Posterior urethral valves in a 6-month-old boy. **A:** Longitudinal scan of the right kidney shows moderate pelvocalyceal dilatation. The renal parenchyma is diffusely echogenic and contains a small cyst (*arrow*) secondary to dysplasia. The left kidney (*cursors*) had a similar appearance. **B:** Transverse view of the pelvis reveals a thick-walled bladder. **C:** Longitudinal view shows a dilated posterior urethra (*PU*). *BL,* bladder.

Prune-Belly (Eagle-Barret) Syndrome

The triad of deficient abdominal musculature, urinary tract anomalies, and cryptorchidism constitutes the prune-belly syndrome. On the basis of radiologic and clinical findings, patients can be divided into three groups (11). Group 1 is the most severe; affected patients have urethral obstruction from valves or even atresia and show bilateral cystic renal dysplasia. Because of pulmonary hypoplasia, these infants are stillborn or die soon after birth. Group 2 patients have less severe urinary tract involvement. They have dilated, enlarged bladders but no evidence of urethral obstruction. The ureters and renal pelves are markedly dilated; the calyces are dysmorphic and often minimally dilated. Group 3 patients have mild involvement with features ranging between those of group 2 and those of a normal urinary tract.

The sonographic features parallel the clinical features. Patients in group 1 have dysplastic kidneys with no visible normal renal parenchyma. In group 2 there is marked ureteral dilatation and mild to moderate pelvocalyceal dilatation (Fig. 12). Patients in group 3 have mildly dilated or even normal urinary tracts (48). Other

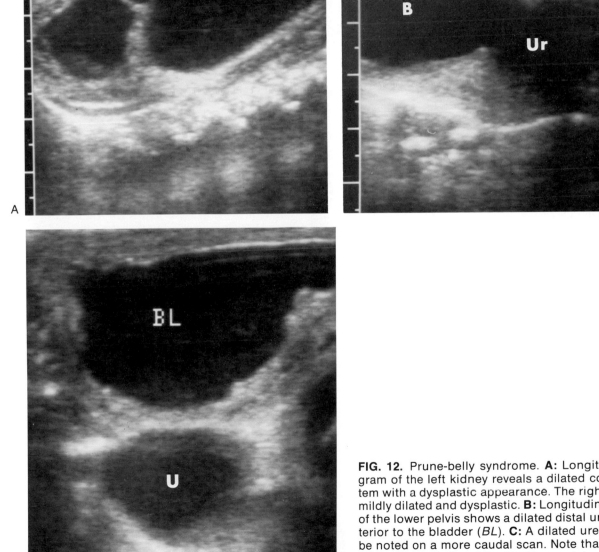

FIG. 12. Prune-belly syndrome. **A:** Longitudinal sonogram of the left kidney reveals a dilated collecting system with a dysplastic appearance. The right kidney was mildly dilated and dysplastic. **B:** Longitudinal sonogram of the lower pelvis shows a dilated distal ureter (*U*) posterior to the bladder (*BL*). **C:** A dilated urethra (*Ur*) can be noted on a more caudal scan. Note that the bladder (*B*) is thin-walled and the bladder neck is wide open, in contrast to the thick-walled bladder and narrow bladder neck seen with posterior urethral valves.

findings include a large distended urinary bladder, patent urachus, and a dilated urethra.

RENAL CYSTIC DISEASE

Cystic diseases of the kidney may be inherited or sporadic, unilateral or bilateral, and symptomatic at birth or detected later in life (Table 1). This section will approach the differential diagnosis from the standpoint of bilateral or unilateral disease.

Autosomal Recessive Polycystic Kidney Disease

Autosomal recessive polycystic kidney disease, frequently referred to as infantile polycystic kidney disease, is a congenital renal abnormality affecting both kidneys. As the name implies, it is inherited as a recessive characteristic, while the adult form is inherited as an autosomal dominant disease. On gross examination, numerous small cysts 1 to 2 mm in diameter are seen in both the cortex and medulla. Microdissection studies have shown that these cysts are predom-

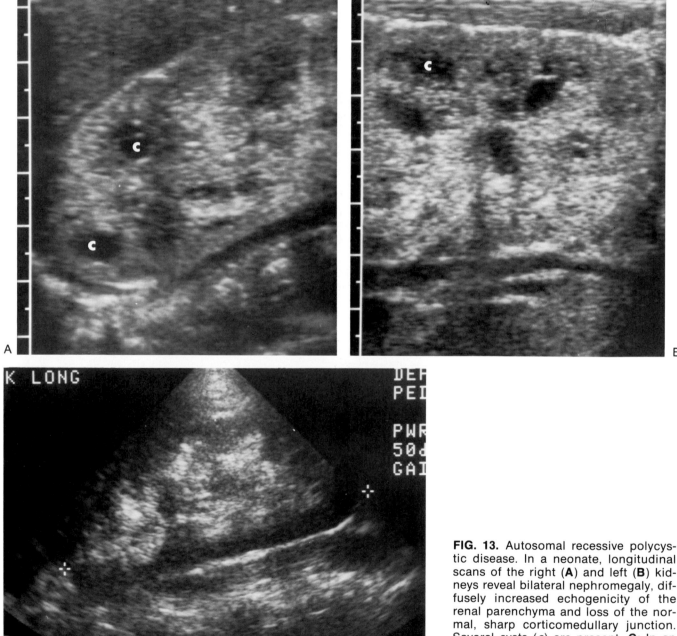

FIG. 13. Autosomal recessive polycystic disease. In a neonate, longitudinal scans of the right (**A**) and left (**B**) kidneys reveal bilateral nephromegaly, diffusely increased echogenicity of the renal parenchyma and loss of the normal, sharp corticomedullary junction. Several cysts (*c*) are present. **C:** In an older child, longitudinal scan demonstrates increased echogenicity, mainly in the medullary region.

TABLE 1. *Cystic diseases of the kidney*

Bilateral Diseases
  Autosomal recessive polycystic kidney disease
  Autosomal dominant polycystic kidney disease
  Glomerulocystic disease
  Cystic disease of renal medulla
  Cysts associated with multiple malformation
    syndromes
  Acquired cystic diseases with chronic hemodialysis

Unilateral Diseases
  Multicystic dysplasia
  Multilocular cyst
  Simple cysts

inantly fusiform dilatations of the collecting tubules; the nephrons are normal or minimally altered (114). Biliary ductal ectasia with a variable degree of periportal fibrosis is seen frequently. Autosomal recessive polycystic kidney disease appears to be a spectrum of abnormality, with the renal disease and hepatic fibrosis varying inversely. Patients presenting in the neonatal period have bilaterally enlarged kidneys and poor renal function; hepatic dysfunction is minimal. In later childhood the liver disease dominates, with portal venous hypertension and esophageal varices being frequent findings. This form of disease is sometimes termed tubular ectasia with congenital hepatic fibrosis or juvenile polycystic disease.

In the neonate, the kidneys are bilaterally enlarged and diffusely echogenic, often with a sonolucent rim. The increased echogenicity is produced by the innumerable fluid-tubular wall interfaces, whereas the sonolucent rim may represent the remnant of compressed normal renal cortex (14,59,71). Occasionally, discrete macroscopic cysts may be seen in the medullary region. In the older child, medullary echogenicity is seen (Fig. 13). Hepatic sonography demonstrates variable findings. In younger children with minimal fibrosis, the liver appears normal or minimally echogenic. With significant periportal fibrosis, diffusely increased parenchymal echogenicity and biliary ductal ectasia may be observed (Fig. 14). The diagnosis of autosomal recessive disease usually can be confirmed by excretory urography, which typically shows nephromegaly and radiating streaks of contrast in dilated collecting tubules.

Autosomal Dominant Polycystic Kidney Disease

Autosomal dominant polycystic kidney disease, also known as adult polycystic renal disease, is a familial disorder. Pathologically, grossly visible cysts of varying size are present throughout the cortex and medulla. Between the cystic areas are islands of normal mesenchymal stroma. Microdissection studies show that

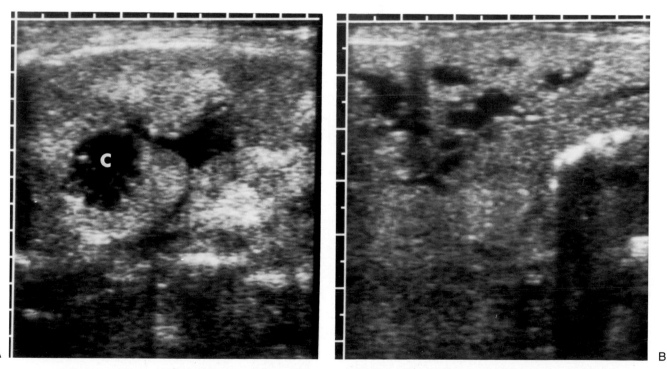

A   B

FIG. 14. Autosomal recessive polycystic disease and hepatic fibrosis. **A:** Longitudinal sonograms of the right flank in a neonate show an echogenic kidney with a large cyst (*C*) and a sonolucent rim. Similar changes were noted in the left kidney. **B:** Transverse sonogram of the liver shows dilated intrahepatic ducts.

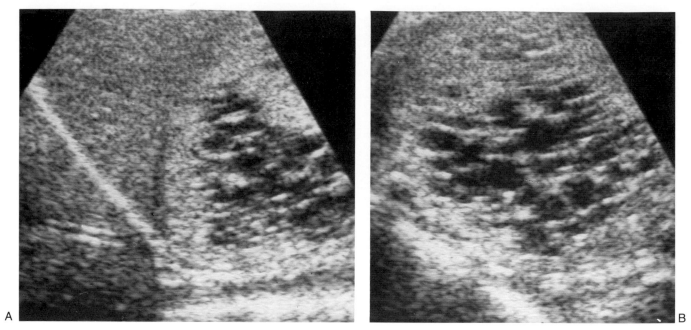

FIG. 15. Autosomal dominant cystic disease in a newborn. **A:** Longitudinal and **B:** transverse scans of the right flank show an enlarged, echogenic kidney with multiple small cysts. The left kidney had a similar appearance.

the cysts communicate with the nephrons as well as with the collecting tubules (114). Hepatic and pancreatic cysts also may be found, but in contrast to infantile polycystic disease there rarely is significant periportal hepatic fibrosis. Typically, the disease presents in the fourth or fifth decade of life with hypertension or hematuria, although rarely it can present in the neonate as abdominal masses.

In the neonate, sonography may demonstrate enlarged, diffusely echogenic kidneys. Occasionally, discrete cysts can be seen within the parenchyma (Fig. 15) (71,179). The sonographic findings in the neonate of the dominant form of polycystic kidney disease are similar to those of the autosomal recessive form of polycystic kidney disease. Diagnosis needs to be based on family history or tissue sampling. In older children,

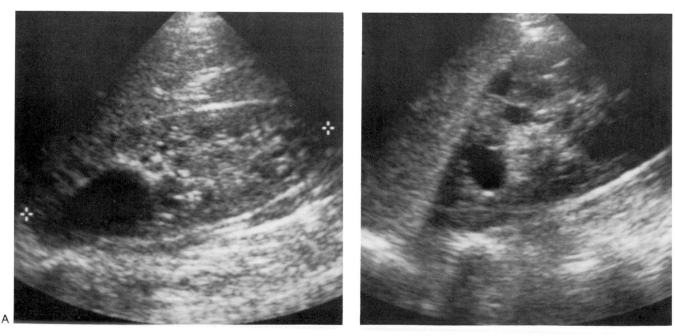

FIG. 16. Autosomal dominant polycystic kidney disease in a young girl. Longitudinal sonograms of the right (**A**) and left (**B**) kidneys reveal cysts in the renal parenchyma bilaterally.

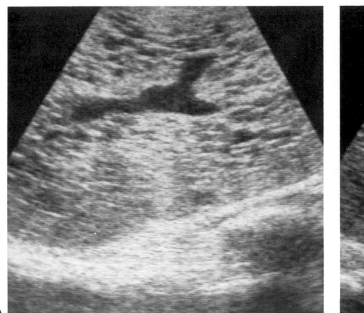
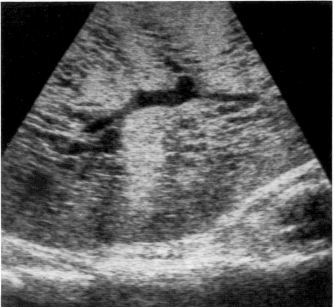

FIG. 17. Glomerulocystic disease in a neonate. Sagittal scans of the right (**A**) and left (**B**) flanks show large, echogenic kidneys containing multiple cysts ranging from 2 to 8 mm in diameter.

the sonographic findings of dominant disease include renal enlargement and multiple anechoic cysts of variable size in the cortex and medulla (Fig. 16) (59,71). These more classic changes permit a specific diagnosis of autosomal dominant disease to be made.

Glomerulocystic Disease

Glomerulocystic disease is a rare condition that is typically sporadic with no familial pattern. Patholog-

ically, the disease is characterized by cystic dilatation of Bowman's space of the glomeruli (107). Periportal hepatic fibrosis, bile duct hyperplasia and dilatation, and hepatic cysts also may be seen. Most affected patients present with palpable abdominal masses and renal failure early in life. The sonographic findings are indistinguishable from those of autosomal dominant or recessive polycystic disease occurring in the neonate. The kidney is echogenic and contains cysts of variable size (Fig. 17) (179).

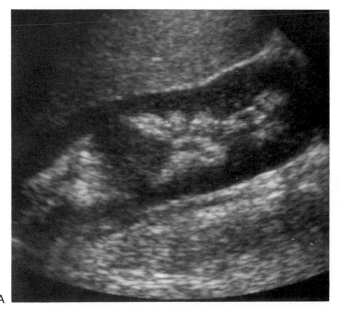
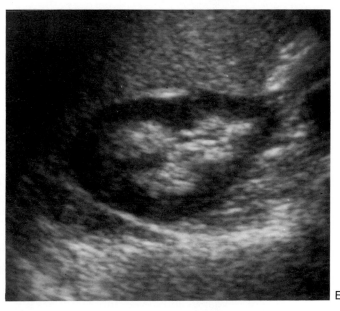

FIG. 18. Medullary sponge kidney. **A:** Longitudinal and **B:** transverse sonograms of the right kidney reveal hyperechoic renal pyramids due to multiple small calculi.

Cystic Disease of the Renal Medulla

Two forms of medullary cystic disease can be encountered in pediatric patients: medullary sponge kidney and juvenile nephronophthisis. Medullary sponge kidney, also referred to as renal collecting tubular ectasia, is not an inherited disease. Pathologically, there is dilatation of the collecting tubules associated with numerous cysts. Although the disease is usually present at birth, it does not become apparent until adulthood. Rarely, it presents in children with complications of infection, calculi, or hematuria. The sonogram usually is normal, although occasionally enlarged, echogenic pyramids due to calcium deposition may be noted (Fig. 18) (131).

Juvenile nephronophthisis or uremic medullary cystic disease is inherited as an autosomal recessive trait. Pathologically, the kidneys are small or normal-sized, the cortex is thin, and macroscopic cysts are seen in the medulla and at the corticomedullary junction. Clinically, nephronophthisis is characterized by polyuria, polydypsia, salt-wasting, and progressive uremia. Sonography demonstrates loss of corticomedullary differentiation, increased parenchymal echogenicity, and a variable number of cysts in the medulla or at the corticomedullary junction (47,59,71). The sonographic findings of uremic medullary cystic disease are similar to those of medullary cystic disease, which is an au-

tosomal dominant disorder occurring in young adults. Diagnosis is based on family history and clinical data.

Renal Cysts Associated with Multiple Malformation Syndromes

The malformation syndromes associated with renal cysts in children include tuberous sclerosis, Meckel's syndrome (microcephaly, polydactyly, posterior encephalocele), Jeune's asphyxiating thoracic dystrophy (small chest, respiratory failure, renal dysplasia), and Zelweger's syndrome (hypotonia, hepatomegaly). Renal cysts also have been associated with von Hippel-Lindau disease. However, this disease is infrequent in childhood, usually presenting in early or middle adulthood. Sonography of these various syndromes demonstrates multiple cysts in the cortex, medulla, or in both areas. In some cases, the cysts may be quite large and have an appearance similar to that of autosomal recessive polycystic kidney disease. Correlation with clinical findings usually permits the correct diagnosis.

Acquired Cystic Diseases

Cystic disease of the kidney occurs in a large percentage of patients on chronic intermittent hemodi-

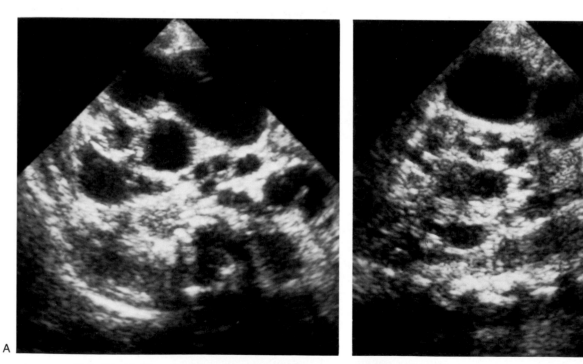

FIG. 19. Multicystic dysplastic kidney. **A:** Longitudinal and **B:** transverse sonograms of the right flank reveal multiple oval and round cysts with a random distribution in the area of the right kidney; there is no central renal pelvis or normal renal parenchyma noted.

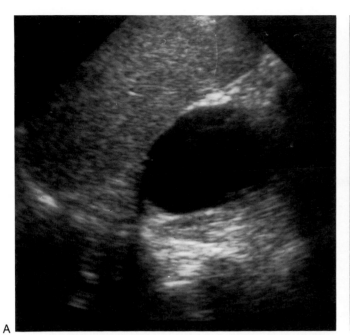 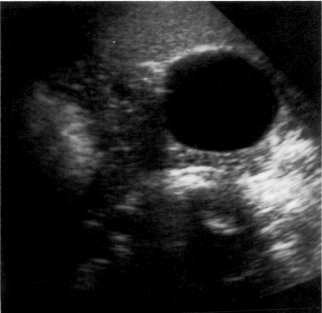

A   B

FIG. 20. Multicystic dysplastic kidney appearing as a solitary cyst. **A:** Longitudinal and **B:** transverse scans through the right renal fossa demonstrate a solitary cystic mass. Renal scintigraphy showed nonfunction of the right kidney. The cyst completely disappeared on a follow-up examination 1 year later.

alysis. The incidence increases with the years on dialysis, and is particularly high after the third year (51). The etiology is unclear, but it is believed to be secondary to ischemia or fibrosis. The cysts in this entity are multiple and may remain small or become markedly enlarged. Complications include hemorrhage within the cyst as well as subcapsular or perinephric hematomas. In addition, the incidence of adenomas and carcinomas of the kidney is increased in chronic hemodialysis patients who have acquired renal cystic disease (51).

Multicystic Dysplastic Kidney

Multicystic dysplastic kidney is the second most common cause of an abdominal mass in the newborn, following hydronephrosis, and is believed to be secondary to atresia of the upper ureter during the metanephric stage of intrauterine development. If the atresia involves the renal pelvis as well as the ureter, the usual form of pelvoinfundibular atresia results (58). If only the upper ureter is atretic, the more unusual hydronephrotic-type multicystic dysplastic kidney develops (39). In both cases the ureter may be absent, atretic, or hypoplastic, and the renal vessels are small or atretic. Histologically, the cysts are separated by tissue containing primitive dysplastic elements.

The sonographic features of the usual multicystic dysplastic kidney are anechoic masses of variable size with a random distribution, no connections between the cysts, no medial location of the largest cyst, absence of an identifiable renal pelvis, and absent or dysplastic renal parenchyma (Fig. 19) (146,164). Rarely, multicystic dysplastic kidney may appear as a solitary cystic mass in the renal fossa (Fig. 20). In the hydronephrotic form of multicystic dysplastic kidney, a renal pelvis can be seen. Radionuclide renal scanning usually demonstrates little or no activity and therefore is useful in differentiating the multicystic dysplastic kidney from mild to moderate hydronephrosis. It should be noted, however, that severe hydronephrosis with nearly absent renal function may be indistinguishable from a multicystic dysplastic kidney. It also is important to examine the contralateral kidneys since at least 10% to 15% of patients with multicystic dysplastic kidney will have abnormalities of the contralateral kidney, most frequently a ureteropelvic junction obstruction.

There is some controversy regarding the need for nephrectomy in cases of multicystic kidney. The diagnosis can be established with a high degree of accuracy by sonography followed by renal scintigraphy. Nonoperative management has, therefore, been advocated by some pediatric urologists. Other urologists prefer nephrectomy, claiming that infection, hyperten-

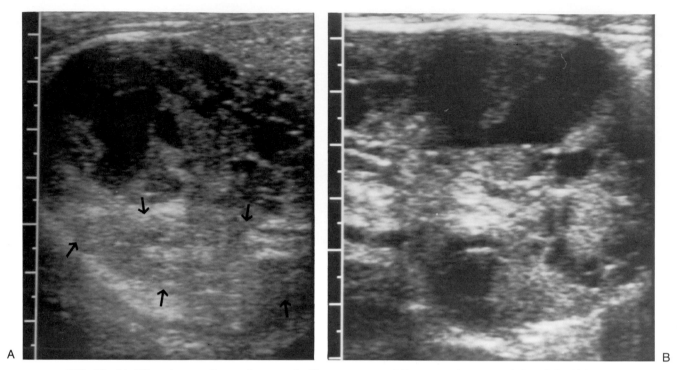

FIG. 21. Multilocular cystic nephroma. **A:** Transverse and **B:** coronal scans of the right kidney show a number of anechoic locules separated by echogenic septa. Normal renal tissue (*arrows*) is seen posteriorly.

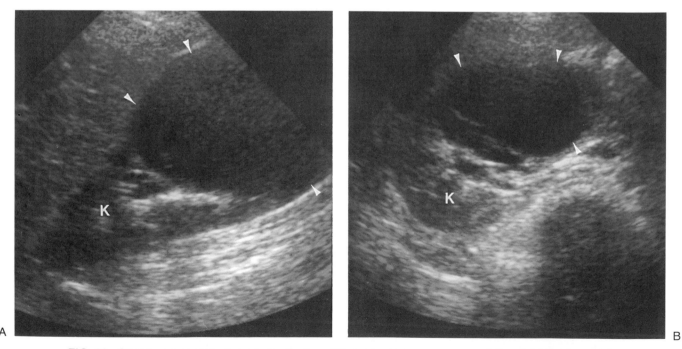

FIG. 22. Simple renal cyst. **A:** Longitudinal and **B:** transverse sonograms of the right flank reveal a well-marginated anechoic mass (*arrowheads*) arising from the lower pole of the right kidney (*K*). A simple cyst was removed surgically.

sion, and rarely malignancy of the multicystic kidney are possibilities (68). In those instances where the decision is made to leave a multicystic dysplastic kidney in place, serial imaging studies are mandatory. Early experience with serial sonography has shown that approximately 70% of multicystic kidneys remain relatively stable in size; the remainder either increase or decrease in size or disappear (174).

Multilocular Cystic Nephroma

Multilocular cystic nephroma, also termed benign cystic nephroma, cystic hamartoma, cystic Wilms' tumor, cystic lymphangioma, and partially polycystic kidney, is an uncommon renal mass with a peak incidence in children under 2 years of age. Grossly, the tumor is a well-circumscribed, encapsulated mass containing a number of noncommunicating fluid-filled cysts that are separated by fibrous septa. Microscopic foci of Wilms' tumor occasionally are found in the cyst wall. Affected patients are evaluated predominantly because of a nonpainful abdominal mass and less commonly hematuria. On sonography, the lesion appears as a well-defined mass with large, multiple anechoic or hypoechoic cysts separated by echogenic septa (Fig. 21) (8). When the cysts are small or contain mucoid material, the multilocular nature may not be apparent and the appearance will be nonspecific and, similar to that of other solid renal tumors (22,113). In these instances, CT may be helpful for diagnosis (129).

Simple Cysts

Simple cysts have been estimated to occur in more than half of adults over 50 years of age, but are rare in children. Pathologically, they are unilocular, solitary masses lined by a single layer of flattened epithelium and containing clear serous fluid; communication between the cyst and the collecting system is absent. The most common presenting feature is a palpable abdominal mass, but they may present with hematuria or be found incidentally during urography (55,156). On sonography, cysts appear as spherical or slightly ovoid, thin-walled anechoic masses with through-transmission (Fig. 22) (163). Internal echoes are absent. Occasionally, simple cysts may be complicated by hemorrhage, infection, or calcification. In these instances, sonography demonstrates a thick-walled mass with internal echoes or shadowing from calcifications in the cyst wall. In the older child, percutaneous aspiration with sonographic guidance may be diagnostic and therapeutic.

RENAL NEOPLASMS

Because of its high accuracy and ease of performance, sonography remains the procedure of choice for initial evaluation of suspected or known renal masses. If the sonogram shows a benign condition such as a hydronephrotic kidney or renal cystic disease, renal scintigraphy or excretory urography should be performed to evaluate function or to confirm the diagnosis, especially in cases of renal cystic disease. If the mass is solid and a malignant neoplasm is suspected, computerized tomography (CT) or magnetic resonance (MR) imaging should be performed to delineate better the extent of the disease.

Malignant Tumors

Wilms' Tumor

Wilms' tumor is the most common renal neoplasm in childhood, accounting for about one-fourth of urologic masses in children older than 1 year of age (85). Approximately 80% of these tumors occur in children under 5 years of age, with a mean age at presentation of 3 years. A palpable abdominal mass is the most frequent presentation, occurring in about 70% of affected patients. Less frequently, children present with abdominal pain (30%), hematuria (25%), or fever (20%). Hypertension is found in up to 90% of patients and has been attributed to an increase in renin activity (133,153). Rarely, associated anomalies such as Beckwith-Wiedemann syndrome, aniridia, and hemihypertrophy may prompt evaluation.

The typical Wilms' tumor is a bulky mass replacing most of the involved kidney. On section, Wilms' tumor is sharply marginated by a pseudocapsule of compressed renal tissue and frequently contains areas of liquefaction necrosis and hemorrhage. Histologically, the tumor usually has a triphasic pattern consisting of blastemal, stromal, and epithelial elements. Infrequently, calcification or fat is identified (133).

The diagnosis of Wilms' tumor by sonography depends on identification of an intrarenal mass. Diagnostic criteria include the following: (a) a mass with a heterogeneous or homogeneous center and an echogenicity similar to or slightly less than that of normal renal parenchyma (Fig. 23); (b) sharp parenchymal inferface; (c) a hypo- or hyperechoic rim representing compressed renal parenchyma at the tumor interface; and (d) secondary characteristics, such as renal vein or inferior vena caval enlargement or invasion, enlarged lymph nodes, metastases, and parenchymal cal-

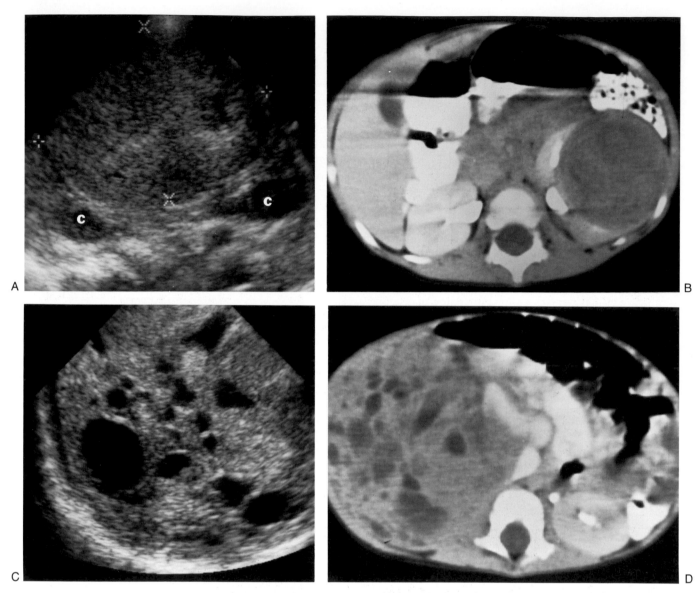

FIG. 23. Wilms' tumor. **A:** Coronal image of the left kidney shows a large, homogeneous echogenic mass arising from the midpole of the left kidney and distorting mildly dilated calyces (*C*). **B:** Contrast enhanced CT scan shows a large, low-density mass displacing the calyces. **C:** Longitudinal scan in another patient demonstrates a heterogeneous echogenic mass with areas of necrosis. **D:** CT reveals a soft tissue mass with areas of necrosis in the upper pole of the right kidney.

cifications (Fig. 24) (28,64,67,79,137). On the basis of these criteria, sonography is extremely accurate in the diagnosis of Wilms' tumor (137). Rarely, Wilms' tumor may arise in an abnormally positioned kidney, such as a horseshoe kidney, or in an extrarenal teratoma (1,112). Extrarenal Wilms' tumor exhibits features similar to those of intrarenal Wilms' tumor (44).

Knowledge of the system for staging Wilms' tumor is important for understanding the many appearances of this tumor and for patient management (Table 2). Tumor extension through the capsule into the perinephric space usually is very difficult to visualize by sonography because of the minute size of the perirenal

infiltration. Since radical nephrectomy with *en bloc* resection of the kidney, perirenal fat, and Gerota's fascia is the surgical treatment of choice, failure to visualize this extension does not affect treatment. Spread to lymph nodes of the renal hilum or to the perinephric

TABLE 2. *Second National Wilms' Tumor Study: Staging of Wilms' Tumor*

I.	Encapsulated tumor, completely excised
II.	Extends beyond the kidney, completely excised
III.	Residual tumor confined to the abdomen or nodes
IV.	Hematogeneous metastases
V.	Bilateral tumors at diagnosis

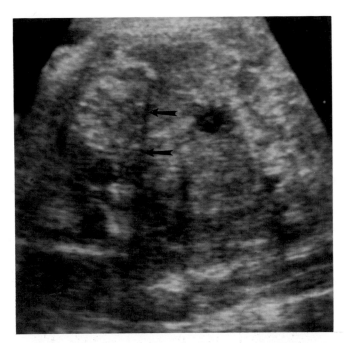

FIG. 24. Wilms' tumor. Longitudinal image of the right kidney demonstrates a heterogeneous mass with focal areas of increased echogenicity, with distal acoustic shadowing (*arrows*) representing calcifications.

lymph nodes occurs in about 20% of cases. The presence of lymph node metastases is important, since it implies a poorer prognosis. Lymph nodes normally are not seen in the retroperitoneum of young children. The demonstration of hilar, periaortic, or paracaval nodes by sonography should be considered abnormal and suspicious for tumor metastases (Fig. 25). Occasionally, enlarged lymph nodes are due to reactive hyperplasia and are a cause of false positive interpretations.

Intrarenal venous invasion by tumor is not visible by sonography, but main renal vein and inferior vena caval involvement can be detected. Vascular invasion occurs in 5% to 10% of children with Wilms' tumor and does not adversely affect prognosis if treatment is appropriate. The diagnosis of venous thrombosis depends on the demonstration of a focally enlarged vein with an echogenic, intraluminal mass (Fig. 26) (160). When venous occlusion is complete, perivertebral collaterals may be identified. The liver is the most common intraabdominal site of hematogeneous spread of Wilms' tumor; hepatic metastases are evident in about 10% of patients at diagnosis. Bilateral synchronous Wilms' tumors occur in 5% to 10% of patients, making it mandatory to evaluate both kidneys prior to surgery. Although sonography can assess local extension of tumor, lymph node involvement, and bilateral tumors, it is not as sensitive as CT or MR imaging for this determination. In one study of patients with Wilms' tumor, the total tumor extent was determined correctly by CT scanning in about 75% of patients and by sonography in approximately 25% of patients (137).

Following therapy, sonography can be used to detect

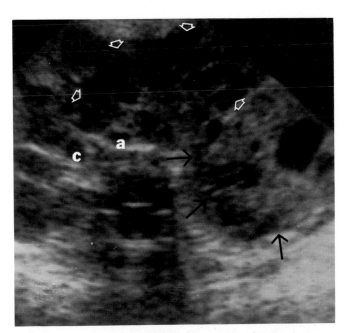

FIG. 25. Wilms' tumors with local nodal spread. A transverse scan of the retroperitoneum demonstrates a heterogeneous echogenic mass (*black arrows*) with areas of necrosis in the left kidney. Also noted is extensive retroperitoneal lymphadenopathy (*open arrows*). *C,* inferior vena cava; *a,* aorta.

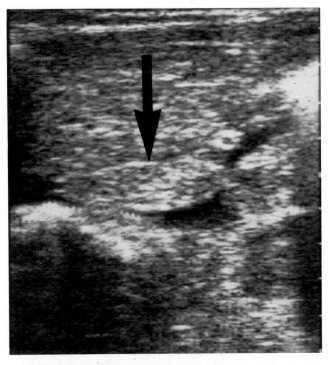

FIG. 26. Wilms' tumor with invasion of the inferior vena cava. Longitudinal sonogram demonstrates a large tumor thrombus in the inferior vena cava (*arrow*).

local recurrence in the renal fossa and hepatic metastases. Patients with incomplete resection of tumor, lymph node involvement, and vascular invasion are at the highest risk for postoperative recurrence. The features that suggest tumor recurrence are a soft tissue mass in the evacuated renal fossa and ipsilateral psoas muscle enlargement.

Nephroblastomatosis

Nephroblastomatosis is a congenital renal lesion that is believed to be a precursor of Wilms' tumor (18,108,109,145). It has been found in 12% to 33% of kidneys with Wilms' tumors as well as in conditions with a high incidence of Wilms' tumor, such as Beckwith-Wiedemann syndrome, sporadic aniridia, and hemihypertrophy. Pathologically, the tumor is characterized by bilateral, subcapsular aggregates of primitive metanephric blastema that range in size from microscopic foci to large confluent masses replacing most of the renal parenchyma (15,42). In general, the smaller tumor foci are referred to as multifocal nephroblastomatosis, and the diffuse confluent aggregates are termed pancortical or diffuse nephroblastomatosis. Diffuse nephroblastomatosis generally affects children under 2 years of age and presents as bilateral

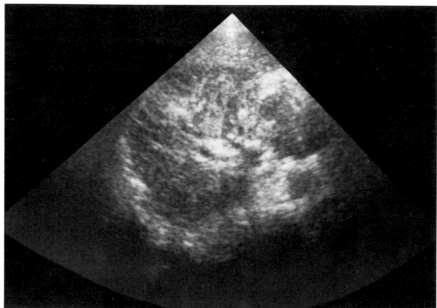

A

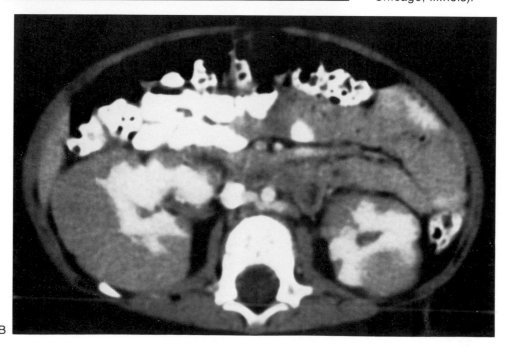

B

FIG. 27. Nephroblastomatosis. **A:** Transverse scan through the right kidney. The echotexture is minimally heterogeneous with loss of the normal corticomedullary differentiation. No discrete masses are seen on sonography. **B:** CT shows cortical soft tissue masses clearly demarcated from the enhanced adjacent renal parenchyma. (Courtesy of Dr. James Donaldson, Chicago, Illinois).

flank masses. Multifocal nephroblastomatosis occurs in children of all ages and usually is clinically silent. The diagnosis in these cases is established at autopsy or at operation for Wilms' tumor.

The sonographic findings vary with the size and distribution of the embryonic rests. The kidneys usually are of normal size in multifocal nephroblastomatosis, although the borders may be lobulated. With diffuse disease there are minimal abnormalities of renal size, contour, and corticomedullary differentiation. In general, the echogenicity of nephroblastomatosis is similar to that of normal parenchyma (40,123). Because of the similar echogenicity, sonography is not sensitive enough to detect discrete nodules. Computerized tomography, however, is capable of showing subcapsular nodular masses because of its superior ability to distinguish small tissue density differences (Fig. 27).

Renal Cell Carcinoma

Less than 0.5% of renal cell carcinomas occur in the first 2 decades of life. The age of peak occurrence during childhood is approximately 9 years, in contrast to Wilms' tumor which has a peak incidence at 3 years of age. Patients with renal cell carcinoma present with abdominal or flank pain (50% to 60%), a palpable abdominal mass (50% to 60%), or hematuria (30% to 60%). Pathologically the tumor may be well-circumscribed by a pseudocapsule, or unencapsulated and infiltrating. Renal vascular invasion is present in about 25% of cases (32,64).

On sonography, renal cell carcinoma appears as a hypoechoic or echogenic intrarenal mass (Fig. 28) (25). The average diameter of the tumor at the time of diagnosis is 4 cm. Calcifications occur in approximately 25% of tumors and appear as echogenic foci, usually centrally located, within the intrarenal mass. Spread of tumor into the retroperitoneum and lymph nodes or invasion of the renal vein also may be identified by sonography. In general, differentiation between renal cell carcinoma and Wilms' tumor usually is not possible on the basis of the sonographic findings, but the age of the patient usually is helpful in providing the correct diagnosis.

Lymphoma

Renal lymphoma usually is discovered at autopsy, rather than during the course of the disease, because it rarely causes symptoms. Approximately 15% of patients with renal lymphoma will have metastatic spread diagnosed antemortem. In this group of patients, clinical findings include flank or abdominal pain, a palpable flank mass, hypertension, hematuria, and azotemia. When renal involvement is present in patients with lymphoma, it is more often associated with non-Hodgkin's lymphoma rather than Hodgkin's disease. Affected children usually are over 5 years old.

On sonography, lymphomatous infiltration usually is bilateral rather than unilateral. The most common appearance of renal lymphoma is multiple hypoechoic

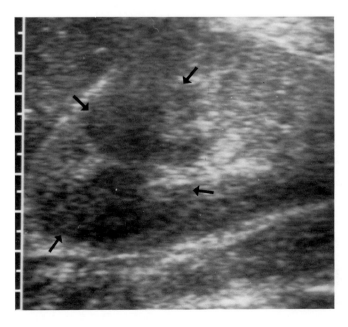

FIG. 28. Renal cell carcinoma. Coronal scan of the right kidney demonstrates a 4 cm hypoechoic mass (*arrows*). The mass is poorly differentiated from adjacent normal parenchyma.

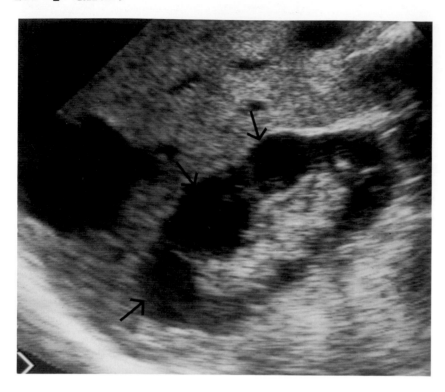

FIG. 29. Lymphoma. Longitudinal images through the right flank demonstrate anechoic masses in the right kidney (*arrows*) and right lobe of the liver.

or anechoic nodules (Fig. 29) (152). Some degree of through-transmission is present, although the extent is less than that of cystic masses (154). Uncommonly, renal lymphoma may appear hyperechoic and be confused with other solid renal tumors (Fig. 30). Other patterns of involvement that have been encountered with renal lymphoma include direct invasion from contiguous retroperitoneal lymph node masses, a single large mass, and diffuse infiltration (63,73). Associated findings that may be demonstrated include lymphomatous involvement of the liver, spleen, or lymph nodes. The pattern of renal lymphomatous involvement may be mimicked by polycystic renal disease, tuberous sclerosis, or leukemia.

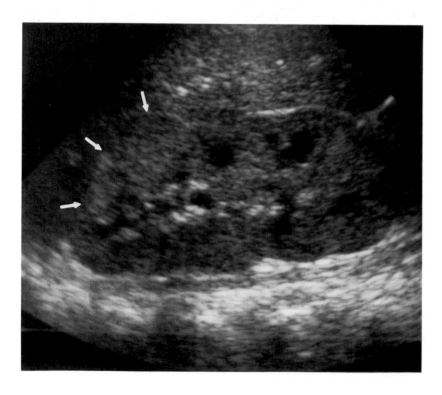

FIG. 30. Lymphoma. Coronal image of the right kidney shows an echogenic mass (*arrows*) distorting the renal contour.

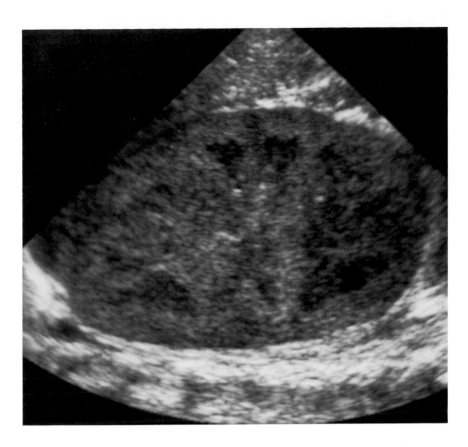

FIG. 31. Leukemia. Longitudinal sonogram of the right flank demonstrates a markedly enlarged kidney measuring 10 cm in diameter. The renal parenchyma is of normal echogenicity but there is loss of corticomedullary differentiation. The left kidney had a similar appearance.

Leukemia

The kidneys may be involved by leukemia during active stages of acute disease and also may act as a sanctuary during bone marrow remission. Leukemic renal infiltration usually is asymptomatic, although it may result in abdominal pain, hematuria, hypertension, or renal failure (52). Sonographic findings of renal leukemic involvement include nephromegaly, altered parenchymal architecture, and hydronephrosis (Fig. 31) (56). Occasionally multiple hypoechoic nodules are seen within the kidneys (52).

Renal Metastases

Renal metastases in children are unusual and result from either hematogenous or direct spread of malignant tumors. Hematogenous metastases occur most often in patients with undifferentiated sarcomas (41). Direct extension of tumor into the kidney usually is found in association with retroperitoneal tumors, such as neuroblastoma or lymphoma. Sonographically, renal metastases appear as hypoechoic intrarenal masses.

Rare Renal Tumors

Clear cell sarcoma and malignant rhabdoid tumor are rare renal masses. The presenting signs are non-specific and similar to those of Wilms' tumor. On sonography, either tumor may appear as a solid intrarenal mass, resembling Wilms' tumor. Malignant rhabdoid tumor also may appear as an echogenic mass, replacing or compressing the remaining normal kidney in association with a thickened renal capsule and subcapsular fluid collection with tumor implants (Fig. 32) (158). Concomitant primary tumors of the posterior cranial fossa, soft tissues, and thymus frequently occur in association with malignant rhabdoid tumor. Clear cell sarcoma not uncommonly metastasizes to bone.

Benign Tumors

Angiomyolipoma

Angiomyolipoma is a rare benign renal tumor composed of angiomatous, myomatous, and lipomatous tissue. It occurs infrequently in the general population, but is present in as many as 80% of children with tuberous sclerosis. The lesions usually are small and asymptomatic, although occasionally renal failure may develop in children with extensive involvement by multiple tumors. The sonographic appearance ranges from marked parenchymal heterogeneity with multiple small echogenic foci corresponding to fat, to uniform echogenicity due to nearly total replacement of the

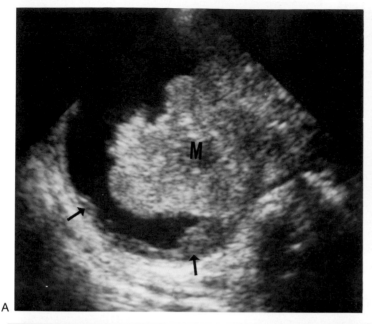

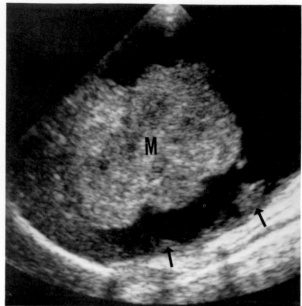

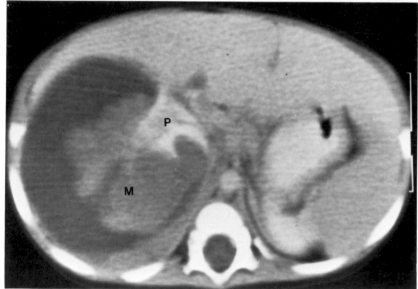

FIG. 32. Malignant rhabdoid tumor. **A:** Transverse and **B:** coronal sonograms of the right kidney demonstrate an irregular echogenic mass (*M*) replacing the renal parenchyma. Subcapsular fluid collection with tumor nodules (*arrows*) surrounds the mass. **C:** Contrast-enhanced CT scan shows a lobulated soft tissue mass (*M*) of lower attenuation than the adjacent compressed parenchyma (*P*). Subcapsular fluid collection and tumor implants are noted again.

renal substance by angiomyolipomas (Fig. 33). In the latter instance, CT is useful to differentiate between solid, cystic, and lipomatous tissues (Fig. 33). Rarely, angiomyolipomas appear as solitary, large, hyperechoic, or complex intrarenal masses (65,171).

Mesoblastic Nephroma

Mesoblastic nephroma, also termed fetal renal hamartoma, is a benign neoplasm accounting for the majority of renal masses in infants under 1 year of age. Children are evaluated predominantly because of a painless mass. On gross section, the tumor is a solid, unencapsulated mass, replacing most if not all of the renal parenchyma. Histologically, it is composed of a fibrous or mesenchymal stroma with scattered dysplastic tubules and glomeruli (15,16,66). Hemorrhage and necrosis are infrequent.

Sonographically, most mesoblastic nephromas are large, well-defined, homogeneous masses with low-level echoes (Fig. 34) (96). Rarely, the center is heterogeneous with anechoic areas representing necrosis or hemorrhage (24,57). Occasionally concentric hypo- and hyperechoic rings surround the mass (i.e., "ring sign") (24). Mesoblastic nephroma may invade the perinephric connective tissue, but typically does not infiltrate the vascular pedicle, extend into the renal pelvis, or metastasize. The vast majority can be cured by nephrectomy alone (9). Differentiation between mesoblastic nephroma and the rare neonatal Wilms' tumor is not possible based on sonographic findings.

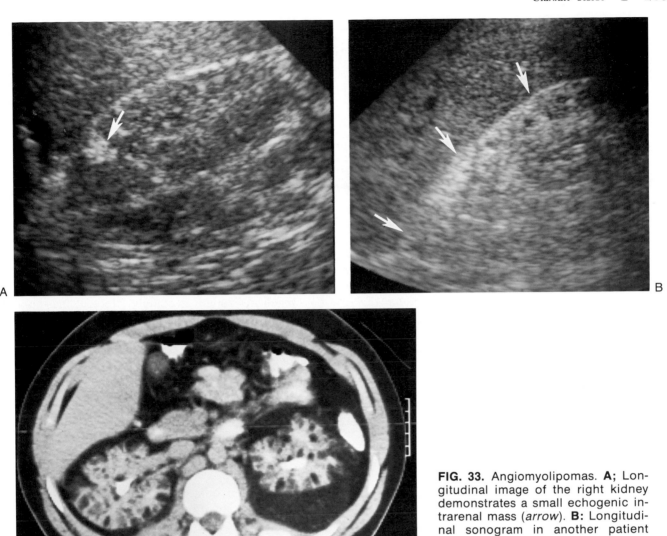

FIG. 33. Angiomyolipomas. **A;** Longitudinal image of the right kidney demonstrates a small echogenic intrarenal mass (*arrow*). **B:** Longitudinal sonogram in another patient shows a diffusely echogenic right kidney (*arrows*). **C:** CT in this patient shows multiple fatty masses replacing most of the renal parenchyma.

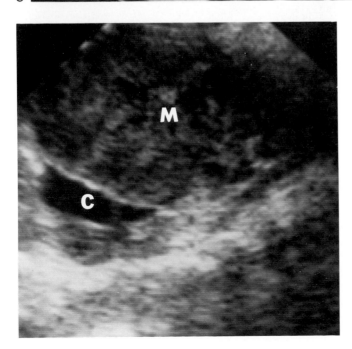

FIG. 34. Mesoblastic nephroma. Longitudinal sonograms show a homogeneous, hypoechoic mass (*M*) distorting dilated calyces (*C*) in the lower pole of the left kidney.

INFECTION

Urinary tract infection (UTI) is one of the most common indications for radiologic investigation of the kidneys and bladder. About 40% of children with proved urinary tract infections will have some type of abnormality that has a potential for causing renal damage. Of the 40%, 20% will show vesicoureteral reflux and 20% will have other conditions ranging from relatively insignificant abnormalities such as congenitally misplaced kidneys to more important conditions such as duplication associated with obstruction (176).

There is general agreement that all children should be studied radiographically after the first well-documented UTI. For children who are not acutely ill and do not have an active infection, the initial examination generally is a voiding cystourethrogram (VCUG) to determine the presence or absence of reflux (13,99, 100,118,119). The radiographic VCUG is preferred to the isotopic or sonographic cystogram because it allows assessment of bladder wall, urethra, and low-grade reflux. Scintigraphic studies are better suited for the follow-up evaluation of reflux because these studies have a lower radiation dose and the ability to quantitate the volume at which reflux occurs. Sonography with microbubbles also has no radiation, but it is technically difficult and less sensitive than conventional VCUG. Microbubbles are produced by shaking contrast medium or saline. Following catheterization, the fluid is infused. Dilatation of the collecting system during the course of bladder filling or visualization of microbubbles in the renal pelvis indicates reflux (91,150). Sonography has a sensitivity of 87%

for detecting reflux into the collecting system, but it detects only 50% of reflux into the distal ureter and has a false positive rate of 10% (91,150). Because sonographic cystography does not predict the presence or degree of reflux accurately, it has not gained widespread acceptance.

If vesicoureteral reflux is absent, a sonogram usually is performed to evaluate the upper urinary tracts for unsuspected renal disease, such as obstruction (3,81,83,84,102,118,119). If the sonogram is normal, no further evaluation is needed. If the VCUG shows reflux, the upper tracts need to be evaluated by excretory urography or renal scintigraphy to determine the presence or absence of cortical scarring and duplicated ureters (3,83,100,118,119). Sonography can identify areas of scarring, but it is not as sensitive as scintigraphy (121,166,172).

When the patient is acutely infected, the initial examination of choice is a sonogram to investigate the possibility of obstruction predisposing to urinary tract infection or complications, such as a focal inflammatory mass or abscess. If sonography is abnormal, then excretory urography or CT should be performed. Voiding cystourethrography is contraindicated until the acute infection has subsided.

Acute Infection

Acute renal inflammatory disease encompasses a broad spectrum of conditions, including diffuse pyelonephritis, acute focal bacterial nephritis, renal abscess, and pyonephrosis (10).

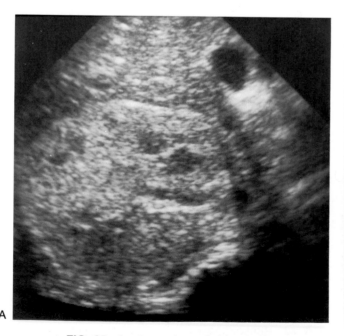
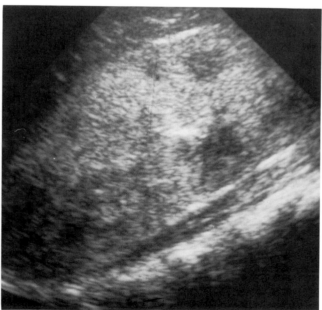

FIG. 35. Acute pyelonephritis. **A:** Transverse and **B:** longitudinal sonograms show a heterogeneously echogenic kidney with prominent pyramids.

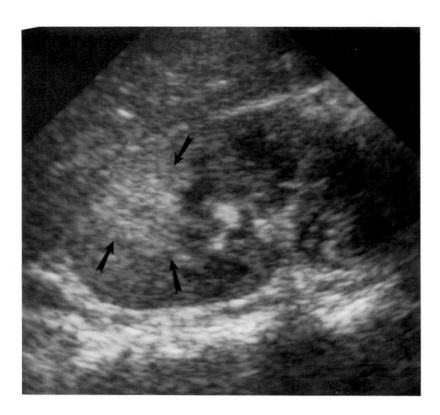

FIG. 36. Acute focal bacterial nephritis. Longitudinal sonogram of the right kidney demonstrates a focal area of increased echogenicity without evidence of liquefaction. The patient was treated for a urinary tract infection and follow-up sonography 6 weeks later showed almost total resolution of the abnormality.

Acute Pyelonephritis

Acute pyelonephritis is an infection of the uroepithelium of the collecting system and renal interstitium, usually caused by gram-negative organisms. Generally, the sonogram is normal. Severe infection, however, can cause diffuse renal enlargement, decreased or increased echogenicity with loss of corticomedullary junction definition, and calyceal distortion (Fig. 35) (33,34,124). Thickening of the renal pelvis and ureteral wall, reflecting mucosal edema and infiltration by inflammatory cells, also may be noted (5,6,125).

On occasion, acute infection results in a focal mass or masses. Acute focal bacterial nephritis, also termed acute lobar nephronia, refers to the early edematous or solid phase of focal renal infection (155). The typical sonographic findings of acute focal bacterial nephritis are an ill-defined hypoechoic mass, without increased through-transmission (101,124). Uncommonly, sonography demonstrates a wedge-shaped echogenic area, thought to represent a hemorrhagic form of acute bacterial nephritis (Fig. 36). The differential diagnostic considerations for a focal mass include tumor and infarct. Clinical history and results of urinalysis should be helpful in providing the correct diagnosis.

Abscess

Infrequently, acute pyelonephritis progresses into a suppurative mass, requiring percutaneous or surgical drainage. On sonography, renal abscess appears as a well-defined hypoechoic mass with thin or thick and well-defined or irregular walls (Fig. 37). Other findings are increased through-transmission and internal echoes indicative of necrotic debris or gas. Once diagnosed, percutaneous aspiration under sonographic

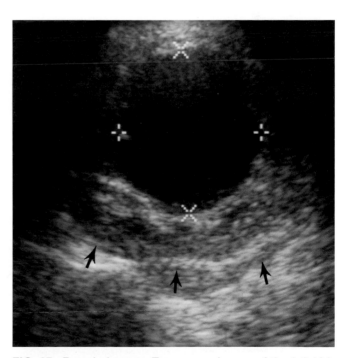

FIG. 37. Renal abscess. Transverse image of the left kidney (*arrows*) shows a large, hypoechoic mass (*calipers*), consistent with an abscess.

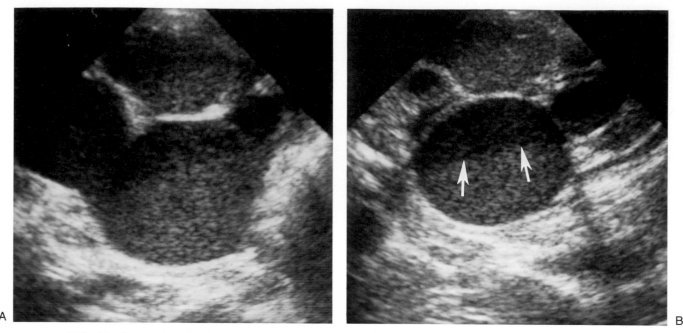

FIG. 38. Pyonephrosis. **A:** Longitudinal sonogram of the left kidney shows a dilated collecting system containing debris. **B:** On a decubitus scan, the dependent debris (*arrows*) shifts in position.

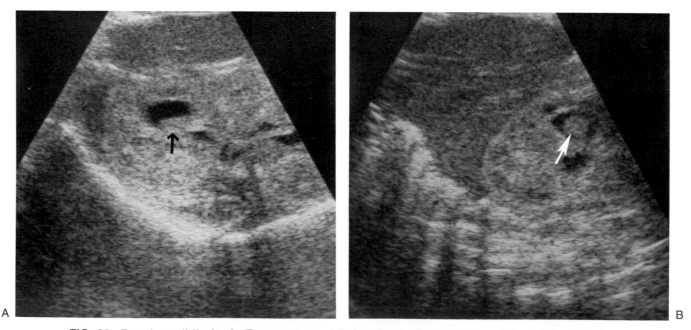

FIG. 39. Renal candidiasis. **A:** Transverse and **B:** longitudinal sonograms of the left flank demonstrate an enlarged, echogenic left kidney. The calyces are dilated and contain echogenic masses (*black and white arrows*), which shift position with changes in patient positioning, representing fungal balls. Percutaneous nephrostomy confirmed the hydronephrosis and filling defects in the collecting system.

guidance can be performed for both diagnosis and therapy.

Pyonephrosis

Pyonephrosis refers to infection proximal to an obstructing lesion, most commonly a congenital anomaly such as a ureteropelvic junction obstruction. Highly reliable findings of pyonephrosis are a dilated collecting system containing medium-amplitude echoes or fluid-fluid levels representing layered debris (Fig. 38) (27,80,167). Rarely, the collecting system may be anechoic, poorly transonic with low-level echoes, or very echogenic with shadowing due to a gas-forming organism (27,80). The specificity for diagnosing pyonephrosis is greater than 95%, and sensitivity varies between 62% and 90% (80,167).

Fungal Infection

Patients with indwelling catheters, hyperalimentation, immunodeficiency states, prolonged antibiotic or immunosuppressive therapy, and premature infants with decreased cellular immunity are particularly susceptible to fungal infection, most commonly caused by *Candida albicans* (130). Pathologically, the initial lesions are microabscesses and inflammatory infiltrates in the renal parenchyma; later complications include mycelia collections in the tubules, necrotizing papillitis, and fungal balls resulting in hydronephrosis (78). Sonographic changes of renal candidiasis include diffusely increased echogenicity, intra- and juxtarenal abscesses, hydronephrosis with echogenic debris (pyonephrosis), and large fungal balls within the renal

pelvis or calyces (Fig. 39) (26,92,93,142). Fungal balls typically appear as echogenic masses without acoustic shadowing (165).

Chronic Infection

Moderate or severe changes of chronic pyelonephritis can be seen with sonography, although milder scarring may be missed. Sonographic findings of chronic inflammation include a small echogenic kidney with irregular contours reflecting focal parenchymal scars.

JUXTARENAL PROCESSES

Major processes that affect the extraperitoneal peri- or paranephric spaces are infection, hemorrhage, or urine leakage. Perinephric inflammatory disease usually is an extension of underlying renal disease. The sonographic appearance of a perinephric abscess is similar to that of abscesses elsewhere. It may be hypoechoic or contain internal echoes indicative of debris or gas; the walls may be thick or thin and smooth or irregular. Rarely, an extrinsic inflammatory process, like a pancreatic pseudocyst, insinuates itself within the anterior perirenal fascia or perinephric space (136).

Hemorrhage into peri- or paranephric spaces usually is due to blunt trauma or a penetrating injury, such as renal biopsy or percutaneous nephrolithotomy. Less frequently it is associated with a bleeding diathesis. The appearance of the hematoma varies with the age of injury. Acute hematomas may appear hyperechoic or complex (Fig. 40). Subacute hematomas are heterogeneous or hypoechoic masses with a variable de-

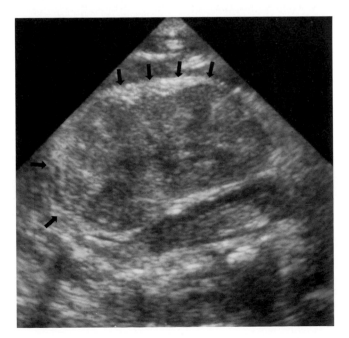

FIG. 40. Acute subcapsular and perinephric hematoma in a patient on heparin. Longitudinal scan of the left flank shows an echogenic, fluid collection (*arrows*) surrounding the left kidney.

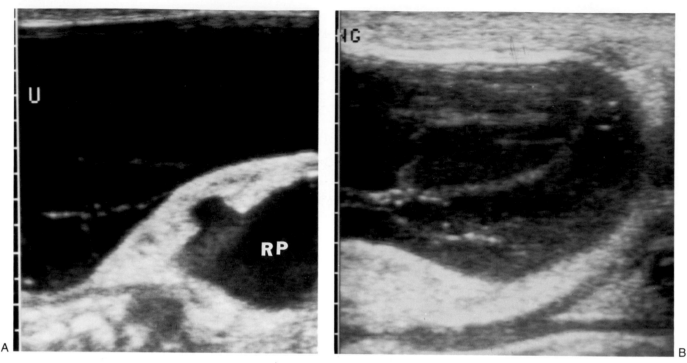

FIG. 41. Perinephric urinoma secondary to ureteropelvic junction obstruction. **A:** Longitudinal sonogram of the left kidney shows a dilated renal pelvis (*RP*) and calyx surrounded by echogenic parenchyma. The anechoic fluid collection with septations lateral to the kidney represents a urinoma (*U*). **B:** Numerous septations are noted in the inferior aspect of the urinoma.

gree of internal echogenicity depending on the extent of fibrin and clot lysis. As the blood clots and retracts, the hematomas may again become echogenic.

Urine extravasation into the perirenal spaces can occur secondary to urinary tract obstruction or after renal trauma. Urinomas usually are hypoechoic and may contain septations or debris (Fig. 41).

RENAL VASCULAR DISEASE

Renal Vein Thrombosis

Renal vein thrombosis in children is predominantly a disease of the newborn. Usually it results from dehydration and associated hemoconcentration, secondary to blood loss, diarrhea, or sepsis. Infants of diabetic mothers also are prone to thrombosis because they are relatively water-depleted. Occasionally, renal vein thrombosis occurs in association with the nephrotic syndrome. Typical clinical signs include a flank mass, hematuria, and transient hypertension. Most cases of renal vein thrombosis are unilateral, but bilateral involvement does occur.

Sonography in the appropriate clinical setting should provide the diagnosis without the need for additional contrast studies. Immediately after obstruction of the renal vein, the kidney becomes enlarged with a diffuse increase in echogenicity secondary to edema and hemorrhage. Over the next 1 to 2 weeks the kidney becomes hypoechoic, with blurring of the corticomedullary junction (128). As cellular infiltration and fibrosis develop, it appears echogenic and of variable size. At any stage, echogenic filling defects representing thrombus may be identified in the renal vein or inferior vena cava (Fig. 42).

The fate of the kidney depends to some extent on the degree and rapidity of venous occlusion. Formation of collateral channels or venous recanalization diminishes intrarenal edema and allows continued arterial perfusion with a more favorable outcome. Thus, the end result is a variable degree of parenchymal damage ranging from complete recovery to severe renal atrophy. The end-stage kidney is small and easily demonstrable with follow-up sonography. At this stage the kidney may contain calcifications. These typically are lacelike and radiate outward from the pelvis into the parenchyma, reflecting the intravascular distribution of thrombi.

Renal Artery Occlusion

Renal artery thrombosis is much rarer than venous thrombosis. It is found in infants of diabetic mothers and in infants with sepsis, dehydration, hemoconcentration, and indwelling umbilical artery catheters. In the acute phase the kidney does not enlarge, but remains of normal size and is often echogenic. Occlusion of the main renal artery can be suspected when echogenic thrombus is identified within the lumen of the affected vessel. The absence of signal from the main renal artery on Doppler sonography supports the diagnosis of occlusion. As with renal vein thrombosis, the end result depends on the extent of the insult and

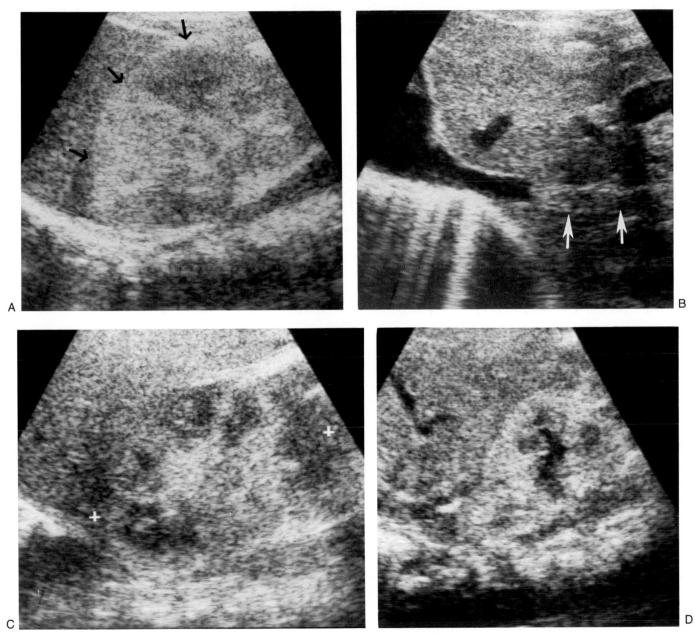

FIG. 42. Renal vein thrombosis in an infant of a diabetic mother. **A:** Longitudinal sonogram shows an enlarged echogenic right kidney (*black arrows*). Note poor definition of the pyramids. **B:** Longitudinal sonogram shows thrombus within the lumen of the inferior vena cava (*white arrows*). **C:** A sonogram 2 weeks later shows a slightly hypoechoic cortex. The pyramids remain poorly defined and there is loss of definition of corticomedullary differentiation. (*cursors,* renal margins). **D:** A follow-up sonogram 1 month later demonstrates a small, intensely echogenic kidney consistent with end-stage fibrosis. This patient subsequently developed hypertension and underwent a nephrectomy.

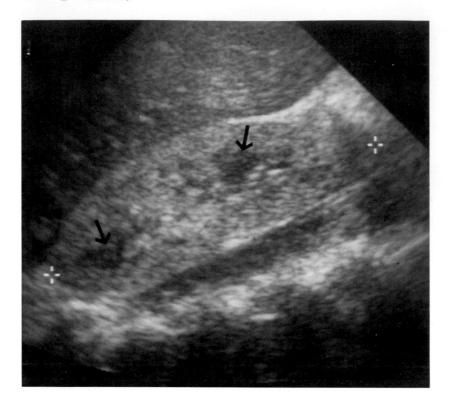

FIG. 43. Acute cortical necrosis in a child with hemolytic uremic syndrome. Longitudinal sonogram of the right kidney demonstrates a markedly echogenic kidney with sonolucent renal pyramids (*arrows*).

the presence or absence of recanalization and collateral channels. An end-stage small kidney caused by arterial thrombosis is indistinguishable from that caused by renal vein thrombosis.

Cortical and Medullary Necrosis

Renal cortical necrosis is a more common problem than renal artery thrombosis in infancy and childhood. In neonates it results from dehydration due to sepsis or blood loss and from severe hypoxia. In older children, sickle cell disease, glomerulonephritis, amyloidosis, or hemolytic uremic syndrome are causes of acute cortical necrosis. The sonographic findings are a normal-size kidney with increased cortical echogenicity and prominent sonolucent pyramids (Fig. 43) (89,132).

Acute tubular or medullary necrosis secondary to drug-induced (such as gentamicin) nephrotoxicity, or myoglobinuria following trauma, produces renal enlargement and a hyperechoic cortex. The renal pyramids often are enlarged and hypoechoic. On the other hand, acute tubular necrosis due to ischemic injury to the kidney usually produces no change in cortical or medullary echogenicity (144).

NEPHROCALCINOSIS AND UROLITHIASIS

Nephrocalcinosis represents a pathologic deposition of calcium in the renal parenchyma. The usual etiologies are primary hyperparathyroidism, renal tubular acidosis, and primary oxaluria (115). Other causes include hypercalcemic states such as sarcoidosis, hypervitaminosis D, milk-alkali syndrome, malignancy, Cushing's syndrome, and hyperthyroidism; parenchymal renal diseases include chronic glomerulonephritis, tuberculosis, mycoses, and medullary sponge kidney; and vascular conditions such as acute cortical or tubular necrosis. Nephrocalcinosis usually affects both kidneys, but involvement occasionally may be unilateral. Sonographically, nephrocalcinosis appears as diffuse or focal echogenicity with or without acoustic shadowing (120). The medullary type is more frequent than the cortical variety (Fig. 44).

Urolithiasis represents calculus formation within the collecting system of the kidneys and distal urinary tract. In children it most often is associated with an underlying urinary tract obstruction and infection. Other causes of urolithiasis include renal tubular syndromes including renal tubular acidosis, cystinuria, and glycinuria; enzyme disorders such as hyperoxaluria and xanthinuria; uric acid lithiasis due to hered-

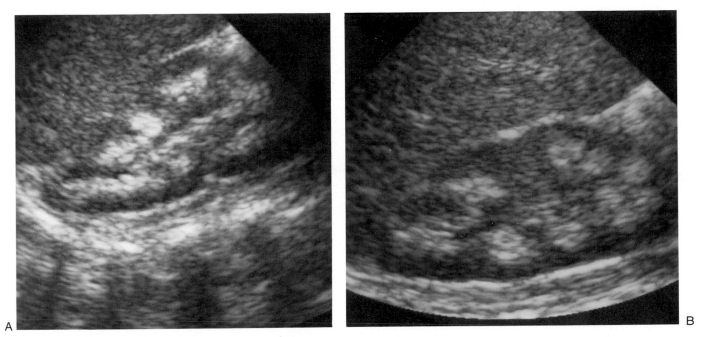

FIG. 44. Nephrocalcinosis. **A, B:** Longitudinal views of the left kidney show increased echogenicity in the medullary portion of the kidney, reflecting changes of nephrocalcinosis. The patient had underlying renal tubular acidosis.

itary hyperuricosuria and myeloproliferative states; the hypercalcemic states mentioned above; and furosemide therapy (50,77,115). Sonographically, a renal calculus appears as a highly reflective structure within the collecting system in association with acoustic shadowing (Fig. 45). Differentiation of the various types of renal calculi usually is not possible on the basis of their sonographic appearance, since nonopaque stones such as uric acid calculi may produce as much acoustical shadowing as opaque or calcium-containing renal calculi. Acoustic shadowing usually can be demonstrated with any calculus greater than 5 mm in diameter.

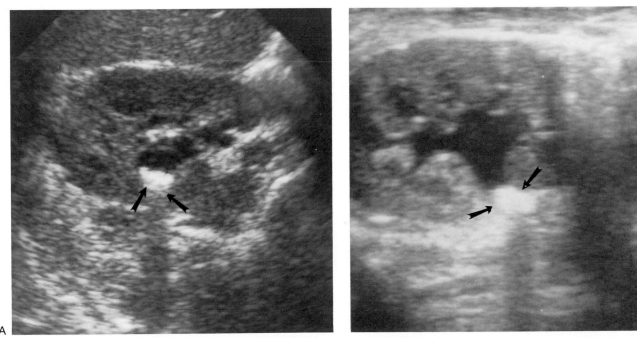

FIG. 45. Urolithiasis. **A:** Transverse and **B:** coronal sonograms of the right kidney show a dilated renal pelvis. An echogenic area (*arrows*) with distal acoustic shadowing is noted within the dilated pelvis. At surgery, this proved to be a ureteral calculus.

TRAUMA

The kidney is the third most frequently injured organ in blunt abdominal trauma, after the liver and spleen. In patients who are clinically stable and suspected of having serious renal injuries, usually on the basis of gross hematuria, CT is generally the study of choice (86,135,169). Although sonography is capable of identifying renal and perirenal hematomas as well as the integrity of the main renal vessels, particularly with duplex Doppler imaging, it is inferior to CT in revealing the extent of injury. Technical problems such as bandages, ileus, and broken ribs also make it difficult to obtain high-quality sonograms. Sonography, however, may be of value in following the course of an intrarenal hematoma or perirenal fluid collection and in identifying preexisting renal disease predisposing to injury, such as obstructive uropathy or tumor (104,169).

Renal injuries can be divided into three categories: (a) minor lesions, consisting of hematomas or contusions and small corticomedullary lacerations that do not extend to the collecting system; (b) major injuries, including parenchymal lacerations that extend into the collecting system or through the cortex and fractures; and (c) catastrophic injuries, consisting of shattered kidneys or laceration of the renal pedicle. On sonography, hematomas are round or ovoid parenchymal le-sions. Lacerations appear as linear hypo- or hyperechoic defects or as a deformity of the renal contour. Perirenal hematomas frequently accompany major and catastrophic injuries, and are recognizable as crescentic fluid collections. Hematomas vary in their echogenicity, depending on age and on the relationship of the examination to the time of injury (46,87). A more detailed description of the sonographic features of hematomas is found earlier in this chapter under "Juxtarenal Processes."

RENAL TRANSPLANT

Normal Anatomy

Sonography, particularly with duplex Doppler scanning, has a major role in the evaluation of patients with renal transplants (2,21,35,43,49,75,139,140,141,162). The sonographic appearance of the normal transplant is similar to that of a normal native kidney, although morphology may be more clearly identified in the transplanted kidney because of its closer proximity to the body's surface. The normal allograft has a smooth contour, distinct corticomedullary differentiation, and minimally hypoechoic medullary pyramids (Fig. 46).

Duplex Doppler sonography combined with the resistive index is the most widely utilized method of ana-

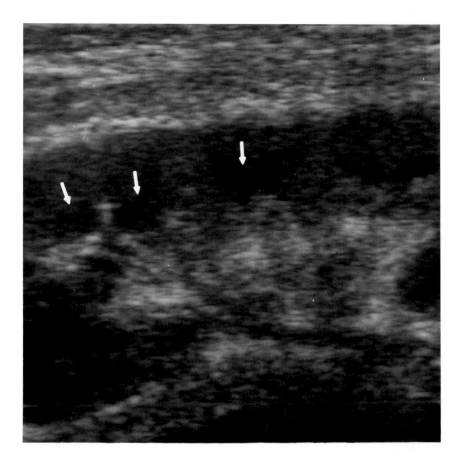

FIG. 46. Normal renal allograft. Longitudinal sonogram of a renal allograft in the right iliac fossa shows hypoechoic parenchyma and an echogenic renal sinus. The renal pyramids (*arrows*) are slightly decreased in echogenicity relative to the adjacent parenchyma.

lyzing renal vascular resistance. The normal renal allograft has a low impedance capillary bed so that antegrade flow is continuous throughout the cardiac cycle (140,141). In normal allografts, the resistive index varies from 0.4 to 0.8 with a mean of 0.6. On duplex Doppler sonography, vascular signals from the anastomosed main renal artery show a rapid rise in systolic frequency shift followed by a gradual decline in diastole. Intrarenal arterial signals are similar to those of the main renal artery, although they are dampened in amplitude. Doppler signals from the main renal vein are in a direction opposite to that of arterial flow. Venous flow is continuous, although minimal variation

may be noted with respiratory and cardiac motion (Fig. 47). Significant venous pulsations can occur with right heart failure or fluid overload. Color flow imaging can provide rapid demonstration of arterial and venous flow (Colorplate 9).

Pathology

There are multiple causes of allograft failure, including acute and chronic rejection, acute tubular necrosis, drug toxicity, renal vascular lesions, infection, obstruction of the collecting system, and occasionally peritransplant fluid collections.

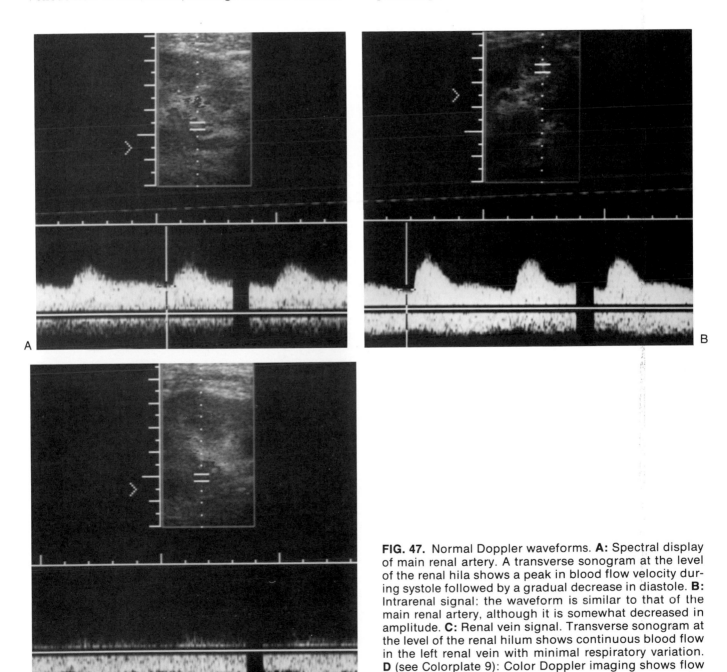

FIG. 47. Normal Doppler waveforms. **A:** Spectral display of main renal artery. A transverse sonogram at the level of the renal hila shows a peak in blood flow velocity during systole followed by a gradual decrease in diastole. **B:** Intrarenal signal: the waveform is similar to that of the main renal artery, although it is somewhat decreased in amplitude. **C:** Renal vein signal. Transverse sonogram at the level of the renal hilum shows continuous blood flow in the left renal vein with minimal respiratory variation. **D** (see Colorplate 9): Color Doppler imaging shows flow in the renal arteries and veins throughout the allograft.

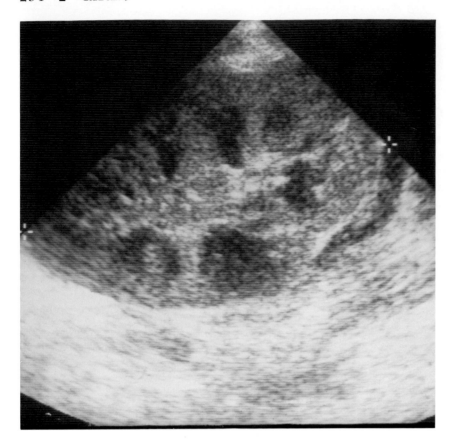

FIG. 48. Acute rejection. The kidney is enlarged, with markedly hypoechoic pyramids.

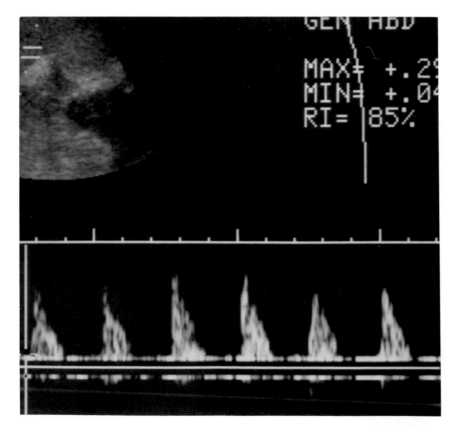

FIG. 49. Severe vascular rejection. Duplex Doppler waveforms obtained from a segmental artery show decreased diastolic flow. The resistive index measured 85%.

Parenchymal Injury

Rejection

Rejection is the most common cause of allograft failure. Clinically, rejection has been subdivided into hyperacute, acute, and chronic forms. Hyperacute rejection occurs within hours of transplantation and is characterized by the presence of fibrin thrombi in arterioles with extensive cortical necrosis. It requires immediate reoperation, and usually is not imaged sonographically. Acute rejection occurs between 24 hr and 3 to 4 months of transplantation and has been subdivided into vascular and interstitial (cellular) forms. In vascular rejection, there is a proliferative endovasculitis characterized by intimal infiltrates of mononuclear cells with vessel thrombosis. In interstitial rejection, there is edema of the interstitium and infiltration with lymphocytes. The lymphocytes are found within capillaries, venules, and lymphatics, but the glomeruli, arterioles, and arteries are spared. Chronic rejection occurs months to years after transplantation. Histologically it is characterized by a sclerosing vasculitis associated with narrowing or obliteration of the vascular lumen and extensive interstitial fibrosis.

Gray-scale findings of both the vascular and interstitial forms of acute rejection include increased renal volume, enlarged hypoechoic medullary pyramids, an indistinct corticomedullary junction, either increased or decreased parenchymal echogenicity, and thickening of the wall of the renal pelvis (Fig. 48) (6,43,75,125,159). Mild dilatation of the collecting system may be observed as well (103).

Duplex sonographic findings of acute vascular rejection are markedly increased vascular resistance, and resistive indexes ranging from 0.7 to 1.0 with a mean of 0.83 (Fig. 49). Acute interstitial rejection causes minimal or no changes in vascular resistance, resulting in resistive indexes varying from 0.4 to 0.85 with a mean of 0.6 (2,140,141). With a resistive index of 0.7 or greater, the sensitivity for diagnosing acute rejection is about 90% and the specificity is approximately 70%. At a resistive index of 0.80 or greater, the specificity for rejection increases to 90% but the sensitivity decreases to 65% (168). In general, values between 0.7 and 0.8 are indeterminate and can be found in patients with pyelonephritis, acute tubular necrosis, and cyclosporine-related toxicity (21,35,49,139,175).

In chronic rejection, the allograft often appears normal or has an irregular surface reflecting areas of old infarct (Fig. 50). Other findings include a decrease in overall allograft size or cortical thickness, decreased pyramidal echogenicity, and increased cortical echogenicity. Resistive indexes range between 0.4 and 0.85 with a mean of 0.61.

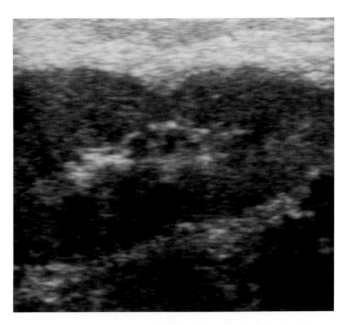

FIG. 50. Chronic allograft rejection. A longitudinal sonogram of the allograft shows an irregular cortical margin consistent with an old infarct. Resistive indexes were normal.

Other Parenchymal Dysfunction

Acute tubular necrosis is the result of renal ischemia and is more commonly seen in patients with cadaveric transplants. The condition occurs early after transplantation and is self-limited, with renal function returning to normal within a few days to weeks. Immunosuppressive drugs to decrease the risk of rejection, such as cyclosporine and antilymphocyte globulin, produce abnormalities of the tubules early and vasculitis later; the changes tend to be patchy and do not affect peripheral resistance. Unlike acute rejection, acute tubular necrosis and drug toxicity produce essentially no change in the echotexture of the cortex or pyramids (75,144); resistive indexes usually are normal, ranging from 0.4 to 0.8 (2,21).

Vascular Complications

Renal allografts are prone to vascular complications, including renal artery thrombosis, stenosis, and arteriovenous fistula. Both duplex Doppler and color flow sonography have been shown to be useful in the diagnosis of vascular complications (170).

Main renal artery thrombosis or occlusion occurs early and can result from twisting or kinking of the renal artery, an intimal flap at the time of surgery, and hyperacute or acute rejection. The end result is infarction and loss of the graft. In the case of an allograft

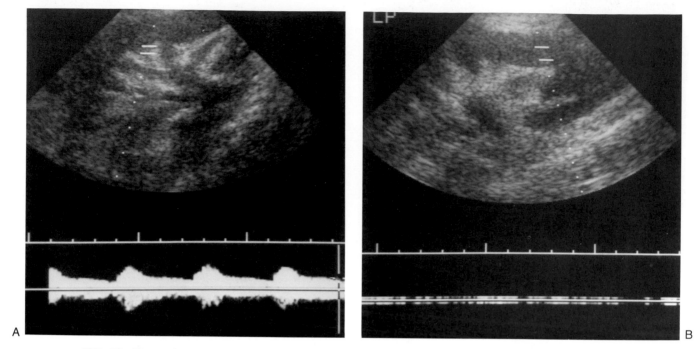

FIG. 51. Transplant, renal artery occlusion. **A:** Longitudinal sonogram from the upper pole of the renal allograft shows normal Doppler waveforms. **B:** No signals could be obtained from the lower pole of the renal allograft. This patient had two renal arteries. At reexploration, the lower pole renal artery was occluded secondary to thrombus.

with more than one artery, the infarction may be segmental rather than global (117). On duplex Doppler sonography, arterial occlusion is characterized by absence of arterial signals from the renal artery or from within the graft parenchyma (Fig. 51).

Renal artery stenosis occurs in approximately 3% to 10% of allografts, typically at the anastomotic site (97). The diagnosis is suspected when patients develop se-

vere hypertension in association with graft dysfunction or an arterial bruit. Duplex Doppler findings of renal artery stenosis include (a) a high peak systolic shift at the stenotic site; (b) diastolic dampening at the stenotic site, (c) turbulence in the poststenotic segment, manifested as forward and reversed flow; and (d) normal or dampened intrarenal arterial waveforms distal to the site of stenosis (170). Color Doppler findings include

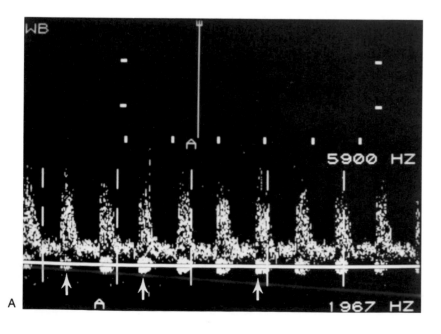

FIG. 52. Transplant, main renal artery stenosis. **A:** Doppler waveform shows elevated frequency shifts at the stenotic site. Flow turbulence causes perivascular soft tissue vibrations which are seen as low-frequency reflection (*white arrows*) on each side of the baseline. **B** (see Colorplate 10): Color flow imaging shows an admixture of red and blue colors, representing perivascular soft tissue vibrations, around the stenotic vessel. The underlying stenosis is obscured by the vibrations.

a narrowed lumen and perivascular soft tissue vibrations appearing as an admixture of arterial and venous flow. These vibrations reflect flow turbulence at the site of the stenosis (Fig. 52). Doppler sonography is incapable of distinguishing between arterial kinking and main renal artery stenosis, so arteriography is required for a definitive diagnosis.

Arteriovenous fistula (AVF) occurs most often after percutaneous renal biopsy. Patients are usually asymptomatic, although they may present with hematuria, bruit, or hypertension. Doppler sonography of the artery supplying the AVF characteristically demonstrates a high-frequency Doppler shift and turbulence, resulting from the large pressure drop from the artery to the vein. Flow within the vein draining the AVF appears as an arterial waveform. Color flow imaging demonstrates increased flow in the feeding arteries and draining veins with a change in color saturation toward white. Localized perivascular soft tissue vibrations (Fig. 53) also may be noted.

Pseudoaneurysms occur either at the anastomotic site, due to breakdown of the anastomosis, or intrarenally, following percutaneous needle biopsy. Sonographic findings include a hypoechoic mass on gray-

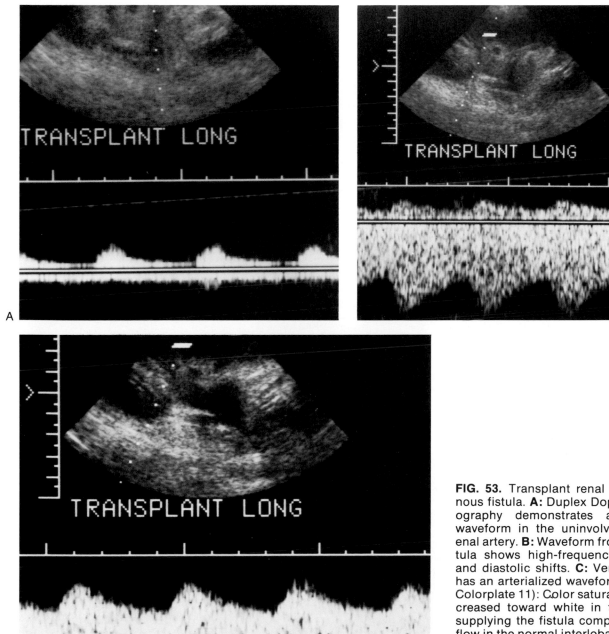

FIG. 53. Transplant renal arteriovenous fistula. **A:** Duplex Doppler sonography demonstrates a normal waveform in the uninvolved intrarenal artery. **B:** Waveform from the fistula shows high-frequency systolic and diastolic shifts. **C:** Venous flow has an arterialized waveform. **D** (see Colorplate 11): Color saturation is increased toward white in the artery supplying the fistula compared with flow in the normal interlobar arteries. *Arrows* indicate perivascular soft tissue vibrations.

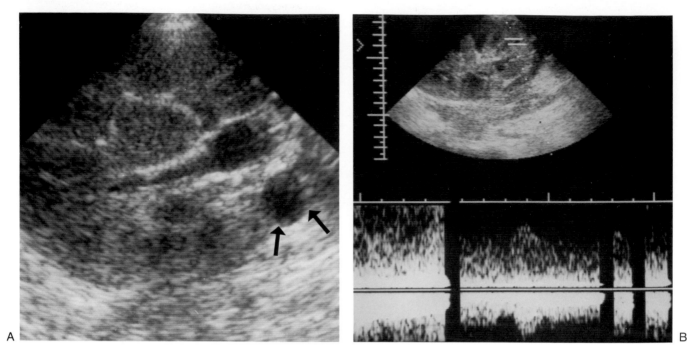

A

B

FIG. 54. Pseudoaneurysm. Longitudinal sonogram (**A**) shows a hypoechoic mass (*arrows*) inferior to the allograft. Doppler waveform (**B**) shows turbulent flow.

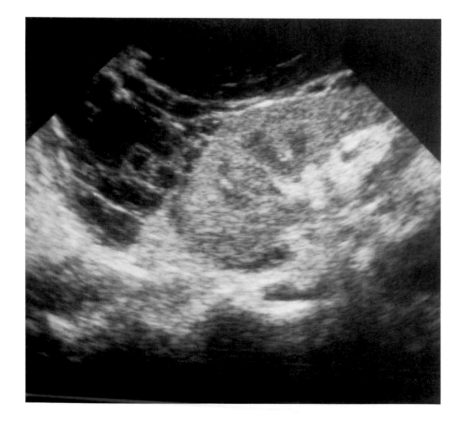

FIG. 55. Perirenal lymphocele. Longitudinal sonogram through the upper pole of the renal allograft demonstrates a well-defined fluid collection with multiple septations.

scale images and turbulence of flow on duplex Doppler and color flow images (Fig. 54). Most pseudoaneurysms regress spontaneously.

Peritransplant Fluid Collections

Perinephric fluid collections may be due to lymphoceles, urinomas, hematomas or abscesses. The sonographic appearances of these fluid collections are largely indistinguishable and final diagnosis requires clinical correlation or needle aspiration.

Lymphoceles are the most common perinephric fluid collections, usually developing 2 to 6 weeks posttransplant (157,180). They represent localized accumulations of lymph around the graft, occurring as a result of seepage of lymph from severed lymphatic vessels in the transplant bed. On sonography, lymphoceles appear as well-defined cystic masses; multiple septations are found in 80% of cases (Fig. 55) (97). Associated hydronephrosis is present if the lymphocele obstructs the ureter.

Urinomas usually occur within the first 2 postoperative weeks, with the site of urinary leakage being most often at the ureteroneocystostomy. Occasionally they occur later secondary to renal biopsy or delayed necrosis of the ureter. Sonographically, urinomas are sonolucent masses interposed between the allograft and bladder; unlike lymphoceles, they rarely contain septations (157). Since urinomas are commonly located near the lower margin of the allograft, they may compress the ureter and lead to hydronephrosis (Fig. 56). Diagnosis of urinary leakage can be confirmed by renal scintigraphy.

Hematomas may be seen in the early postoperative period or develop later as a complication of percutaneous biopsy. The sonographic appearance varies depending on the age of the hemorrhage as well as its location (see earlier discussion under "Juxtarenal Processes," page 287). Perirenal hematomas lie within the confines of the anterior and posterior renal (Gerota's) fascia. They have a "C"-shaped border with the convexity bulging inferiorly. Subcapsular hematomas occupy a smaller space between the renal parenchyma medially and the capsule laterally. They appear as len-

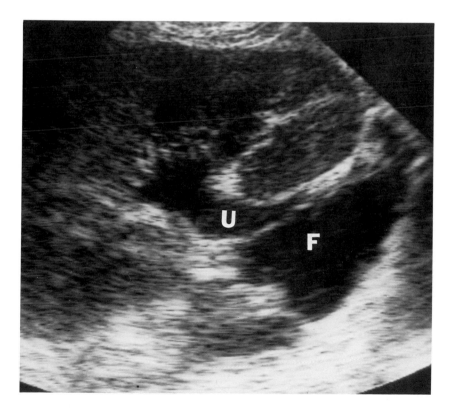

FIG. 56. Perirenal urinoma. Longitudinal sonogram demonstrates dilated intrarenal collecting system and ureter (*U*). A hypoechoic fluid (*F*) collection below the ureter represents a urinoma. Urinary leakage was subsequently demonstrated by renal scintigraphy.

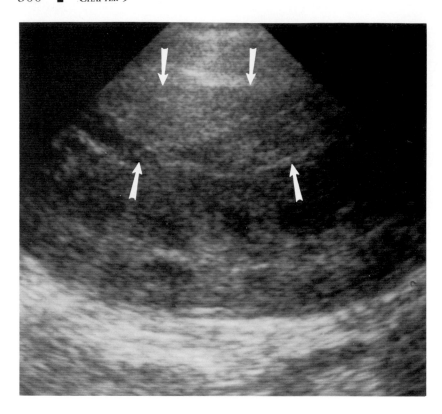

FIG. 57. Subcapsular hematoma. Longitudinal sonogram of the renal allograft shows a minimally echogenic fluid collection (*arrows*) compressing the renal parenchyma. Percutaneous aspiration of the fluid collection revealed blood.

ticular fluid collections compressing the renal parenchyma (Fig. 57) (97). Resistive indexes may become elevated if diastolic flow decreases secondary to the compressive effect of a subcapsular fluid collection.

Abscesses usually occur early in the postoperative period. On sonography, they are hypoechoic fluid collections containing internal echoes caused by debris and septations. The borders may be sharply defined or irregular if there is significant inflammation and edema around the lesion.

Obstructive Uropathy

Obstructive uropathy may be caused by intrinsic lesions, such as ureteral strictures, clots, or calculi, or extrinsic masses, such as lymphoceles, urinomas, or hematomas (see Fig. 56). The dilated intra- and extrarenal collecting system is easily recognized by sonography.

It is important to recognize that mild degrees of dilatation may not represent obstruction. Immediately posttransplant, mild dilatation is a normal occurrence and is due to transient edema at the ureteroneocystostomy site. A distended bladder also may cause dilatation of the collecting system. The dilatation in this instance usually resolves after the patient empties the bladder. Mild dilatation of the collecting system in the absence of anatomical obstruction also has been described in allograft rejection. The musculature of the ureter is infiltrated by edema and mononuclear cells

during acute rejection, leading to decreased ureteral peristalsis and eventual ureteral dilatation. When differentiation between nonobstructive dilatation and obstructive dilatation is a problem, a diuretic renogram can be useful. In the presence of obstruction, the dil-

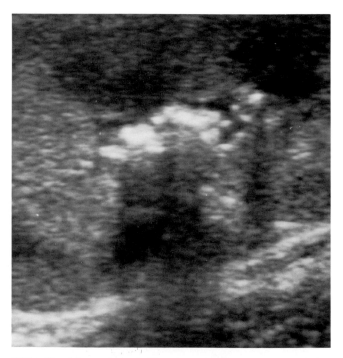

FIG. 58. Allograft calcification. A dense band of increased echogenicity with distal shadowing is consistent with parenchymal calcification, related to prior biopsy.

atation of the collecting system increases after administration of a diuretic agent, whereas in nonobstructive dilatation, there is no significant change in the appearance of the collecting system with diuresis.

Miscellaneous Complications

Calculus formation or nephrocalcinosis and urinary tract infections are unusual complications of transplantation. Calcifications are late complications, usually due to biopsy or recurrent urinary tract infections. On sonography, they appear as echogenic foci with acoustic shadowing (Fig. 58). Infection can be an early or late complication and has a paucity of findings unless the collecting system is dilated. In the presence of hydronephrosis, a debris-fluid level or fungal ball within a dilated calyx or renal pelvis can be identified. Occasionally, severe infection may cause elevated resistive indexes due to intrarenal edema. Renal transplant recipients also are at increased risk for the development of malignancies, particularly lymphomas. On sonography, lymphoma appears as a hypoechoic mass or masses in the renal transplant.

BLADDER AND URETHRA

Technique and Normal Anatomy

Sonography of the bladder requires that the bladder be distended with fluid, either by having the patient not void for several hours prior to the examination or by instilling sterile water into the bladder via catheterization. Depending on the size of the child, a 3.5 or 5 MHz real-time transducer, preferably a sector scanner, is used to obtain transverse and sagittal views of the bladder. The normal bladder wall is smooth and echogenic with a thickness between 3 and 5 mm, depending on the degree of bladder distention. Complete distention of the bladder is important when evaluating bladder tumors because a poorly filled bladder may appear falsely thickened and irregular (Fig. 59) (82).

The distal ureters, with the exception of the submucosal intravesical portion in the trigone of the bladder, are not routinely identified by sonography. The diameter of the submucosal ureter on sonography varies between 1 and 2 mm and the length from 6 to 21 mm. The submucosal tunnel length increases directly with increasing patient age (116). Occasionally, spurts of low-intensity echoes or ureteral jets are visible near the inferior wall of the distended bladder (37,95). The jets may start from either ureteral orifice and flow toward the center of the bladder. Within a few seconds, the low-intensity jets are no longer identifiable. The ureteral jet is attributed to differences in acoustic interfaces between fluids of different specific gravities (95). With high-resolution sonography, the urethra occasionally can be visualized in both girls and boys. If urethral abnormalities are suspected on conventional scans, further evaluation is possible with perineal imaging.

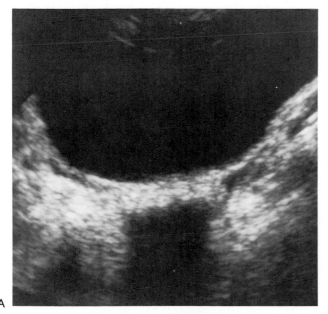
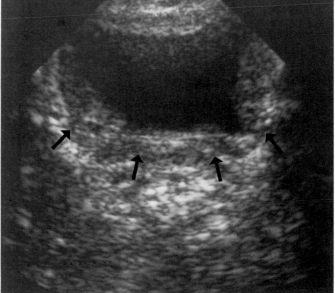

FIG. 59. Normal urinary bladder. **A:** Transverse sonogram through the pelvis demonstrates a thin-walled, fluid-filled bladder. The wall measures less than 3 mm in thickness. **B:** With the bladder incompletely filled, the walls (*arrows*) appear falsely thickened.

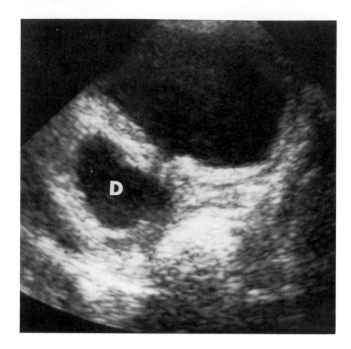

FIG. 60. Congenital bladder diverticulum. Transverse image of the bladder demonstrates a thin-walled diverticulum (*D*), with a narrow neck, arising from the bladder base. Note the smooth bladder wall.

Pathology

Sonography is considered the screening technique for evaluation of a pediatric pelvic mass believed related to the urinary tract. When sonography suggests a malignant mass, or if a pediatric malignancy has been diagnosed, CT or MR imaging may be warranted to detect the extent of pelvic invasion prior to surgery, chemotherapy, or radiation therapy. Most non-neoplastic bladder abnormalities, such as congenital or inflammatory lesions, are usually imaged initially by a voiding cystourethrogram. Sonography has a limited role, but may be a valuable ancillary examination to confirm selected abnormalities, such as diverticula or bladder wall thickening.

Congenital Anomalies

Bladder Diverticula

Diverticula of the bladder are herniations of bladder mucosa through fibers of the detrusor muscle. Most diverticula in childhood are associated with reflux, neurogenic bladders, or obstructed urethras, but congenital diverticula unassociated with these conditions can occur. Diverticula occurring with obstruction tend to be multiple and associated with cellules and severe bladder trabeculation. Congenital diverticula unassociated with obstruction or neurogenic bladder are usually solitary, typically occur at the ureterovesical junction, and are often larger than those caused by obstruction or neurogenic bladder. Occasionally, congenital diverticula occur in association with Menkes' syndrome (an abnormality of copper metabolism), cutis laxa, Williams syndrome and Ehlers-Danlos syndrome. Patients with bladder diverticula present with urinary tract infection, incontinence, or urinary retention.

On sonography, diverticula appear as round or oval anechoic fluid collections arising from the base of the

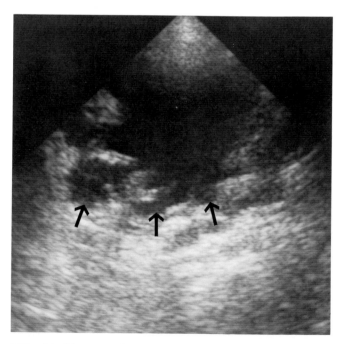

FIG. 61. Neurogenic bladder. Transverse scan of the bladder shows multiple hypoechoic fluid collections (*arrows*), consistent with diverticula, extending from a thickened, irregular bladder wall.

bladder or around the ureteric orifice. A dilated distal ureter also may be seen secondary to ureterovesical obstruction or reflux. Congenital diverticula usually occur with smooth-walled bladders, whereas acquired ones are found with trabeculated bladders (Figs. 60,61).

Neurogenic Bladder

Neurogenic bladder in childhood usually is congenital due to myelomeningocele or sacral agenesis. Acquired causes are rarer and include traumatic paraplegia, encephalitis, or meningitis. On sonography, the bladder is irregularly thickened, often with small diverticula (Fig. 61). Occasionally, complications such as bladder calculi can be identified by sonography. Postvoid images of the bladder are useful in evaluating bladder function and usually demonstrate inability of the patients to empty the bladder completely.

Urethral Obstruction

Urethral obstruction, including posterior or anterior valves, duplication, agenesis, and stricture are causes of bladder outlet obstruction. The sonographic findings are similar to those of posterior urethral valves—an irregular, thickened bladder wall, frequently in association with ureteropyelocaliectasis and a dilated urethra (Fig. 62; see also Fig. 11, p. 266).

Urachal Anomalies

The urachus arises from the anterior bladder wall and extends to the umbilicus. There are four basic disorders of the urachus: patent urachus, urachal sinus, urachal diverticulum, and urachal cyst. A patent urachus arises when there is failure of the urachal lumen to obliterate, resulting in a communication between the bladder and umbilicus. Patent urachus has been reported in association with the prune-belly syndrome. A urachal sinus is the result of persistent communication of the urachal lumen with the umbilicus; a urachal diverticulum implies communication of the urachal lumen with the bladder; and a urachal cyst represents accumulation of fluid within a portion of the urachus that does not communicate with either the bladder or the umbilicus. Patent urachus and urachal sinus manifest as fluid leakage from the umbilicus. Urachal diverticulum is usually asymptomatic and discovered incidentally on imaging studies. Urachal cyst presents as a palpable mass that is often tender due to infection. Urachal cyst and diverticulum can be easily

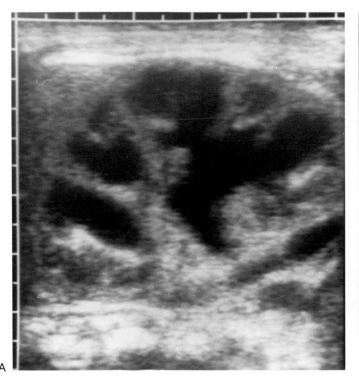
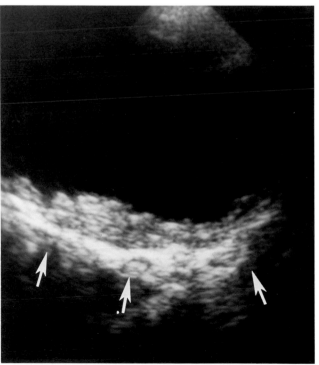

A

B

FIG. 62. Urethral stricture. **A:** Longitudinal view of the left kidney shows moderate dilatation of the renal pelvis and calyces. **B:** Longitudinal scan of the pelvis shows a thickened, irregular bladder wall (*arrows*).

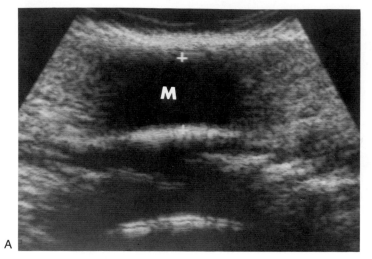

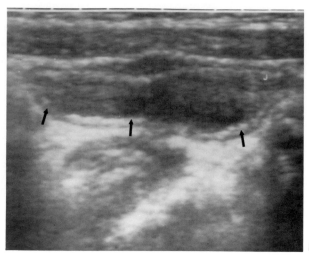

FIG. 63. Urachal cyst. **A:** Transverse sonogram of the anterior abdominal wall demonstrates a well-defined anechoic mass (*M*). At surgery the mass did not communicate with either the bladder or the umbilicus. Pathology of the lesion revealed a lining of transitional cell epithelium, confirming its relationship to the urinary tract. **B:** In another patient, transverse image shows a fluid collection (*arrows*) with through-transmission and internal debris. An infected urachal cyst was found at operation.

identified with high-resolution sonography and appear as fluid-filled masses, either beneath the umbilicus or adjacent to the bladder (19). The presence of debris within the lumen of the cyst suggests infection (Fig. 63).

Neoplasms

Tumors of the bladder in children are rare and more often malignant than benign. Embryonal rhabdomyosarcoma is the most common neoplasm of the lower

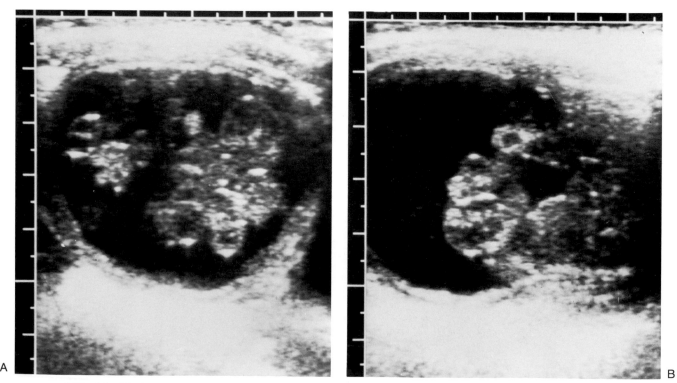

FIG. 64. Rhabdomyosarcoma of the bladder wall. **A:** Transverse and **B:** longitudinal images through the trigone show solid polypoid masses with cystic areas protruding into the bladder lumen.

urinary tract in childhood, usually affecting children under 5 years of age (72). The majority of children present with urinary retention or hematuria. Bladder rhabdomyosarcoma typically involves the region of the trigone, although in about 25% of cases it originates in the dome of the bladder. The tumor arises in the submucosa and infiltrates the wall and mucosa of the bladder, the urethra, and perivesical tissues.

Sonographically, the tumor usually appears as a polypoid mass projecting into the bladder lumen, and less commonly as bladder wall thickening. Polypoid lesions often are complex, with cystic areas representing areas of hemorrhage or necrosis, but they may be homogeneously echogenic (Fig. 64). Infiltrating tumors show few intraluminal components, but they are easily recognized because they produce irregular wall thickening; the echogenicity may be equal to or less than that of the bladder wall. In advanced cases, the bladder wall will be markedly deformed and bladder capacity will be diminished. Hydronephrosis and invasion of

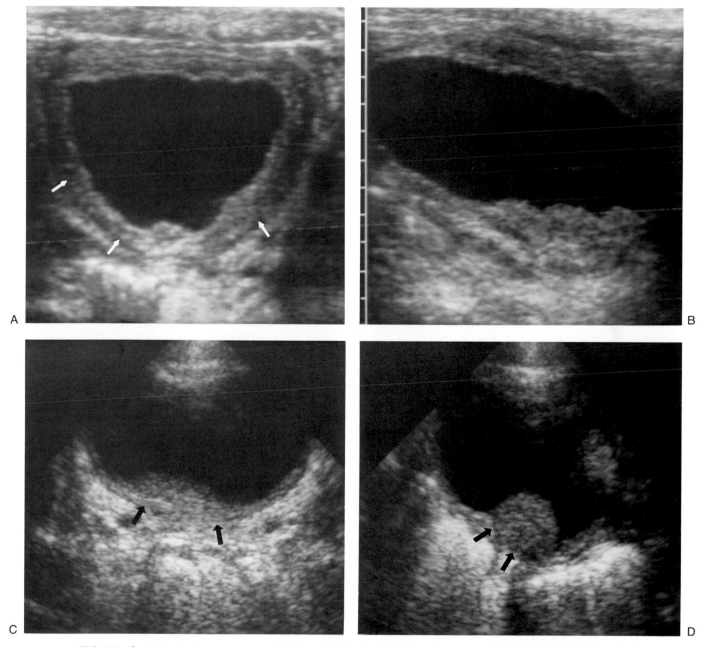

FIG. 65. Cystitis. **A:** Transverse and **B:** longitudinal sonograms demonstrate diffuse bladder wall thickening (*white arrows*). The thickness measured from inner to outer wall is 8 mm. **C:** Transverse and **D:** longitudinal scans in another patient show focal wall thickening (*black arrows*), appearing as a mass lesion. Urine cultures grew *E. coli*. Follow-up sonograms 1 month later demonstrated a normal bladder wall.

perivesical structures also can be noted. When the tumor causes diffuse thickening of the bladder wall, it can be confused with cystitis, although the thickening usually is more uniform in the latter entity.

Benign lesions of the bladder include neurofibroma, hemangioma, pheochromocytoma, transitional cell papilloma, and leiomyoma (17). Neurofibromatosis produces marked localized thickening of the bladder wall or diffuse bladder involvement with a lobulated, irregular wall (122). Invasion of the seminal vesicles, prostate, testicles, and distal urethra is frequent. Other benign tumors present as focal wall thickening or as an echogenic soft tissue mass projecting into the bladder lumen (177). Congenital polyps are the most common benign tumor of the urethra, usually arising from a long stalk near the verumontanum (88). On sonography they appear as echogenic polypoid masses projecting from the bladder neck into the bladder lumen (23,31).

Infection

Inflammation of the bladder or cystitis usually is bacterial in origin, but other etiologies include viral infection, tuberculosis, chemotherapy with cyclophosphamide, and indwelling catheters. Typically, patients present with dysuria and hematuria. The most common sonographic finding is uniform bladder wall thickening; occasionally, cystitis appears as a focal mass with or without associated wall thickening (Fig. 65) (29,53,138). Cystitis cystica particularly may be localized to the trigone and ureteral orifices. When involvement is extensive, focal lesions may protrude into the bladder lumen, mimicking rhabdomyosarcoma. Other findings of cystitis include echogenic debris or a fluid-fluid level within the bladder lumen and intraluminal or intramural gas. The latter appears as echogenic areas with shadowing.

Trauma

Injury to the bladder and urethra in childhood most often occurs with blunt trauma, but it can also be a complication of surgery or penetration by foreign bodies. Sonography has a limited role in evaluating bladder injury, but it can demonstrate the presence of free fluid in the pelvis and abdomen. Following surgery, sonography can be used to evaluate the presence of complications such as seromas, urinomas, hematomas, or abscesses.

REFERENCES

1. Akhtar M, Kott E, Brooks B. Extrarenal Wilms' tumor. Report of a case and review of the literature. *Cancer* 1977;40:3087–3091.

2. Allen KS, Jorkasky DK, Arger PH, et al. Renal allografts: Prospective analysis of Doppler sonography. *Radiology* 1988;169:371–376.

3. Alon U, Pery M, Davidai G, Berant M. Ultrasonography in the radiologic evaluation of children with urinary tract infection. *Pediatrics* 1986;78:58–64.

4. Athey PA, Carpenter RJ, Hadlock RP, Hedrick TD. Ultrasonic demonstration of ectopic ureterocele. *Pediatrics* 1983;71:568–571.

5. Avni EF, Van Gansbeke D, Thoua Y, et al. US demonstration of pyelitis and ureteritis in children. *Pediatr Radiol* 1988;18:134–139.

6. Babcock DS. Sonography of wall thickening of the renal collecting system. A nonspecific finding. *J Ultrasound Med* 1987;6:29–32.

7. Banner MP, Pollack HM, Chatten J, Witzleben C. Multilocular renal cysts: Radiologic-pathologic correlation. *AJR* 1981;136:239–247.

8. Beckwith JB. Mesenchymal renal neoplasms of infancy revisited. (Editorial). *J Ped Surg* 1974;9:803–805.

9. Ben-Ami T. The sonographic evaluation of urinary tract infections in children. *Semin US, CT, MR* 1984;5:19–34.

10. Berdon WE, Baker DH, Wigger HJ, Blanc WA. The radiologic and pathologic spectrum of the prune belly syndrome. *Radiol Clin North Am* 1977;15:83–92.

11. Blane CE, Bookstein FL, DiPietro MA, Kelsch RC. Sonographic standards for normal infant kidney length. *AJR* 1985;145:1289–1291.

12. Blickman JG, Taylor GA, Lebowitz RL. Voiding cystourethrography: The initial radiologic study in children with urinary tract infection. *Radiology* 1985;156:659–662.

13. Boal DK, Teele RL. Sonography of infantile polycystic kidney disease. *AJR* 1980;135:575–580.

14. Bolande RP. Congenital and infantile neoplasia of the kidney. *Lancet* 1974;2:1497–1499.

15. Bolande RP, Brough AJ, Izant RJ Jr. Congenital mesoblastic nephroma of infancy. A report of eight cases and the relationship to Wilms' tumor. *Pediatrics* 1967;40:272–278.

16. Bornstein I, Charboneau JW, Hartman GW. Leiomyoma of the bladder: Sonographic and urographic findings. *J Ultrasound Med* 1986;5:407–408.

17. Bove KE, McAdams AJ. The nephroblastomatosis complex and its relationship to Wilms' tumor: A clinicopathologic treatise. *Perspect Pediatr Pathol* 1976;3:185–223.

18. Boyle G, Rosenberg HK, O'Neill J. An unusual presentation of an infected urachal cyst. *Clin Pediatr* 1988;27:130–134.

19. Brown T, Mandell J, Lebowitz RL. Neonatal hydronephrosis in the era of sonography. *AJR* 1987;148:959–963.

20. Buckley AR, Cooperberg PL, Reeve CE, Magil AB. The distinction between acute renal transplant rejection and cyclosporine nephrotoxicity: Value of duplex sonography. *AJR* 1987;149:521–525.

21. Carlson DH, Carlson D, Simon H. Benign multilocal cystic nephroma. *AJR* 1978;131:621–625.

22. Caro PA, Rosenberg HK, Snyder HM III. Congenital urethral polyp. *AJR* 1986;147:1041–1042.

23. Chan HSL, Cheng M-Y, Mancer K, et al. Congenital mesoblastic nephroma: A clinicoradiologic study of 17 cases representing the pathologic spectrum of the disease. *J Pediatr* 1987;111:64–70.

24. Chan HSL, Daneman A, Gribbin M, Martin DJ. Renal cell carcinoma in the first two decades of life. *Pediatr Radiol* 1983;13:324–328.

25. Cohen HL, Haller JO, Schechter S, Slovis T, Merola R, Eaton DH. Renal candidiasis of the infant: Ultrasound evaluation. *Urol Radiol* 1986;8:17–21.

26. Coleman BG, Arger PH, Mulhern CB Jr., Pollack HM, Banner MP. Pyonephrosis: Sonography in the diagnosis and management. *AJR* 1981;137:939–943.

27. Cremin BJ. Wilms' Tumour: Ultrasound and changing concepts. *Clin Radiol* 1987;38:465–474.

28. Cremin BJ. Radiological imaging of urogenital tuberculosis in children with emphasis on ultrasound. *Pediatr Radiol* 1987;17:34–38.

30. Cremin BJ, Aaronson IA. Ultrasonic diagnosis of posterior urethral valve in neonates. *Br J Radiol* 1983;56:435–438.

31. de Filippi G, Derchi LE, Coppi M, Biggi E. Sonographic diagnosis of urethral polyp in a child. *Pediatr Radiol* 1983;13:351–352.

32. Dehner LP, Leestma JE, Price EB Jr. Renal cell carcinoma in children: A clinicopathologic study of 15 cases and review of the literature. *J Pediatr* 1970;76:358–368.

33. Diard F, Nicolau A, Bernard S. Intra-renal reflux: A new cause of medullary hyperechogenicity? *Pediatr Radiol* 1987;17:154–155.

34. Dinkel E, Orth S, Dittrich M, Schulte-Wissermann H. Renal sonography in the differentiation of upper from lower urinary tract infection. *AJR* 1986;146:775–780.

35. Don S, Kopecky KK, Filo RS, et al. Duplex Doppler US of renal allografts: Causes of elevated resistive index. *Radiology* 1989;171:709–712.

36. Dremsek PA, Kritscher H, Bohm G, Hochberger O. Kidney dimensions in ultrasound compared to somatometric parameters in normal children. *Pediatr Radiol* 1987;17:285–290.

37. Dubbins PA, Kurtz AB, Darby J, Goldberg BB. Ureteric jet effect: The echographic appearance of urine entering the bladder. *Radiology* 1981;140:513–515.

38. Feinstein DA, Fernbach SK. Septated urinomas in the neonate. *AJR* 1987;149:997–1000.

39. Felson B, Cussen LJ. The hydronephrotic type of unilateral congenital multicystic disease of the kidney. *Semin Roentgenol* 1975;10:113–123.

40. Fernbach SK, Feinstein KA, Donaldson JS, Baum ES. Nephroblastomatosis: Comparison of CT with US and urography. *Radiology* 1988;166:153–156.

41. Filiatrault D, Hoyoux C, Benoit P, Garel L, Esseltine D. Renal metastases from neuroblastoma. Report of two cases. *Pediatr Radiol* 1987;17:137–138.

42. Franken EA Jr, Yiu-Chiu V, Smith WL, Chiu LC. Nephroblastomatosis: Clinicopathologic significance and imaging characteristics. *AJR* 1982;138:950–952.

43. Frick MP, Feinberg SB, Sibley R, Idstrom ME. Ultrasound in acute renal transplant rejection. *Radiology* 1981;138:657–660.

44. Fried AM, Hatfield DR, Ellis GT, Fitzgerald KW. Extrarenal Wilms' tumor: Sonographic appearance. *JCU* 1980;8:360–362.

45. Friedman AP, Haller JO, Schulze G, Schaffer R. Sonography of vesical and perivesical abnormalities in children. *J Ultrasound Med* 1983;2:385–390.

46. Furtschegger A, Egender G, Jakse G. The value of sonography in the diagnosis and follow-up of patients with blunt renal trauma. *Br J Urol* 1988;62:110–116.

47. Garel LA, Habib R, Pariente D, Broyer M, Sauvegrain J. Juvenile nephronophthisis: Sonographic appearance in children with severe uremia. *Radiology* 1984;151:93–95.

48. Garris J, Kangarloo H, Sarti D, Sample WF, Smith LE. The ultrasound spectrum of prune-belly syndrome. *JCU* 1980; 8:117–120.

49. Genkins SM, Sanfilippo FP, Carroll BA. Duplex Doppler sonography of renal transplants: Lack of sensitivity and specificity in establishing pathologic diagnosis. *AJR* 1989;152:535–539.

50. Glasier CM, Stoddard RA, Ackerman NB Jr, McCurdy FA, Null DM Jr, deLemos RA. Nephrolithiasis in infants: Association with chronic furosemide therapy. *AJR* 1983;140:107–108.

51. Glassberg KI, Filmer RB. Renal dysplasia, hypoplasia, and cystic disease of the kidney. In: Kellalis PP, King LR, Belman (eds). *Clinical Pediatric Urology,* 2nd ed. Philadelphia: W.B. Saunders, 1985;948–971.

52. Goh TS, LeQuesne GW, Wong KY. Severe infiltration of the kidneys with ultrasonic abnormalities in acute lymphoblastic leukemia. *Am J Dis Child* 1978;132:1204–1205.

53. Gooding GAW. Varied sonographic manifestations of cystitis. *J Ultrasound Med* 1986;5:61–63.

54. Goodman JD, Norton KI, Carr L, Yeh H-C. Crossed fused renal ectopia: Sonographic diagnosis. *Urol Radiol* 1986;8:13–16.

55. Gordon RL, Pollack HM, Popky GL, Duckett JW Jr. Simple serous cysts of the kidney in children. *Radiology* 1979;131:357–361.

56. Gore RM, Shkolnik A. Abdominal manifestations of pediatric leukemias: Sonographic assessment. *Radiology* 1982;143:207–210.

57. Grider RD, Wolverson MK, Jagannadharao B, Graviss ER, O'Connor DM. Congenital mesoblastic nephroma with cystic component. *JCU* 1981;9:43–45.

58. Griscom NT, Vawter GF, Fellers FX. Pelvoinfundibular atresia: The usual form of multicystic kidney: 44 unilateral and two bilateral cases. *Semin Roentgenol* 1975;10:125–131.

59. Grossman H, Rosenberg ER, Bowie JD, Ram P, Merten DF. Sonographic diagnosis of renal cystic diseases. *AJR* 1983;140:81–85.

60. Haller JO, Berdon WE, Friedman AP. Increased renal cortical echogenicity: A normal finding in neonates and infants. *Radiology* 1982;142:173–174.

61. Han BK, Babcock DS. Sonographic measurements and appearance of normal kidneys in children. *AJR* 1985;145:611–616.

62. Hantman SS. Sonographic diagnosis of vaginal ectopic ureter. *J Ultrasound Med* 1983;2:523–524.

63. Hartman DS, Davis CJ Jr, Goldman SM, Friedman AC, Fritzsche P. Renal lymphoma: Radiologic-pathologic correlation of 21 cases. *Radiology* 1982;144:759–766.

64. Hartman DS, Davis CJ Jr, Madewell JE, Friedman AC. Primary malignant renal tumors in the second decade of life: Wilms' tumor versus renal cell carcinoma. *J Urol* 1982;127:888–891.

65. Hartman DS, Goldman SM, Friedman AC, Davis CJ Jr, Madewell JE, Sherman JL. Angiomyolipoma: Ultrasonic-pathologic correlation. *Radiology* 1981;139:451–458.

66. Hartman DS, Lesar MSL, Madewell JE, Lichtenstein JE, Davis CJ Jr. Mesoblastic nephroma: Radiologic-pathologic correlation of 20 cases. *AJR* 1981;136:69–74.

67. Hartman DS, Sanders RC. Wilms' tumor versus neuroblastoma: Usefulness of ultrasound in differentiation. *J Ultrasound Med* 1982;1:117–122.

68. Hartman GE, Smolik LM, Shochat SJ. The dilemma of the multicystic dysplastic kidney. *AJDC* 1986;140:925–928.

69. Hayden CK Jr, Santa-Cruz FR, Amparo EG, Brouhard B, Swischuk LE, Ahrendt DK. Ultrasonographic evaluation of the renal parenchyma in infancy and childhood. *Radiology* 1984;152:413–417.

70. Hayden CK Jr, Swischuk LE, Davis M, Brouhard BH. Puddling: A distinguishing feature of adult polycystic kidney disease in the neonate. *AJR* 1984;142:811–812.

71. Hayden CK Jr, Swischuk LE, Smith TH, Armstrong EA. Renal cystic disease in childhood. *Radiographics* 1986;6:97–116.

72. Hays DM. Pelvic rhabdomyosarcomas in childhood: Diagnosis and concepts of management reviewed. *Cancer* 1980;45:1810–1814.

73. Heiken JP, Gold RP, Schnur MJ, King DL, Bashist B, Glazer HS. Computed tomography of renal lymphoma with ultrasound correlation. *J Comput Assist Tomogr* 1983;7:245–250.

74. Hoffer FA, Hanabergh AM, Teele RL. The interrenicular junction: A mimic of renal scarring on normal pediatric sonograms. *AJR* 1985;145:1075–1078.

75. Hricak H, Cruz C, Eyler WR, Madrazo BL, Romanski R, Sandler MA. Acute post-transplantation renal failure: Differential diagnosis by ultrasound. *Radiology* 1981;139:441–449.

76. Hricak H, Slovis TL, Callen CW, Callen PW, Romanski RN. Neonatal kidneys: Sonographic anatomic correlation. *Radiology* 1983;147:699–702.

77. Hufnagle KG, Khan SN, Penn D, Cacciarelli A, Williams P. Renal calcifications: A complication of long-term furosemide therapy in preterm infants. *Pediatrics* 1982;70:360–363.

78. Hurley R, Winner HI. Experimental renal moniliasis in the mouse. *J Pathol* 1963;86:75–82.

79. Jaffe MH, White SJ, Silver TM, Heidelberger KP. Wilms tumor: Ultrasonic features, pathologic correlation, and diagnostic pitfalls. *Radiology* 1981;140:147–152.

80. Jeffrey RB, Laing FC, Wing VW, Hoddick W. Sensitivity

of sonography in pyonephrosis: A reevaluation. *AJR* 1985; 144:71–73.

81. Jequier S, Forbes PA, Nogrady MB. The value of ultrasonography as a screening procedure in a first-documented urinary tract infection in children. *J Ultrasound Med* 1985;4:393–400.

82. Jequier S, Rousseau O. Sonographic measurements of the normal bladder wall in children. *AJR* 1987;149:563–566.

83. Johnson CE, DeBaz BP, Shurin PA, DeBartolomeo R. Renal ultrasound evaluation of urinary tract infections in children. *Pediatrics* 1986;78:871–878.

84. Kangarloo H, Gold RH, Fine RN, Diament MJ, Boechat MI. Urinary tract infection in infants and children evaluated by ultrasound. *Radiology* 1985;154:367–373.

85. Kasper TE, Osborne RW Jr, Semerdjian HS, Miller HC. Urologic abdominal masses in infants and children. *J Urol* 1976;116:629–633.

86. Kaufman RA. CT of blunt abdominal trauma in children: A five-year experience. In: Siegel MJ, ed. *Pediatric Body CT.* New York: Churchill-Livingstone, 1988;313–347.

87. Kay CJ, Rosenfield AT, Armm M. Gray-scale ultrasonography in the evaluation of renal trauma. *Radiology* 1980;134:461–466.

88. Kearney GP, Lebowitz RL, Retik AB. Obstructing polyps of the posterior urethra in boys: Embryology and management. *J Urol* 1979;122:802–804.

89. Kenney PJ, Brinsko RE, Patel DV, Spitzer RE, Farrar FM. Sonography of the kidneys in hemolytic uremic syndrome. *Invest Radiol* 1986;21:547–550.

90. Kenney IJ, Wild SR. The renal parenchymal junctional line in children: Ultrasonic frequency and appearances. *Br J Radiol* 1987;60:865–868.

91. Kessler RM, Altman DH. Real-time sonographic detection of vesicoureteral reflux in children. *AJR* 1982;138:1033–1036.

92. Kintanar C, Cramer BC, Reid WD, Andrews WL. Neonatal renal candidiasis: Sonographic diagnosis. *AJR* 1986;147:801–805.

93. Kirpekar M, Abiri MM, Hilfer C, Enerson R. Ultrasound in the diagnosis of systemic candidiasis (renal and cranial) in very low birth weight premature infants. *Pediatr Radiol* 1986;16:17–20.

94. Kountz PD, Siegel MJ, Shapiro E. Flank mass in a newborn. *Urol Radiol* 1989;11:61–64.

95. Kremer H, Dobrinski W, Mikyska M, Baumgartner M, Zollner N. Ultrasonic *in vivo* and *in vitro* studies on the nature of the ureteral jet phenomenon. *Radiology* 1982;142:175–177.

96. Kremer SM, Rosenberg HK, Sherman NH, Tarry W, Duckett JW, Snyder HM III. Rapidly expanding mass in a neonate. *JCU* 1986;14:569–573.

97. Kumar R, Wilson DD, Santa-Cruz FR. Postoperative urological complications of renal transplantation. *Radiographics* 1984;4:531–546.

98. Laing FC, Burke VD, Wing VW, Jeffrey RB Jr, Hashimoto B. Postpartum evaluation of fetal hydronephrosis: Optimal timing for follow-up sonography. *Radiology* 1984;152:423–424.

99. Lebowitz RL. The detection of vesicoureteral reflux in the child. *Invest Radiol* 1986;21:519–531.

100. Lebowitz RL, Mandell J. Urinary tract infection in children: Putting radiology in its place. *Radiology* 1987;165:1–9.

101. Lee JKT, McClennan BL, Melson GL, Stanley RJ. Acute focal bacterial nephritis: Emphasis on gray scale sonography and computed tomography. *AJR* 1980;135:87–92.

102. Leonidas JC, McCauley RGK, Klauber GC, Fretzayas AM. Sonography as a substitute for excretory urography in children with urinary tract infection. *AJR* 1985;144:815–819.

103. Letourneau JG, Day DL, Feinberg SB. Ultrasound and computed tomographic evaluation of renal transplantation. *Radiol Clin North Am* 1987;25:267–279.

104. Livne PM, Gonzales ET Jr. Genitourinary trauma in children. *Urol Clin North Am* 1985;12:53–65.

105. Lubat E, Hernanz-Schulman M, Genieser NB, Ambrosino MM, Teele RL. Sonography of the simple and complicated ipsilateral fused kidney. *J Ultrasound Med* 1989;8:109–114.

106. McAlister WH. Demonstration of the dilated prostatic urethra in posterior urethral valve patients. *J Ultrasound Med* 1984;3:189–190.

107. McAlister WH, Siegel MJ, Shackelford G, Askin F, Kissane JM. Glomerulocystic kidney. *AJR* 1979;133:536–538.

108. Machin GA. Persistent renal blastema (nephroblastomatosis) as a frequent precursor of Wilms' tumor; A pathological and clinical review. Part 2. Significance of nephroblastomatosis in the genesis of Wilms' tumor. *Am J Pediatr Hematol Oncol* 1980;2:253–261.

109. Machin GA. Persistent renal blastema (nephroblastomatosis) as a frequent precursor of Wilms' tumor; A pathological and clinical review. Part 3. Clinical aspects of nephroblastomatosis. *Am J Pediatr Hematol Oncol* 1980;2:353–362.

110. Macpherson RI, Gordon L, Bradford BF. Neonatal urinomas: Imaging considerations. *Pediatr Radiol* 1984;14:396–399.

111. Macpherson RI, Leithiser RE, Gordon L, Turner WR. Posterior urethral valves: An update and review. *Radiographics* 1986;6:753–791.

112. Madanat F, Osborne B, Cangir A, Sutow WW. Extrarenal Wilms' tumor. *J Pediatr* 1978;93:439–443.

113. Madewell JE, Goldman SM, Davis CJ Jr, Hartman DS, Feigin DS, Lichtenstein JE. Multilocular cystic nephroma: A radiographic-pathologic correlation of 58 patients. *Radiology* 1983;146:309–321.

114. Madewell JE, Hartman DS, Lichtenstein JR. Radiologic-pathologic correlation in cystic diseases of the kidney. *Radiol Clin North Am* 1979;17:261–279.

115. Malek RS. Urolithiasis. In: Kelalis PP, King LR, Belman AB, eds. *Clinical Pediatric Urology.* 2nd ed. Philadelphia: W.B. Saunders Co., 1985;1093–1124.

116. Marchal GJ, Baert AL, Eeckels R, Proesmans W. Sonographic evaluation of the normal ureteral submucosal tunnel in infancy and childhood. *Pediatr Radiol* 1983;13:125–129.

117. Martin KW, McAlister WH, Shackelford GD. Acute renal infarction: Diagnosis by Doppler ultrasound. *Pediatr Radiol* 1988;18:373–376.

118. Mason WG Jr. Urinary tract infections in children: Renal ultrasound evaluation. *Radiology* 1984;153:109–111.

119. Mason WG Jr, Stevens PS. Options in the evaluation of pediatric urinary tract infections: The role of radiography and ultrasound. *Semin US, CT, MR* 1986;7:234–245.

120. Matsumoto J, Han BK, de Rovetto CR, Welch TR. Hypercalciuric Bartter syndrome: Resolution of nephrocalcinosis with Indomethacin. *AJR* 1989;152:1251–1253.

121. Merrick MV, Uttley WS, Wild SR. The detection of pyelonephritic scarring in children by radioisotope imaging. *Br J Radiol* 1980;53:544–556.

122. Miller WB Jr, Boal DK, Teele R. Neurofibromatosis of the bladder: Sonographic findings. *JCU* 1983;11:460–462.

123. Montgomery P, Kuhn JP, Berger PE, Fisher J. Multifocal nephroblastomatosis: Clinical significance and imaging. *Pediatr Radiol* 1984;14:392–395.

124. Morehouse HT, Weiner SN, Hoffman JC. Imaging in inflammatory disease of the kidney. *AJR* 1984;143:135–141.

125. Nicolet V, Carignan L, Dubuc G, Hebert G, Bourdon F, Paquin F. Thickening of the renal collecting system: Nonspecific findings at US. *Radiology* 1988;168:411–413.

126. Nussbaum AR, Dorst JP, Jeffs RD, Gearhart JP, Sanders RC. Ectopic ureter and ureterocele: Their varied sonographic manifestations. *Radiology* 1986;159:227–235.

127. Nussbaum AR, Hartman DS, Whitley N, McCauley RGK, Sanders RC. Multicystic dysplasia and crossed renal ectopia. *AJR* 1987;149:407–410.

128. Paling MR, Wakefield JA, Watson LR. Sonography of experimental acute renal vein occlusion. *JCU* 1985;13:647–653.

129. Parienty RA, Pradel J, Imbert M, Picard JD, Savart P. Computed tomography of multilocular cystic nephroma. *Radiology* 1981;140:135–139.

130. Patriquin H, Lebowitz R, Perreault G, Yousefzadeh D. Neonatal candidiasis: Renal and pulmonary manifestations. *AJR* 1980;135:1205–1210.

131. Patriquin HB, O'Regan S. Medullary sponge kidney in childhood. *AJR* 1985;145:315–319.

132. Patriquin HB, O'Regan S, Robitaille P, Paltiel H. Hemolyticuremic syndrome: Intrarenal arterial Doppler patterns as a useful guide to therapy. *Radiology* 1989;172:625–628.

133. Pizzo PA, Miser JS, Cassady JR, Filler RM. Wilms' Tumor. In: Devita VT, Hellman S, Rosenberg SA, eds. *Cancer Principles and Practice of Oncology*, 2nd ed. London: J.B. Lippincott Co., 1985;1516–1525.

134. Platt JF, Rubin JM, Ellis JH, DiPietro MA. Duplex Doppler US of the kidney: Differentiation of obstructive from nonobstructive dilatation. *Radiology* 1989;171:515–517.

135. Pollack HM, Wein AJ. Imaging of renal trauma. *Radiology* 1989;172:297–308.

136. Raptopoulos V, Kleinman PK, Marks S Jr, Snyder M, Silverman PM. Renal fascial pathways: Posterior extension of pancreatic effusions within the anterior pararenal space. *Radiology* 1986;158:367–374.

137. Reiman TH, Siegel MJ, Shackelford GD. Wilms' tumor in children: Abdominal CT and US evaluation. *Radiology* 1986; 160:501–505.

138. Rifkin MD, Kurtz AB, Pasto ME, Goldberg BB. Unusual presentations of cystitis. *J Ultrasound Med* 1983;2:25–28.

139. Rifkin MD, Needleman L, Pasto ME, et al. Evaluation of renal transplant rejection by duplex Doppler examination: Value of the resistive index. *AJR* 1987;148:759–762.

140. Rigsby CM, Burns PN, Weltin GG, Chen B, Bia M, Taylor KJW. Doppler signal quantitation in renal allografts: Comparison in normal and rejecting transplants, with pathologic correlation. *Radiology* 1987;162:39–42.

141. Rigsby CM, Taylor KJW, Weltin G, et al. Renal allografts in acute rejection: Evaluation using duplex sonography. *Radiology* 1986;158:375–378.

142. Robinson PJ, Pocock RD, Frank JD. The management of obstructive renal candidiasis in the neonate. *Br J Urol* 1987;59:380–382.

143. Rosenbaum DM, Korngold E, Teele RL. Sonographic assessment of renal length in normal children. *AJR* 1984;142:467–469.

144. Rosenfield AT, Zeman RK, Cicchetti DV, Siegel NJ. Experimental acute tubular necrosis: US appearance. *Radiology* 1985;157:771–774.

145. Rosenfield NS, Shimkin P, Berdon W, Barwick K, Glassman M, Siegel NJ. Wilms' tumor arising from spontaneously regressing nephroblastomatosis. *AJR* 1980;135:381–384.

146. Sanders RC, Hartman DS. The sonographic distinction between neonatal multicystic kidney and hydronephrosis. *Radiology* 1984;151:621–625.

147. Sanders RC, Nussbaum AR, Solez K. Renal dysplasia: Sonographic findings. *Radiology* 1988;167:623–626.

148. Schaffer RM, Shih YH, Becker JA. Sonographic identification of collecting system duplications. *JCU* 1983;11:309–312.

149. Schlesinger AE, Hedlund GL, Pierson WP, Null DM. Normal standards for kidney length in premature infants: Determination with US. *Radiology* 1987;164:127–129.

150. Schneider K, Jablonski C, Wiessner M, Kohn M, Fendel H. Screening for vesicoureteral reflux in children using real-time sonography. *Pediatr Radiol* 1984;14:400–403.

151. Share JC, Lebowitz RL. Ectopic ureterocele without ureteral and calyceal dilatation (ureterocele disproportion): Findings on urography and sonography. *AJR* 1989;152:567–571.

152. Shawker TH, Dunnick NR, Head GL, Magrath IT. Ultrasound evaluation of American Burkitt's lymphoma. *JCU* 1979;7:279–283.

153. Sheth KJ, Tang TT, Blaedel ME, Good TA. Polydipsia, polyuria, and hypertension associated with renin-secreting Wilms' tumor. *J Pediatr* 1978;92:921–924.

154. Shirkhoda A, Staab EV, Mittelstaedt CA. Renal lymphoma imaged by ultrasound and gallium-67. *Radiology* 1980;137:175–180.

155. Siegel MJ, Glasier CM. Acute focal bacterial nephritis in children: Significance of ureteral reflux. *AJR* 1981;137:257–260.

156. Siegel MJ, McAlister WH. Simple cysts of the kidney in children. *J Urol* 1980;123:75–78.

157. Silver TM, Campbell D, Wicks JD, Lorber MI, Surace P, Turcotte J. Peritransplant fluid collections. *Radiology* 1981; 138:145–151.

158. Sisler CL, Siegel MJ. Malignant rhabdoid tumor of the kidney: Radiologic features. *Radiology* 1989;172:211–212.

159. Slovis TL, Babcock DS, Hricak H, et al. Renal transplant rejection: Sonographic evaluation in children. *Radiology* 1984;153:659–665.

160. Slovis TL, Philippart AI, Cushing B, et al. Evaluation of the inferior vena cava by sonography and venography in children with renal and hepatic tumors. *Radiology* 1981;140:767–772.

161. Snyder HM, Lebowitz RL, Colodny AH, Bauer SB, Retik AB. Ureteropelvic junction obstruction in children. *Urol Clin North Am* 1980;7:273–290.

162. Steinberg HV, Nelson RC, Murphy FB, Chezmar JL, Baumgartner BR, Delaney VB, Whelchel JD, Bernardino ME. Renal allograph rejection: Evaluation by Doppler US and MR imaging. *Radiology* 1987;162:337–342.

163. Steinhardt GF, Slovis TL, Perlmutter AD. Simple renal cysts in infants. *Radiology* 1985;155:349–350.

164. Stuck KJ, Koff SA, Silver TM. Ultrasonic features of multicystic dysplastic kidney: Expanded diagnostic criteria. *Radiology* 1982;143:217–221.

165. Stuck KJ, Silver TM, Jaffe MH, Bowerman RA. Sonographic demonstration of renal fungus balls. *Radiology* 1981;142:473–474.

166. Sty JR, Wells RG, Starshak RJ, Schroeder BA. Imaging in acute renal infection in children. *AJR* 1987;148:471–477.

167. Subramanyam BR, Raghavendra BN, Bosniak MA, Lefleur RS, Rosen RJ, Horii SC. Sonography of pyonephrosis: A prospective study. *AJR* 1983;140:991–992.

168. Surratt JS, Siegel MJ, Middleton WM. Sonography of pediatric renal allografts RadioGraphics 1990;10:687–699.

169. Taylor GA, Eichelberger MR, Potter BM. Hematuria, A marker of abdominal injury in children after blunt trauma. *Ann Surg* 1988;208:688–693.

170. Taylor KJW, Morse SS, Rigsby DM, Bia M, Schiff M. Vascular complications in renal allografts: Detection with duplex Doppler US. *Radiology* 1987;162:31–38.

171. Totty WG, McClennan BL, Melson GL, Patel R. Relative value of computed tomography and ultrasonography in the assessment of renal angiomyolipoma. *J Comput Assist Tomogr* 1981;5:173–178.

172. Traisman ES, Conway JJ, Traisman HS, et al. The localization of urinary tract infection with ^{99m}Tc glucoheptonate scintigraphy. *Pediatr Radiol* 1986;16:403–406.

173. Vade A, Lau P, Smick J, Harris V, Ryva J. Sonographic renal parameters as related to age. *Pediatr Radiol* 1987;17:212–215.

174. Vinocur L, Slovis TL, Perlmutter AD, Watts FB Jr, Chang C-H. Follow-up studies of multicystic dysplastic kidneys. *Radiology* 1988;167:311–315.

175. Warshauer DM, Taylor KJW, Bia MJ, et al. Unusual causes of increased vascular impedance in renal transplants: Duplex Doppler evaluation. *Radiology* 1988;169:367–370.

176. Whitaker RH, Sherwood T. Another look at diagnostic pathways in children with urinary tract infection. *Br Med J* 1984;288:839–841.

177. Williams JL, Cumming WA, Walker RD, Hackett RL. Transitional cell papilloma of the bladder. *Pediatr Radiol* 1986; 16:322–323.

178. Wood BP, Ben-Ami T, Teele RL, Rabinowitz R. Ureterovesical obstruction and megaloureter: Diagnosis by real-time US. *Radiology* 1985;156:79–81.

179. Worthington JL, Shackelford GD, Cole BR, Tack ED, Kissane JM. Sonographically detectable cysts in polycystic kidney disease in newborn and young infants. *Pediatr Radiol* 1988; 18:287–293.

180. Yap R, Madrazo B, Oh HK, Dienst SG. Perirenal fluid collection after renal transplantation. *Am Surg* 1981;47:287–290.

10

Female Pelvis

Marilyn J. Siegel

In recent years, sonography has become an important imaging study for evaluating girls suspected of having pelvic diseases. Before the introduction of sonography, it was impossible to visualize the female reproductive organs unless contrast agents were placed within the vagina or uterine canal, or gas was introduced into the peritoneal cavity. With the advent of sonography, however, a wide variety of abnormalities of the ovary and uterus, as well as abnormalities of adjacent structures which mimic gynecologic disease, can be delineated (5,21,36,45,52,64,71,104).

TECHNIQUE

An adequately distended urinary bladder is essential for pelvic sonography. A distended bladder allows for transmission of sound into deeper structures of the pelvis and displaces the gas-filled bowel, allowing easier visualization of the ovaries and uterus. If the bladder is inadequately filled, gas-filled loops of bowel may interpose themselves between the bladder and ovaries and uterus, leading to a nondiagnostic study. An overdistended bladder, however, causes patient discomfort and can distort the uterine shape and displace ovarian masses from the pelvis into the lower abdomen. In the latter location, a mass may become obscured by overlying gas-filled loops of bowel, creating imaging problems.

Adequate bladder distention can be achieved by having the patient drink large volumes of fluid, or if the patient is not allowed oral intake, the bladder can be distended with sterile fluid through a Foley catheter. Most pelvic imaging in children can be performed with a 5 MHz transducer. Once the bladder is adequately distended, longitudinal and transverse sonograms should be obtained through the pelvis. Occasionally, oblique positioning of the patient may improve visualization of the ovaries. This position allows the sound beam to be more perpendicular to the ovary.

In cases where there is a question of a pseudotumor (i.e., fluid or fecal material within the bowel, masquerading as a gynecologic or other pelvic mass) a water enema can be useful. With this technique, the rectosigmoid colon can be easily identified and differentiated from masses or fluid collections.

Transvaginal scanning, in which a transducer is placed within the vagina, has been shown to be useful in the evaluation of obstetrical and gynecological abnormalities in adults (19). There has been limited experience with this technique in younger children, although this approach can be useful in older adolescents when findings with the transabdominal approach are equivocal or confusing. The greatest advantage of transvaginal over transabdominal scanning is the high-resolution imaging of adnexal, uterine, and cul-de-sac masses with superb tissue characterization. The transvaginal technique also can facilitate identification and localization of loculated fluid collections and can guide diagnostic needle aspiration (67,69,82,83).

INDICATIONS FOR SONOGRAPHY

There are two common reasons for pelvic sonography in childhood. The first is the evaluation of a palpable mass and the second is to exclude a pelvic abnormality in a girl with right lower quadrant pain. Other indications include ambiguous genitalia, amenorrhea or delayed sexual development, and premature menarche. This chapter will review some of the common abnormalities of the female pediatric pelvis with attention to clinical and pathologic findings as well as sonographic features.

OVARIES

Normal Prepubertal Anatomy

At birth, the ovaries usually have descended from the upper abdomen into the pelvis and lie within the superior margin of the broad ligament, although in some patients, descent is arrested and the ovaries may be anywhere from the inferior edge of the kidney down to the broad ligament. Rarely, the ovaries will descend further inferiorly into the inguinal canal.

At birth, the ovary is approximately 15 mm long, 3 mm wide and 2.5 mm thick (53). Throughout childhood, thickness and width increase more than length. Since the normal ovary may vary in configuration, ovarian volume is a more reproducible method of evaluating size. Ovarian volume is determined using the simplified formula for a prolate ellipsoid ($\frac{1}{2} \times$ width $\times$ thickness $\times$ length) (122). Normal mean ovarian volume is less than 0.7 cm^3 in girls under 2 years of age, increasing to between 0.75 to 3.80 cm^3 in girls 2 to 12 years of age (64,102,122).

Because they are small and relatively high in the pelvis, the normal ovaries can be difficult to identify in children under 5 years of age. When visualized, they almost always have a solid, homogeneous appearance. Occasionally the ovaries of neonates and young infants contain small follicles which are thought to reflect maternal hormonal stimulation. The vast majority of these follicles undergo spontaneous regression, but a few fail to involute and instead undergo growth and development, producing a palpable abdominal mass.

At least one ovary is identified in about 90% of pediatric patients over 5 years of age, while both ovaries are seen in 80% of patients (102). The vast majority of normal ovaries in younger girls demonstrate a finely, heterogeneous echotexture (Fig. 1). Occasionally small follicles, under 9 mm in diameter, are visualized and are of no particular consequence (Fig. 1). After 6 years of age, the ovaries begin to enlarge and as adolescence approaches, they become more heterogeneous due to an increase in the number of primordial follicles (102).

Normal Postpubertal Anatomy

With activation of the hypothalamic-pituitary-ovarian axis at puberty, the ovary acquires an ovoid shape and descends deeper into the pelvis. Ultimately, the ovaries will lie lateral or posterolateral to the uterus, although not necessarily at the same horizontal level. Occasionally the ovaries may be located high in the pelvis or behind the uterus because of mobile ligamentous attachments. They also may be located dorsal or cephalad to the uterus, especially when the bladder is full (50). In postpubertal and ovulatory patients, the ovaries measure 2.5 to 5 cm in length, 1.5 to 3.0 cm in width and 0.6 to 1.5 cm in thickness, with a volume of 1.8 to 5.7 cm^3 (50,71,122). Multiple cysts representing stimulated and unstimulated follicles usually can be seen during each menstrual cycle (see below) (Fig. 2).

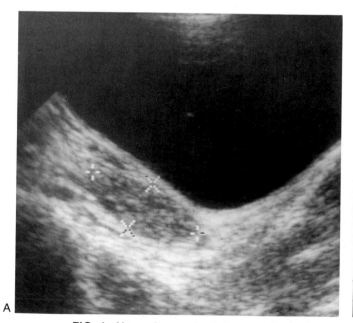
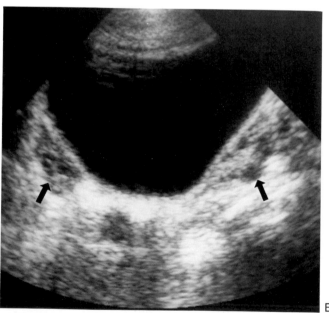

FIG. 1. Normal prepubertal ovary. **A:** Sagittal image through the pelvis of a 7-year-old girl demonstrates a normal right ovary (*calipers*) lying behind the distended bladder. The ovarian size is 12 × 10 mm with an estimated volume of 2.0 cm^3. The echotexture of the ovary is slightly heterogeneous. **B:** Transverse sonogram in an 8-year-old girl shows small cysts in both ovaries (*arrows*).

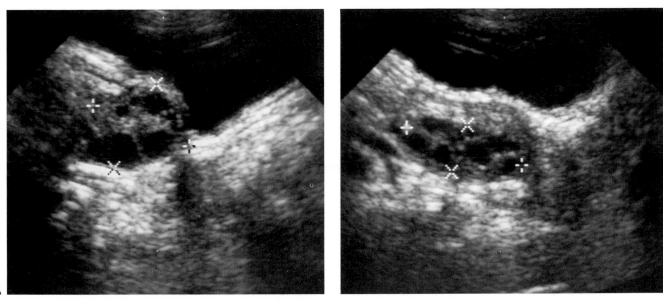

FIG. 2. Normal postpubertal ovary. **A:** Transverse and **B:** longitudinal scans of a 13-year-old girl demonstrate multiple developing follicles within the right ovary (*calipers*). The ovarian size is 26 × 24 × 15 mm with an estimated volume of 4.6 cm³.

Physiology

Under the influence of pituitary gonadotropins, the ovary goes through three phases during each menstrual cycle: the follicular phase, ovulation, and the luteal phase (33,49,50,116). The follicular phase begins on the first day of the menstrual cycle and continues until ovulation, which is usually day 14 of a 28-day cycle. This phase typically begins with the development of the primordial follicle, consisting of an oocyte surrounded by a single layer of epithelium. The unstimulated primordial follicles often are too small to resolve sonographically. In response to follicle-stimulating hormone, a number of previously dormant primordial follicles begin to mature and increase in size, eventually forming antral follicles (116). Antral follicles measuring 0.5 to 1.0 cm in diameter can be imaged within the ovary, appearing as circular or oval anechoic spaces surrounded by ovarian parenchyma. By day 8 or 9, the dominant follicle destined for eventual ovulation emerges and continues to develop under the influence of estrogen (Fig. 3). The other stimulated follicles that do not progress to ovulation undergo replacement by fibrous tissue and become atretic. By the

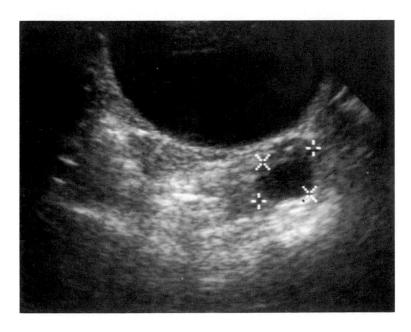

FIG. 3. Dominant ovarian follicle. Transverse section of the left ovary of a 15-year-old girl demonstrates a single developing follicle (*calipers*) measuring 17 × 12 × 10 mm. This examination was obtained on day 10 of the menstrual cycle.

time of ovulation, the diameter of the dominant follicle, now called the graafian follicle, ranges from 17 to 29 mm (mean, 20 to 23 mm) (33,65,100,101,110). A dominant follicle can be demonstrated sonographically in approximately 80% of cases (33).

As ovulation approaches, a zone of decreased echogenicity develops around the follicle and the follicular wall becomes indistinct (108). With follicular rupture and extrusion of the ovum, there is a sudden decrease in follicular size and the appearance of intrafollicular echoes representing collapse of the follicle, crenation of the walls, and accumulation of blood within the antrum (25). Almost simultaneous with ovulation, sonography can reveal fluid in the cul-de-sac in 25% to 45% of women (23,50,109,116).

After ovulation the luteal phase begins, with filling in of the antrum with blood and lymph to form a corpus hemorrhagicum. The developing corpus hemorrhagicum may be present as early as 1 hr postovulation. Next, the remaining granulosa cells enlarge and accumulate lipid and lutein, and vascularization of the granulosa occurs to form the corpus luteum which remains for 14 days, after which it rapidly degenerates unless the ovum is fertilized. The mature corpus luteum can be seen on sonography in about 50% of individuals. It varies between 1.6 to 2.4 cm in diameter and appears cystic, with scattered echoes representing retained follicular fluid and blood (50). Eventually the follicle atrophies with regression of vessels (retrogressive corpus). The corpus albicans is the final stage of the menstrual cycle. During this stage the corpus is replaced by collagen-rich cicatricial tissue. This remnant of follicular development is not detectable by sonography.

ADNEXAL LESIONS

Congenital Anomalies

Polycystic Ovary Disease

Polycystic ovary disease is one of the most frequent anatomic and physiologic abnormalities of the ovary. Also known as the Stein-Leventhal syndrome, it is associated with amenorrhea, infertility, and hirsutism. The endocrine profile of affected patients reveals low levels of follicle-stimulating hormone and elevated levels of luteinizing hormone.

The typical sonographic appearance of polycystic ovary disease is bilateral ovarian enlargement, occurring in up to 70% of affected patients. The mean volume of the enlarged ovary is 14 cm³, which is significantly larger than normal. In the remaining patients, the ovaries are normal in size (55,92,149). The shape of the ovaries may be oval or round. Multiple small cysts (0.5 to 0.8 cm in diameter) are present in the majority of cases (Fig. 4), but occasionally the ovaries may be isoechoic or hypoechoic in comparison to the uterus, without definable cysts (55,103,106,149). Maturing follicles are rarer in patients with polycystic ovary disease than they are in healthy patients. Long-

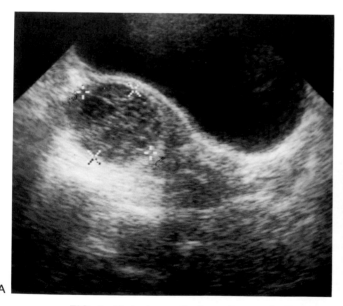
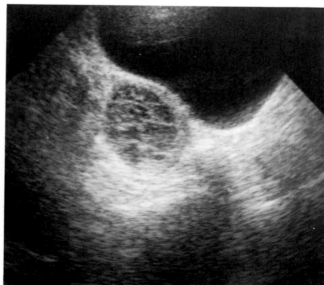

FIG. 4. Stein-Leventhal syndrome. **A:** Transverse and **B:** longitudinal sonograms of the pelvis of a 17-year-old girl demonstrate an enlarged right ovary (*calipers*) measuring 4 × 4 × 8 cm. Multiple small follicles are present.

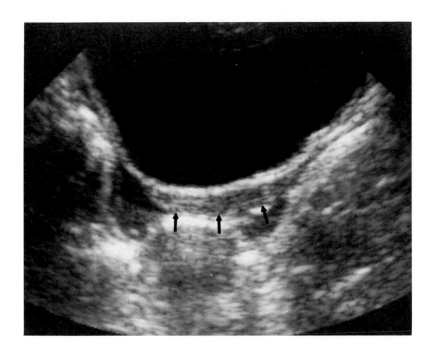

FIG. 5. Turner's syndrome. Longitudinal scan of the pelvis shows a prepubertal size uterus (*arrows*) in a 16-year-old girl with a 45XO karyotype. The ovaries were not identifiable.

term follow-up of patients with polycystic ovary disease is important since there is an increased incidence of endometrial carcinoma in this disease, presumably secondary to unopposed estrogenic stimulation.

Multiple ovarian cysts have been described in association with acquired primary hypothyroidism and cystic fibrosis (60,70,114,128). In addition, bilateral ovarian enlargement with discrete cysts has been seen in children with McCune-Albright syndrome (fibrous dysplasia, patchy cutaneous pigmentation, and sexual precocity) (115).

Gonadal Dysgenesis

Gonadal dysgenesis, or Turner's syndrome, is typically characterized by streak ovaries and a 45XO karyotype. Occasionally patients have chromosomal mosaics and a small percentage of patients with this syndrome have a Y chromosome in their karyotype and are at risk for developing gonadoblastoma. Clinically, classic or mosaic Turner's syndrome results in primary amenorrhea and sexual infantilism. Characteristic physical findings include short stature, webbed neck, shield chest, scoliosis, and cubitus valgus deformities. Other anomalies include renal duplication, horseshoe kidney, coarctation of the aorta, bicuspid aortic valve, and lymphatic obstruction.

In patients with a 45XO karyotype, the ovaries are not recognizable by sonography, reflecting absence or small size. Uterine size and configuration remain prepubertal with increasing age (Fig. 5). Individuals with chromosomal mosaics have a spectrum of findings on sonography, ranging from nonvisualized ovaries and an infantile uterus to normal-size gonads and uterus (79,126). Ovarian enlargement or a mass may be encountered in some patients, particularly those with Y-bearing dysgenic gonads.

Ovarian Masses

Although pediatric ovarian masses are uncommon, they account for 80% of female genital tumors in childhood (22). In the newborn female infant, these masses are almost always non-neoplastic cysts. Ovarian cysts also occur frequently in older girls, but there is an increased prevalence of solid tumors, ectopic pregnancies, pelvic inflammatory disease, and torsion. Sonography can afford an accurate assessment of the presence, size, location, and internal consistency of ovarian masses (35,87,142,148) and also can provide a specific histologic diagnosis in about 50% of cases. A specific diagnosis usually is possible in selected patients with simple ovarian cysts, cystadenomas, dermoids, and ectopic pregnancy (148).

Non-Neoplastic Lesions

Follicular and Corpus Luteum Cysts

Functional cysts are the most common cause of an ovarian mass in infant and adolescent girls and usually result from exaggerated development of follicular or corpus lueum cysts (13,53,54,78,84). The origin of follicular cysts in neonates is thought to be excessive stimulation by maternal hormones. In adolescent girls,

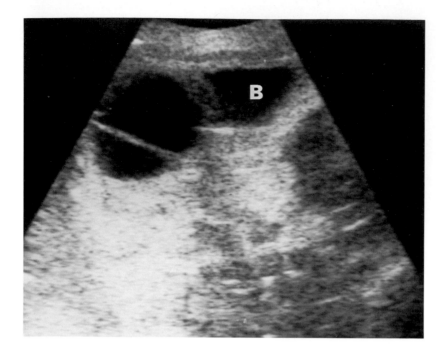

FIG. 6. Ovarian cyst in a 2-month-old girl with a palpable lower abdominal mass. Transverse sonogram demonstrates a 2.0 cm well-defined cystic lesion with a single thin septation to the right of the bladder (*B*). Exploratory laparotomy revealed a follicular ovarian cyst.

follicular cysts result when a mature follicle fails to ovulate or to involute. Follicular cysts usually vary in size between 3 cm and 20 cm. Pathologically, most are smooth with clear serous fluid. Corpus luteum cysts are caused by excessive bleeding into the corpus luteum or failure of absorption. They range from 5 to 11 cm in diameter and may contain serous or hemorrhagic fluid.

The majority of follicular cysts are discovered incidentally on pelvic sonograms. However, if extremely large, the cyst may produce a palpable abdominal mass and be the reason for presentation. Pelvic pain from hemorrhage, rupture, or torsion also may occur. Corpus luteum cysts tend to be more symptomatic than follicular cysts and typically present with pain secondary to hemorrhage or rupture.

The sonographic appearance of an ovarian cyst varies, depending on whether it is uncomplicated or complicated by torsion or hemorrhage. Sonographically, uncomplicated follicular and corpus luteum cysts are anechoic and thin-walled. Internal septations occasionally are present (50,96) (Figs. 6,7). Specific differentiation between follicular and corpus luteum cysts is not possible on sonography, but this is not critical

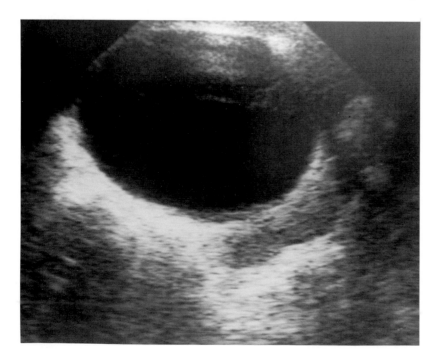

FIG. 7. Ovarian cyst in a 14-year-old girl with lower abdominal pain. Transverse sonogram of the pelvis shows a 4 cm anechoic mass in the expected region of the right ovary. The mass is homogeneously cystic and has well-defined, thin walls with increased through-transmission. No normal right ovary was identified. Operation revealed a corpus luteum cyst.

since the goal of diagnosis is to exclude neoplastic lesions. Serial sonography is recommended since the majority of functional cysts in adolescent girls change in appearance or regress spontaneously within days or weeks. There also have been a few reported cases of spontaneous resolution of neonatal cysts (97). Cysts that persist for several cycles need percutaneous or surgical aspiration for further investigation in order to exclude a neoplasm (44).

Hemorrhagic Ovarian Cysts

Hemorrhage may be a complication of follicular or corpus luteum cysts. Classically, patients present with acute lower quadrant or pelvic pain. Blood has a spectrum of sonographic findings, primarily related to the temporal sequence of clot formation and lysis. At the time of diagnosis, the most common appearance of a hemorrhagic ovarian cyst on sonography, occurring in about 85% of patients, is that of a heterogeneous mass with predominantly anechoic or hypoechoic contents with a fluid-debris level or internal echoes (Fig. 8). The remaining cysts are completely homogeneous, either hypo- or hyperechoic (6,9). The vast majority (more than 90%) have increased sound transmission, reflecting the underlying cystic nature of the mass. Other sonographic features of hemorrhagic ovarian cysts in-

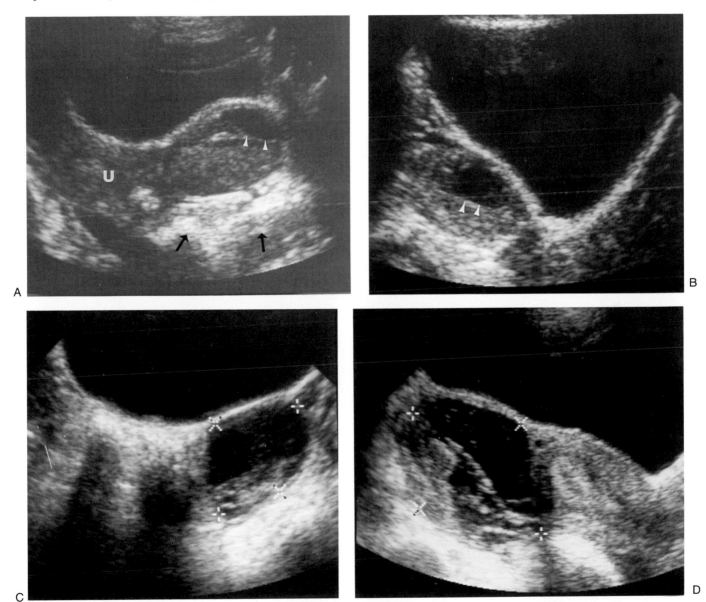

FIG. 8. Hemorrhagic ovarian cyst. **A:** Transverse and **B:** longitudinal images demonstrate a cystic mass with increased through-transmission (*black arrows*) and a fluid-debris level (*white arrowheads*) in the expected location of the left ovary. *U*, uterus. **C:** Transverse and **D:** longitudinal scans of another girl show an enlarged left ovary (*calipers*) containing a large anechoic area with scattered internal echoes. Normal ovarian parenchyma with tiny follicles is noted posterior to the cystic lesion. Follow-up sonogram a few weeks later demonstrated resolution of the mass.

clude a thick rim, septations, and associated cul-de-sac fluid.

The sonographic appearance of a hemorrhagic ovarian cyst is nonspecific and may be similar to that of an ovarian teratoma, abscess, torsion, malignancy, or ectopic pregnancy. If acute surgical conditions such as adnexal torsion, ectopic pregnancy, and appendicitis can be excluded, an adnexal mass in a patient with acute pelvic pain can be followed conservatively with serial sonography. The appearance and size of a hemorrhagic ovarian cyst would be expected to change with time and eventually resolve, while other lesions would remain unaltered or increase in size (Fig. 9).

Theca-Lutein Cysts

A rare form of a functional cyst is the theca-lutein cyst. Theca-lutein cysts are found in association with elevated levels of human chorionic gonadotropin and are believed to be the result of hyperstimulation of follicular cysts (116). They generally are associated with gestational trophoblastic disease but also can be seen as a complication of medication given for ovulation induction. In contrast to follicular and corpus luteum cysts, theca-lutein cysts are large, bilateral, and multiloculated. The ovaries of affected patients are often markedly enlarged and exceed 25 cm in diameter.

Parovarian Cysts

Parovarian cysts are neoplasms of paramesonephric or mesothelial origin that are found in the broad ligament or fallopian tubes (4,53). They usually are discovered incidentally after the fourth decade of life, but occasionally they may present in childhood as a palpable mass or with acute pelvic pain after undergoing torsion, rupture, or hemorrhage. Unlike functional

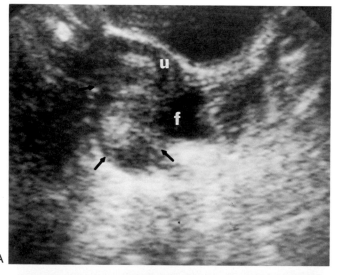

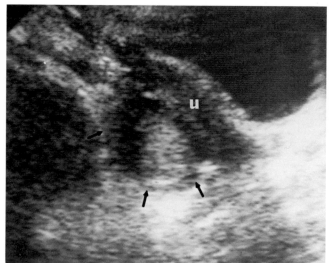

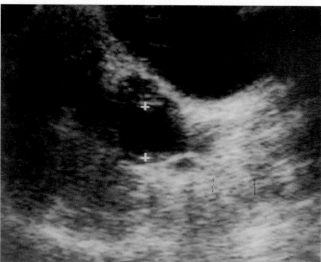

FIG. 9. Hemorrhagic ovarian cyst. **A, B:** Two longitudinal sonograms of the pelvis show a moderately well-defined, complex mass (*arrows*) with acoustic enhancement in the region of the right ovary. The mass cannot be clearly separated from the ovary. A small amount of fluid (*f*) is present in the cul-de-sac. *u,* uterus. **C:** Transverse sonogram 7 days later demonstrates a large cystic area (*calipers*) in the lesion. These sequential sonographic findings are typical of a hemorrhagic ovarian cyst.

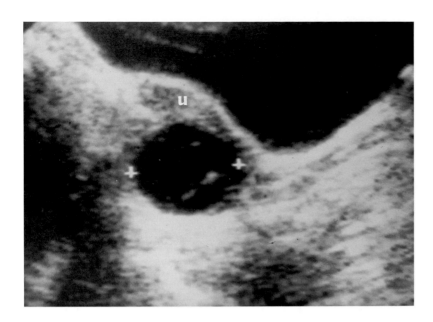

FIG. 10. Cystadenoma. A longitudinal sonogram through the right pelvis demonstrates a 4 cm cystic lesion (*calipers*) with several smooth septations. *u*, uterus.

ovarian cysts, parovarian cysts show no cyclic changes.

Most uncomplicated parovarian cysts are anechoic with an appearance indistinguishable from that of a simple ovarian cyst (4,35,112). If hemorrhage occurs, internal echoes are noted. Parovarian cysts cannot be differentiated from ovarian cysts unless a normal ovary is visualized separately from the cyst.

Benign Neoplastic Lesions

Two-thirds of all ovarian tumors in childhood are true neoplasms. Approximately 65% of these are benign and 35% are malignant (16,29,46).

Cystadenoma

Although cystadenomas are rare under the age of 20 years, occasionally they may be found in childhood (16). The serous type is slightly more frequent than the mucinous type. Both forms usually present as pelvic masses ranging in size from 4 to 20 cm. Sonographically the lesions may be entirely cystic and unilocular, but they more often contain fine internal echoes or septations (87,149) (Fig. 10). Hemorrhage and ascites secondary to rupture are infrequent complications. Rarely, malignant transformation is present.

Germ Cell Tumors

Ovarian germ cell tumors, either dermoids or teratomas, make up between one-third and one-half of all benign ovarian tumors (16,29,46). Dermoids contain two cell layers, mesoderm and ectoderm, while teratomas contain elements from all three germ cell layers: ectoderm, mesoderm, and endoderm. Almost all dermoids and teratomas are benign, with an incidence of malignancy between 2% and 10% (75,138). The majority of affected children are between 6 and 11 years of age. Very rarely, teratomas are found in children under 2 years of age (75). About two-thirds of teratomas are discovered incidentally, presenting as palpable masses, but they may present with acute abdominal signs corresponding to torsion and tumor rupture. The average diameter is 10 cm, with a range between 5 and 25 cm (16). Germ cell tumors are bilateral in up to 20% of cases.

The sonographic appearance is extremely variable, depending on the relative amounts of fluid, calcium, and fat within the lesion (66,123,129). Approximately two-thirds of dermoids or teratomas appear as complex lesions on sonography, with echogenic and hypoechoic components (133) (Fig. 11). The hypoechoic components correspond to sebum, known to be liquid at body temperature, or to serous fluid, whereas the echogenic foci represent an admixture of soft tissue, hair, fat, and calcification. The echogenic components have a variable sonographic appearance, ranging from a single

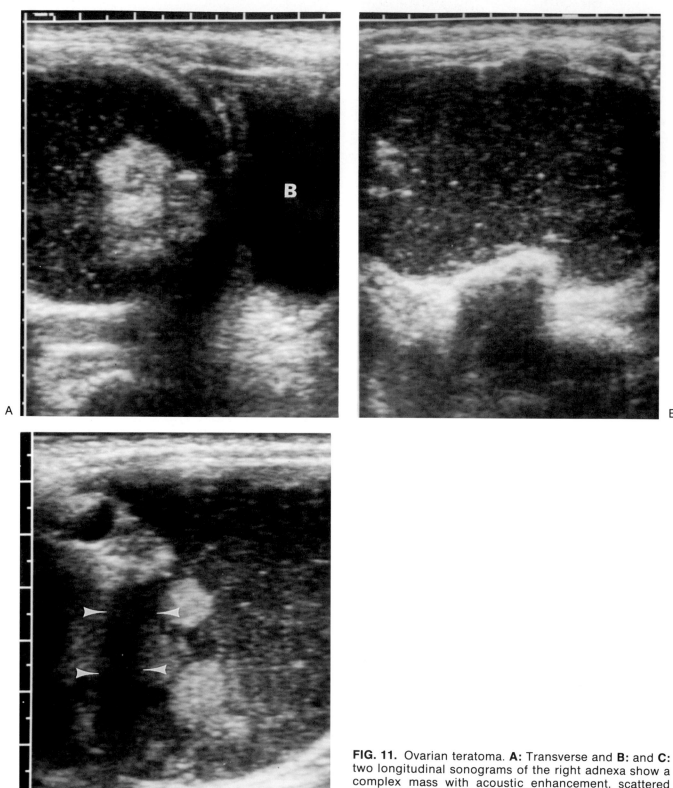

FIG. 11. Ovarian teratoma. **A:** Transverse and **B:** and **C:** two longitudinal sonograms of the right adnexa show a complex mass with acoustic enhancement, scattered low-level echoes, and large central echogenic components. Acoustic shadowing (*arrowheads*) is noted. *B,* bladder. At histopathologic examination, the teratoma contained sebum, hair, fat, and calcification.

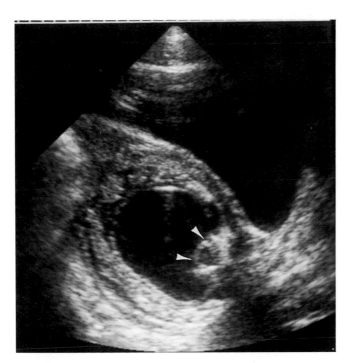

FIG. 12. Ovarian teratoma with a mural nodule. Longitudinal sonogram of the right ovary shows a cystic mass with a peripheral echogenic nodule (*arrowheads*).

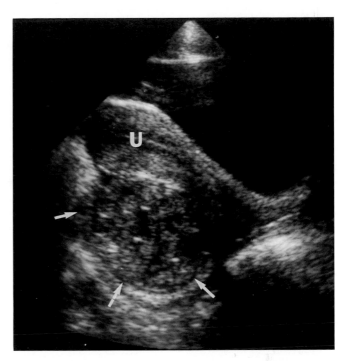

FIG. 14. Echogenic ovarian teratoma discovered incidentally in a 14-year-old girl. Longitudinal sonogram of the right adnexa shows a solid mass (*arrows*) containing multiple echogenic foci. Surgical exploration confirmed a benign ovarian teratoma containing predominantly fat and calcification. *U,* uterus.

mural nodule projecting from the cyst wall to large, central, soft tissue masses. Mural nodules typically are round, form an acute angle with the cyst wall, and tend to be predominantly hyperechoic (111) (Fig. 12).

Probably the most characteristic and specific finding of a benign cystic teratoma is the presence of acoustic shadowing, either in the mural nodule or central mass, occurring in about 25% of cases (123). Acoustic shadowing does not necessarily imply calcified material such as teeth, but may rather represent a matted mixture of sebum and hair. At times posterior shadowing from hair may impair visualization of the back wall of the tumor, the so-called "iceberg" sign (48). Occasionally a fat-fluid or fluid-fluid level may be noted.

Approximately one-third of benign dermoid cysts or teratomas are purely anechoic or predominantly echogenic (133). The purely anechoic lesions contain primarily serous fluid or sebum. Small mural nodules, less than 4 mm in diameter, usually are found on pathologic examination. In general, these are too small to be detected by sonography (Fig. 13). Predominantly solid tumors contain primarily hair and fat and a sparse amount of fluid or sebaceous material (Fig. 14).

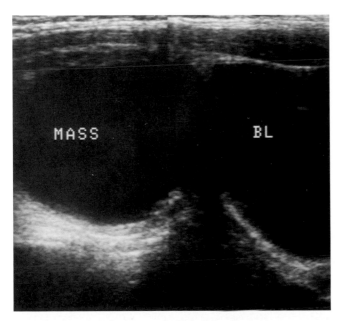

FIG. 13. Cystic ovarian teratoma. A transverse sonogram through the right adnexa shows a large predominantly cystic mass (*MASS*) with a thin wall. At surgery, the lesion contained a 4 mm mural nodule not visible by sonography. *BL,* bladder.

Malignant Ovarian Lesions

Primary Neoplasms

Ovarian germ cell tumors account for 60% to 90% of malignant ovarian neoplasms in childhood, with stromal tumors (Sertoli-Leydig, granulosa-theca, and

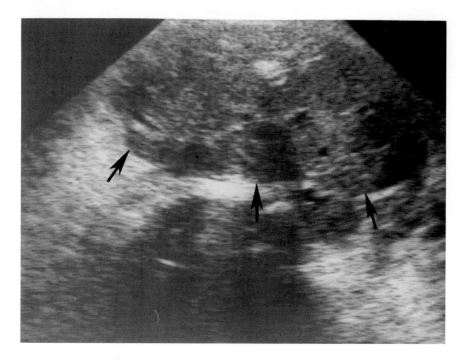

FIG. 15. Malignant ovarian tumor. Longitudinal scan of the right adnexa shows a large complex mass (*arrows*) containing irregular hypo- and hyperechogenic areas. Malignant dysgerminoma was identified pathologically.

undifferentiated neoplasms) having a 10% to 13% incidence and epithelial carcinomas comprising some 5% to 11% of gonadal tumors (16,22,75). The most common germ cell tumors in order of decreasing frequency are dysgerminoma, endodermal sinus tumor, immature teratoma, embryonal carcinoma, and choriocarcinoma. Most malignant tumors occur in postpubertal children just after 13 years of age. Symptoms are nonspecific and include abdominal pain, mass, or disten-

tion, followed by gastrointestinal symptoms such as nausea, vomiting, and anorexia (28,29).

Sonography cannot provide a specific histologic diagnosis, but it can be useful in determining the origin, size, and internal characteristics of the mass. Malignant solid ovarian tumors have variable sonographic appearances, being usually solid or mixed solid-cystic (Fig. 15). Other features of malignancy include irregular margins, papillary masses, or thickened or irreg-

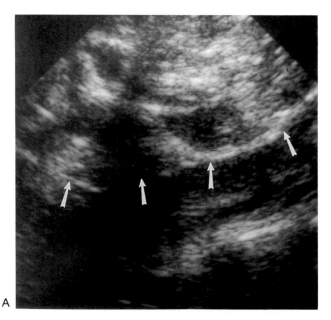

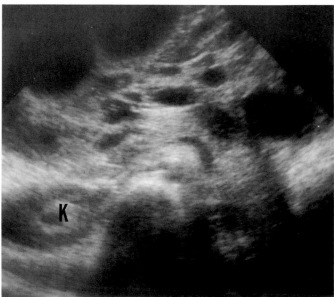

FIG. 16. Malignant ovarian teratoma. **A:** Longitudinal scan demonstrates a poorly defined predominantly echogenic mass (*arrows*) in the anterior pelvis. **B:** On a transverse scan at a higher level the mass is more heterogeneous with multiple cystic areas separated by thick septae. *K,* kidney.

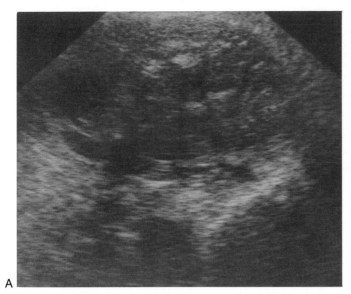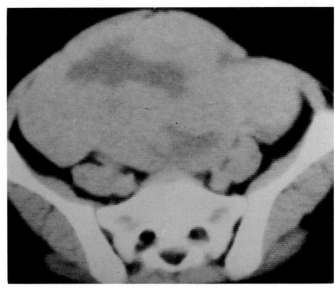

FIG. 17. Ovarian dysgerminoma. **A:** Longitudinal scan shows a predominantly hypoechoic mass with a few echogenic areas within the pelvis. **B:** CT scan shows a large inhomogeneous mass occupying almost the entire pelvis. Several areas of necrosis are present. Although sonography showed the tumor, CT is superior in demonstrating the extent of spread and the relationship of the tumor to surrounding structures.

ular septa in a multicystic mass (138) (Fig. 16). Fluid is present in the cul-de-sac in 50% of malignant ovarian tumors. In advanced cases, ascites, peritoneal implants, pelvic and retroperitoneal adenopathy, and hepatic metastases may be detected by sonography (105).

Secondary Neoplasms

Neuroblastoma, lymphoma, and leukemia may all involve the ovaries during childhood. Patients are usually asymptomatic and the diagnosis is rarely made prior to autopsy. Rarely, the tumors grow large enough to produce a palpable mass. The sonographic appearance may be that of diffuse ovarian enlargement or a poorly marginated mass with smooth or irregular margins (12,68,130). The echotexture ranges from cystic to solid with areas of decreased echogenicity representing necrosis or hemorrhage.

Comparative Imaging of Gynecologic Masses

Sonography is used for the initial evaluation of patients suspected of having gynecologic masses because it does not involve ionizing radiation. However, it is not the procedure of choice in preoperative staging. Ovarian tumors may spread by local extension, by peritoneal seeding, or by dissemination through the lymphatics and blood vessels. Because they better demonstrate the extent of disease in the presacral space, pelvic side walls, retroperitoneum, and peritoneal surfaces, CT and MR imaging are more accurate than sonography for staging ovarian malignancy (Fig. 17).

PELVIC INFLAMMATORY DISEASE

Pelvic inflammatory disease occurs almost exclusively in sexually active postpubertal patients and is rare in premenopausal girls. The infection spreads in a retrograde fashion from the vagina and cervix to the endometrium. Eventually the fallopian tubes become infected and as the disease progresses, purulent material exudes from the fimbria to involve the ovaries, parametrium, and peritoneal cavity. The inflammatory process is usually bilateral, but occasionally only one adnexa is involved. The majority of cases are caused by *Neisseria gonorrhoeae, Chlamydia trachomatis,* and endogeneous anaerobic organisms. Rarely, pelvic inflammation is due to ruptured appendiceal or postsurgical abscesses. These disorders, however, are not usually referred to as pelvic inflammatory disease.

The classical signs and symptoms of acute pelvic inflammatory disease include pelvic pain, vaginal discharge, fever, cervical motion tenderness, and adnexal tenderness. Unfortunately, these findings occur in only 20% of affected patients (59). Other conditions that can produce findings similar to pelvic inflammatory disease include ruptured ectopic pregnancy or cystic teratoma, hemorrhagic ovarian cyst, and appendiceal abscess. Sonography in conjunction with the history, physical examination, and laboratory studies often can differentiate these diseases.

The sonographic findings in pelvic inflammatory disease are variable (136). Early in the course of infection, there are minimal if any abnormalities on sonography. Occasionally, the uterine outline becomes indistinct,

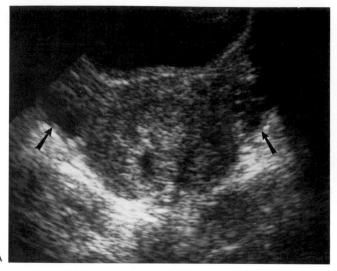

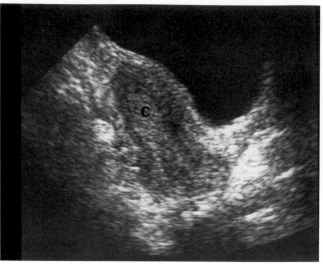

FIG. 18. Pelvic inflammatory disease. **A:** Transverse and **B:** longitudinal images of the pelvis show an enlarged uterus with an echogenic central canal (*C*). The planes between the uterus and ovaries are poorly defined. Small cysts are noted in both ovaries (*arrows*). *N. gonorrhoeae* was cultured from vaginal secretions.

a finding known as the "indefinite uterus" sign (Fig. 18). The uterus also may appear more hyperechoic than normal and contain a small amount of fluid centrally. With adequate treatment, the uterus returns to normal.

Recurrent, acute infection leads to more significant involvement of the uterus and fallopian tubes and produces a wider range of abnormalities on the pelvic sonogram. Indicative of more serious infection, pyosalpinx appears on sonography as hypoechoic tubular masses, containing internal echoes representing pu-

rulent debris. Tubo-ovarian abscess is another sign of significant infection and has been reported in 20% of adolescents with pelvic inflammatory disease (39). Early in its course it can appear predominantly solid, similar to inflammatory masses elsewhere in the body. Later the abscess becomes more cystic as necrosis and liquefaction occur, and occasionally contains fluid-debris levels and septations. Typically, the walls are thick, irregular, and shaggy (10,134) (Fig. 19).

Large amounts of fluid in the cul-de-sac also indicate extraadnexal extension of inflammation. If the fluid

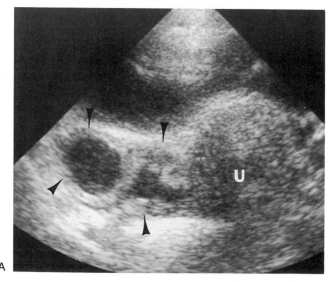

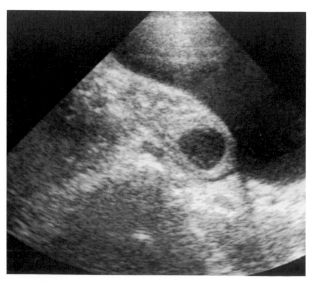

FIG. 19. Tubo-ovarian abscess. **A:** Transverse and **B:** longitudinal scans of the right adnexa show an irregular, thick-walled mass (*arrowheads*) with several cystic areas representing a tubo-ovarian abscess. The margins between the mass and the uterus (*U*) are poorly defined.

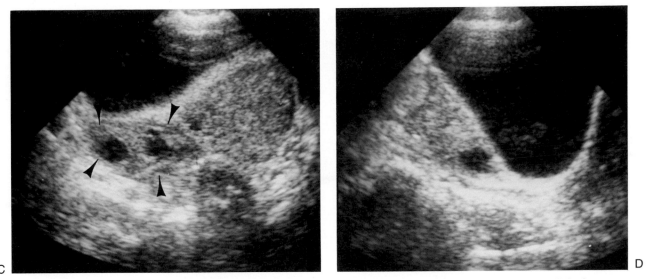

FIG. 19. *Continued.* **C:** Transverse and **D:** longitudinal scans of the pelvis 1 week after antibiotic therapy show decreased size of the adnexal mass (*arrowheads*) and of the fluid-filled areas.

becomes loculated, a peritoneal abscess may form which typically is poorly defined and appears as a complex mass with solid and cystic areas posterior to the uterus. With extensive involvement, pelvic anatomy may be so distorted that the uterus is not identifiable. Multiple abscesses can be found within the peritoneal cavity if the disease process extends outside of the cul-de-sac.

Although the diagnosis of pelvic inflammatory disease is usually made clinically, sonography can be valuable not only in confirming the diagnosis, but also in assessing response to treatment. Following appropriate antibiotic treatment, pelvic inflammatory disease may resolve or may leave chronic residua, such as hydrosalpinx, inflammatory cysts, or adhesions. Hydrosalpinx usually appears as unilateral or bilateral fusiform or round, sonolucent adnexal masses (Fig. 20), while inflammatory cysts frequently appear as spherical masses. Differentiation between hydrosalpinx and ovarian cysts may not be possible sonographically.

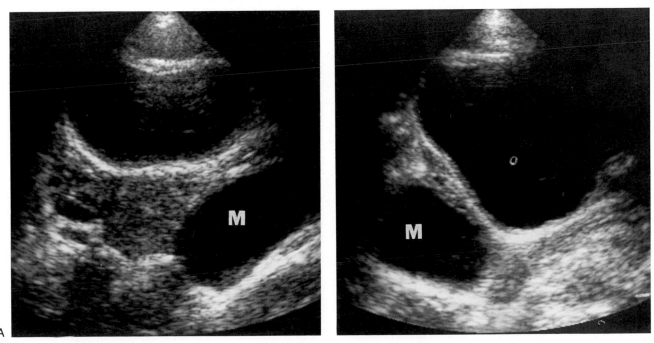

FIG. 20. Hydrosalpinx. **A:** Transverse and **B:** longitudinal sonograms demonstrate a tubular sonolucent mass (*M*) in the left adnexa, which was laparoscopically confirmed to be a hydrosalpinx.

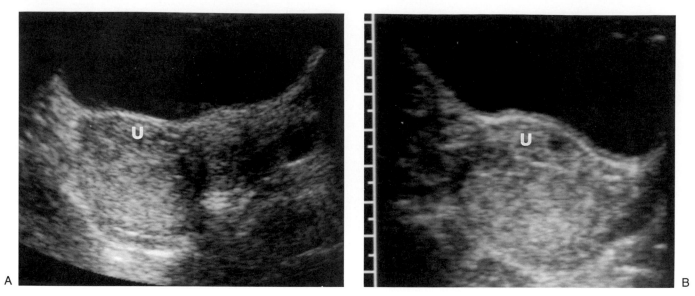

FIG. 21. Ovarian torsion. **A:** Transverse and **B:** longitudinal sonograms show a large mass with slight acoustic enhancement behind the uterus (*U*). The planes between the uterus and the mass are poorly defined. At operation, the right adnexa contained a hemorrhagic cyst that had undergone torsion.

OVARIAN TORSION

Torsion of the ovary and fallopian tube is the result of partial or complete rotation of the ovarian pedicle on its axis, producing vascular impairment, congestion of the ovarian parenchyma, and ultimately hemorrhagic infarction. The underlying adnexa most often is abnormal, containing a cyst or tumor that acts as a fulcrum to potentiate torsion (31,42,47). Torsion of a normal adnexa occurs less frequently. The most likely explanation for the latter event is that the adnexae of young patients are normally very mobile and move with changes in intraabdominal pressure or body position (61). Rarely, adnexal torsion is bilateral (147).

Torsion of the ovary and fallopian tube is more common during the first 2 decades of life, usually in the premenarchal age group (56). The typical presentation of torsion is acute lower abdominal pain often associated with nausea, vomiting, and leukocytosis (47,61). A palpable mass is present in about 50% of children.

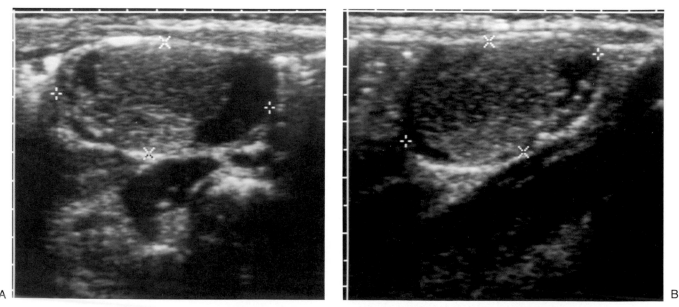

FIG. 22. Torsion of normal adnexa. **A:** Transverse and **B:** longitudinal sonograms show an enlarged right ovary (*calipers*) with peripheral cysts. At operation, the right ovary had undergone torsion and contained numerous dilated follicles.

A history of previous episodes of similar pain is found in at least half of the patients.

The sonographic findings of adnexal torsion are non-specific and include a relatively echogenic mass in a midline location, free fluid in the cul-de-sac, and other adnexal pathology such as cysts or tumors (31,42,43,143,147) (Fig. 21). The torsed ovary and tube usually demonstrate good sound transmission, reflecting the pathologic findings of vascular engorgement and stromal edema (31). The only sign considered relatively specific for ovarian torsion is the presence of multiple, small (8–12 mm in size), peripherally located cysts. These cystic changes are attributed to transudation of fluid into follicles secondary to vascular congestion and have been found in up to 74% of torsed normal ovaries (42,43) (Fig. 22). In the absence of prominent follicles, the diagnostic considerations must include other conditions such as appendiceal abscess, hemorrhagic ovarian cyst, and dermoid cyst.

UTERUS AND VAGINA

Normal Development

Prepubertal

The normal fetal uterus increases in size late in gestation as the result of maternal hormonal stimulation. During the first week of life, the uterus can be identified in almost 90% of full-term infant girls by sonography (95). The normal neonatal uterus is a prominent structure with a length ranging from 2.3 to 4.6 cm (mean, 3.4 cm), fundal width ranging from 0.8 to 2.1 cm (mean, 1.2 cm), and cervical width ranging from 0.8 to 2.2 cm (mean, 1.4 cm) (95). During the neonatal period, the uterus regresses in size because of falling levels of maternal hormones, so that the corpus or fundus eventually becomes smaller than the cervix. From infancy until approximately 7 years of age, uterine size shows little change, with a length ranging between 2.5 and 3.3 cm, a fundal width between 0.4 and 1.0 cm, and cervical width between 0.6 and 1.0 cm (58, 102,122).

In the neonate, the uterus has a tubular or spade shape. The endometrial cavity is visualized in almost all infants (97%) as a thin, highly echogenic line in the center of the uterus (Fig. 23). This linear echo is caused either by mucus or secretions within the uterine cavity or by the endometrium itself. A hypoechoic halo surrounding the endometrial canal will be noted in about 30% of neonatal uteri. This halo is believed to represent the inner third of the myometrium, which is hypoechoic because of vascular engorgement (95). A small amount of endometrial fluid is present in about 25% of neonatal uteri.

After 7 years of age, the uterus undergoes an increase in length and width, with the corpus growing faster than the cervix. In the sagittal plane the endometrial canal can be visualized as a thin echogenic line in almost all patients. It is continuous with the vagina, which also appears as a bright, midline, echogenic line, corresponding to apposed mucosal linings.

Postpubertal

As puberty approaches, the uterus descends with the adnexa deeper into the pelvis. Typically, the fundus elongates and thickens and ultimately becomes larger

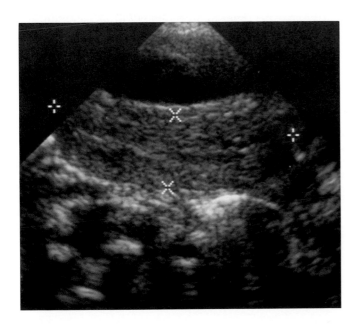

FIG. 23. Normal uterus of a 2-month-old girl. A longitudinal sonogram shows a normal tubular uterus (*calipers*) with no clear-cut separation between cervix and fundus. A thin, central echogenic line is present, representing the endometrial canal. Uterine length is 2.3 cm.

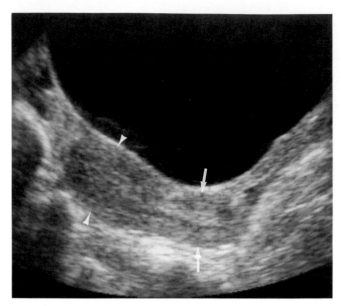

FIG. 24. Normal uterus in a 14-year-old girl. A longitudinal sonogram shows a pear-shaped configuration. The anterior-posterior (AP) diameter of the fundus (*arrowheads*) is larger than the AP diameter of the cervix (*arrows*).

than the cervix, producing the adult pear-shaped uterus (Fig. 24). After puberty, the uterus measures 5 to 8 cm in length, 1.6 to 3 cm in maximum anteroposterior diameter, and 3.5 cm in width (71,122).

Physiology

The sonographic appearance of the uterus after puberty can be correlated with cyclic changes in the endometrium (34,49,109,116). There are two main layers of the endometrium: the functionalis layer which thickens and sheds with each menses, and the basalis layer which remains intact throughout the cycle and contains the vessels which supply the endometrium as it thickens. The endometrial changes can be divided into three phases: menstrual, proliferative, and secretory (Fig. 25). In the menstrual phase, lasting about 5 days, the functionalis layer of the endometrium is shed, leaving only the basal layer subjacent to the myometrium. During this phase, the endometrium appears as a thin, slightly irregular, echogenic line on sonography, presumably reflecting blood and sloughed tissue in the uterine canal. During the proliferative phase, lasting about 9 days, the endometrium increases in thickness as ovulation approaches. In the first few days of the phase, the endometrium may appear hypoechoic, probably reflecting the straight and orderly arrangement of glands within the functionalis layer. By the time of ovulation, the endometrium is moderately thick, measuring 3 to 5 mm in diameter, and quite echogenic, a reflection of the increased tortuosity of the

glandular elements. Immediately after ovulation, the innermost part of the endometrium becomes hypoechoic and is surrounded by echogenic tissue. This appearance, best appreciated on transverse sonograms, has been referred to as a ring sign and is probably a reflection of stromal edema in the functionalis (49). In the secretory phase, lasting 14 days, the endometrium reaches maximal echogenicity and thickness, measuring 5 to 6 mm. The increase in endometrial echogenicity and thickness reflects distention of the endometrial glands with mucin and glycogen. This appearance persists until the onset of menses (34,116).

Congenital Abnormalities

Uterine Agenesis and Hypoplasia

Uterine malformations are relatively infrequent, occurring in 0.1% to 0.5% of all women. The spectrum of anomalies includes agenesis, hypoplasia, and duplication (26,85). The most common causes of an absent uterus are the testicular feminization and Mayer-Rokitansky-Küster-Hauser syndromes. Patients with testicular feminization have a 46XY karyotype and typically female external genitalia. The vagina ends blindly in a pouch, and the uterus is absent. The gonads are testes which produce normal male levels of testosterone, but there is end organ insensitivity to androgens. In adolescents, amenorrhea is the usual presenting symptom. A uterus cannot be identified on sonography, but testes may be noted in the inguinal area.

In patients with the Mayer-Rokitansky-Küster-Hauser syndrome, the uterus is rudimentary or absent while the ovaries and fallopian tubes are normal. There is a high rate of association with vaginal absence or hypoplasia, renal abnormalities (50%) including renal agenesis, ectopia, fusion anomalies, and duplication, and skeletal (12%) anomalies. Affected patients have a normal female karyotype and secondary sexual development, and present with primary amenorrhea. The sonographic findings of Mayer-Rokitansky-Küster-Hauser syndrome are uterine or vaginal absence or a severely atretic uterus or vagina with absence of the midline echoes (36,140).

Uterine hypoplasia may be an isolated finding, although more frequently it is associated with Turner's syndrome. An acquired cause of a hypoplastic uterus is exposure to diethylstilbestrol *in utero* (141). The most common features of diethylstilbestrol exposure on sonography are a small T-shaped uterus, lacking the normal bulbous expansion of the uterine body. Other significant genital anomalies associated with diethylstilbestrol relate to the vagina and include adenosis and clear cell carcinoma.

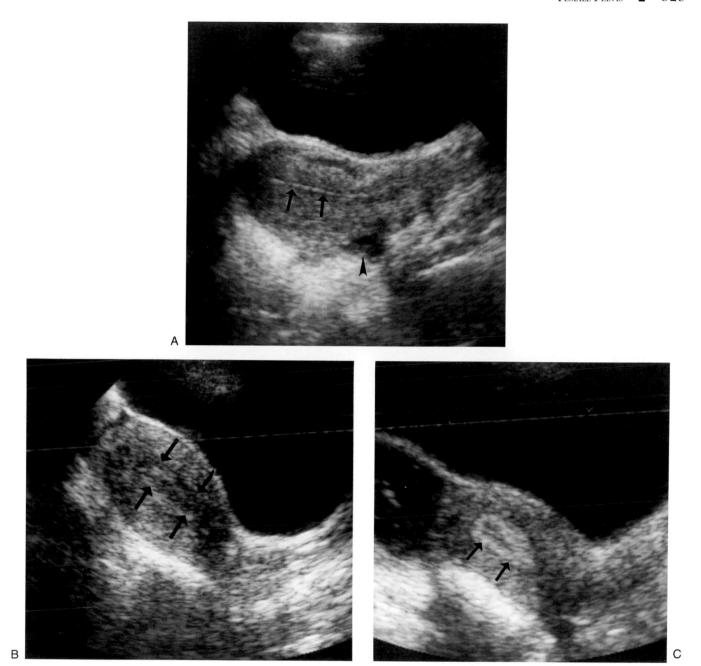

FIG. 25. Phases of endometrial development. **A:** In the menstrual phase, the endometrial canal is seen as a thin, echogenic interface (*arrows*). A small amount of fluid is seen in the cul-de-sac (*arrowhead*). **B:** Longitudinal scan in the proliferative phase shows a relatively hypoechoic endometrium surrounded by a thin rim of echogenic tissue (*arrows*). **C:** Longitudinal scan in the secretory phase demonstrates a thickened, echogenic endometrium (*arrows*).

Uterine Duplication

The uterus and upper two-thirds of the vagina arise from fused portions of the müllerian ducts, while the lower vagina and vestibule arise from the urogenital sinus. A multiplicity of anomalies can occur from total or partial absence of müllerian duct fusion during prenatal life (85). Complete absence of union results in two vaginas, two cervices, and two uterine corpora (uterine didelphys). This anomaly often is associated with cloacal exstrophy. Partial absence of fusion may result in a single vagina; two cervices and two uteri (uterus duplex bicollis); or one vagina, one cervix, and two uteri (uterus duplex unicollis or bicornuate uterus). Rarely, there may be a single uterus, single cervix, and single vagina, with a septum dividing the

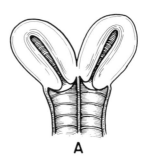
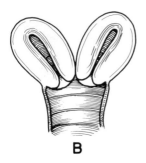
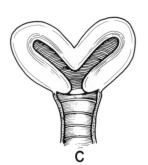
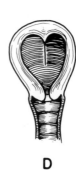

FIG. 26. Müllerian duct fusion anomalies. **A:** Uterus didelphys. Two uteri, two cervices, two vaginas. **B:** Uterus duplex bicollis. Two uteri, two cervices, one vagina. **C:** Uterus duplex unicollis. Two uteri, one cervix, one vagina. **D:** Uterus septus. Single uterus divided by a septum. (Adapted from ref. 20.)

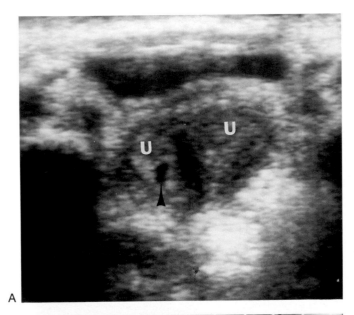

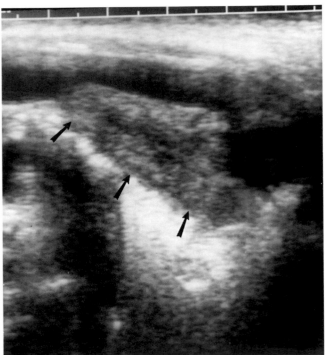

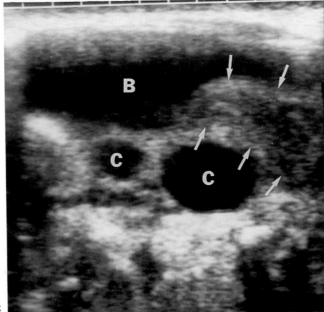

FIG. 27. Bicornuate uterus in a neonate. **A:** Transverse image shows two separate uteri (*U*) with flared fundi. Also noted is fluid in the right (*black arrowhead*) uterine cavity. **B:** Longitudinal parasagittal image shows the left uterine horn (*black arrows*). **C:** Right parasagittal image shows the uterine horn (*white arrows*) and a multicystic (*C*) structure that at operation was a multicystic dysplastic kidney. *B,* bladder.

uterus into two compartments (uterus septus) (20) (Fig. 26). The clinical presentation of uterine duplication in neonates is a lower abdominal or pelvic mass. Occasionally the diagnosis is delayed until menarche when the patient presents with hematocolpos, or the condition may be detected later as an incidental finding during obstetrical sonography (11,89,107,119,135). On sonography, bicornuate uterus or uterus duplex bicollis can be suggested when two separate uterine cornua with flared margins are identified (Fig. 27). The diagnosis of uterine didelphys is suggested when a bilobed uterine shape and two distinct vaginas are seen (Fig. 28). Obstruction of one or both components of the uterus, as well as unilateral renal anomalies, also may be encountered (Fig. 29). The septate uterus is characterized by a nearly normal external contour, in contradistinction to the bicornuate uterus which has a flared fundus and a midline echogenic septum (113).

Vaginal Obstruction

Congenital vaginal obstruction may be encountered in the neonatal period or at the time of menarche. If only the vagina is dilated, the obstruction is termed hydrocolpos, while if both the uterus and the vagina are involved, it is termed hydrometrocolpos. If the discharge is bloody, the condition is termed hematometrocolpos. In infancy, vaginal obstruction may be due to vaginal atresia, high-grade stenosis, transverse septum, or an imperforate membrane. The maternal sex hormones to which the fetus is exposed *in utero* can persist in the infant in the early postnatal period, causing production and excessive accumulation of secretions in the vagina or in the uterus and vagina. The end result clinically is a palpable, firm, midline mass in the pelvis and/or abdomen. If the obstruction is low in the vagina, the accumulated secretions may evert the obstructing membrane or septum, giving rise to a bulging mass at the introitus (94). Almost all patients with vaginal or cervical stenosis or atresia have severe and often multiple congenital anomalies, particularly fistulaes, bicornuate uterus, urogenital sinus, unilateral renal agenesis, imperforate anus, esophageal or duodenal atresia, and congenital heart disease (62,118).

If vaginal distention is not present at birth, recognition of the problem may be delayed until menarche. Vaginal obstruction in pubertal girls is most often the result of a simple imperforate membrane or hymen, rather than vaginal atresia. Most patients present with recurrent lower abdominal pain or a lower abdominal mass. There is no increased association of congenital anomalies in patients with imperforate hymen, in contrast to the higher incidence of such anomalies in neonates with vaginal atresia.

The sonographic findings of hydrometrocolpos are those of a tubular, predominantly cystic, midline mass,

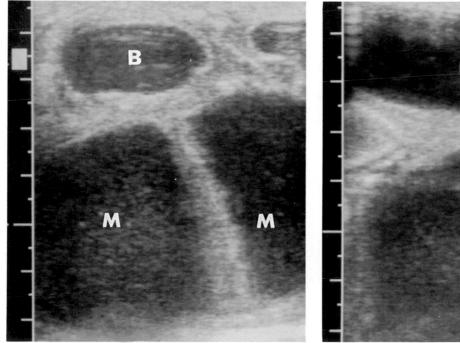
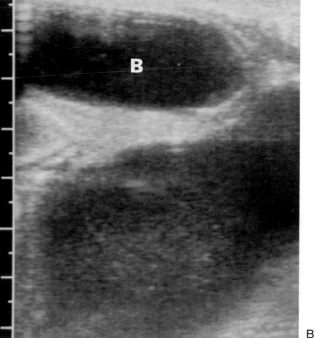

FIG. 28. Uterus didelphys. **A:** Transverse image shows two thin-walled, fluid-filled masses (*M*) representing dilated vaginas, in the pelvis of a newborn girl. Operation revealed two separate vaginas, cervices, and uterine corpora. *B,* bladder. **B:** On a longitudinal scan, the right vagina extends to the top of the bladder (*B*).

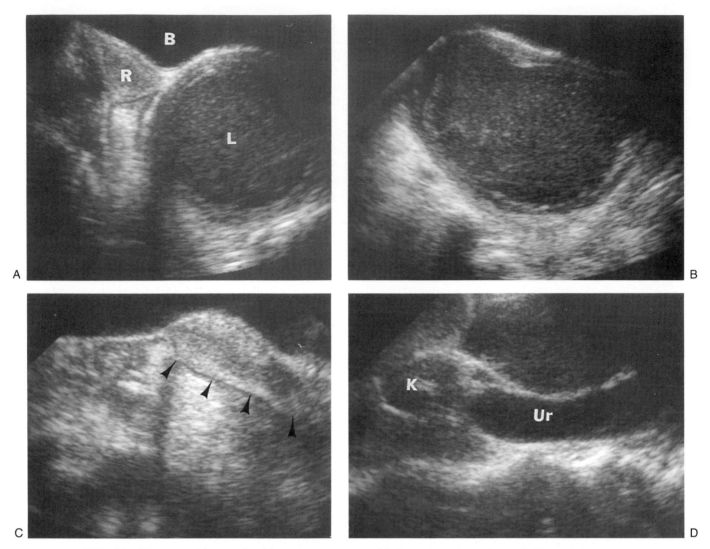

FIG. 29. Obstructed horn of a bicornuate uterus with hematometrocolpos. **A:** Transverse sonogram through the midpelvis demonstrates a normal right (*R*) uterine fundus posterior to the bladder (*B*). The obstructed left (*L*) uterine fundus appears as a hypoechoic mass indenting the left lateral aspect of the bladder. **B:** Left parasagittal image shows the dilated left uterine horn. **C:** Right parasagittal image shows a normal right horn (*arrowheads*). **D:** Longitudinal scan through the left flank demonstrates a hypoplastic kidney (*K*) with a dilated left ureter (*Ur*).

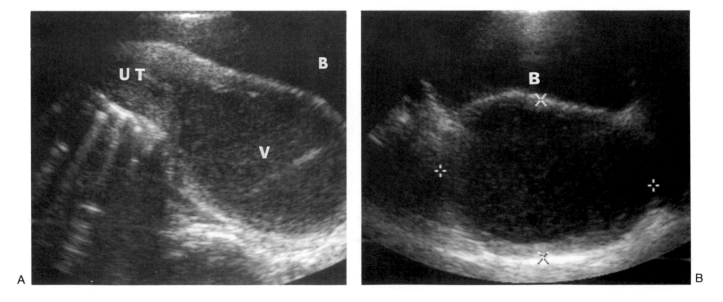

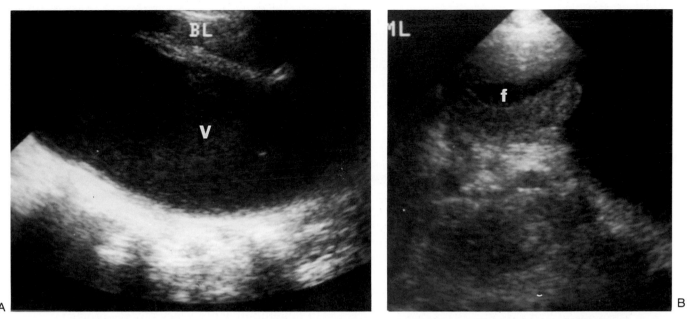

FIG. 31. Hydrometrocolpos in a 13-year-old girl. **A:** Longitudinal sonogram shows a markedly dilated vagina (*V*); *BL,* bladder. **B:** A much smaller uterus is identified on a longitudinal scan at a higher level. Fluid (*f*) is noted in the uterine cavity.

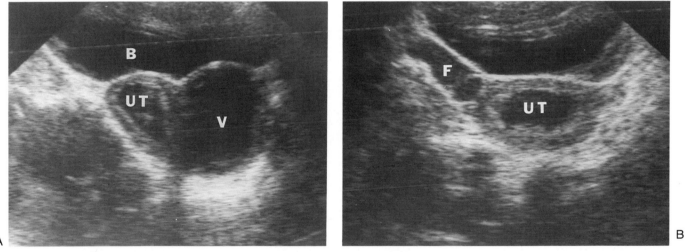

FIG. 32. Hematometrocolpos in a 14-year-old girl. **A:** Longitudinal pelvic sonogram shows a distended bladder (*B*) anterior to a dilated, fluid-filled vagina (*V*) and thick-walled uterus (*UT*). Low-level echoes, representing blood, are noted in the uterine cavity. **B:** On a transverse scan, the dilated, thick-walled uterus (*UT*) is contiguous with a dilated right fallopian tube (*F*).

representing the dilated vagina and uterus, between the bladder and rectum (72,120,145) (Fig. 30). The vagina contains most of the blood and is about five to nine times larger than the uterus (1) (Fig. 31). Not infrequently, scattered internal echoes representing cellular debris or a fluid-debris level will be present within the

uterus or vagina. Occasionally, the fallopian tubes also will be filled with blood, particularly in the pubertal girl (Fig. 32). If large enough, the mass can displace and obstruct the ureters, giving rise to hydronephrosis.

Fluid within the vagina occasionally can be seen as a normal finding in infants and younger children. It

FIG. 30. Hydrometrocolpos in an 11-year-old girl. **A:** Longitudinal pelvic sonogram shows a dilated, fluid-filled vagina (*V*) posterior to the bladder (*B*). The uterus (*UT*) is identified superior to the vagina. **B:** On a transverse sonogram, the dilated vagina (*calipers*) indents the posterior wall of the bladder (*B*). An obstructing transverse vaginal septum was confirmed at surgery.

occurs when urine refluxes from the bladder into the vagina during voiding because the patient is in a supine position. In older girls and adolescents, it can occur during sonography when the bladder is overdistended and a small amount of urine refluxes into the vagina (124). Differentiation from obstructive hydrocolpos is made by rescanning the patient after having her stand erect (80).

Tumor

Rhabdomyosarcoma

Rhabdomyosarcoma is the most common malignant tumor of the vagina and uterus in childhood, usually occurring in girls under 4 years of age. The typical clinical presentation of vaginal rhabdomyosarcoma is a vaginal mass, discharge, or bleeding. If the mass is of sufficient size, it may present as a grapelike cluster of gray masses prolapsing through the vagina, known as sarcoma botryoides (94). Uterine rhabdomyosarcoma presents predominantly as an abdominal mass (146). Pathologically, rhabdomyosarcoma is an aggressive tumor that tends to metastasize early by direct extension and hematogeneous and lymphatic dissemination. Distant metastases are to liver, lung, and bone.

On sonography, rhabdomyosarcoma appears as a soft tissue mass enlarging the vagina or uterus (54,81,146) (Fig. 33). Central areas of decreased echogenicity are present if the tumor undergoes necrosis or ulceration. In some cases the primary tumor may occlude the cervical os, resulting in uterine enlargement and fluid collections in the endometrial cavity. Lymph node metastases can also be detected if the involved nodes are enlarged.

The role of imaging in patients with a suspected vaginal or uterine tumor is to determine the presence or absence of local invasion into pelvic fat, adjacent viscera, or pelvic lymph nodes, and distant metastatic disease. Accurate determination of the tumor extent is important in planning treatment and assessing prognosis. Sonography is a good screening examination and can detect the presence of tumor and occasionally lymph nodes, but it cannot accurately determine distant extent of tumor outside the uterus or vagina. Once the diagnosis has been established, CT or MR imaging is required for precise evaluation of tumoral extension in order to plan treatment (38,132).

Adenocarcinoma of the Vagina

Carcinoma of the vagina is much less common than rhabdomyosarcoma. Typically, this neoplasm is found in children under 2 years of age, producing vaginal bleeding or a polypoid growth resembling sarcoma botryoides (131). It also has been reported in adolescent girls who have been exposed to diethylstilbestrol *in utero*. Histologically, the most common type is clear cell carcinoma (93). Sonographically, the appearance is identical to that of rhabdomyosarcoma (54).

PRECOCIOUS PUBERTY

Precocious puberty in females is almost always isosexual and characterized by the premature development of secondary sex characteristics, gonadal development, and ovulation before 8 years of age. Over 80% of cases of true sexual precocity are due to idiopathic activation of the hypothalamic-pituitary-gonadal axis.

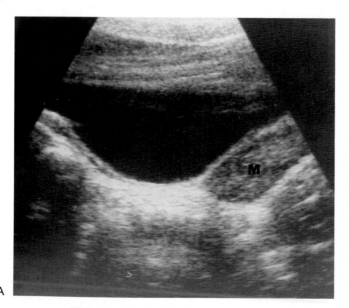

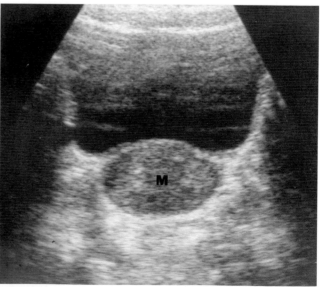

A

B

FIG. 33. Vaginal rhabdomyosarcoma. **A:** Longitudinal and **B:** transverse scans demonstrate an echogenic mass (*M*) in the vagina. Surgery confirmed a rhabdomyosarcoma arising from the cervix.

Occasionally lesions of the central nervous system, located in the pituitary gland or hypothalamus, are demonstrated (115). In true precocious puberty, levels of luteinizing hormones increase in response to the gonadotropin-releasing factor stimulation test.

In contrast to true precocious puberty, pseudoprecocious puberty is caused by lesions outside the hypothalamic-pituitary axis. Patients with pseudoprecocious puberty may have iso- or heterosexual sexual characteristics. Gonadal enlargement may be present, but there is no ovulation. Ovarian tumors, including granulosa-theca cell tumors, arrhenoblastomas, cysts, thecomas and choriocarcinomas, and rarely adrenal tumors such as adenomas and carcinomas, are causes of pseudoprecocious puberty (8,27,71,73,127). Levels

of luteinizing hormone remain prepubertal in response to gonadotropin-releasing factor.

The primary role of sonography is to determine ovarian and uterine size. This information may be valuable in distinguishing between true precocious and pseudoprecocious puberty. In patients with true precocious puberty, adult-size ovaries and uterus are present, with a prevalence of the corpus over the cervix. Ovarian and uterine sizes may be normal or enlarged in patients with pseudoprecocious puberty. Occasionally large ovaries or cysts are encountered in patients with pseudoprecocious puberty, often in association with the McCune-Albright syndrome (fibrous dysplasia, cutaneous pigmentation, and sexual precocity) and neurofibromatosis (8,30,121,127) (Fig. 34).

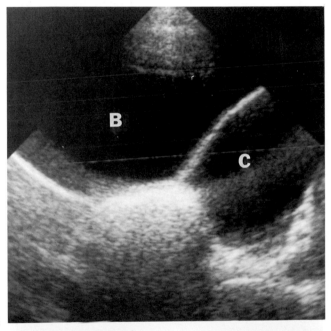

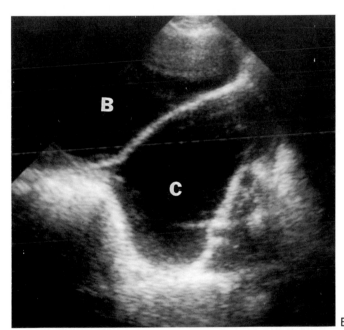

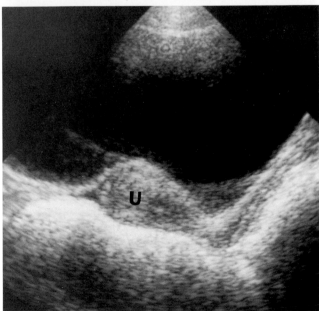

FIG. 34. Functioning follicular ovarian cyst in a 3-year-old girl with pseudoprecocious puberty. **A:** Transverse and **B:** longitudinal scans of the pelvis show a 4 cm cyst (*C*) in the area of the left ovary, displacing the urinary bladder (*B*) to the right. **C:** The uterus (*U*) has an adult size and shape.

Sonography also can be used to evaluate the effect of treatment of precocious puberty. With appropriate therapy, the ovaries and uterus decrease and revert to prepubertal volumes and configuration (51).

AMENORRHEA

Primary amenorrhea is characterized by the failure of menses by age 16 years. The etiology of primary amenorrhea is varied and includes hypothalamic and pituitary lesions, androgen-producing adrenal tumors, and primary abnormalities of the ovary (gonadal dysgenesis, Stein-Leventhal syndrome, or neoplasm), the uterus (intersex syndromes, agenesis, testicular feminization syndrome), or the vagina (imperforate hymen, vaginal atresia, or stenosis). The appearance of most of these lesions has been discussed previously in this chapter.

INTERSEX STATES

Based on gonadal histology, the intersex state may be classified as female pseudohermaphrodite, male pseudohermaphrodite, true hermaphrodite, and mixed gonadal dysgenesis (2). The clinical findings of intersex states are ambiguous genitalia including cryptorchidism, labial fusion, clitoromegaly, epispadius, and hypospadius. When external genitalia are ambiguous, knowledge of internal genital anatomy can be determined by sonography. Such information can be important in assigning a sex to the individual.

Female pseudohermaphrodites have a normal karyotype (46XX); normal ovarian, uterine, and vaginal anatomy; and masculinized external genitalia. The etiology of this condition is believed to be exposure to excessive androgens at some point in the first trimester, often in association with the adrenogenital syndrome. Sonography confirms the female gender by identifying the presence of ovaries and uterus.

Male pseudohermaphroditism is characterized by the presence of testes, feminized or ambiguous external genitalia, and an XY karyotype. This disorder is due to a deficiency of testicular secretions or an abnormal response by target organs. Sonography is useful in excluding the presence of ovaries and a uterus and in some patients may locate undescended testes (40).

True hermaphrodites, having both ovarian and testicular tissue, and, hence, either an XX or XY karyotype, account for less than 10% of the intersex states. They usually have an ovary on one side and a testis on the other side or an ovary opposite an ovotestis. A uterus typically is present but it may be hypoplastic. Histologically, the ovary is often normal but the testicular tissue is primitive, or if normal initially, may develop degenerative changes at puberty. The anatomy of the external genitalia is variable, ranging from feminine with slight clitoral prominence to nearly com-

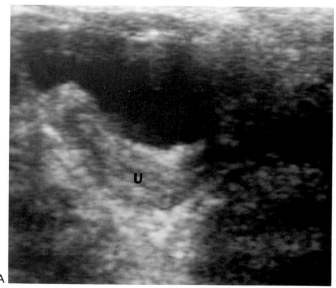
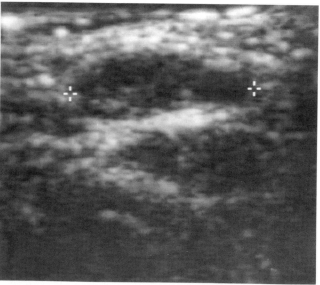

FIG. 35. True hermaphrodite. A 2-year-old child with ambiguous external genitalia and a palpable mass in the left inguinal area. **A:** A longitudinal sonogram through the midline of the pelvis demonstrates a small uterus (*U*) posterior to a fluid-filled bladder. **B:** A transverse sonogram through the palpable mass in the left inguinal area demonstrates a homogeneous, ovoid structure (*cursors*). Biopsy of the left inguinal mass revealed both ovarian and testicular tissue and the diagnosis of true hermaphrodite was established.

plete masculinization. Sonography can demonstrate the uterus if present and may be successful in identifying a gonad for biopsy (Fig. 35).

Patients with mixed gonadal dysgenesis have both a testis and a gonadal streak with an XO/XY karyotype. Although the external genitalia are nearly always ambiguous, gonads are usually palpable on one or both sides and may even be located within the scrotum. The streak gonad is composed of tissue resembling ovarian stroma, but without oocytes. A uterus, sometimes bicornuate, is generally present. Sonography is useful to visualize the uterus and to confirm the position of the gonad for biopsy.

NONGYNECOLOGIC PELVIC MASSES

Presacral Masses

Neoplasms arising from the presacral space or sacrum may extend into the anterior pelvis and be confused with adnexal masses. However, the close association of these lesions with the bony pelvis usually allows the correct diagnosis to be made. The vast majority of presacral tumors are sacrococcygeal teratomas, neuroblastomas, and lymphomas. Most sacrococcygeal teratomas are benign and noted at birth, but those encountered beyond the neonatal period are more likely to contain malignant elements. Patients with teratomas generally present with a large soft tissue mass in the sacrococcygeal region. The tumor, however, can be predominantly presacral or extrapelvic. Sonography can readily detect the lesion, but the features are nonspecific and include a cystic, solid, or mixed mass (24). Nevertheless, sonography may be valuable in determining the extent of mass and the presence of obstructive hydronephrosis.

Neuroblastoma is a disease of the young child with a mean age of 2 years. Most presacral neuroblastomas present as palpable masses or produce constipation. Symptoms and signs of ureteral obstruction, spinal cord compression, or metastases also may be present. Sonographically, neuroblastoma appears either as a heterogeneously echogenic tumor or as a complex mass with anechoic areas representing hemorrhage and necrosis (144).

Lymphoma most frequently presents as enlargement of the internal or external pelvic lymph nodes and occasionally as a presacral mass. On sonography, lymphomatous nodes in the presacral space or lateral pelvis typically appear as homogeneous sonolucent masses indenting the bladder, although occasionally they may be heterogeneous or solid. Lymphomatous infiltration of various intraabdominal organs such as the liver, spleen, and kidneys also can be seen by sonography.

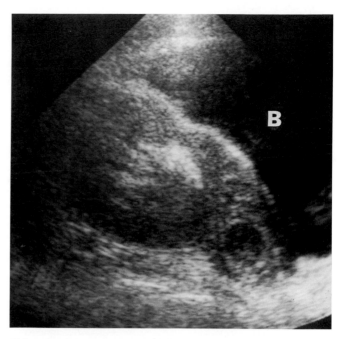

FIG. 36. Appendiceal abscess in a 4-year-old girl. Longitudinal sonogram shows a large, complex, predominantly solid mass displacing the bladder (*B*) anteriorly. Several nonshadowing, echogenic foci are noted within the lesion. Since the right ovary was not identified as a separate structure, the diagnostic considerations included an ovarian teratoma as well as an appendiceal abscess. Surgery confirmed an appendiceal abscess.

Inflammatory Masses

Pelvic abscesses in children generally are related to appendicitis or Crohn's disease, or are a postoperative complication. Typically, abscesses appear as ovoid or irregular fluid collections, usually with internal echoes representing pus and necrotic debris. In the presence of gas, bright echoes with shadowing may occur. Occasionally, thickened bowel wall may be present. Abscesses that occur in the adnexal area or cul-de-sac may be indistinguishable from primary adnexal masses on sonography (Fig. 36). In such instances, clinical findings coupled with the sonographic findings should lead to the correct diagnosis.

OBSTETRICAL APPLICATION

Pregnancy is one of the most common causes of a pelvic mass in postpubertal girls. Sonography is the procedure of choice in imaging the gravid uterus. Its real-time capability combined with its ability to provide images in multiple planes allows demonstration of fetal anatomy in any axis. The primary role of sonography is to recognize the presence of the gravid uterus so that the patient can be appropriately referred

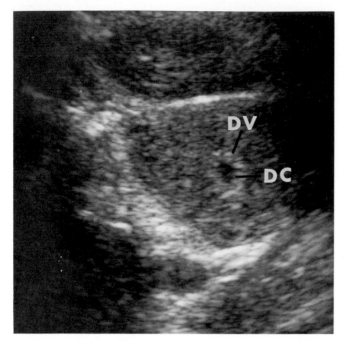

FIG. 37. Early gestational sac. Transverse sonogram shows an intrauterine fluid collection surrounded by a double decidual sac, indicating an intrauterine pregnancy. The double decidual sign is composed of the decidua vera (*DV*) surrounding decidua capsularis (*DC*).

the transabdominal sonographic features of the normal pregnancy and ectopic pregnancy so that appropriate steps in patient management can be taken. For more detailed information about sonography in pregnancy, the reader is referred to standard textbooks (17).

Normal First Trimester Anatomy

The earliest sonographic finding of an intrauterine pregnancy is the gestational sac, appearing as an intrauterine fluid collection surrounded by a rim of moderate echoes, representing the decidua (Fig. 37). The size of the gestational sac when first observed is approximately 2 to 3 mm in diameter. There is some controversy regarding the exact time at which transabdominal sonography can first detect a gestational sac, but it ranges between 3.5 to 5 weeks following the last menstrual period. By 6 weeks the yolk sac becomes consistently visible within the developing gestational sac, and by 7 menstrual weeks, an embryo can be detected (Fig. 38). With modern equipment, fetal cardiac activity is visible concurrently with the visualization of the embryo. From this time forward, the embryonic structures undergo differentiation and variable parts of the fetus can be recognized.

to an obstetrician. In patients who present with abdominal pain it is also important to determine whether the embryo is viable and whether the pregnancy is intrauterine. The following discussion will review briefly

Ectopic Pregnancy

The diagnosis of ectopic pregnancy is important because of its associated morbidity and mortality. Clin-

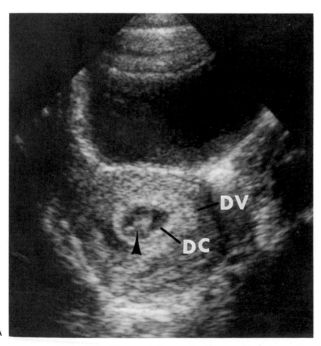

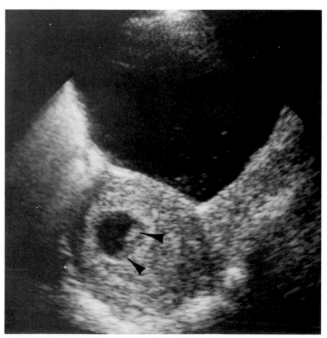

FIG. 38. Normal intrauterine pregnancy. **A:** Transverse and **B:** longitudinal scans of an early pregnancy show an intrauterine fluid collection containing an embryo (*arrowheads*). The double decidual sac sign, consisting of the decidua capsularis (*DC*) and the decidua vera (*DV*), is seen.

ical findings include abdominal pain, a missed menstrual period, and irregular vaginal bleeding. In the extreme case, the patient may present with hypotension or overt shock (150). A serum beta human chorionic gonadotropin (hCG) assay is essential for diagnosis, since it has been shown to be an extremely sensitive test for diagnosis of an early gestation (63,99,125). If the test is negative, the diagnosis of ectopic pregnancy is virtually excluded. If the result is positive, the differential diagnosis includes intrauterine or ectopic pregnancy. Pelvic sonography often can be useful in distinguishing between these entities (32,125).

The vast majority of ectopic pregnancies are tubal in location. Because of the small size of the fallopian tube, tubal pregnancies present clinically at 5 to 8 weeks after the last menstrual period. An absolutely specific sign for ectopic pregnancy is visualization of an intact extrauterine gestational sac with a living fetus. This is a rare finding, however, occurring in less than 5% of ectopic pregnancies. In the majority of cases of ectopic pregnancy, sonography demonstrates only nonspecific signs including adnexal fluid collections, complex or solid-appearing adnexal masses, cul-de-sac fluid, and an empty uterus lacking a gestational sac (74,76,150) (Fig. 39). Free cul-de-sac fluid in a patient at risk for an ectopic pregnancy is especially significant since it suggests that the pregnancy is leaking or rupturing. Cul-de-sac fluid has a spectrum of sonographic appearances ranging from echogenic to sonolucent with septations, reflecting hemorrhage in varying stages of maturation. Although nonspecific, these findings may strongly suggest ectopic pregnancy, especially in conjunction with clinical data.

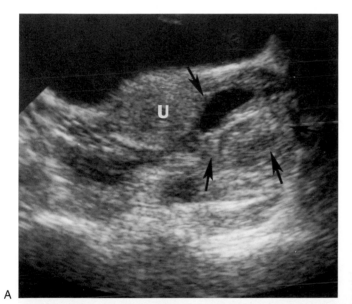

A

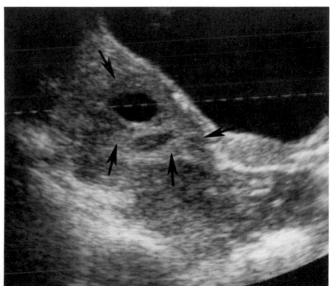

B

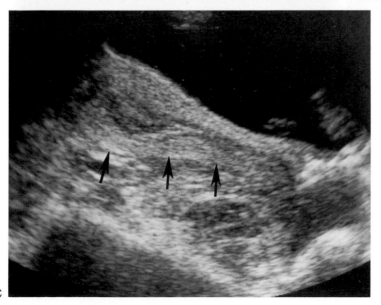

C

FIG. 39. Ectopic pregnancy in a 15-year-old girl who presented with sudden onset of lower abdominal pain and bleeding. A positive pregnancy test was obtained. **A:** Transverse and **B:** longitudinal sonograms of the left adnexal region show a poorly defined, complex mass (*arrows*) with echogenic and hypoechoic regions. A normal left ovary could not be identified. *U,* uterus. **C:** A longitudinal scan through the uterus (*arrows*) shows no evidence of a fetus. The sonographic findings in conjunction with the positive pregnancy test are consistent with ectopic gestation, subsequently confirmed at surgery.

Other sonographic findings of ectopic pregnancy include uterine enlargement (60%) and an intrauterine fluid collection with a rim of echogenic endometrium, often referred to as the pseudogestational sac of an ectopic pregnancy (77,150). The false or pseudogestational sac, occurring in up to 20% of ectopic pregnancies, is characterized by a single ring of echoes, representing only decidual parietalis, surrounding an intrauterine fluid collection. In contradistinction, a normal early intrauterine pregnancy has a "double decidual sac sign" which consists of two concentric rings, the decidua capsularis and decidua vera, surrounding the gestational sac. The double-ring sign is highly reliable in distinguishing an intrauterine from ectopic pregnancy, but does not absolutely confirm that an intrauterine pregnancy is normal (14,32,74,99).

Twenty percent of women with ectopic pregnancies will have a virtually normal sonogram because the pregnancy is small in size and hemorrhage or rupture has not occurred (32,74,150). In this group of patients who are clinically suspected of having an ectopic pregnancy, serial hCG measurements can be helpful in diagnosis. Women with ectopic pregnancies will show a subnormal increase in circulating hCG levels over a 48 hr span (32).

Extrauterine or ectopic pregnancies rarely may be abdominal in location. They usually are secondary to tubal extrusion or rupture of a viable pregnancy into the peritoneal cavity. The sonographic appearance of an abdominal pregnancy can resemble that of an intrauterine pregnancy, but usually the detection of an empty uterus in the pelvis, absence of myometrium around the fetus, and relative oligohydramnios can separate these entities (3,41).

Trophoblastic Disease

The adolescent female carries a higher risk of developing trophoblastic disease than does the young adult (7). Trophoblastic disease is a spectrum of proliferative diseases of the trophoblast with biological behavior varying from a relatively benign form, hydatidiform mole, to the more malignant invasive mole and choriocarcinoma (18). Hydatidiform moles may be classified as complete or incomplete. Complete or classical mole is characterized by edematous chorionic villi with trophoblastic proliferation, and absence of fetal parts. The partial mole demonstrates edematous chorionic villi with little or no trophoblastic proliferation, a gestational sac containing identifiable fetal tissue, and a high incidence of gross fetal and chromosomal abnormalities. Clinical features of trophoblastic disease are vaginal bleeding in the first or second trimesters and elevated levels of serum human chorionic gonadotropin. Sonography may give useful preoperative information about the extent of tumor and the presence or absence of hydronephrosis.

The typical sonographic appearance of a classic hydatidiform mole is that of an enlarged-for-dates uterus containing an echogenic soft tissue mass with multiple small anechoic spaces (Fig. 40). This typical appearance is recognized during the second trimester. In the first trimester, a molar pregnancy may appear relatively solid with few or no vesicles visualized and resemble a solid adnexal or uterine mass (88). In these cases, a high index of clinical suspicion in conjunction with elevated serum levels of human chorionic gonadotropin usually allows the correct diagnosis of molar pregnancy to be suggested. In equivocal cases, Dop-

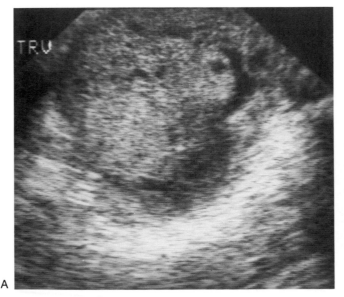
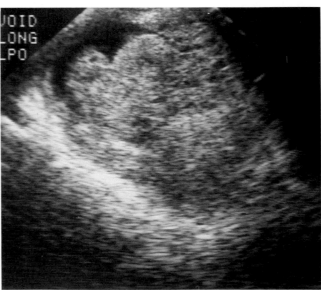

FIG. 40. Classical hydatidiform mole. **A:** Transverse and **B:** longitudinal scans show a large, echogenic mass with small cystic spaces filling the uterine cavity. A small amount of fluid is noted at the periphery of the mass.

pler sonography may be useful. Doppler interrogation of the uterine artery shows higher systolic and diastolic Doppler shifts in patients with trophoblastic neoplasia, when compared with signals from the uterine artery of gravid, nongravid, and postabortal patients (139).

A partial hydatidiform mole may be similar in appearance to a complete or classic mole, with an admixture of solid echogenic material and fluid-filled cysts filling the uterus. More often, however, patients with partial moles demonstrate an intrauterine gestational sac surrounded by a very thick placenta in which there are multiple well-defined cystic spaces (15,57,88,90). The gestational sac itself may be empty or contain a small fetal pole or immature fetus. Often the uterus is small for dates, which can help differentiate this condition from the classic hydatidiform mole in which the uterus is markedly enlarged.

About 80% of patients diagnosed as having hydatidiform mole have resolution of their disease after tumor evacuation. In approximately 12% to 15% of patients, invasive mole develops, and in 5% to 8%, the most malignant form of trophoblastic disease, metastatic choriocarcinoma, occurs (18). Differentiation among the various forms of trophoblastic disease may be difficult, although the presence of extension into the myometrium and parametrium suggests invasion, while the presence of distant metastases in combination with a molar pregnancy should make one suspect choriocarcinoma.

REFERENCES

1. Ali GM, Kordorff R, Franke D. Ultrasound volumetry in hematometrocolpos. *JCU* 1988;17:257–259.
2. Allen TD. Disorders of sexual differentiation. In: Kelalis PP, King LR, Belman AB, eds. *Clinical Pediatric Urology*. Philadelphia: W.B. Saunders Co., 1985;904–921.
3. Allibone GW, Fagan CJ, Porter SC. The sonographic features of intra-abdominal pregnancy. *JCU* 1981;9:383–387.
4. Alpern MB, Sandler MA, Madrazo BL. Sonographic features of parovarian cysts and their complications. *AJR* 1984;143:157–160.
5. Babcock DS, Han BK. The pediatric pelvis. *Clin Diag Ultrasound* 1984;15:27–46.
6. Baltarowich OH, Kurtz AB, Pasto ME, Rifkin MD, Needleman L, Goldberg BB. The spectrum of sonographic findings in hemorrhagic ovarian cysts. *AJR* 1987;148:901–905.
7. Bandy LC, Clarke-Pearson DL, Hammond CB. Malignant potential of gestational trophoblastic disease at the extreme ages of reproductive life. *Obstet Gynecol* 1984;64:395–399.
8. Baran GW, Alkema RC, Barkett GK, Frisch KM. Autonomous ovarian cyst in isosexual precocious pseudopuberty. *JCU* 1988;16:58–60.
9. Bass IS, Haller JO, Friedman AP, Twersky J, Balsam D, Gotteman R. The sonographic appearance of the hemorrhagic ovarian cyst in adolescents. *J Ultrasound Med* 1984;3:509–513.
10. Berland LL, Lawson TL, Foley WD, Albarelli JN. Ultrasound evaluation of pelvic infections. *Radiol Clin North Am* 1982;20:367–382.
11. Berman L, Stringer DA, St Onge O, Daneman A, Smith C. Case report: Unilateral haematocolpos in uterine duplication associated with renal agenesis. *Clin Radiol* 1987;38:545–547.
12. Bickers GH, Siebert JJ, Anderson JC, Golladay S, Berry DL. Sonography of ovarian involvement in childhood acute lymphocytic leukemia. *AJR* 1981;137:399–401.
13. Bower R, Dehner LP, Ternberg JL. Bilateral ovarian cysts in the newborn. A triad of neonatal abdominal masses, polyhydramnios, and maternal diabetes mellitus. *Am J Dis Child* 1974;128:731–733.
14. Bradley WG, Fiske CE, Filly RA. The double sac sign of early intrauterine pregnancy: use in exclusion of ectopic pregnancy. *Radiology* 1982;143:223–226.
15. Bree RL, Silver TM, Wicks JD, Evans E. Trophoblastic disease with coexistent fetus: A sonographic and clinical spectrum. *JCU* 1978;6:310–314.
16. Breen JL, Bonamo JF, Maxson WS. Genital tract tumors in children. *Pediatr Clin North Am* 1981;28:355–367.
17. Callen PW. *Ultrasonography in Obstetrics and Gynecology*, 2nd ed. Philadelphia: W.B. Saunders Co., 1988.
18. Callen PW. Ultrasound evaluation of gestational trophoblastic disease. In: Callen PW, ed. *Ultrasonography in Obstetrics and Gynecology*. Philadelphia: W.B. Saunders, Co., 1988;412–422.
19. Coleman BG, Arger PH, Grumbach K, Menard MK, Mintz MC, Allen KS, Arenson RL, Lamon KA. Transvaginal and transabdominal sonography: Prospective comparison. *Radiology* 1988;168:639–643.
20. Colodny AH. Disorders of the female genitalia. In: Kelalis PP, King LR, Belman AB, eds. *Clinical Pediatric Urology*. Philadelphia: W.B. Saunders, Co., 1985;888–903.
21. Comstock CH, Boal DK. Pelvic sonography of the pediatric patient. *Semin Ultrasound CT, NMR* 1984;5:54–67.
22. Copeland LJ. Malignant gynecologic tumors. In: Sutow WW, Fernbach DJ, Vieth TJ, eds. *Clinical Pediatric Oncology*. St. Louis: C.V. Mosby Co., 1984;744–760.
23. Davis JA, Gosink BB. Fluid in the female pelvis: Cyclic patterns. *J Ultrasound Med* 1986;5:75–79.
24. Davidson AJ, Hartman DS, Goldman SM. Mature teratoma of the retroperitoneum: Radiologic, pathologic, and clinical correlation. *Radiology* 1989;172:421–425.
25. de Crespigny LC, O'Herlihy C, Robinson HP. Ultrasonic observation of human ovulation. *Am J Obstet Gynecol* 1981;139:636–639.
26. Deutsch AL, Gosink BB. Nonneoplastic gynecologic disorders. *Semin Roentgenol* 1982;17:269–283.
27. Eberlein WR, Bongiovanni AM, Jones IT, Yakovac WC. Ovarian tumors and cysts associated with sexual precocity. Report of 3 cases and review of the literature. *J Pediatr* 1960;57:484–497.
28. Ehren IM, Mahour GH, Isaacs H. Benign and malignant ovarian tumors in children and adolescents. *Am J Surg* 1984;147:339–344.
29. Ein SH, Darte JMM, Stephens CA. Cystic and solid ovarian tumors in children: A 44-year review. *J Pediatr Surg* 1970;5:148–156.
30. Fakhry J, Koury A, Kotval PS, Noto RA. Sonography of autonomous follicular ovarian cysts in precocious pseudopuberty. *J Ultrasound Med* 1988;7:597–603.
31. Farrell TP, Boal DK, Teele RL, Ballantine TV. Acute torsion of normal uterine adnexa in children: Sonographic demonstration. *AJR* 1982;139:1223–1225.
32. Filly RA. Ectopic pregnancy: The role of sonography. *Radiology* 1987;162:661–668.
33. Fleischer AC, Daniell JF, Rodier J, Lindsay AM, James AE Jr. Sonographic monitoring of ovarian follicular development. *JCU* 1981;9:275–280.
34. Fleischer AC, Kalemeris GC, Entman SS. Sonographic depiction of the endometrium during normal cycles. *Ultrasound Med Biol* 1986;12:271–277.
35. Fleischer AC, James A, Millis JB, Julian C. Differential diagnosis of pelvic masses by gray scale sonography. *AJR* 1978;131:469–476.
36. Fleischer AC, Shawker TH. The role of sonography in pediatric gynecology. *Clin Obstet Gynecol* 1987;30:735–746.
37. Friedman AP, Haller JO, Schulze G, Schaffer R. Sonography of vesical and perivesical abnormalities in children. *J Ultrasound Med* 1983;2:385–390.

38. Goeffray A, Couanet D, Montagne JP, Leclere J, Flamant F. Ultrasonography and computed tomography for diagnosis and follow-up of pelvic rhabdomyosarcomas in children. *Pediatr Radiol* 1987;17:132–136.

39. Golden N, Cohen H, Gennari G, Neuhoff S. The use of pelvic ultrasonography in the evaluation of adolescents with pelvic inflammatory disease. *Am J Dis Child* 1987; 141:1235–1238.

40. Goske MJ, Emmens RW, Rabinowitz R. Inguinal ovaries in children demonstrated by high resolution real-time ultrasound. *Radiology* 1984;151:635–636.

41. Graham D, Johnson TRB Jr, Sanders RC. Sonographic findings in abdominal pregnancy. *J Ultrasound Med* 1982;1:71–74.

42. Graif M, Itzchak Y. Sonographic evaluation of ovarian torsion in childhood and adolescence. *AJR* 1988;150:647–649.

43. Graif M, Shalev J, Strauss S, Engelberg S, Mashiach S, Itzchak Y. Torsion of the ovary: Sonographic features. *AJR* 1984;143:1331–1334.

44. Granberg S, Crona N, Enk L, Hammarberg K, Wikland M. Ultrasound-guided puncture of cystic tumors in the lower pelvis of young women. *JCU* 1989;17:107–111.

45. Grimes CK, Rosenbaum DM, Kirkpatrick JA Jr. Pediatric gynecologic radiology. *Semin Roentgen* 1982;17:284–301.

46. Groeber WR. Ovarian tumors during infancy and childhood. *Am J Obstet Gynec* 1963;86:1027–1035.

47. Grossman JA, Filtzer HS, Aliapoulios MA. Torsion and infarction of cystic ovaries in children. *Am J Dis Child* 1974;128:713–714.

48. Guttman PH. In search of the elusive benign cystic ovarian teratoma: Application of the ultrasound "tip of the iceberg" sign. *JCU* 1977;5:403–406.

49. Hackeloer BJ. The role of ultrasound in female infertility management. *Ultrasound Med Biol* 1984;10:35–50.

50. Hall DA. Sonographic appearance of the normal ovary, of polycystic ovary disease, and of functional ovarian cysts. *Semin Ultrasound* 1983;4:149–165.

51. Hall DA, Crowley WF, Wierman ME, Simeone JF, McCarthy KA. Sonographic monitoring of LHRH analogue therapy in idiopathic precocious puberty in young girls. *JCU* 1986;14:331–338.

52. Haller JO, Fellows RA. The pelvis. *Clin Diag Ultrasound* 1981;8:165–185.

53. Haller JO, Friedman AP, Schaffer R, Lebensart DP. The normal and abnormal ovary in childhood and adolescence. *Semin Ultrasound* 1983;4:206–225.

54. Haller JO, Schneider M, Kassner ED, et al. Ultrasonography in pediatric gynecology and obstetrics. *AJR* 1977;128:423–429.

55. Hann LE, Hall DA, McArdle CR, Seibel M. Polycystic ovarian disease: Sonographic spectrum. *Radiology* 1984;150:531–534.

56. Helvie MA, Silver TM. Ovarian torsion: Sonographic evaluation. *JCU* 1989;17:327–332.

57. Hertzberg BS, Kurtz AB, Wapner RJ, Blocklinger A, Davis G, Roberts N, Needleman L. Gestational trophoblastic disease with coexistent normal fetus: Evaluation by ultrasound-guided chorionic villus sampling. *J Ultrasound Med* 1986;5:467–469.

58. Ivarsson S-A, Nilsson KO, Persson P-H. Ultrasonography of the pelvic organs in prepubertal and postpubertal girls. *Arch Dis Child* 1983;58:352–354.

59. Jacobson L, Westron L. Objectivized diagnosis of acute pelvic inflammatory disease. *Am J Obstet Gynecol* 1969;105:1088–1096.

60. Jafri SZH, Bree RL, Silver TM, Ouimette M. Fetal ovarian cysts: Sonographic detection and association with hypothyroidism. *Radiology* 1984;150:809–812.

61. James DF, Barber HRK, Graber EA. Torsion of normal uterine adnexa in children. Report of three cases. *Obstet Gynecol* 1970;35:226–230.

62. Janus C, Godine L. Newborn with hydrometrocolpos and ambiguous genitalia: Clinical significance. *JCU* 1986;14:739–741.

63. Kadar N, Taylor KJW, Rosenfield AT, Romero R. Combined use of serum HCG and sonography in the diagnosis of ectopic pregnancy. *AJR* 1983;141:609–615.

64. Kangarloo H, Sarti DA, Sample WF. Ultrasound of the pediatric pelvis. *Semin Ultrasound* 1980;1:51–60.

65. Kerin JF, Edmonds DK, Warnes GM, et al. Morphological and functional relations of graafian follicle growth to ovulation in women using ultrasonic, laparoscopic and biochemical measurements. *Br J Obstet Gynaecol* 1981;88:81–90.

66. Laing FC, Van Dalsem VF, Marks WM, Barton JL, Martinez DA. Dermoid cysts of the ovary: Their ultrasonographic appearances. *Obstet Gynecol* 1981;57:99–104.

67. Lande IM, Hill MC, Cosco FE, Kator NN. Adnexal and cul-de-sac abnormalities: Trasvaginal sonography. *Radiology* 1988;166:325–332.

68. Lane DM, Birdwell RL. Ovarian leukemia detected by pelvic sonography. *Cancer* 1986;58:2338–2342.

69. Leibman AJ, Kruse B, McSweeney MB. Transvaginal sonography: Comparison with transabdominal sonography in the diagnosis of pelvic masses. *AJR* 1988;151:89–92.

70. Lindsay AN, Voorhess ML, MacGillivray MH. Multicystic ovaries in primary hypothyroidism. *Obstet Gynecol* 1983;61:433–437.

71. Lippe BM, Sample WF. Pelvic ultrasonography in pediatric and adolescent endocrine disorders. *J Pediatr* 1978;92:897–902.

72. Little HK, Crawford DB, Meister K. Hemotocolpos: Diagnosis made by ultrasound. *JCU* 1978;6:341–342.

73. Lyon AJ, de Bruyn R, Grant DB. Transient sexual precocity and ovarian cysts. *Arch Dis Child* 1985;60:819–822.

74. Mahony BS, Filly RA, Nyberg DA, Callen PW. Sonographic evaluation of ectopic pregnancy. *J Ultrasound Med* 1985;4:221–228.

75. Mahour GH, Woolley MM, Landing BH. Ovarian teratomas in children. A thirty-three year experience. *Am J Surg* 1976;132:587–589.

76. Manor WF, Zwiebel WJ, Hanning RV, Raymond HW. Ectopic pregnancy and other causes of acute pelvic pain. *Semin US CT MR* 1985;6:181–206.

77. Marks WM, Filly RA, Callen PW, Laing FC. The decidual cast of ectopic pregnancy: A confusing ultrasonographic appearance. *Radiology* 1979;133:451–454.

78. Marshall JR. Ovarian enlargements in the first year of life: Review of 45 cases. *Ann Surg* 1965;161:372–377.

79. Massarano AA, Adams JA, Preece MA, Brook CGD. Ovarian ultrasound appearances in Turner's syndrome. *J Pediatr* 1989;114:568–573.

80. McCarthy S, Taylor KJW. Sonography of vaginal masses. *AJR* 1983;140:1005–1008.

81. McLeod AJ, Lewis E. Sonographic evaluation of pediatric rhabdomyosarcomas. *J Ultrasound Med* 1984;3:69–73.

82. Mendelson EB, Böhm-Vélez M, Neiman HL, Russo J. Transvaginal sonography in gynecologic imaging. *Semin US CT MR* 1988;9:102–121.

83. Mendelson EB, Böhm-Vélez M, Joseph N, Neiman HL. Gynecologic imaging: Comparison of transabdominal and transvaginal sonography. *Radiology* 1988;166:321–324.

84. Miles PA, Penney LL. Corpus luteum formation in the fetus. *Obstet Gynecol* 1983;61:525–529.

85. Mintz MC, Grumbach K. Imaging of congenital uterine anomalies. *Semin US CT MR* 1988;9:167–174.

86. Mitchell DG, Mintz MC, Spritzer CE, et al. Adnexal masses: MR imaging observations at 1.5T, with US and CT correlation. *Radiology* 1987;162:319–324.

87. Moyle JW, Rochester D, Sider L, Shrock K, Krause P. Sonography of ovarian tumors: Predictability of tumor type. *AJR* 1983;141:985–991.

88. Munyer TP, Callen PW, Filly RA, Braga CA, Jones HW. Further observations on the sonographic spectrum of gestational trophoblastic disease. *JCU* 1981;9:349–358.

89. Musante F, Derchi LE. Spontaneous resolution of unilateral hematometra in a patient with bicornuate uterus: Sonographic findings. *Clin Ultrasound* 1986;14:307–309.

90. Naumoff P, Szulman AE, Weinstein B, Mazer J, Surti U. Ultrasonography of partial hydatidiform mole. *Radiology* 1981;140:467–470.

91. Neiman HL, Mendelson EB. Ultrasound evaluation of the ovary. In: Callen PW, ed. *Ultrasonography in Obstetrics and Gynecology.* Philadelphia: W.B. Saunders, Co. 1988;423–446.

92. Nicolini U, Ferrazzi E, Bellotti M, Travaglini P, Elli R, Scaperrotta RC. The contribution of sonographic evaluation of ovarian size in patients with polycystic ovarian disease. *J Ultrasound Med* 1985;4:347–351.

93. Norris HJ, Bagley GP, Taylor HB. Carcinoma of the infant vagina. *Arch Path* 1970;90:473–479.

94. Nussbaum AR, Lebowitz RL. Interlabial masses in little girls: Review and imaging recommendations. *AJR* 1983;141:65–71.

95. Nussbaum AR, Sanders RC, Jones MD. Neonatal uterine morphology as seen on real-time US. *Radiology* 1986;160:641–643.

96. Nussbaum AR, Sanders RC, Hartman DS, Dudgeon DL, Parmley TH. Neonatal ovarian cysts: Sonographic-pathologic correlation. *Radiology* 1988;168:817–821.

97. Nussbaum AR, Sanders RC, Benator RM, Haller JA Jr, Dudgeon DL. Spontaneous resolution of neonatal ovarian cysts. *AJR* 1987;148:175–176.

98. Nyberg DA, Filly RA, Mahony BS, Monroe S, Laing FC, Jeffrey RB Jr. Early gestation: Correlation of HCG levels and sonographic identification. *AJR* 1985;144:951–954.

99. Nyberg DA, Laing FC, Filly RA, Uri-Simmons M, Jeffrey RB Jr. Ultrasonographic differentiation of the gestational sac of early intrauterine pregnancy from the pseudogestational sac of ectopic pregnancy. *Radiology* 1983;146:755–759.

100. O'Herlihy C, de Crespigny LC, Lopata A, Johnston I, Hoult I, Robinson H. Preovulatory follicular size: A comparison of ultrasound and laparoscopic measurements. *Fertil Steril* 1980;34:24–26.

101. O'Herlihy C, de Crespigny LJC, Robinson HP. Monitoring ovarian follicular development with real-time ultrasound. *Br J Obstet Gynaecol* 1980;87:613–618.

102. Orsini LF, Salardi S, Pilu G, Bovicelli L, Cacciari E. Pelvic organs in premenarcheal girls: Real-time ultrasonography. *Radiology* 1984;153:113–116.

103. Orsini LF, Venturoli S, Lorusso R, Pluchinotta V, Paradisi R, Bovicelli L. Ultrasonic findings in polycystic ovarian disease. *Fertil Steril* 1985;43:709–714.

104. Ouimette MV, Bree RL. Sonography of pelvoabdominal cystic masses in children and adolescents. *J Ultrasound Med* 1984;3:149–153.

105. Paling MR, Shawker TH. Abdominal ultrasound in advanced ovarian carcinoma. *JCU* 1981;9:435–441.

106. Parisi L, Tramonti M, Derchi LE, Casciano S, Zurli A, Rocchi P. Polycystic ovarian disease: Ultrasonic evaluation and correlations with clinical and hormonal data. *J Clin Ultrasound* 1984;12:21–26.

107. Pennes DR, Bowerman RA, Silver TM. Congenital uterine anomalies and associated pregnancies: Findings and pitfalls of sonographic diagnosis. *J Ultrasound Med* 1985;4:531–538.

108. Picker RH, Smith DH, Tucker MH, Saunders DM. Ultrasonic signs of imminent ovulation. *JCU* 1983;11:1–2.

109. Pupols AZ, Wilson SR. Ultrasonographic interpretation of physiological changes in the female pelvis. *J Assoc Can Radiol* 1984;35:34–39.

110. Queenan JT, O'Brien GD, Bains LM, Simpson J, Collins WP, Campbell S. Ultrasound scanning of ovaries to detect ovulation in women. *Fertil Steril* 1980;34:99–105.

111. Quinn SF, Erickson S, Black WC. Cystic ovarian teratomas: The sonographic appearance of the dermoid plug. *Radiology* 1985;155:477–478.

112. Ralls PW, Rotter AJ, Halls JM. Non-ovarian adnexal pathology. *Semin Ultrasound* 1983;4:193–205.

113. Reuter KL, Daly DC, Cohen SM. Septate versus bicornuate uteri: Errors in imaging diagnosis. *Radiology* 1989;172:749–752.

114. Riddlesberger MM Jr, Kuhn JP, Munschauer RW. The association of juvenile hypothyroidism and cystic ovaries. *Radiology* 1981;139:77–80.

115. Rieth KG, Comite F, Shawker TH, Cutler GB Jr. Pituitary and ovarian abnormalities demonstrated by CT and ultrasound in children with features of the McCune-Albright syndrome. *Radiology* 1984;153:389–393.

116. Ritchie WGM. Sonographic evaluation of normal and induced ovulation. *Radiology* 1986;161:1–10.

117. Rosenberg HK, Sherman NH, Tarry WF, Duckett JW, Synder HM. Mayer-Rokitansky-Küster-Hauser syndrome: US aid to diagnosis. *Radiology* 1986;161:815–819.

118. Rosenberg HK, Udassin R, Howell C, Betts J, Schnauffer L. Duplication of the uterus and vagina, unilateral hydrometrocolpos, and ipsilateral renal agenesis: Sonographic aid to diagnosis. *J Ultrasound Med* 1982;1:289–291.

119. Russ PD, Zavitz WR, Pretorius DH, Manco-Johnson ML, Rumack CM, Pfister RR, Greenholz SK. Hydrometrocolpos, uterus didelphys, and septate vagina: An antenatal sonographic diagnosis. *J Ultrasound Med* 1986;5:211–213.

120. Sailer JF. Hematometra and hematocolpos: Ultrasound findings. *AJR* 1979;132:1010–1011.

121. Salardi S, Orsini LF, Cacciari E, et al. Pelvic ultrasonography in girls with precocious puberty, congenital adrenal hyperplasia, obesity, or hirsutism. *J Pediatr* 1988;112:880–887.

122. Sample W, Lippe B, Geypes M. Gray scale ultrasonography of the normal female pelvis. *Radiology* 1977;125:477–483.

123. Sandler MA, Silver TM, Karo JJ. Gray-scale ultrasonic features of ovarian teratomas. *Radiology* 1979;131:705–709.

124. Schaffer RM, Taylor C, Haller JO, Friedman AP, Shih YH. Nonobstructive hydrocolpos: Sonographic appearance and differential diagnosis. *Radiology* 1983;149:273–278.

125. Schwartz RO, Di Pietro DL. B-hCG as a diagnostic aid for suspected ectopic pregnancy. *Obstet Gynecol* 1980;56:197–203.

126. Shawker TH, Garra BS, Loriaux DL, Cutler GB, Ross JL. Ultrasonography of Turner's syndrome. *J Ultrasound Med* 1986;5:125–129.

127. Shawker TH, Comite F, Rieth KG, Dwyer AJ, Cutler GB, Loriaux L. Ultrasound evaluation of female isosexual precocious puberty. *J Ultrasound Med* 1984;3:309–316.

128. Shawker TH, Hubbard VS, Reichert CM, Guerreiro de Matos OM. Cystic ovaries in cystic fibrosis: An ultrasound and autopsy study. *J Ultrasound Med* 1983;2:439–444.

129. Sheth S, Fishman EK, Buck JL, Hamper UM, Sanders RC. The variable sonographic appearances of ovarian teratomas: Correlation with CT. *AJR* 1988;151:331–334.

130. Shirkhoda A, Eftekhari F, Frankel LS, Lewis E. Diagnosis of leukemic relapse in the pelvic soft tissues of juvenile females. *JCU* 1986;14:191–195.

131. Siegel HA, Sagerman R, Berdon WE, Wigger HJ. Mesonephric adenocarcinoma of the vagina in a 7-month-old infant simulating sarcoma botryoides successful control with supervoltage radiotherapy. *J Pediatr Surg* 1970;5:468–470.

132. Siegel MJ. Pelvic organs and soft tissues. In: Siegel MJ, ed. *Pediatric Body CT*. New York: Churchill Livingstone, 1988;219–251.

133. Sisler CL, Siegel MJ. Ovarian teratomas: A comparison of the sonographic appearance in prepubertal and postpubertal girls. *AJR* 1990;154:139–141.

134. Spiegel RM, Ben-Ora A. Ultrasound of inflammatory disease in the pelvis. *Semin Ultrasound* 1980;1:41–50.

135. Stangl W, Frank RC, Frank W, Nelli S. Sonographic findings in a case of uterine and vaginal duplication (didelphys) with unilateral hematocolpometrasalpinx. *JCU* 1983;11:40–41.

136. Swayne LC, Love MB, Karasick SR. Pelvic inflammatory disease: Sonographic-pathologic correlation. *Radiology* 1984;151:751–755.

137. Swayne LC, Rubenstein JB, Mitchell B. The Mayer-Rokitansky-Küster-Hauser syndrome: Sonographic aid to diagnosis. *J Ultrasound Med* 1986;5:287–289.

138. Taylor CR, Taylor KJW. Malignant ovarian teratomas. *Clin Diag Ultrasound* 1984;15:61–72.

139. Taylor KJW, Schwartz PE, Kohorn EI. Gestational trophoblastic neoplasia: Diagnosis with Doppler US. *Radiology* 1987;165:445–448.

140. Valdes C, Malini S, Malinak LR. Sonography in the surgical management of vaginal and cervical atresia. *Fertil Steril* 1983;40:263–265.

141. Viscomi GN, Gonzalez R, Taylor KJW. Ultrasound detection of uterine abnormalities after diethylstilbestrol (DES) exposure. *Radiology* 1980;136:733–735.

142. Walsh JW, Taylor KJW, Wasson JFM, Schwartz PE, Rosenfield AT. Gray-scale ultrasound in 204 proved gynecologic masses: Accuracy and specific diagnostic criteria. *Radiology* 1979;130:391–397.

143. Warner MA, Fleischer AC, Edell SL, Thieme GA, Bundy AL, Kurtz AB, James AE. Uterine adnexal torsion: Sonographic findings. *Radiology* 1985;154:773–775.

144. White SJ, Stuck KJ, Blane CE, Silver TM. Sonography of neuroblastoma. *AJR* 1983;141:465–468.

145. Wilson DA, Stacy TM, Smith EI. Ultrasound diagnosis of hydrocolpos and hydrometrocolpos. *Radiology* 1978;128:451–454.

146. Woodring JH, Halberg DH, Duff DE. Sarcoma botryoides of the uterus presenting as an abdominal mass. *JCU* 1982;10:347–349.

147. Worthington-Kirsch RL, Raptopoulos V, Cohen IT. Sequential bilateral torsion of normal ovaries in a child. *J Ultrasound Med* 1986;5:663–664.

148. Wu A, Siegel MJ. Sonography of pelvic masses in children: Diagnostic predictability. *AJR* 1987;148:1199–1202.

149. Yeh H-C, Futterweit W, Thornton JC. Polycystic ovarian disease: US features in 104 patients. *Radiology* 1987;163:111–116.

150. Zwiebel WJ, Haning RV Jr. A rational approach to diagnosis and management in ectopic pregnancy. *Semin Ultrasound* 1983;4:235–253.

Male Genital Tract

William H. McAlister

Sonography has become an essential imaging tool for evaluating the scrotal contents because it is non-invasive, nonionizing, rapid, and without discomfort and risk to the patient. Current indications for its use include evaluation of scrotal masses, assessment of scrotal trauma, evaluation of scrotal pain, localization of the undescended testis, and follow-up of patients with tumors and infections. This chapter will highlight the use of sonography in diagnosing a variety of scrotal abnormalities and will also provide general guidelines to aid in appropriately selecting imaging tests.

TECHNIQUES

Sonographic examination of the scrotal contents requires real-time equipment with high-frequency linear array transducers. Routinely 5 to 10 MHz transducers are used. Direct contact of the transducer on the scrotum usually produces excellent images, but occasionally a standoff pad placed between the transducer and scrotum is needed to improve resolution in the near field. For the diagnosis of torsion or infarction, color flow Doppler is essential.

Examination of the testicles is performed with the patient supine. The scrotum should be elevated from between the legs and supported by a rolled towel; the penis should be placed on the lower abdomen and draped with a towel. Both transverse and longitudinal scans of each testis are performed.

TESTICULAR DEVELOPMENT AND ANATOMY

The testis descends from the peritoneum into the scrotum at about 8 weeks gestation. As the testis descends it becomes invested with a portion of peritoneum, termed the process vaginalis. After birth the process vaginalis closes proximally; the lower portion remains as a closed sac around the testis and epididymis, termed the tunica vaginalis (Fig. 1). The tunica encircles the testis except posteriorly and superiorly in the area of the head of the epididymis. The tunica vaginalis is composed of two layers: an outer parietal and inner visceral layer which are separated by 1 to 2 ml of fluid (Fig. 1). The visceral layer of the tunica vaginalis is closely adherent to the tunica albuginea, a fibrous capsule that surrounds the testis (36).

The innermost aspect of the tunica albuginea gives off numerous minute septa which converge posteriorly to form a mass of fibrous tissue called the mediastinum testis. The mediastinum testis provides support for the veins, arteries, and ducts of the testis as they enter and exit the testis.

The testis is composed of over 250 lobules. Each lobule contains tortuous seminiferous tubules which are estimated to total 840 per testis. These tubules course centrally to join with other seminiferous tubules to form 20 to 30 larger straight ducts, termed tubuli recti. The tubuli recti enter the mediastinum testis where they form a network of channels known as the rete testis. The rete testis drains into 12 to 20 efferent ductules which proceed to the head of the epididymis where they drain into a single duct referred to as the ductus epididymis.

Both testes are of similar size and shape. At birth the testes measure 1.5 cm in length and 1.0 cm in width. The length increases to 2.0 cm and the width to 1.2 cm by 3 months of age due to a normal rise of testosterone in young infants (8,12). By the time the patient is 6 months old the testes have regressed slightly and remain relatively constant in size until the patient is about 6 years old when the testes again increase in size. Postpubescent testes measure 3 to 5 cm in length and 2 to 3 cm in both anteroposterior diameter and in width (38,46). The testes lie in the scrotum with their long axes upright and tilted forward and slightly lateral. The left testis usually is slightly lower than the right.

The normal infant testis is ovoid and demonstrates uniform low-level echoes throughout. Testicular echogenicity increases from age 8 years until puberty, at which time the testis has a medium-level echogenicity.

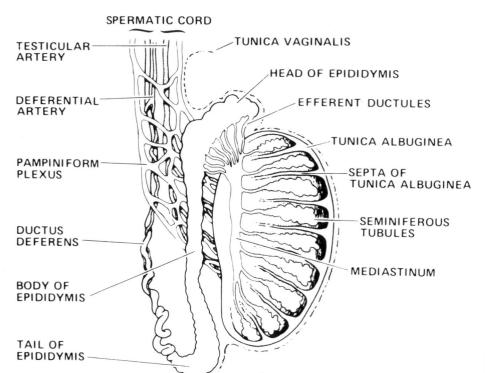

SPERMATIC CORD

TESTICULAR ARTERY

DEFERENTIAL ARTERY

PAMPINIFORM PLEXUS

DUCTUS DEFERENS

BODY OF EPIDIDYMIS

TAIL OF EPIDIDYMIS

TUNICA VAGINALIS

HEAD OF EPIDIDYMIS

EFFERENT DUCTULES

TUNICA ALBUGINEA

SEPTA OF TUNICA ALBUGINEA

SEMINIFEROUS TUBULES

MEDIASTINUM

FIG. 1. Normal anatomy of the scrotum. Adapted from Krone and Carroll, ref. 46.

The change in sonographic appearance correlates with the histologic development of germ cell elements and tubular maturation. The tunicas are not routinely seen as discrete structures in the absence of a hydrocele, but the mediastinum testis is often seen as a highly echogenic line along the superior-inferior axis of the testis in postpubertal patients. Arteries and veins coursing within the testis can be seen easily with color flow imaging (Fig. 2).

Posterolateral to the testis lies the epididymis, composed of a head, body, and tail (Fig. 3). The head is the largest portion and is attached to the superior pole of the testis. It is triangular in shape and as echogenic or slightly more echogenic than the testis. The body is located along the posterolateral aspect of the testis; the tail lies at the inferior aspect of the testis. The body has an echogenicity equal to or slightly less than that of the testis; the tail normally is not seen on sonography.

The spermatic cord contains the vas deferens, spermatic and ductus deferens arteries, and a pampiniform plexus of veins, nerves, and lymphatics. It courses

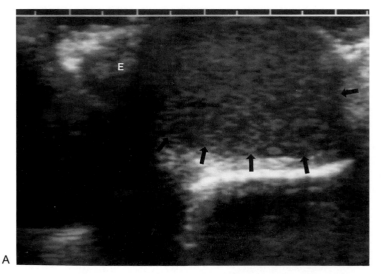

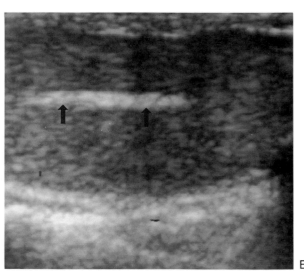

FIG. 2. Normal testes. **A:** Longitudinal scan of the left testis (*arrows*) of a 14-year-old boy showing the normal homogeneous medium-level echotexture and ovoid shape. Note epididymis (*E*) above superior pole of testis. **B:** Longitudinal scan demonstrates the echogenic mediastinum testis (*arrows*) in another boy. **C** (see Coloplate 12): Color flow Doppler showing arteries and veins within the testis.

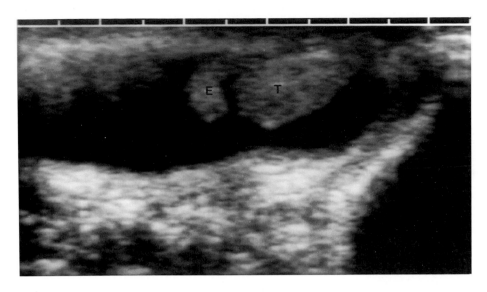

FIG. 3. Normal epididymis in a 1-month-old boy. Longitudinal scan of left hemiscrotum reveals equal echogenicity of the epididymis (*E*) and testis (*T*). There is a surrounding hydrocele.

from the superior pole of the testis through the inguinal canal to enter into the abdomen. Duplex or color flow Doppler sonography can frequently demonstrate venous and arterial flow within the spermatic cord.

The layers of tissue covering the testis, starting from the outermost layer, are the scrotal skin, dartos muscle (which is responsible for wrinkling of the scrotal skin), external spermatic fascia, cremasteric fascia and muscle, internal spermatic fascia, and tunica vaginalis. The thickness of the scrotal wall in older children measures between 3 to 6 mm. Scrotal thickness measurements vary, however, depending on transducer pressure, and are of limited value.

CONGENITAL ANOMALIES

Anomalies of Number, Size, and Position

Anorchidism or testicular absence occurs in 1 in 5,000 to 1 in 20,000 male newborns (43). Monorchidism is four times as common as testicular absence, occurring in 1 in 5,000 boys, and is usually left sided. Monorchid patients have been shown to have blind-ending spermatic vessels and spermatic cords, suggesting intrauterine torsion or vascular accident as an etiology for the anomaly (81).

Polyorchidism is a rare condition in which more than one testis is present on one side of the scrotum. The accessory testes are separate structures and each may have a separate epididymis and vas deferens, or they may show common ducts. They are unequal in size and smaller than the normal-sized contralateral testis. The condition is usually incidentally discovered as an asymptomatic scrotal mass, but rarely may present with torsion (56). Rarely, a bilobed testis may mimic a polyorchid testis. Sonographically, polyorchid and bilobed testes have the same echo-characteristics as the normal testicle (Fig. 4) (53).

A small testis may be congenital in origin or secondary to cryptorchidism, torsion, inflammation,

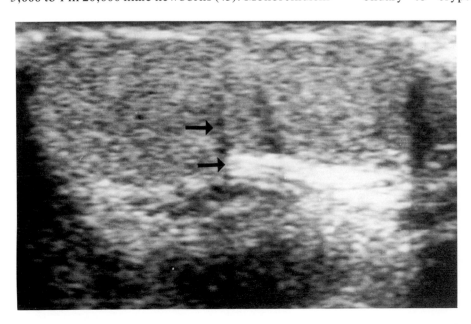

FIG. 4. Bilobed testis in a 14-year-old with a left scrotal mass. Longitudinal scan of the left testis shows a cleft (*arrows*) in its midportion. The echotexture is normal. At surgery, the patient had an enlarged left testicle separated by infolded capsule. Biopsies showed normal testicular parenchyma.

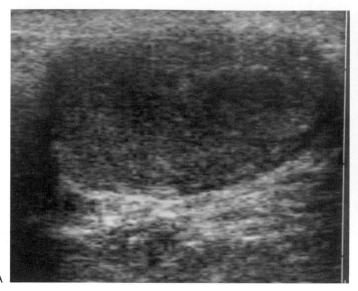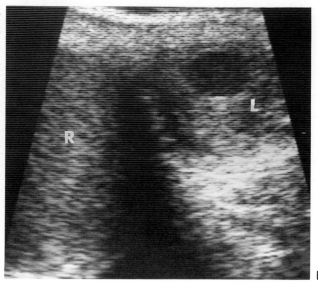

A   B

FIG. 5. Testicular atrophy in a teenager with a small, firm left testis at physical examination. **A:** Longitudinal scan of the left testis demonstrates a hypoechoic, inhomogeneous echopattern. **B:** Transverse scan of both testes shows that the left (*L*) is smaller than the right (*R*). Again noted is the inhomogeneous echotexture. Surgical removal confirmed atrophic parenchyma.

Klinefelter's syndrome, or trauma. Sonographically, it can have normal, increased, or decreased echogenicity and may be confused with a testicular neoplasm (Fig. 5).

Transverse testicular ectopia is an anomaly in which both testes migrate to the same hemiscrotum. Clinically, patients present with a nonpalpable testis and contralateral scrotal masses. Associated anomalies, found in 20% of affected patients, include hypospadias, seminal vesicle cysts, renal dysplasia, ureteropelvic obstruction, ipsilateral inguinal hernia, and testicular tumors (21).

Cystic Dysplasia of the Testes

Cystic dysplasia of the testis is a rare condition believed to be due to a failure of the rete testis tubules to connect to the efferent ducts. It is characterized by multiple cysts in the mediastinum testis, rete testis and adjacent seminiferous tubules, and parenchymal atrophy (10). Cystic dysplasia may be associated with ipsilateral renal agenesis and bilateral renal dysplasia.

Cryptorchidism

Cryptorchidism or incomplete testicular descent is probably related to impairment of the hypothalamic pituitary axis (29). At birth, approximately 33% of premature male infants weighing under 2,500 grams will have undescended testes, in contrast to 3% to 4% of term infants. Testicular descent continues after birth for a few weeks to months, so that at the end of 12

months, only 0.8% of infants have true cryptorchidism (45).

The testes can be arrested anywhere along the course of descent from the retroperitoneum into the scrotum (40). However, approximately 80% of undescended testes are located in the inguinal canal or just proximal to the internal inguinal ring. Rarely, the testis is found in the perineum or at the base of the penis. Cryptorchidism is bilateral in about one-third of patients. Associated urologic anormalities occur in 20% of affected boys (62).

Sonographic findings of cryptorchidism are those of an elliptical mass of uniform echogenicity anywhere along the path of testicular descent (Fig. 6). The undescended testis may be smaller than the contralateral normally located testis and hypoechoic because of atrophy. A small testis may be indistinguishable from a gubernaculum testis or inguinal lymph nodes (84).

Identification of an undescended testis is important because of the increased risks of infertility if the testis remains undescended and because of the increased incidence of malignancy (23,34). Orchiopexy is considered the treatment of choice. Preoperative localization of a nonpalpable, undescended testis by radiologic examination is helpful in directing the surgical approach and shortening anesthesia time. Sonography has a sensitivity of about 90% for detecting an undescended testis, a specificity of 100%, and an accuracy of 91% (85). Because a majority of undescended testes are within the inguinal canal, sonography is the initial examination of choice. However, sonography is not as reliable in detecting undescended testes located higher in the pelvis or in the abdomen, where adjacent structures

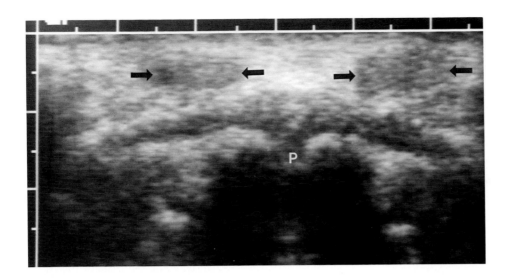

FIG. 6. Cryptorchidism. Transverse scan of the inguinal canals above the symphysis pubis (*P*) demonstrates small, ovoid testes bilaterally (*arrows*).

such as bowel loops are more of a problem. Therefore, if the sonographic examination is equivocal or negative, computerized tomography (CT) or magnetic resonance (MR) imaging should be used for identification of the intraabdominal testis. Sonography can be used for follow-up evaluation of patients who do not have orchiopexies.

SCROTAL MASS

The role of sonography in the evaluation of scrotal masses is to confirm whether or not there is a lesion present, localize its site of origin, and characterize its contents. The most valuable information provided is the separation of intra- and extratesticular pathology. The importance of this distinction is that the vast majority of intratesticular lesions are malignant, while most extratesticular lesions are benign. The accuracy of sonography in providing this determination approaches 90% to 95% (46). The overall accuracy in detecting and characterizing soft tissue masses as cys-

tic or solid also is somewhere in the range of 90% to 100%. However, sonography cannot ascertain whether a solid tumor is benign or malignant (72). At present, MR imaging provides information similar to that obtained with sonography in most cases (80).

Testicular Tumors

Testicular tumors account for approximately 1% of all childhood malignancies; they represent 2% to 3% of malignant tumors in males (19). Approximately 70% of primary testicular neoplasms are of germ cell origin and 30% are nongerminal (14). Yolk sac tumors are the most common of the germ cell tumors, representing 70% of this group. The remainder of the germ cell tumors are usually benign teratomas. Both tumors tend to occur in prepubescent boys. After puberty, germ cell tumors are more likely to be embryonal cell carcinomas, seminomas, choriocarcinomas, and teratocarcinomas. Most often these tumors present with painless, unilateral testicular enlargement. Pain, sec-

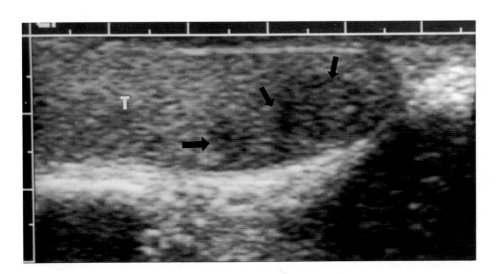

FIG. 7. Embryonal cell carcinoma in a teenage boy. Longitudinal scan shows a hypoechoic mass (*arrows*) in the lower pole of the testis (*T*).

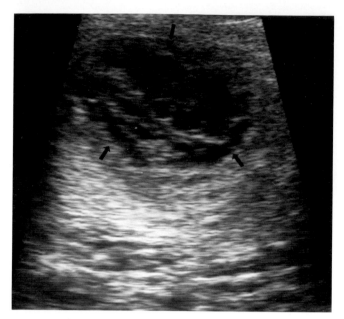

FIG. 8. Seminoma in a teenage boy who presented with metastatic chest disease. Longitudinal scan shows a well-defined, inhomogeneous hypoechoic mass (*arrows*) within the testis.

ondary to torsion or hemorrhage into the tumor, and metastatic disease are infrequent symptoms (19,61).

Nongerminal cell tumors account for about 30% of all testicular tumors in children (64). Leydig cell tumors represent approximately 42% of the nongerminal tumors; Sertoli cell tumors, 20%; and paratesticular rhabdomyosarcoma, 38% (64). Sertoli cell tumors usually appear as a painless mass in the first year of life, whereas Leydig cell tumors are found in patients 3 to 6 years of age who generally present with precocious puberty or gynecomastia. Paratesticular tumors are described below.

Gonadoblastomas are rare tumors composed of germ cell elements and cells similar to immature Sertoli or Leydig cells (74). They usually occur in phenotypic females with streak gonads or testes and a male karyotype. The majority are small and recognizable only at the time of operation to remove dysgenetic gonads.

On sonography, testicular neoplasms usually are solid, well-defined masses; the echogenicity varies from homogeneously hypoechoic to heterogeneous with areas of decreased echogenicity, reflecting hemorrhage or necrosis (Figs. 7,8,9) (3,19,31,54,67). Areas of increased echogenicity also may be present and represent calcifications. Sonographic patterns of the most common histologic types have been reported, although these are not specific and significant overlap occurs. The sonographic appearance of embryonal cell carcinoma is most often a hypoechoic, inhomogeneous mass (Fig. 7). The tunica may be invaded, resulting in irregular tumor margins (65). By contrast, seminoma is usually uniformly hypoechoic and rarely contains necrosis or hemorrhage. Teratomas often are complex tumors containing hypoechoic and highly calcified echogenic components (Fig. 9). Rarely, testicular tumors are primarily echogenic (Fig. 10) (11). A hydrocele may be present with benign or malignant testicular tumors. Besides being used for initial diagnosis, sonography can be used after orchiectomy to assess the status of the contralateral testis (73). Although the frequency is uncertain, patients with testicular cancers are at greater risk for developing a tumor in the opposite testis.

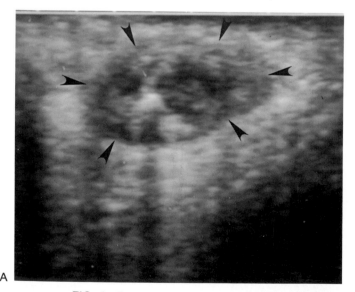
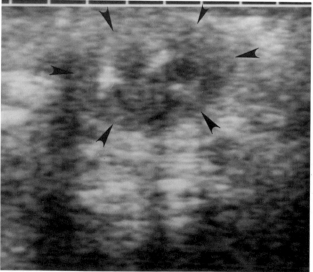

FIG. 9. Benign teratoma in an 18-month-old boy with a hard testicular mass on palpation. **A:** Longitudinal and **B:** transverse scans show a hypoechoic mass (*arrowheads*) with focal areas of increased and decreased echogenicity, representing calcification and cystic degeneration, respectively. Distal acoustic shadowing is associated with the areas of calcification.

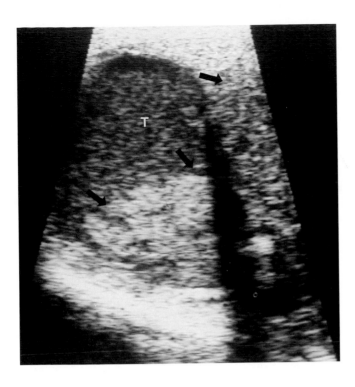

FIG. 10. Teratocarcinoma in a teenage boy. Transverse scan shows a lobulated, hyperechoic mass (*black arrows*) extending from the periphery of the right testis (*T*).

Benign testicular masses include lipoma, hemangioma, neurofibroma, fibroma, and cyst (24,35). Mass lesions in the testes that can simulate a solid neoplasm include adrenal rests and hematomas (76). Most benign lesions appear as solid, hypoechoic masses, but they at times may be complex or hyperechoic.

Secondary Neoplasms

The role of sonography in patients with secondary neoplasms is to identify recurrent tumor or a site for biopsy (79). The testis can act as a sanctuary for leukemic cells during chemotherapy and remission. Although leukemic infiltrates are present in 60% to 90% of children at autopsy, they are less often clinically apparent (14). Occult leukemic infiltrates have been documented by testicular biopsy in 8.5% of children who are in bone marrow remission (1). Testicular infiltrates due to Burkitt's lymphoma are present at autopsy in 5% to 30% of children and clinically in about 5% of children (87). On sonography, the testes are usually diffusely enlarged and hypoechoic (Fig. 11) (63).

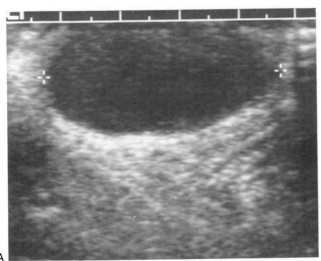

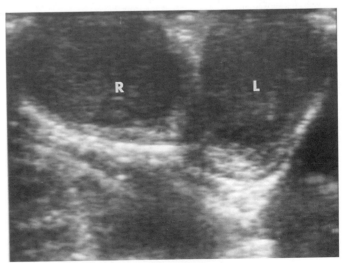

FIG. 11. Leukemia. **A:** Longitudinal scan of a 7-year-old demonstrates an enlarged, markedly hypoechoic right testis (*cursors*), measuring 4 cm in length. **B:** On a transverse scan, the left testis has a similar appearance. *R*, right testis; *L*, left testis.

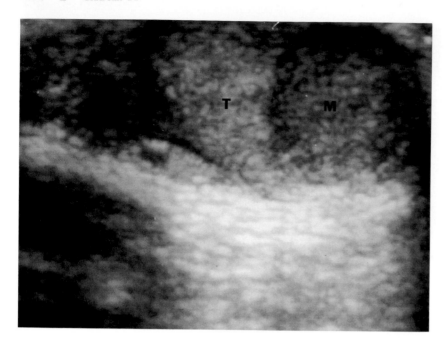

FIG. 12. Metastatic neuroblastoma in a 4-year-old boy. Longitudinal scan shows a hypoechoic mass (*M*) adjacent to testis (*T*). The mass was separate from the testis at surgery.

Metastatic tumors involving the testes include Wilms' tumor, neuroblastoma, histiocytosis X, sinus histiocytosis, retinoblastoma, and rhabdomyosarcoma. On sonography, secondary neoplasms appear as focal or diffuse areas of decreased echogenicity in an enlarged testis.

PARATESTICULAR TUMORS

Paratesticular tumors may arise in the spermatic cord (75% of cases) or in the appendix testis, epididymis, or testicular tunics. About 30% of spermatic cord tumors are malignant (64). The most common malig-

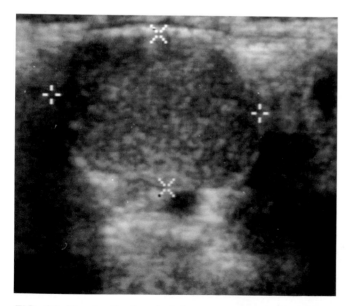

FIG. 13. Paratesticular rhabdomyosarcoma in a 3-year-old boy. Transverse scan of the left lower inguinal canal shows a well-defined mass of uniform echogenicity (*calipers*). The testis was identified as a separate structure in the scrotum.

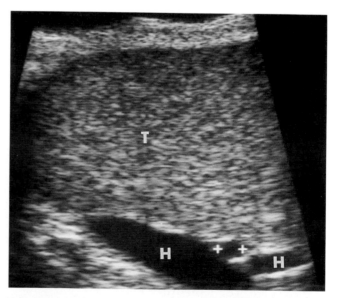

FIG. 14. Cyst of tunica albuginea. Longitudinal scan demonstrates a small cyst (*calipers*) in the periphery of testis (*T*). An adjacent hydrocele (*H*) is seen.

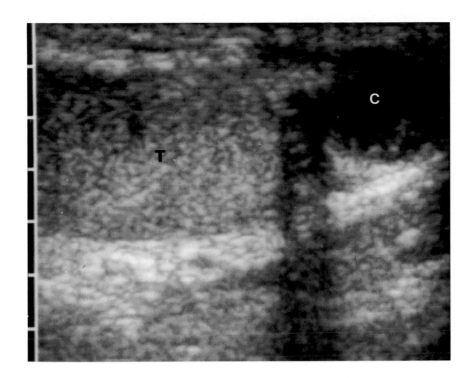

FIG. 15. Spermatocele. Longitudinal scan shows a cystic mass (*C*) in the epididymis. Echogenic debris is seen within the cyst. The testis (*T*) is normal.

nant tumor is embryonal rhabdomyosarcoma. It can occur throughout childhood, but it is most common in boys under 5 years of age. Patients usually present with rapidly growing, painless intrascrotal masses. Approximately 40% have metastatic disease to regional lymph nodes at the time of diagnosis. Other malignant paratesticular tumors include metastatic neuroblastoma (Fig. 12), leiomyosarcoma, and fibrosarcoma. Sonographically, paratesticular tumors are well-defined solid masses, with an echogenicity equal to or greater than that of the testis (Fig. 13); they may have focal anechoic areas of necrosis.

The most frequently encountered benign paratesticular masses are adenomatoid tumors or cysts; the latter include spermatoceles and cysts of the tunica albuginea (Fig. 14) (58). Adenomatoid tumors tend to be hypoechoic relative to normal epididymis, whereas spermatoceles and cysts are anechoic and often septated (Fig. 15). Rarer benign tumors include fibromas, leiomyomas, hemangiomas (Fig. 16), lymphangiomas, and neurofibromas. Differentiation between solid benign and malignant paratesticular tumors usually is not possible by sonography, and tissue sampling is required.

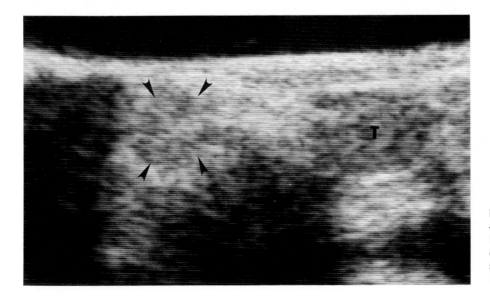

FIG. 16. Hemangioma of cord in a 4-year-old boy with a scrotal mass. Longitudinal scan of the scrotum, obtained with a standoff pad, shows an echogenic mass (*arrowheads*) superior to the testis (*T*).

INFLAMMATORY DISEASE

Causes of an acutely swollen and painful scrotum in childhood include torsion, infarct, trauma, epididymitis, orchitis, acute vasculitis, hemorrhage, and idiopathic scrotal edema. However, testicular torsion and epididymitis occur most frequently and present the greatest diagnostic problems. Differentiation between these two conditions is important because in the former, prompt surgical intervention is necessary to save the testis, whereas in the latter, surgery is not required. Frequently, clinical history and presentation are nonspecific and confusing. In some series, as many as 60% of patients had unnecessary surgery for epididymitis or acute scrotal abnormalities, other than torsion, based on clinical findings alone (61). High-resolution sonography can be valuable in the evaluation of the acute scrotum.

Acute Epididymitis/Orchitis

Infection of the epididymis usually follows infection elsewhere in the urinary tract. In adolescent boys, the sexually transmitted organisms that cause urethritis may also produce acute epididymitis. In many cases, epididymitis is associated with abnormalities of the uri-

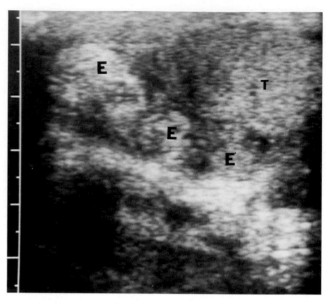

FIG. 18. Acute epididymitis. Longitudinal scan shows an enlarged, inhomogeneous left epididymis (*E*). The left testis (*T*) is normal.

nary tract such as distal urethral obstruction or an ectopic ureter draining into the vas deferens or seminal vesicles. Although bacterial infection is frequent, it also appears that sterile urine can produce an inflammatory response in the epididymis. The clinical picture includes scrotal edema, pain, and tenderness. Sonography demonstrates an enlarged epididymis; the echogenicity of the epididymis can be normal, decreased, or increased (Fig. 18). A reactive hydrocele usually is present, which may be anechoic or have a complex appearance.

Epididymitis will spread to involve the testis in 20% of postpubertal males, producing epididymo-orchitis (28). Testicular involvement may be focal or diffuse. Focal lesions appear as hypoechoic areas at the periphery of the testicle immediately adjacent to the inflamed epididymis (Fig. 19) (49). They gradually merge with the normal parenchyma (28,51). In cases in which the testis is diffusely involved either primarily or in association with epididymitis, it is inhomogeneous, enlarged, and hypoechoic. Color flow Doppler of orchitis or acute epididymis shows increased perfusion of the testes (Fig. 20, Colorplate 13). Orchitis in childhood also may be primary due to viral infections, particularly mumps, although this is less common than a bacterial etiology.

Rarely, acute epididymitis or epididymo-orchitis will go on to testicular infarction, usually the result of compression of the spermatic vessels by an enlarged epididymis or edematous spermatic cord (75). The tes-

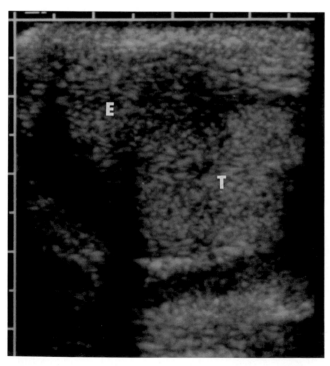

FIG. 17. Acute epididymitis. Longitudinal scan of the epididymis (*E*) shows it to be homogeneously enlarged. The echogenicity is normal and equal to that of the testis (*T*).

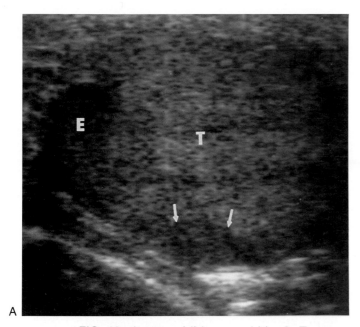
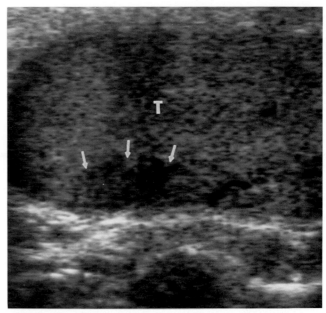

FIG. 19. Acute epididymo-orchitis. **A:** Transverse and **B:** longitudinal scans show an enlarged left testis (*T*). A small hypoechoic area is present along the posterior aspect of the testis (*arrows*), representing focal orchitis. The epididymis (*E*) is hypoechoic compared to the testis.

tis is enlarged, heterogeneous, and contains multiple hypoechoic spaces which enlarge rapidly over several days.

In chronic epididymitis or epididymo-orchitis, the epididymis is enlarged and inhomogeneous and may be hypo- or hyperechoic (Fig. 21). The parietal and visceral layers of the tunica are thickened and appear as an echogenic band around the testicle (20). Calcification, appearing as small echogenic areas with acoustic shadowing, can be present in the epididymis and tunica albuginea. The testis may be atrophic and diffusely or focally hypoechoic.

Abscess

Testicular abscess usually is a complication of orchitis, but it can be secondary to missed testicular torsion, infected hematoma, or primary orchitis. It also can develop from hematogenous or lymphatic dissemination of systemic infection. Conditions associated with testicular abscess include scarlet fever, influenza, typhoid fever, sinusitis, osteomyelitis, appendicitis, and cholecystitis (69). On sonography, a mature abscess appears as an anechoic, hyperechoic, or complex mass with low-level echoes representing

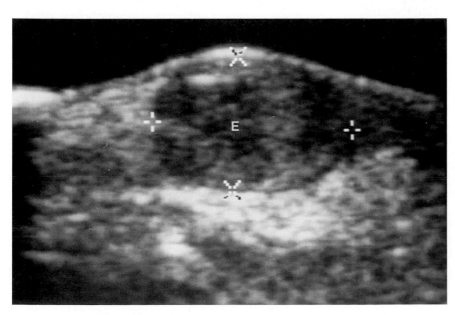

FIG. 21. Chronic epididymitis in a 9-month-old boy with a palpable scrotal mass. Longitudinal scan of the mass (*cursors*) shows that it is an enlarged epididymis (*E*). The entire epididymis is more hypoechoic and inhomogeneous than normal. There were no underlying genitourinary anomalies.

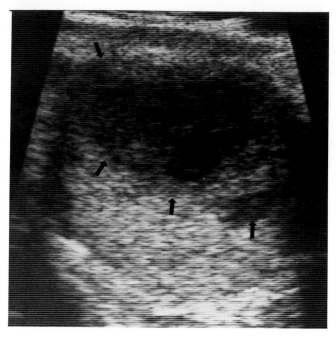

FIG. 22. Testicular abscess. Longitudinal scan of the left testis shows a fairly well-defined hypoechoic mass (*arrows*) with increased through-transmission. Aspiration revealed purulent fluid.

debris (Fig. 22). Increased through-transmission due to liquefaction and areas of intense echogenicity with shadowing due to gas bubbles may be present.

Fournier's Gangrene

Spontaneous gangrene, also known as Fournier's gangrene, is a rare, necrotizing infection of the scrotum, usually affecting neonates (4). Clinically, it is characterized by toxemia and rapid spread of inflammation to the inferior surface of the penis. The perineum, thighs, and abdominal wall usually are not involved. Pathologically, there is edema and necrosis of the scrotal wall with sparing of the testis and cord. The usual organisms involved are both aerobes and anaerobes; the infection can be gas-forming. Sonographically, the scrotal skin and soft tissues are thickened with hypo- and hyperechoic areas reflecting the presence of edema and gas bubbles. The underlying testis and epididymis are normal.

TORSION/INFARCTION

Torsion of the testis, or more correctly, spermatic cord, is of two types: intravaginal and extravaginal, with the former being more common. Intravaginal torsion is believed to be due to an anomalous attachment of the tunica vaginalis. Normally, the tunica vaginalis is strongly attached to the posterolateral wall of the testis. In the intravaginal type of torsion, the testis is completely enveloped by the tunica vaginalis which inserts high on the spermatic cord rather than on the testis. This "bell and clapper" deformity results in a propensity for torsion. Intravaginal torsion can occur in any age group, but it is most common in adolescence. Patients present with sudden onset of scrotal or lower abdominal pain. On examination, the affected testis is swollen and tender and may have a transverse lie. Clinically, intravaginal torsion can be difficult to distinguish from acute epididymitis (61).

In extravaginal torsion the peritoneal investment is normal but weakly attached, leading to torsion of the spermatic cord at the level of the external ring and all the scrotal contents. The condition usually occurs perinatally; affected infants present with a red, swollen scrotum and firm testes. Differential diagnostic considerations include meconium peritonitis, intraperitoneal bleeding tracking through the patent processus vaginalis, and tumor.

In patients with a high clinical suspicion of torsion, imaging studies may be bypassed and the patient taken to surgery. When the diagnosis is unclear or the patient presents with pain of more than 18 hr duration, imaging studies are performed. Because of its 95% accuracy rate, scintigraphy has been the examination of choice for diagnosing torsion (9,57). However, a recent series with a small number of patients suggests that sonography with color flow Doppler may be as sensitive as scintigraphy (59).

Torsion is divided into acute torsion with symptoms lasting less than 24 hr; subacute, lasting more than 24 hr but less than 10 days; and chronic, lasting greater than 10 days. The sonographic appearance of the testis in both intra- and extravaginal torsion is related to the duration of the torsion. In the first few hours, the testis may appear normal. After 4 to 6 hr and possibly earlier, the testis usually is enlarged and hypoechoic (Fig. 23) (39). It rarely may be hyperechoic. The epididymis also may enlarge and be hypoechoic or may have an inhomogeneous echo pattern. After 24 hr, the testis appears heterogeneous because of necrosis and hemorrhage (Fig. 24). A hydrocele, scrotal wall thickening, and large extratesticular hematoma may be present (83).

Continuous wave and duplex Doppler sonography have been used to examine flow in the vessels of the spermatic cord and testis (7,47). Unfortunately, there are pitfalls in diagnosis associated with the use of Doppler sonography (48,70). The testicular vessels are small and detection of arterial flow may be difficult even in normal testes. Additionally, Doppler sonography cannot reliably distinguish between paratesticular and intratesticular arterial pulsations, so that scrotal hyperemia associated with torsion may be mistaken for normal flow to the affected testis. The overall accuracy of continuous wave Doppler sonography in

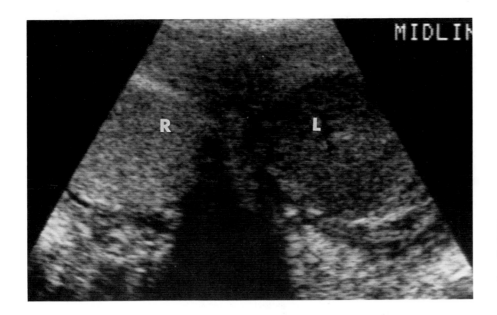

FIG. 23. Acute torsion in a patient with 4 hr of scrotal pain. Transverse scan shows the left testis to be enlarged and hypoechoic. The testis was viable at surgery. *L,* left testis; *R,* right testis.

diagnosing torsion is about 80% (70). Color flow Doppler sonography is capable of reliably demonstrating testicular arteries in normal individuals and is more sensitive than duplex Doppler sonography in assessing abnormalities that affect scrotal blood flow, such as torsion (Fig. 25, Colorplate 14) (59,60).

Treatment for intravaginal testicular torsion is immediate detorsion and fixation of the testis to the scrotal wall. A clearly necrotic testis is removed because it has been shown that it can adversely affect the contralateral testis by a presumed immunologic process (57). Orchiopexy is simultaneously performed on the contralateral normal testis at the time of operation on the torsed testis, because an abnormal attachment of the tunica vaginalis is believed frequently to exist bilaterally. Surgery for extravaginal torsion is controversial since the testis is rarely viable at the time of diagnosis. The duration of the torsion determines the success rate of surgery in salvaging the testis. Viable testes are found in 80% to 100% of patients who are operated on within 6 hr of the symptoms' onset, in 70% of those operated on between 6 and 12 hr, and in 20% of patients with symptoms for over 12 hr (18). Thus, early diagnosis is important.

If surgery is not performed, the infarcted testis will begin to atrophy after 14 days. It may remain hypoechoic or it may increase in echogenicity as fibrosis or calcification develops. The epididymis may be enlarged in chronic torsion.

In addition to torsion, other causes of testicular infarction include epididymitis, orchitis, trauma, polyarteritis nodosa, and subacute bacterial endocarditis.

Torsion of Testicular Appendages

Torsion of the appendix testis or appendix epididymis can mimic acute testicular torsion. Differentiation is important because the former does not need surgery, whereas immediate surgical intervention is required for the latter condition (36). The normal appendix testis is a remnant of the müllerian duct and is attached to the tunica albuginea, whereas the appendix epididymis is a mesonephric vestige. Both appendices are pedunculated, making them prone to torsion. Peak clinical incidence is in boys between 6 and 12 years of age who present with pain which often is localized to the upper pole of the testis. On physical examination, a small, firm, tender nodule may be palpated in the

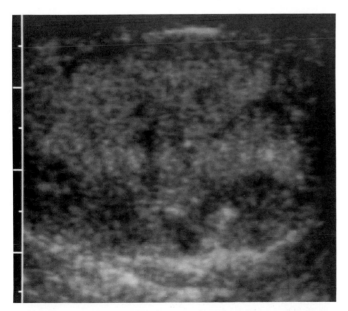

FIG. 24. Subacute torsion. Longitudinal scan reveals an enlarged, inhomogeneous left testis. Patient had symptoms more than 24 hr. At operation testis was infarcted and was removed.

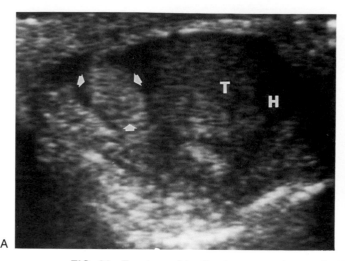

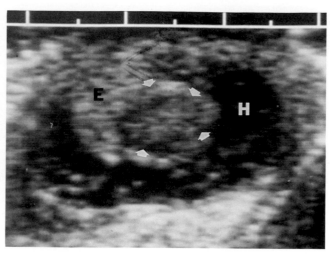

FIG. 26. Torsion of testicular appendages. **A:** Torsed appendix testis in a 13-year-old boy with left scrotal pain and blue discoloration of the scrotum. Longitudinal scan shows a 9 mm mass (*arrows*) next to the upper pole of the testis (*T*). A normal epididymis was identified separate from the mass. A small hydrocele (*H*) also is noted. At surgery the appendix testis was necrotic and attached to the upper pole of the testis. **B:** Torsion of appendix epididymis in a 5-year-old boy with a 5-day history of right scrotal pain. Longitudinal scan shows a hypoechoic mass (*arrows*) projecting from the right epididymis(*E*). A surrounding hydrocele (*H*) is noted. At operation, the appendix epididymis was necrotic. The underlying epididymis and testis were edematous but viable without evidence of torsion.

upper scrotum (77). The infarcted appendage appears blue or black with transillumination. Complications rarely follow cases of torsion of the appendix testis. Atrophy of the appendage and resolution of symptoms is the usual outcome.

The torsed appendix is not always seen by sonography. When visualized, it is a small hyper- or hypoechoic mass adjacent to the testis or epididymis (Fig. 26). The testis and epididymis may be enlarged and hypoechoic due to edema. A reactive hydrocele usually is present.

TRAUMA

Blunt injuries to the scrotum usually are the result of child abuse, motor vehicle accidents, athletic injuries, fighting, or a straddle injury (compression of the scrotum against the pubic rami). Physical examination of the scrotum is often limited by pain and swelling. Sonography can be useful in determining the presence or absence of hematoma, hematocele, and testicular rupture; the latter is particularly important because it requires immediate surgical intervention. Ninety percent of ruptured testes can be salvaged if the surgery is performed within the first 72 hr (71). Sequelae of delayed diagnosis include ischemic necrosis, epididymitis, abscess, and loss of spermatogenesis or hormonal function (51). Surgery is unnecessary if a hematocele or hematoma is present, as long as the testis is intact.

Testicular rupture leads to extrusion of the testicular contents into the scrotal sac. Sonographically, the rup-

tured testis is inhomogeneous with irregular, poorly defined borders. Occasionally a fracture line, appearing as a linear echolucency in the testicular parenchyma, may be seen (Fig. 27). An associated hematocele is frequent (71).

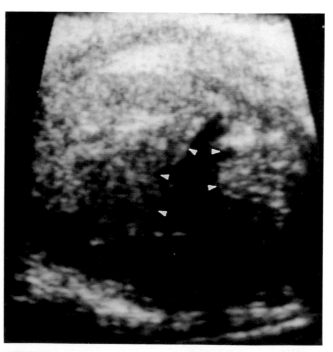

FIG. 27. Testicular rupture with hematocele. Longitudinal scan shows a hypoechoic fracture line (*white arrowheads*) extending through the testis. The inferior testicular surface is poorly defined.

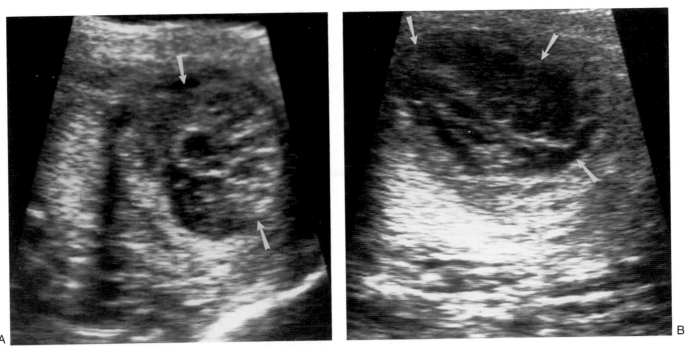

FIG. 28. Testicular hematoma: **A:** Transverse and **B:** longitudinal scans show a well-defined, hypoechoic mass (*arrows*) in the left testis. The hematoma has a complex echotexture containing anechoic areas and septations.

Testicular hematoma unassociated with rupture produces an enlarged testis with focal areas of increased or decreased echogenicity, depending on the age of the hematoma. Acutely, the lesion may appear complex, or hyperchoic (54). With later liquefaction, it develops more cystic areas and septations (Fig. 28). Associated scrotal wall thickening is frequently seen. Extratesticular hematoma involving the scrotal wall or

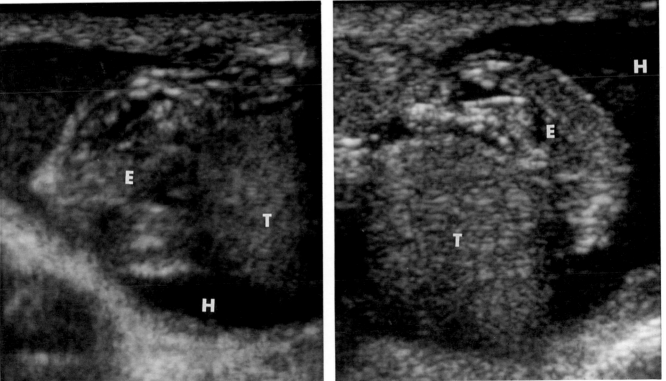

FIG. 29. Epididymal hematoma. **A:** Longitudinal and **B:** transverse scans of the right epididymis (*E*) shows it to be enlarged and heterogeneous. The right testis (*T*) is normal. A moderate-size hematocele (*H*) is seen.

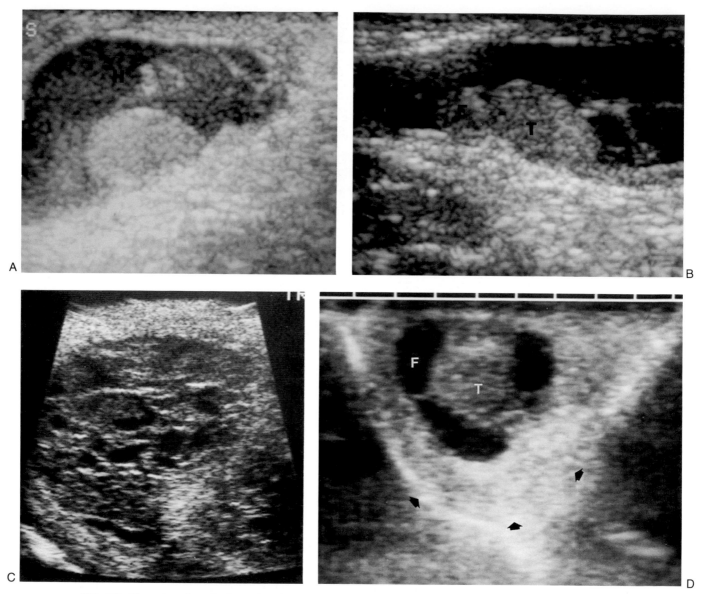

FIG. 30. Hematoceles. **A:** Longitudinal scan of the right scrotum immediately following trauma reveals a large echogenic hematocele (*H*). **B:** One month later the fluid has become anechoic with several septations. The epididymis (*E*) and testis (*T*) are more clearly defined. **C:** In another patient with scrotal trauma, transverse scan shows a complex fluid collection within the scrotal sac containing cystic areas and septations. **D:** Transverse scan in another patient demonstrates a testis (*T*) surrounded by hypoechoic fluid (*F*) containing septations. The scrotal wall (*arrows*) is thickened. Scrotal blood was secondary to adrenal hemorrhage and hemoperitoneum.

epididymis and hematocele also have a variable appearance depending on the length of time that the hematoma has been present (Fig. 29). Hematoceles often contain septations and loculations and have thick walls (Fig. 30). In the presence of large hematomas, identification of discrete intrascrotal structures may be difficult. In this instance, color flow Doppler is valuable to localize the testis and evaluate blood flow.

Sonography can be used to localize foreign bodies in the testicle, such as bullet fragments (22), and to detect scrotal urinomas. Urinoma usually occurs when there is rupture of the bulbous urethra with leakage of

urine into the soft tissues of the scrotum (28). Rarely, scrotal urinoma may result from bladder rupture. Sonographically, urinoma appears as diffuse scrotal thickening or as an anechoic intrascrotal fluid collection that is distinguishable from a hydrocele.

HYDROCELE

A hydrocele is a collection of fluid between the two layers of the tunica vaginalis. In infants and young children, virtually all hydroceles represent collections of peritoneal fluid that have entered the scrotal sac by way of a patent processus vaginalis. The majority of congenital hydroceles undergo spontaneous resolution by 18 months of age (46). In older children and adolescents, hydroceles are more frequently due to torsion, trauma, inflammation, or tumor (33).

Sonography allows evaluation of the testis and epididymis when a large hydrocele makes the physical examination difficult. Most hydroceles are anechoic collections with strong through-transmission and thin walls (Fig. 31) (36). Septations are present in cases due to prior hemorrhage or infection. Scattered echos caused by cholesterol crystals, hemorrhage, infection, or calculi also may be observed. With chronic hydroceles, variable thickening of the scrotal wall may occur (Fig. 32). Measurements of hydrocele size have been published, but are of little clinical significance (65).

Additional causes of hydroceles are ventriculoperitoneal shunts and lymphoceles. If the processus vaginalis is patent, cerebrospinal fluid from a ventriculoperitoneal shunt may tract into the scrotum. At times, the catheter tip may actually enter the scrotum. Scrotal lymphoceles have been associated with ipsilateral renal transplantation. They usually are secondary to lymphatic disruption with seepage of lymph fluid into the tunica vaginalis, or to direct extension of a periallograft lymphocele around the transplanted kidney through the inguinal canal into the scrotum (16). Sonographically, sonolucent scrotal fluid collections with multiple septations can be observed (Fig. 33). Associated hydroceles are common.

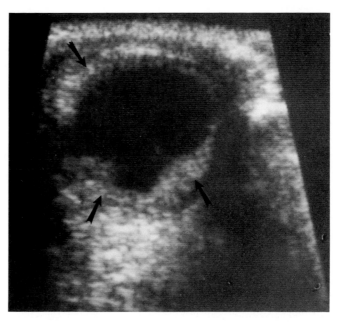

FIG. 32. Chronic hydrocele. Transverse scan above testis shows a hydrocele surrounded by a thickened wall (*arrows*).

Hematoceles are complicated hydroceles containing predominantly hemorrhagic fluid. Most are secondary to trauma or surgery, but other causes include malignant tumors and bleeding disorders. The sonographic appearance has been described earlier in the trauma section. The tunica vaginalis becomes thick in association with chronic hematoceles.

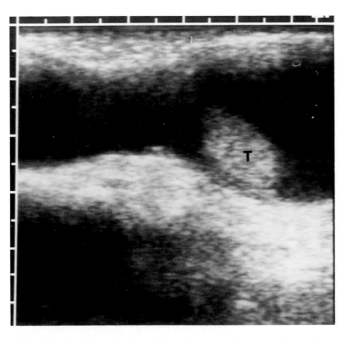

FIG. 31. Hydrocele involving the scrotum and inguinal canal of a 2-month-old boy. Longitudinal scan shows anechoic fluid surrounding the testis (*T*).

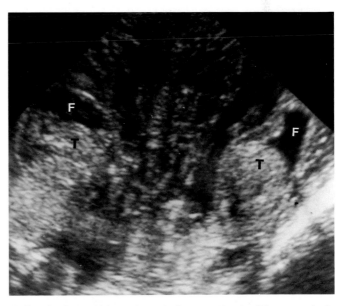

FIG. 33. Scrotal lymphocele in a patient with a renal allograft. Transverse scan shows septated fluid collections dissecting along tissue planes of the scrotum and around the testes (*T*). Extratesticular fluid (*F*) collections represent small hydroceles.

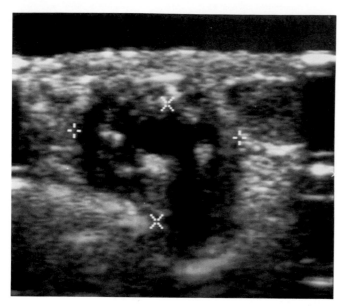

FIG. 34. Inguinal hernia. Transverse scan of lower inguinal area shows a bowel loop (*cursors*) in the inguinal canal. The bowel exhibited peristalsis on real-time imaging.

INGUINAL AND SCROTAL HERNIA

Although the vast majority of hernias are usually clinically obvious, sonography can be valuable in patients with small, painful hernias in whom physical examination is difficult. When fluid-filled loops of bowel are observed in the inguinal canal or scrotum,

the diagnosis of a hernia can be made easily (Fig. 34). If peristalsis is observed on real-time sonography the bowel is viable; absence of peristalsis suggests incarceration. When omentum or gas-filled intestine lie in the inguinal canal, a complex echogenic mass is observed. Demonstration of peristalsis confirms that the scrotal mass is bowel (51). The underlying testicle and epididymis are normal, but often are difficult to image because of the presence of adjacent bowel or omentum (27). Inguinal hernias may coexist with a hydrocele because both are associated with patent processus vaginalis. Complex hydrocele, hematocele, scrotal abscess, or urinoma can simulate a hernia, but differentiation is possible when peristalsis is identified on a real-time examination.

VARICOCELE

Varicocele is an acquired malformation due to dilatation of the pampiniform plexus and is a cause of scrotal swelling (68). It may be primary or secondary to an intraabdominal or pelvic mass. The majority of primary varicoceles involve the left hemiscrotum. The mechanism postulated for the development of a varicocele involves the presence of incompetent venous valves which permit retrograde blood flow through the internal spermatic vein, leading to dilatation of the pampiniform plexus. On physical examination, varicoceles increase in size when the patient is upright or performs Valsalva's maneuver. Such varices may im-

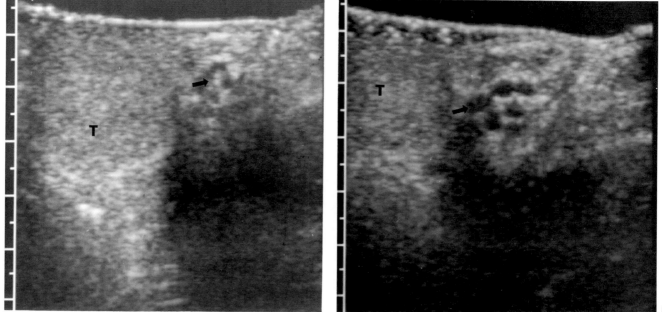

FIG. 35. Left varicocele. **A:** Longitudinal scan showing multiple tortuous tubular structures (*arrow*) adjacent to the testis (*T*). **B:** The veins increase in size (*arrow*) during Valsalva's maneuver.

pair sperm motility and be associated with infertility (2). The testis on the affected side may be smaller than the one on the uninvolved side (32).

On sonography, varicoceles appear as tortuous, tubular structures just superior to the testis (Fig. 35). Their individual diameters range from 2 to 7 mm or greater; by contrast, normal veins have a diameter of 0.5 to 2 mm (36). The veins increase in size during Valsalva's manuever or with pressure on the base of the scrotum. Duplex Doppler examination can demonstrate venous flow and can evaluate the degree of venous reflex into the spermatic veins (37). Blood flow is slow in comparison to normal and at times may be almost absent. Because of the tortuosity of the veins, flow occurs in different directions in adjacent veins and there may even be flow reversal. Direction and flow speed also can be affected by the pressure of the transducer. Heavy compression may cause flow to slow or cease. Occasionally, areas of intense echogenicity with associated shadowing are seen within the varicosities, corresponding to calcifications or phleboliths (25).

MISCELLANEOUS

Scrotal Calcifications

Scrotal calcifications may be secondary to chronic hematoma or inflammation, phleboliths, metastatic neuroblastoma, scrotal calculi, or meconium peritonitis. Scrotal calculi lie between the membranes of the tunica vaginalis and are believed to result from either torsion of the appendix testis or epididymis, or from inflammation of the tunica vaginalis (50,82). In the for-

mer cases, infarcted tissues slough and calcify, whereas in the latter instance, desquamated epithelial cells and fibrous debris calcify. Scrotal calculi may be single or multiple and vary in size from 4 to 10 mm (36). On sonography, they are round, mobile, and highly echogenic, with associated acoustic shadowing (50). Testicular microlithiasis is a rare cause of scrotal calcification and has been reported with cryptorchidism and Klinefelter's syndrome. The sonographic pattern is one of tiny bright echos with attenuation of the sound beam (17).

Meconium peritonitis follows antenatal perforation of the bowel in the second or third trimester of pregnancy. Sterile intestinal contents leak into the peritoneal cavity producing an inflammatory reaction which subsequently calcifies (41). The extruded meconium may extend into the scrotum through a patent processus vaginalis to produce a calcified scrotal mass. On sonography, meconium peritonitis appears as a complex mass with highly echogenic areas which produce acoustic shadowing (Fig. 36) (6). The extent of calcification may be so great that it precludes evaluation of the underlying testis. Meconium peritonitis can be mistaken for a solid neoplasm, particularly a teratoma. The diagnosis can be confirmed if abdominal radiographs show concomitant peritoneal calcifications.

Idiopathic Scrotal Edema

Acute idiopathic scrotal wall edema is an uncommon condition involving one or both hemiscrota (42). Patients are usually about 5 years of age and present with

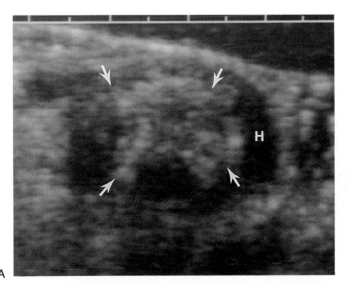
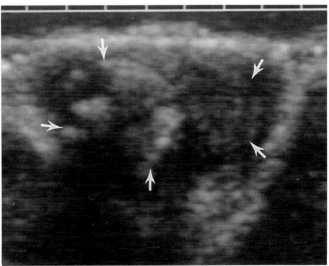

FIG. 36. Meconium peritonitis in an infant with a right scrotal mass. **A:** Longitudinal and **B:** transverse scans demonstrate a mass (*arrows*) containing multiple echogenic areas representing calcifications. The testis could not be identified as a discrete structure. An adjacent hydrocele (*H*) is seen.

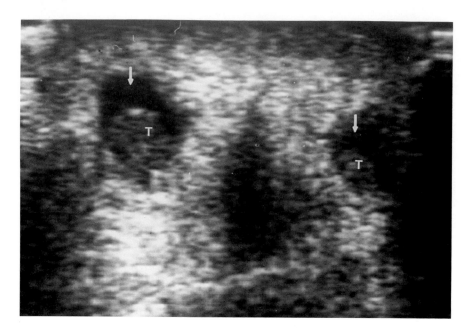

FIG. 37. Idiopathic scrotal edema. Transverse scan shows diffuse thickening of the scrotal wall which is echogenic. Small bilateral hydroceles (*arrows*) surround the testes (*T*).

a painful, edematous, and discolored scrotum and peripheral eosinophilia. The underlying scrotal contents are nontender and not swollen on palpation. On sonography there usually is thickening of the scrotal soft tissues without testicular involvement (Fig. 37). Acute scrotal edema resolves spontaneously without treatment and without sequelae. The major differential diagnostic consideration is nonaccidental trauma.

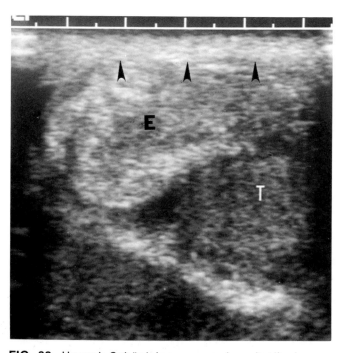

FIG. 38. Henoch-Schönlein purpura. Longitudinal sonogram shows an enlarged and echogenic epididymis (*E*), hypoechoic testis (*T*), and echogenic thickened scrotal wall (*arrowheads*).

Acute Vasculitis

Acute vasculitis of the scrotal wall due to Henoch-Schönlein purpura is an unusual entity, occurring in children 2 to 8 years of age. The skin, gastrointestinal tract, joints, and kidneys are affected most often, but the testis and scrotum may be involved in up to 15% of cases; genital involvement may occur prior to other organ involvement (42,44). On sonography, the testicle and occasionally the epididymis are diffusely enlarged with an inhomogeneous echo pattern (Fig. 38). A reactive hydrocele and swelling of the scrotal wall often are observed. The clinical and sonographic findings may be difficult to distinguish clinically from torsion or orchitis (78). A high index of suspicion is needed to make the diagnosis.

PROSTATE AND SEMINAL VESICLES

The prostate and seminal vesicles can be examined through an anterior abdominal approach using the distended bladder as an acoustic window or by transrectal transducers. The incidence of disease of these structures in the pediatric population is small, although congenital prostatic cysts, prostatic utricles and seminal vesicle cysts have been reported (26,30). Prostatic cysts and utricles represent residual müllerian duct structures and are seen in association with hypospadias, intersex problems, cryptorchidism, and renal dysgenesis (26). Seminal vesical cysts arise from the mesonephric (wolffian) duct and approximately two-thirds are associated with ipsilateral renal agenesis. Most cysts are asymptomatic but they may present with signs and symptoms of cystitis, epididymitis, or prostatitis. Sonography can accurately define the size

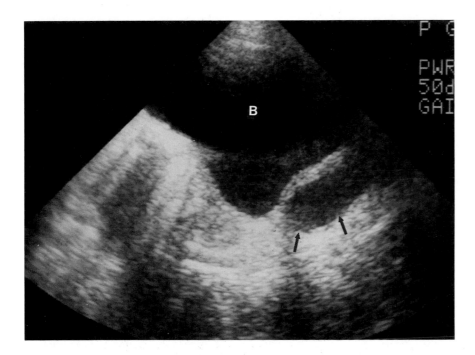

FIG. 39. Prostatic utricle in a male infant with hypospadias at the peno-scrotal junction. Longitudinal scan shows a cystic structure (*arrows*) posterior to the bladder (*B*).

of the cyst or utricle, its fluid nature, and its relationship to adjacent organs (Fig. 39).

Rhabdomyosarcoma is the most common prostatic malignancy in children. It tends to extend early outside the capsule of the prostate and infiltrate bladder neck, posterior urethra, and adjacent soft tissues. Affected children usually present with urinary retention and less frequently with infection. Sites of distant metastases are the lungs, bone, liver, and bone marrow. Sonographically, prostatic rhabdomyosarcoma often appears as a complex pelvic mass with cystic areas, representing foci of hemorrhage or necrosis (Fig. 40). The mass often indents or displaces the bladder and may cause localized bladder wall thickening if there is intramural extension.

Urethra

The posterior urethra is imaged through the bladder, perineum, or transrectally, while the anterior urethra is studied with a linear array transducer placed directly

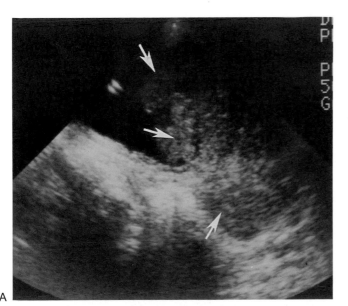
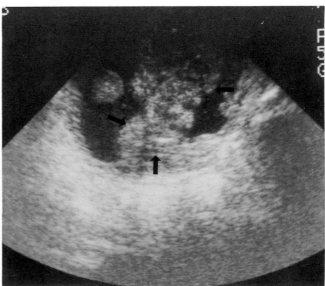

FIG. 40. Rhabdomyosarcoma of the prostate in a 23-month-old boy. **A:** Longitudinal midline scan shows an inhomogeneous mass (*arrows*) arising from the prostate and extending into the bladder. **B:** Transverse scan shows polypoid masses (*arrows*) within the bladder lumen. (Courtesy of Dr. L. Magill, Memphis, Tennessee).

on the penis. After the bladder is filled, voiding sonourethrography can demonstrate strictures, calculi, anterior or posterior valves, foreign bodies, bladder neck dyssynergia, diverticuli, and trauma (5,13, 15,52,55).

REFERENCES

1. Askin FB, Land VJ, Sullivan M, et al. Occult testicular leukemia: Testicular biopsy at three years continuous complete remission of childhood leukemia: A southwest oncology group study. Cancer 1981;47:470–475.
2. Basile-Fasolo C, Izzo PL, Canale D, Menchini Fabris GF. Doppler sonography, contact scrotal thermography, and venography. A comparative study in the evaluation of subclinical varicocele. Int J Fertil 1986;30:62–64.
3. Batata MA, Chu FCH, Hilaris BS, et al. Cryptorchidism and testicular cancer in cryptorchids. Cancer 1982;49:1023–1039.
4. Begley MG, Shawker TH, Robertson CN, et al. Fournier gangrene: Diagnosis with scrotal US. Radiology 1988;169:387–389.
5. Benson CB, Doubilet PM, Richie JP. Sonography of the male genital tract. AJR 1989;153:705–713.
6. Berdon WE, Baker DH, Becker J, de Sanctis P. Scrotal masses in healed meconium peritonitis. N Engl J Med 1967;277:585–587.
7. Bickerstaff KI, Sethia K, Murie JA. Doppler ultrasonography in the diagnosis of acute scrotal pain. Br J Surg 1988;75:238–239.
8. Cassorla FG, Golden SM, Johnsonbaugh RD, et al. Testicular volume during early infancy. J Pediatr 1981;99:742–743.
9. Chen DC, Holder LE, Kaplan GN. Correlation of radionuclide imaging and diagnostic ultrasound in scrotal diseases. J Nucl Med 1986;27:1774–1781.
10. Cho CS, Kosek J. Cystic dysplasia of the testis: Sonographic and pathologic findings. Radiology 1985;156:777–778.
11. Cooper SG, Richman AH, Carpenter TO, Rosenfeld AT. Scrotal ultrasonography in Leydig cell hyperplasia. J Ultrasound Med 1989;8:689–692.
12. Daniels WA Jr, Feinstein RA, Howard-Peebles P, et al. Testicular volumes of adolescents. J Pediatr 1982;101:1010–1012.
13. de Filippi G, Derchi LE, Coppi M, Biggi E. Sonographic diagnosis of a urethral polyp in a child. Pediatr Radiol 1983;13:351–352.
14. Dehner LP. The male reproductive system. In: Pediatric Surgical Pathology, 2nd ed. St. Louis: C.V. Mosby, 1987;712–742.
15. Dierks PR, Hawkins H. Sonography and penile trauma. J Ultrasound Med 1983;2:417–419.
16. Dierks PR, Moore PT. Scrotal lymphocele: A complication of renal transplant surgery. J Ultrasound Med 1986;4:91–92.
17. Doherty FJ, Mullins TL, Sant GR, Drinkwater MA, Ucci AA. Testicular microlithiasis. A unique sonographic appearance. J Ultrasound Med 1987;6:389–392.
18. Donohue RE, Utley WLF. Torsion of spermatic cord. Urology 1978;11:33–36.
19. Finkelstein MS, Rosenberg HK, Snyder HM, Duckett JW. Ultrasound evaluation of scrotum in pediatrics. Urology 1986;27:1–9.
20. Fowler RC, Chennells PM, Ewing R. Scrotal ultrasonography: A clinical evaluation. Br J Radiol 1987;60:649–654.
21. Gauderer MWL, Grisoni ER, Stellato TA, Ponsky JL, Izant RJ, Jr. Transverse testicular ectopia. J Pediatr Surg 1982;17:43–47.
22. Gavant ML, Smith WC, Parks FD. Ultrasonic evaluation of gun shot injury to testicle. JCU 1984;12:355–356.
23. Gibbons MD, Cromie WJ, Duckett JW, Jr. Management of the abdominal undescended testicle. J Urol 1979;122:76–79.
24. Gooding GAW, Leonhardt W, Stein R. Testicular cysts: US finding. Radiology 1987;163:537–538.
25. Gottlieb RH, Poster R, Subudhi MK. Computed tomographic, ultrasound, and plain film appearance of phleboliths in varicoceles. J Ultrasound Med 1989;8:329–331.
26. Gregg DC, Sty JR. Sonographic diagnosis of enlarged prostate utricle. J Ultrasound Med 1989;8:51–52.
27. Gutman H, Golimbu M, Subramanyam BR. Diagnostic ultrasound of scrotum. Urology 1986;27:72–75.
28. Haddick WK, Hricak H, Jeffrey RB. Scrotal sonography. Semin Urol 1985;3:146–157.
29. Hadziselimovic F. Cryptorchidism. In: Retik AB, Cukier J, eds. Pediatric Urology. Baltimore: Williams and Wilkins, 1987; 271–281.
30. Hamilton S, Fitzpatrick JM. Ultrasound diagnosis of a prostatic cyst causing acute urinary retention. J Ultrasound Med 1987;6:385–387.
31. Hamm B, Fobbe F, Loy V. Testicular cysts: Differentiation with US and clinical findings. Radiology 1988;168:19–23.
32. Hamm B, Fobbe F, Sörensen R, Felsenberg D. Varicoceles: Combined sonography and thermography in diagnosis and posttherapeutic evaluation. Radiology 1986;160:419–424.
33. Han BK. Uncommon causes of scrotal and inguinal swelling in children: Sonographic appearance. JCU 1986;14:421–427.
34. Hederstrom E, Forsberg L, Kullendorff CM. Ultrasonography of the undescended testis. Acta Radiol Diag 1985;26:453–456.
35. Hertzberg BS, Mahoney BS, Bowie JO, Anderson EE. Sonography of an intratesticular lipoma. J Ultrasound Med 1985;4:619–621.
36. Hill MC, Sanders RC. Sonography of benign disease of the scrotum. In: Sanders RC, Hill M, eds. Ultrasound Annual. New York: Raven Press, 1986;197–237.
37. Hirsh AV, Kellett MJ, Robertson G, Pryor JP. Doppler flow studies, venography and thermography in the evaluation of varicoceles of fertile and subfertile men. Br J Urol 1980;52:560–565.
38. Hricak H, Filly RA. Sonography of the scrotum. Invest Radiol 1983;18:112–121.
39. Hricak H, Lue T, Filly RA, Alpers CE, Zeineh SJ. Tanagho EA. Experimental study of the sonographic diagnosis of testicular torsion. J Ultrasound Med 1983;2:349–356.
40. Johansen TEB, Larmo A. Ultrasound in the evaluation of retractile and truly undescended testes. Scan J Urol Nephrol 1988;22:245–250.
41. Kenney PJ, Spirt BA, Ellis DA, Patil U. Scrotal masses caused by meconium peritonitis: Prenatal sonographic diagnosis. Radiology 1985;154:362.
42. Khan AU, Williams TH, Malek RS. Acute scrotal swelling in Henoch-Schönlein syndrome. Urology 1977;10:139–141.
43. Kirschner MA, Jacobs JB, Fraley EE. Bilateral anorchia with persistent testosterone production. N Engl J Med 1970;282:240–244.
44. Klauber GT, Grannum RS. Disorders of the male external genitalia. In: Kelalis PP, King LR, Belman AB. Clinical Pediatric Urology, 2nd ed. New York: W.B. Saunders, 1985;825–861.
45. Kogan SJ. Cryptorchidism. In: Kelalis PP, King LR, Belman AB. Clinical Pediatric Urology, 2nd ed. New York: W.B. Saunders, 1985;864–887.
46. Krone KD, Carroll BA. Scrotal ultrasound. Radiol Clin North Am 1985;23:121–139.
47. Leahy PF. Diagnosis of testicular torsion using Doppler ultrasonic examination. Br J Urol 1986;58:696–697.
48. Lee LM, Wright JE, McLoughlin MG. Testicular torsion in the adult. J Urol 1983;130:93–94.
49. Lentini JF, Benson CB, Richie JP. Sonographic features of focal orchitis. J Ultrasound Med 1989;8:361–365.
50. Linkowski GD, Avellone A, Gooding GAW. Scrotal calculi: Sonographic detection. Radiology 1985;156:484.
51. Martin B, Conte J. Ultrasonography of the acute scrotum. JCU 1987;15:37–44.
52. McAlister WH. Demonstration of the dilated prostatic urethra in posterior urethral valve patients. J Ultrasound Med 1984;14:91–93.
53. McAlister WH, Manley CB. Bilobed testicle. Pediatr Radiol 1987;17:82.
54. McAlister WH, Sisler CL. Scrotal sonography in infants and children. Current Problems in Radiology. Chicago: Year Book Medical Publishers (in press).

55. McAninch JW, Laing FC, Jeffrey RB. Sonourethrography in the evaluation of urethral strictures: A preliminary report. *J Urol* 1988;139:294–297.

56. Mehan DJ, Chehval J, Ullah S. Polyorchidism. *J Urol* 1976;116:530–532.

57. Mendel JB, Taylor GA, Treves S, Cheng TH, Retik A, Bauer S. Testicular torsion in children: Scintigraphic assessment. *Pediatr Radiol* 1985;15:110–115.

58. Mevorach RA, Lerner RM, Linke C, DiSant'Agnese PA. Ultrasound diagnosis of tunica albuginea cyst: Clinical perspective. *Urology* 1985;5:551–553.

59. Middleton WD, Melson GL. Testicular ischemia: Color Doppler sonographic findings in five patients. *AJR* 1989;152:1237–1239.

60. Middleton WD, Thorne DA, Melson GL. Color Doppler ultrasound of the normal testis. *AJR* 1989;152:293–297.

61. Mueller DL, Amundson GM, Rubin SZ, Wesenberg RL. Acute scrotal abnormalities in children: Diagnosis by combined sonography and scintigraphy. *AJR* 1988;150:643–646.

62. Pappis CH, Argianas SA, Bousgas D, Athanasiades E. Unsuspected urological anomlies in asymptomatic cryptorchid boys. *Pediatr Radiol* 1988;18:51–53.

63. Phillips G, Kumari-Subaiya S, Sawitsky A. Ultrasonic evaluation of the scrotum in lymphoproliferative disease. *J Ultrasound Med* 1987;6:169–175.

64. Raney RB Jr, Duckett JW, Donaldson MH. Malignant genitourinary tumors. In: Sutow WW, Fernback DJ, Vietti TJ, eds. *Clinical Pediatric Oncology*. St. Louis: C.V. Mosby, 1984;734–743.

65. Rifkin MD. Scrotal ultrasound. *Urol Radiol* 1987;9:119–126.

66. Rifkin MD, Kurtz AB, Pasto ME, Goldberg BB. Diagnostic capabilities of high-resolution scrotal ultrasonography: Prospective evaluation. *J Ultrasound Med* 1985;4:13–19.

67. Rifkin MD, Kurtz AB, Pasto ME, et al. The sonographic diagnosis of focal and diffuse infiltrating intrascrotal lesions. *Urol Radiol* 1984;6:20–26.

68. Rifkin MD, Foy PM, Kurtz AB, Pasto ME, Goldberg BB. The role of diagnostic ultrasonography in varicocele evaluation. *J Ultrasound Med* 1983;2:271–275.

69. Rockey KE, Cusack TJ. Ultrasound imaging of the scrotum. A pictorial guide to its varied capabilities. *Postgrad Med* 1987;82:219–227.

70. Rodríquez DD, Rodríguez WC, Rivera JJ, Rodríguez S, Otero AA. Doppler ultrasound versus testicular scanning in the evaluation of the acute scrotum. *J Urol* 1981;125:343–346.

71. Schaffer RM. Ultrasonography of scrotal trauma. *Urol Radiol* 1985;7:245–249.

72. Schwerk WB, Schwerk WN, Rodeck G. Testicular tumors: Prospective analysis of realtime US findings and abdominal staging. *Radiology* 1987;164:369–374.

73. Scott RF, Bayless AP, Calder JF, Garvie WHH. Indications for ultrasound in the evaluation of the pathological scrotum. *Br J Urol* 1986;58:178–182.

74. Scully RE. Gonadoblastoma. Review of 74 cases. *Cancer* 1970;25:1340–1356.

75. See WA, Mack LA, Krieger JN. Scrotal ultrasonography: A predictor of complicated epididymitis requiring orchiectomy. *J Urol* 1988;139:55–56.

76. Seidenwurm D, Smathers RL, Kan P, Hoffman A. Intratesticular adrenal rests diagnosed by ultrasound. *Radiology* 1985;155:479–481.

77. Skoglund RW, McRoberts JW, Ragde H. Torsion of testicular appendages: Presentation of 43 new cases and a collective review. *J Urol* 1970;104:598–604.

78. Stein BS, Kendell AR, Harke HT, et al. Scrotal imaging in Henoch-Schönlein. *J Urol* 1980;124:568–569.

79. Tackett RE, Ling D, Catalona WJ, Melson GL. High resolution sonography in diagnosing testicular neoplasms: Clinical significance of false positive scans. *J Urol* 1986;135:494–496.

80. Thurnher S, Hricak H, Carroll PR, Pobiel RS, Filly RA. Imaging the testis: Comparison between MR imaging and US. *Radiology* 1988;167:631–636.

81. Tibbs SJ. Unilateral absence of the testis: Eight cases of true monorchism. *Br J Surg* 1961;48:601–608.

82. Török P, Perjés G, Rosdy E. Intrascrotal calcification. *Int Urol Nephrol* 1981;13:167–173.

83. Vick CW, Bird K, Rosenfield AT, Klein FA, Schneider V, Walsh JW, Bewer WH. Extratesticular hemorrhage associated with torsion of the spermatic cord: Sonographic demonstration. *Radiology* 1986;158:401–404.

84. Weiss RM, Carter AR, Rosenfield AT. High resolution real-time ultrasonogaphy in the localization of the undescended testis. *J Urol* 1986;135:936–938.

85. Wolverson MK, Houttuin E, Heiberg E, Sundaram M, Shields JB. Comparison of computed tomography with high-resolution realtime ultrasound in the localization of the impalpable undescended testis. *Radiology* 1983;146:133–136.

86. Worthy L, Miller EI, Chinn DH. Evaluation of extratesticular findings in scrotal neoplasms. *J Ultrasound Med* 1986;5:261–263.

87. Zwanger-Mendelson S, Schneck EH, Doshi V. Burkitt lymphoma involving the epididymis and spermatic cord: Sonographic and CT findings. *AJR* 1989;153:85–86.

12

Musculoskeletal System and Spine

William H. McAlister

Sonography has many advantages as a musculoskeletal imaging technique. These include its display of cross-sectional anatomy and spatial relationship, its ability to image both sides of the body for comparison purposes, and its ability to provide a dynamic component to the evaluation. Because it can penetrate cartilage and soft tissues, which are major components of the immature skeleton, sonography is particularly well-suited for pediatric applications. It has become accepted as a primary method for imaging localized soft tissue masses and for evaluating hip abnormalities in newborns and infants. It also has been employed to evaluate the integrity of the cartilage in patients with skeletal deformities and arthritis and to evaluate tendons and ligaments. The first part of this chapter will review the techniques and applications of sonography in the pediatric musculoskeletal system; a discussion of spinal sonography will follow.

TECHNIQUE

High-frequency transducers are required for musculoskeletal imaging to provide resolution of structures close to the skin surface. Generally, a 5.0 or 7.5 MHz transducer will be adequate. Rarely, a 3.5 MHz is required to visualize deep lesions in a large or muscular patient. Either a linear array or sector transducer may be used, although linear array transducers are preferred because they permit a larger field of view. The use of an acoustic standoff pad is helpful for obtaining satisfactory images of superficial structures. The pad improves contact between the surface of the transducer and the anatomic structures and allows visualization of skin and immediate subcutaneous tissues. Both longitudinal and transverse images of the area of interest should be obtained.

NORMAL ANATOMY

Normal muscle imaged in longitudinal planes has a brightly echogenic outer border, corresponding to connective tissue fascia, and medium-level echoes internally, representing the muscle fiber bundles (Fig. 1). Within the muscle fibers are fine, oblique, parallel echoes corresponding to fibroadipose septa. On cross-section, the muscles have a more circular appearance with areas of increased echogenicity, corresponding to fibrous septa, scattered throughout. Contracted muscle has a decreased echogenicity compared with that of relaxed muscle (45). Typically the surrounding subcutaneous tissue is more echogenic than muscle, but it may be nearly isoechoic with muscle, especially in obese patients. Although generally not necessary for accurate recognition of abnormality, measurements of muscle and soft tissue thickness have been established for some areas of the body (30). Arteries and veins appear as anechoic, ovoid, or tubular structures coursing between muscles.

Tendons are bundles of collagen oriented in a longitudinal plane. The normal tendon is echogenic with fine, hypoechoic, parallel echoes (15). However, it may appear falsely hypoechoic when it is obliquely imaged in relationship to the sonographic beam. This artifact tends to occur at the bony attachments of the tendons where the latter have a slightly curved course. Recognition of this pitfall is important so that it is not mistaken as tendonitis. Placing the probe parallel to the tendon will result in demonstration of the normal echogenicity of the tendon.

Bone appears as a highly echogenic structure with distal acoustic shadowing. Cartilage, on the other hand, is hypoechoic compared with adjacent soft tissue. Fine, speckled echoes often are noted within the cartilage. Ossification centers appear as bright reflections within the cartilage (27).

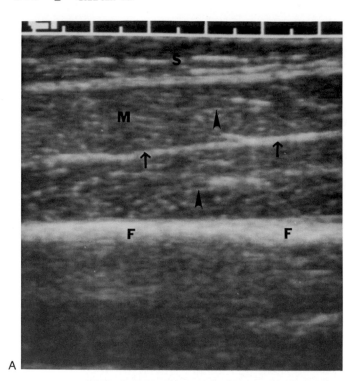

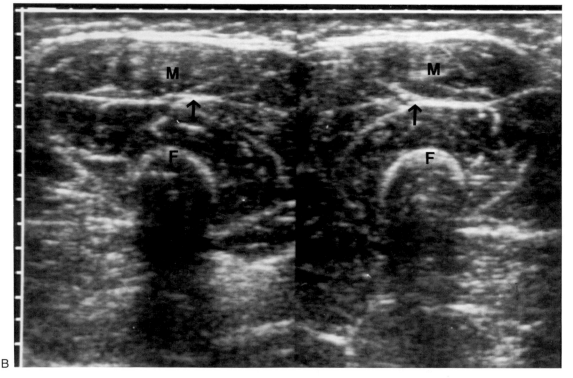

FIG. 1. Normal muscle. **A:** Coronal scan of the left thigh shows echodense, linear fibroadipose septa (*arrowheads*) within muscle (*M*) which has a medium-level echogenicity. The muscle groups are separated by brightly echogenic connective tissue fascia (*arrows*). **B:** On transverse views of left and right thighs, the fibroadipose septae appear as small foci of echogenicity scattered throughout the muscle (*M*). Again noted is brightly echogenic intermuscular connective tissue fascia (*arrows*). *F*, femur; *S*, subcutaneous tissue.

HIP

Congenital Hip Dysplasia

Congenital hip dislocation has an incidence of 1 to 10 to 1 in 1,000 neonates. The discrepancy is presumably due to the inclusion of mild ligamentous laxity at birth that resolves spontaneously within days. In true hip dislocation, the femoral head is entirely displaced from the acetabulum. A dislocatable hip is one that may be manually dislocated, but is reducible. A subluxable hip has significant movement but cannot be displaced out of the acetabulum. Teratogenic or dysplastic hips are infrequent and are found in association with other congenital anomalies such as caudal regression, myelodysplasia, or arthrogryposis.

Early diagnosis of congenital hip dysplasia is important because even a short delay in diagnosis can lead to abnormal hip development. Conventional radiography has been the gold standard for the diagnosis of congenital hip dislocation (68). In the newborn or very young infant, however, radiography is somewhat limited because the femoral epiphysis is unossified (58). Between 3 and 6 months of age, when the femoral head begins to ossify, the relationship of the proximal femur with the acetabulum and the amount of acetabular coverage can be determined by plain radiography. With sonography, the cartilage and associated soft tissues of the hip can be imaged directly before radiographic ossification is apparent. Sonography, thus, provides information that had previously been inferred subjectively from radiographs and leads to an earlier diagnosis of congenital hip dysplasia. Currently accepted usages of sonography are to evaluate infants with a high likelihood of hip dysplasia, and to follow patients who are under treatment for hip dislocation. Mass screening of congenital hip dislocation has been performed by some physicians, but its practical value has not been established in large series (6).

There are two basic methods of sonographic evaluation of the hip. The technique reported by Graf is based on a coronal image of the hip obtained with the transducer positioned lateral to the femur, which is extended (21). This is a static B-scan method which emphasizes the position of the femoral head, appearance of the bony acetabulum, configuration of the acetabular rim, position of the cartilaginous labrum, and the shape of the cartilaginous roof. Objective measurements are made and the depth of the bony acetabulum and the position of the labrum are determined (3,46,73).

The more widely accepted technique is a dynamic approach using transverse and coronal images with the transducer positioned directly over the lateral aspect of the hip (4,26,57). In contradistinction to the Graf technique which emphasizes actual measurements, the dynamic technique favors visual assessment of morphology, position, and mobility of the femoral head. Images are obtained with the femur in neutral and frog-leg positions as well as during dislocation maneuvers (40). The normal femoral head appears hypoechoic with fine, stippled echoes scattered throughout (Fig. 2). On transverse views, it sits in the center of a V-shaped acetabulum formed by the larger ischial portion posteriorly, the smaller pubic portion anteriorly, and the triradiate cartilage centrally. The ossified portions of the acetabulum are echogenic and cast an acoustic shadow, while the triradiate cartilage is nonossified and permits sound transmission. In most normal neonates, 3 to 4 mm of posterior movement of the femoral head can be seen with abduction-adduction and flexion-stress maneuvers (40). On the coronal view, half the diameter of the femoral head lies on either side of the ileum. The cartilaginous limbus can be identified superolateral to the femoral head (Fig. 2) (38,70).

The transverse view is important in determining an-

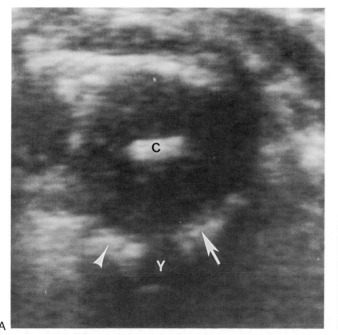
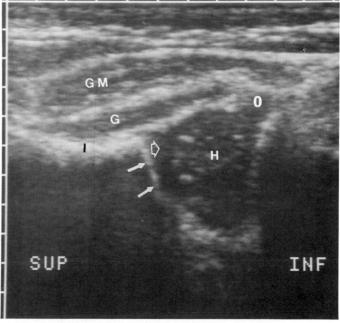

A   B

FIG. 2. Normal hips. **A:** Transverse scan showing the hypoechoic femoral head with an echogenic ossification center (*C*) seated within the bony acetabulum, formed by the ischium (*arrow*) posteriorly, triradiate cartilage (*Y*), and pubic bone (*arrowhead*) anteriorly. **B:** Coronal scan shows the femoral head (*H*) seated within the acetabulum (*white arrows*). *I,* ilium; *open arrow,* limbus; *G,* gluteus minimus; *GM,* gluteus medius.

terior, posterior, or lateral displacement of the femoral head, whereas the coronal view is important in determining lateral, superior, or rarely inferior dislocation (Figs. 3 and 4). On transverse views, a subluxed or dislocated femoral head no longer relates to the center of the acetabulum. Most often, when the hip is subluxable or dislocatable but reducible, the acetabulum

appears normal. A dysplastic acetabulum may contain soft tissue (the pulvinar) in association with a dislocated hip. More than 4 mm of posterior femoral head displacement may be noted with abduction-adduction. In the coronal plane, findings of subluxation or dislocation include superior and lateral displacement of the femoral head and a shallow acetabulum. Occa-

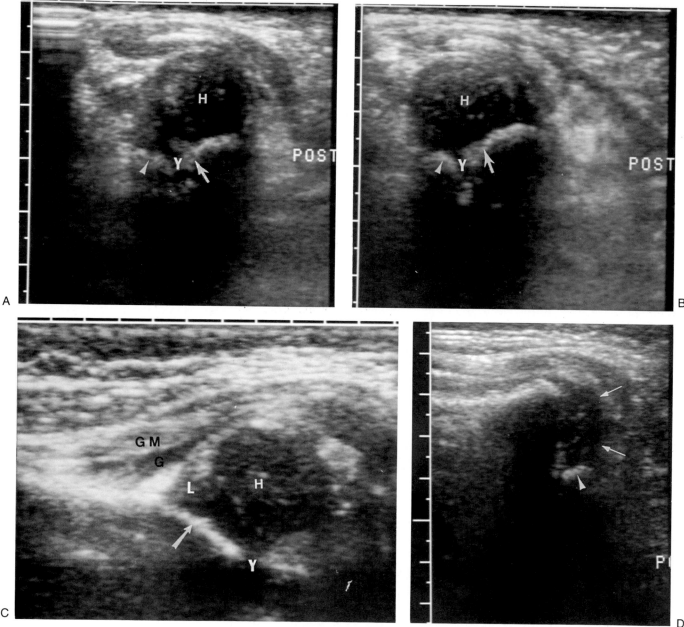

FIG. 3. Hip subluxation. **A:** Transverse scan with the leg flexed and adducted (Barlow maneuver). The femoral head (*H*) has moved slightly posterior onto the ischium. **B:** Transverse scan with the hip abducted and internally rotated (Ortolani maneuver) shows the femoral head (*H*) to be seated in the center of the triradiate cartilage. *Y*, triradiate cartilage; *arrow*, posterior ischium; *arrowhead*, anterior pubic bone. **C:** Coronal scan of another patient shows a shallow acetabulum (*arrow*) with the femoral head (*H*) incompletely covered and slightly laterally subluxed so that it no longer lies against the triradiate cartilage (*Y*); the limbus (*L*) is interposed between the head and acetabulum. *G*, gluteus minimus; *GM*, gluteus medius. **D:** Transverse scan with the hip flexed shows the femoral head (*arrows*) subluxed posterior to the acetabular lip (*arrowhead*).

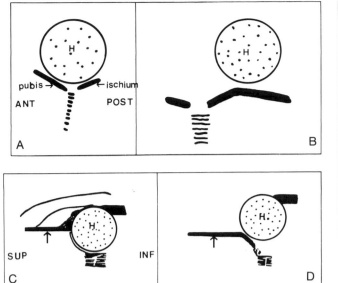
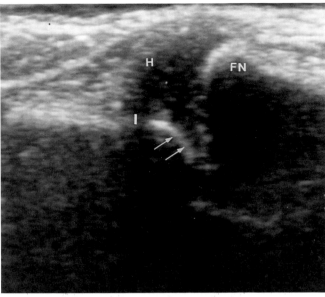

FIG. 4. Hip dislocation. **A:** Diagram of transverse sonogram of a normal hip; **B:** posteriorly dislocated femoral head; **C:** diagram of a coronal scan of a normal hip; **D:** lateral and superiorly dislocated femoral head. *H*, femoral head; *Ant*, anterior; *Post*, posterior, *Sup*, superior; *Inf*, inferior; *arrow*, ilium. **E:** Dislocated hip. Coronal scan showing femoral head (*H*) completely displaced superiorly and laterally out of the acetabulum (*arrows*) onto the flatter part of the ilium (*I*). *FN*, femoral neck.

sionally abnormal soft tissue will be seen within the acetabulum, or the labrum will be inverted and interposed between the head and acetabulum. Flexion-stress maneuvers may be needed to provoke instability or dislocation (40).

In experienced hands sonography of the hip is a sensitive procedure for detecting hip dysplasia, with false-negative and false-positive results of 1.8% and 2.4%, respectively. In patients older than 7 months of age sonography usually is no longer needed to establish the relationship of the femoral head to the acetabulum, since at this age the epiphysis is ossified in 95% of infants and visible on plain radiographs.

When the child is in an abduction splint or Pavlik harness for treatment of dislocation, serial sonography is an excellent method to monitor the position of the femoral head with respect to the acetabulum (Fig. 5) (24). If the femoral head remains posteriorly displaced while the patient is in a Pavlik harness, posterior and lateral acetabular underdevelopment can ensue (33). In contrast to the normal examination, the anterior acetabular lip normally is not seen by sonography with the hip flexed in a harness.

When a spica cast is used for treatment, determination of the femoral head placement by sonography requires that a window be cut in the side of the cast and replaced after scanning is complete. However, this practice may allow too much motion within the cast and increase the risk of redislocation. Computerized tomography is currently the preferred method for ver-

ifying the femoral head position with the patient in a spica cast. Although it is not very useful once the hip has been casted, sonography can be valuable intraoperatively to ensure adequate seating of the femoral head prior to casting (33,39).

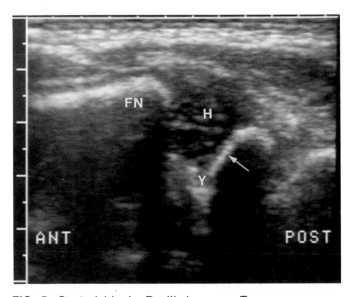

FIG. 5. Seated hip in Pavlik harness. Transverse scan shows the speckled femoral head (*H*) in the center of the acetabulum. Only the posterior lip of the acetabulum (*arrow*) and a portion of triradiate cartilage (*Y*) are seen. The anterior acetabular lip is obscured by the femoral neck (*FN*) which lies anteriorly when the hip is positioned in a harness. *ANT*, anterior; *POST*, posterior.

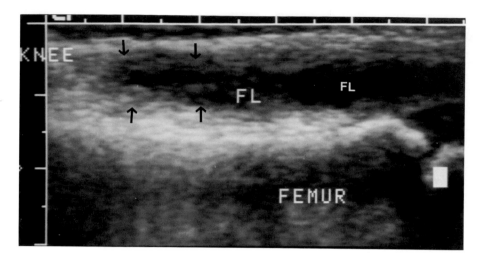

FIG. 13. Knee effusion. Longitudinal scan of left knee in a 7-year-old with rheumatoid arthritis shows fluid (*FL*) in an enlarged suprapatellar bursa. The bursa has ill-defined margins superiorly (*arrows*), representing associated synovial thickening.

With tenosynovitis or tendonitis, the tendons appear enlarged and hypoechoic (19). Chronic tendonitis shows diffuse or focal enlargement as well as focal areas of increased echogenicity representing fibrosis or calcification. Acute partial tears of the tendon appear as focal hypoechoic areas, while complete ruptures produce discontinuity of the tendon. Fragmentation of the tibial tubercle associated with Osgood-Schlatter disease or the patella in Sinding-Larsen-Johansson disease also can be observed in addition to tendon swelling (9).

Fluid Collections

Effusions

Although seldom needed to detect the presence of joint effusion in the knee, sonography can be useful in patients in whom there is difficulty in differentiating effusion from synovial thickening. Suprapatellar bursa fluid is easy to recognize sonographically with the patient supine and the knee extended; images are obtained in a longitudinal plane. The effusion appears as a well-defined anechoic space superior and posterior to the patella (Fig. 13). Synovial thickening also can be seen, especially in the presence of a large effusion.

Popliteal Cysts

Popliteal cysts are fluid collections in the gastrocnemiosemimembranous bursa. In young children most occur in the absence of underlying disease; occasionally they are associated with rheumatoid arthritis or

trauma. Patients may present with an asymptomatic mass behind the knee or with knee pain and abnormal knee mobility. Infrequently the cysts rupture or dissect into the calf. Sonography is useful in separating a cyst from a soft tissue mass. Popliteal cysts are seen best with the patient in the prone position, the knee extended, and the transducer placed posteromedially on the popliteal fossa. They appear as sonolucent fluid collections posterior to the joint (Fig. 14); infrequently extension of fluid superiorly into the thigh or inferiorly into the calf is noted. Although most cysts communicate with the joint space, the communication may be small and not identified. The treatment for popliteal cysts in children is conservative since most resolve spontaneously. The differential diagnosis includes a capacious gastrocnemiosemimembranous bursa which can be seen with the knee in flexion but decreases or disappears with the knee extended.

Miscellaneous

Sonography has been employed to evaluate tibial hemimelia and torsion, congenital subluxation, and hyperextension of the knees, and bone mineral content (29). Tibial hemimelia is characterized by partial or total absence of the tibia and fibula. Sonography can demonstrate the presence or absence of the cartilaginous anlage not seen on plain radiographs and can establish the relationship of the rudimentary bones to the femoral condyle (Fig. 15). Such information is important in determining the level of amputation. Congenital subluxation or hypertension of the knee can occur with or without tibial subluxation or dislocation. In young infants, sonography can assess the relation of the

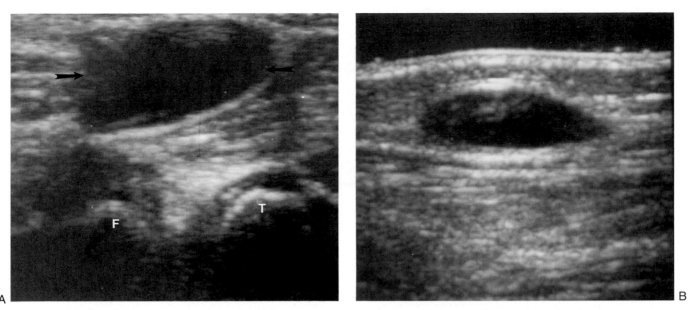

FIG. 14. Popliteal cyst. **A:** Longitudinal posterior scan through the popliteal fossa of a 4-year-old boy shows a hypoechoic fluid collection (*arrows*) posterior to the knee joint, representing a cyst. *F*, femur; *T*, tibia. **B:** Longitudinal scan more inferiorly demonstrates extension of the cyst into the proximal calf.

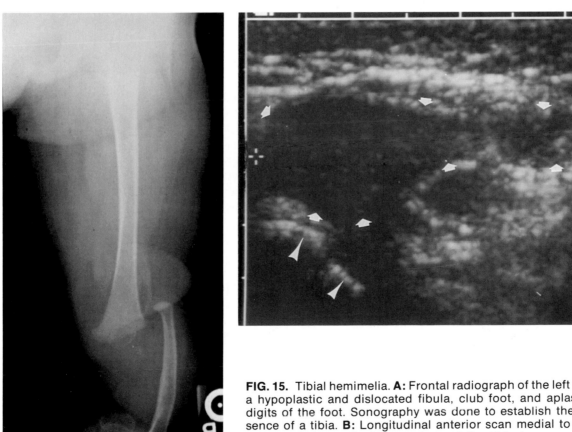

FIG. 15. Tibial hemimelia. **A:** Frontal radiograph of the left lower limb shows a hypoplastic and dislocated fibula, club foot, and aplasia of the medial digits of the foot. Sonography was done to establish the presence or absence of a tibia. **B:** Longitudinal anterior scan medial to the fibula shows a hypoechoic cartilaginous anlage of the tibia (*cursors* and *arrows*). The tibia is dislocated anteriorly and superiorly relative to the femur (*arrowheads*).

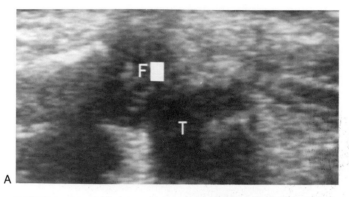

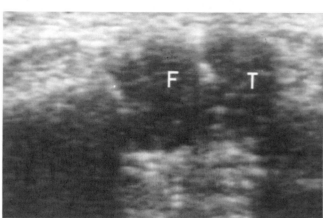

FIG. 16. Bilateral genu recurvatum with dislocations. **A:** Longitudinal scan through lateral aspect of popliteal fossa with the leg hyperextended beyond 90° shows the tibial epiphysis (*T*) dislocated anteriorly and superiorly relative to the femoral epiphysis (*F*). **B:** With leg straightening, the tibia (*T*) and femur (*F*) remain dislocated. **C:** Comparison view of opposite knee shows normal alignment of the tibia (*T*) and femoral (*F*) epiphyses with leg straightening.

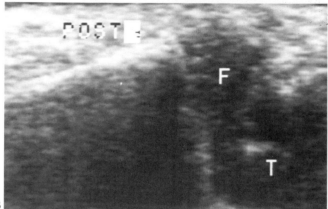

femur and tibia at rest and with motion (Fig. 16). If dislocation is present and not reducible with flexion maneuver, surgical treatment may be required. If mild instability is present, the treatment is usually casting. Use of sonography to evaluate tibial torsion and bone mineral content has not been widely accepted because measurements are less accurate than with other imaging studies (34,42).

SHOULDER AND UPPER EXTREMITY

Rotator Cuff Injuries

The major use of sonography in the shoulder has been the detection of rotator cuff tears (28,51,52). These generally are encountered in adults and result from acute trauma superimposed on chronic degeneration of the cuff, but occasionally they may occur in adolescents following sports injuries. The examination is performed with the patient seated with the elbow flexed, the upper arm held in a neutral, adducted position, and the forearm resting on the thigh. Initially, transverse scans along the anterior aspect of the shoulder at the level of the biceps tendon groove are obtained. Longitudinal scans are then performed along

the lateral aspect of the shoulder from the level of the insertion of the rotator cuff to the greater tuberosity. Comparison views of the contralateral side are obtained routinely (51). The normal rotator cuff appears as a well-marginated band of homogeneous echogenicity extending from the acromion to its insertion on the greater tuberosity (Fig. 17). The echogenicity is greater or equal to that of the overlying deltoid muscle (14).

Rotator cuff tears can be partial or complete. Sonographic findings of rotator cuff tear include: (a) discontinuity of the normal homogeneous echogenicity of the cuff muscles on static and dynamic images; (b) replacement of the normal cuff by a central echogenic band; (c) thinning and irregularity of the cuff; (d) focal cuff thickening with increased or decreased echogenicity; and (e) nonvisualization of the cuff (Fig. 17) (51). Joint or bursal fluid may be noted.

The biceps tendon is evaluated in transverse and longitudinal planes at the same time that the rotator cuff is examined. On transverse views, it appears as an echogenic oval structure within the biceps tendon groove, often surrounded by a small amount of hypoechoic fluid; on longitudinal views it is seen as an echogenic band. Abnormalities of the biceps tendon include effusion in the tendon sheath resulting from an

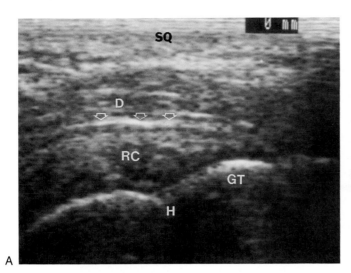 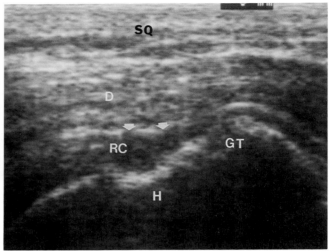

FIG. 17. Rotator cuff tear. **A:** Longitudinal scan of normal shoulder shows a well-defined echogenic interface (*open arrows*) between deltoid muscle (*D*) and rotator cuff (*RC*) muscle. **B:** Longitudinal scan of abnormal shoulder shows thinning and disruption (*closed arrows*) of the rotator cuff (*RC*), consistent with a complete tear. *SQ*, subcutaneous tissues; *H*, humerus; *GT*, greater tuberosity.

associated shoulder effusion or from synovitis of the tendon sheath itself, irregularity of the tendon sheath due to tendonitis, and interruption of the tendon sheath.

Miscellaneous

In addition to evaluating the painful shoulder in adolescents, sonography has been used in younger children to detect sternoclavicular dislocation (Fig. 18), separation of the proximal humeral epiphysis (71), and clavicular fractures (36).

Sonography is occasionally helpful in evaluating congenital anomalies of the upper extremity. It can show the presence of an omo-vertebral bone in patients with Sprengel's deformity before radiographic ossification is present. Such information is important because these anomalous bones may require surgical resection. In radial hemimelia, sonography can show the presence or absence of rudimentary cartilage. This information may help the surgeon decide whether or not to amputate. Sonography also has been used to detect tenosynovitis of the hand and wrist in rheumatoid arthritis (13).

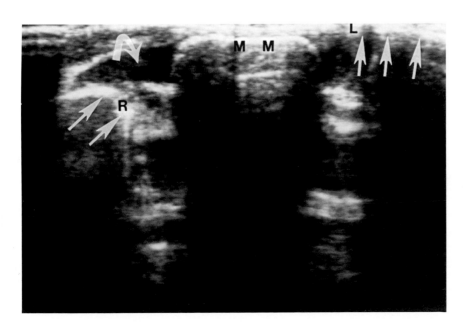

FIG. 18. Sternoclavicular dislocation. Transverse dual image scan over upper chest shows posterior displacement of the medial end of the right clavicle (*R*) (*arrows*). The left clavicle (*L*) (*arrows*) is normally positioned. The hypoechoic triangle (*curved arrow*) is believed to represent blood in the periosteal sleeve of the right clavicle. *MM*, manubrium. (Courtesy of J. Donaldson, Chicago, Illinois)

ANKLE AND FOOT

Achilles Tendon

The use of sonography in the ankle has been limited to evaluation of the Achilles tendon and the detection of joint fluid. A painful Achilles tendon may result from trauma or inflammation. When there is a history of trauma, it is mandatory to establish the integrity of the Achilles tendon because tears of the tendon are managed differently from soft tissue injuries, which may have similar clinical findings. The patient is usually scanned in the prone position with the foot in plantar and dorsiflexion; images are obtained in longitudinal and transverse planes. The normal Achilles tendon in adolescents and adults is 4 to 6 mm thick and 5 to 6 cm long. It is characterized by fine, parallel, internal echoes, similar to those seen in other tendons, and well-defined echogenic margins (Fig. 19).

Sonographic findings of Achilles tendon tears include discontinuity of the tendon, or an actual gap, which is noted in complete tears; thinning of the tendon in incomplete tears; and focal areas of swelling with decreased or increased echogenicity, depending on the age of the injury (14,44). With acute tendonitis, the tendon is diffusely or focally thickened and hypoechoic; the peritendinous structures also may be thickened and hypoechoic. Dystrophic calcification can be seen with chronic tendonitis or following trauma; ankle effusions also can be observed.

Miscellaneous Anomalies

Sonography has been used to detect congenital tarsal abnormalities. It can demonstrate a vertical talus and dislocation of the talonavicular joint before ossification is apparent, thus leading to earlier surgery.

SOFT TISSUE MASSES

Sonography is well-suited for detecting, localizing, and characterizing a variety of soft tissue masses and for defining the relationship of a mass to adjacent muscle. With Doppler sonography, it is possible to separate vascular from soft tissue masses. Sonography also is valuable for guiding needle placement for tissue sampling.

Although sonography cannot suggest a specific tissue type, it can separate cystic from solid lesions and can define the margins of these abnormalities. An aggressive mass typically has irregular margins and infiltrates adjacent structures, whereas a classic benign mass usually has a well-defined periphery and displaces but does not invade tissues. However, it is important to recognize that both benign and malignant masses may appear as either well-defined or infiltrating masses. Aggressive characteristics may be noted with benign processes such as acute hematomas, abscesses, and some benign tumors. Therefore, tissue sampling is required for a specific diagnosis.

Neoplasia

Soft tissue tumors may arise in the skin, muscle, fat, or lymph nodes. The most common malignant pediatric soft tissue tumor is rhabdomyosarcoma; less frequent tumors include fibrosarcoma, liposarcoma, and angiosarcoma. On sonography they are relatively indis-

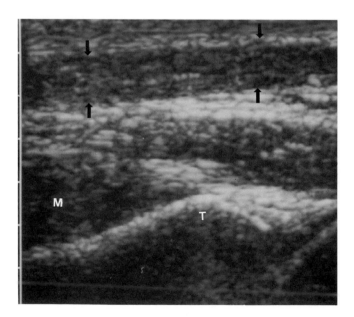

FIG. 19. Normal Achilles tendon. Longitudinal scan shows a well-defined tendon (*arrows*) with fine internal echoes. *T*, tibia; *M*, tibial flexor hallucis longus muscle.

tinguishable and have a variable matrix ranging from hypoechoic to highly echogenic (Fig. 20). The margins range from fairly well-defined to very invasive.

The most common benign soft tissue masses in children are hemangiomas, lymphangiomas, fibrous tu-

mors, nerve sheath tumors, and lipomas. On sonography, small hemangiomas may be diffusely hyper- or hypoechoic or of mixed attenuation with irregular or sharp margins (10). Large hemangiomas are characteristically hypoechoic. Septations, a feeding or drain-

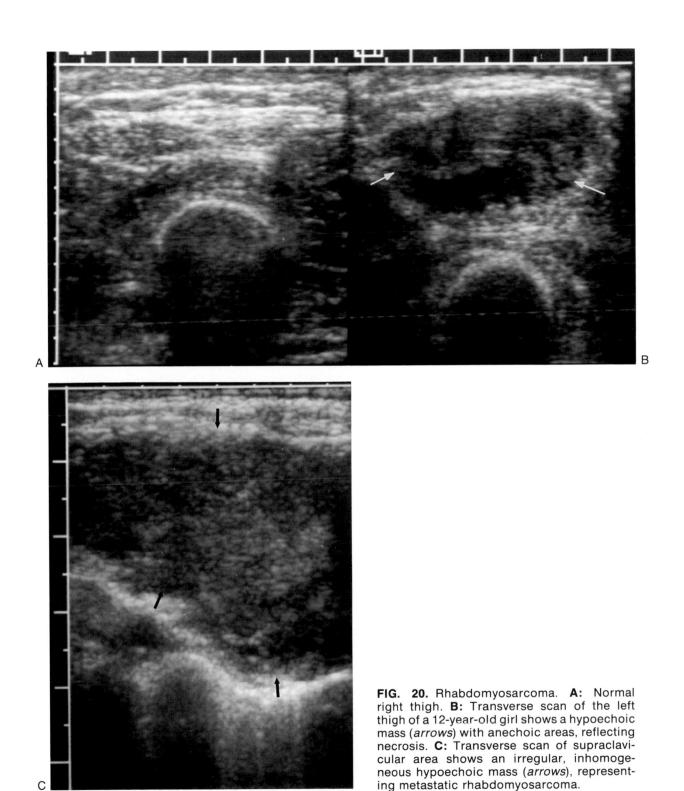

FIG. 20. Rhabdomyosarcoma. **A:** Normal right thigh. **B:** Transverse scan of the left thigh of a 12-year-old girl shows a hypoechoic mass (*arrows*) with anechoic areas, reflecting necrosis. **C:** Transverse scan of supraclavicular area shows an irregular, inhomogeneous hypoechoic mass (*arrows*), representing metastatic rhabdomyosarcoma.

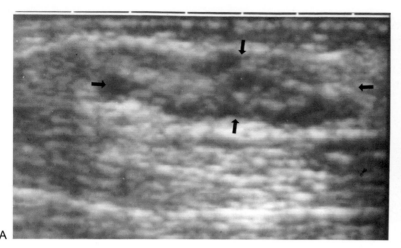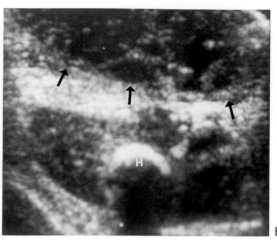

FIG. 21. Hemangiomas: **A:** Longitudinal scan of upper extremity shows a hypoechoic mass (*arrows*) with small sonolucent areas representing vascular channels. **B:** Transverse scan of upper arm of another patient shows a hypoechoic mass (*arrows*) with large vascular channels and increased through-transmission. *H*, humerus.

ing vessel, and calcifications also may be seen (Fig. 21). Lymphangiomas usually are well-defined, multilocular, cystic structures, although occasionally they may appear as solitary cysts (Fig. 22) (18). Fibrous tumors and tumors of neural sheath origin tend to be round or oval smooth masses; they often are hypoechoic relative to surrounding tissues and may be homogeneous or heterogeneous with echogenic foci related to calcifications (Fig. 23). By contrast, lipomas are usually intensely echoic. Generally the sonographic appearance of these lesions is not specific; however, sonography does help to identify and localize them so that the surgical approach can be planned.

Inflammatory Processes

Inflammatory processes include abscesses, pyomyositis, and cellulitis. Soft tissue abscesses occasionally present as masses. When they do, they usually are elliptical or spherical in shape and predominantly hypoechoic with through-transmission, but occasionally they may contain cellular debris and be hyperechoic. Foci of increased echogenicity with distal shadowing may be seen with gas-forming organisms or foreign bodies. The sonographic appearance of an abscess is nonspecific and may be confused with that of a hematoma or even necrotic tumor (Fig. 24). Clinical

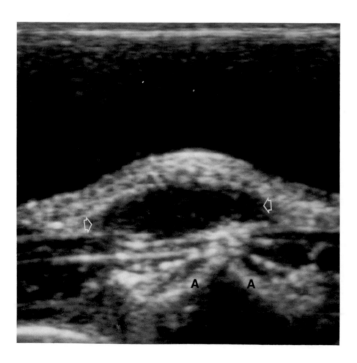

FIG. 22. Lymphangioma. Transverse scan over the midback performed with an acoustic standoff pad shows a well-defined hypoechoic mass (*arrows*) posterior to the neural arches (*A*). Echogenic areas within mass represent septations.

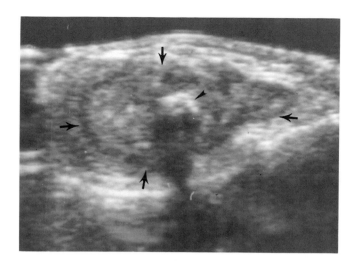

FIG. 23. Fibromyomatosis. Longitudinal scan of the arm demonstrates a well-circumscribed mass (*arrows*) that is hypoechoic relative to surrounding subcutaneous fat. Echogenic focus with acoustic shadowing represents calcification (*arrowhead*).

correlation, and in some cases biopsy, is required for diagnosis.

Pyomyositis is a rapidly progressing infection characterized by edema and necrosis of muscle. Typically, the muscle increases in echogenicity with loss of internal septations (Fig. 25). The surrounding subcutaneous tissues also become echogenic and fluid accumulates along the fascial planes.

In contrast to abscess, cellulitis is an infiltrating process; most often the disease affects subcutaneous fat.

On sonography, the fat is less echogenic than normal and is increased in thickness. Transition from abnormal to normal subcutaneous tissues is usually gradual.

Hematoma

Soft tissue hematoma usually follows trauma, although occasionally it may be associated with bleeding diathesis, or it may occur spontaneously. Intramus-

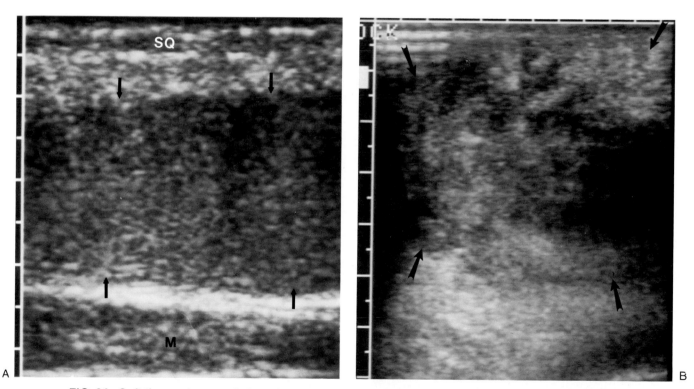

FIG. 24. Soft tissue abscess. **A:** Longitudinal scan along the lateral aspect of the upper leg shows a relatively homogeneous hypoechoic mass (*arrows*) superficial to muscle (*M*). *SQ*, subcutaneous tissue. **B:** Longitudinal scan of buttock of another patient shows an inhomogeneous, poorly defined mass (*arrows*) with hypo- and hyperechoic areas and through-transmission. Purulent material was aspirated from both lesions.

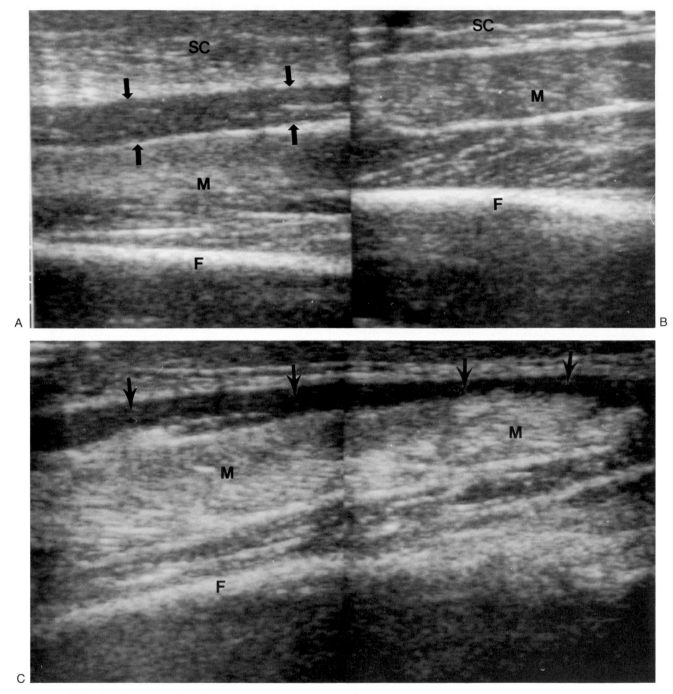

FIG. 25. Pyomyositis. **A:** Longitudinal scan of left and right thighs of an 8-year-old girl with chickenpox and acute right thigh swelling demonstrates thickened subcutaneous tissue (*SC*), an enlarged sonolucent fascial plane (*arrows*), and edematous echogenic muscle (*M*). **B:** Normal left side is presented for comparison. **C:** Longitudinal dual image scan of right thigh 1 day later shows a more sonolucent fascial plane (*arrows*) and markedly echogenic, swollen muscle (*M*) with a disorganized echotexture. At operation, there was pus in the fascial layer and necrotic muscle. *F*, femur.

cular hematoma will cause diffuse or focal enlargement of the muscle that is usually recognized when right and left sides are compared. Fresh hematoma is highly echogenic due to fibrin material, and then as liquefaction occurs, it becomes anechoic (Fig. 26). With subse-

quent retraction and organization, the clot may appear heterogeneous with internal echoes and septations, or echogenic (47). Myositis ossificans or ossification of the hematoma may occur if muscle necrosis accompanies the hemorrhage. Myositis ossificans character-

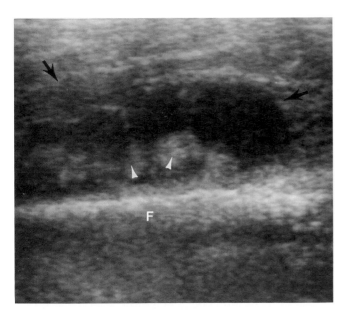

FIG. 26. Hematoma. Longitudinal scan of the thigh in a teenager with sickle cell anemia demonstrates a hypoechoic mass (*arrows*) containing echogenic debris (*arrowheads*). Approximately 50 ml of dark red blood was aspirated from the mass. *F*, femur.

istically appears as a soft tissue mass with multiple echogenic foci with acoustic shadowing (16).

When a hematoma is associated with a torn muscle, it appears as a fluid collection around the echogenic retracted portions of the ruptured muscle, often re-

ferred to as the bell-clapper sign. Differentiation between a retracted, ruptured muscle and a hematoma in an intact muscle is possible by scanning the muscle at rest and contracted. With contraction a torn muscle appears larger, whereas an intramuscular hematoma is compressed.

Rhabdomyolysis is a severe muscle injury, often associated with crush injuries or child abuse, that allows red cells to escape into the extracellular fluid. Sonography of rhabdomyolysis demonstrates a well-defined, hypoechoic mass within the affected muscle. However, this appearance is nonspecific and requires clinical correlation or tissue sampling for definitive diagnosis.

Foreign Bodies

The most common foreign bodies in the soft tissues of children are wood, glass, and metal slivers. While the latter two elements are almost always visible on plain radiographs, wood is seen only 15% of the time. With sonography, all three types of foreign bodies can be identified (20). On sonography, foreign bodies appear as hyperechoic foci with or without associated acoustic shadowing or reverberating "comet-tail" artifacts (Fig. 27). Preoperative localization of a foreign body is valuable in planning the site of surgical excision and in decreasing the extent of soft tissue dissection (17).

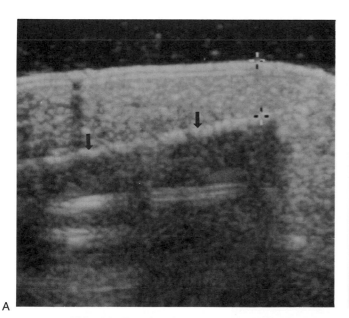

A

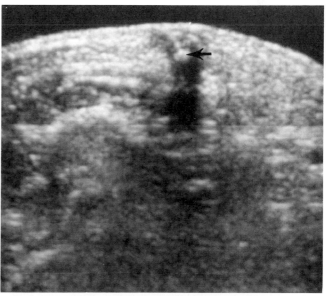

B

FIG. 27. Foreign bodies. **A:** Longitudinal scan, performed with a standoff pad, of the plantar aspect of the foot shows a hyperechoic band (*arrows*) with marked acoustic shadowing. A wooden foreign body was excised at operation. **B:** Transverse scan of the mid calf of another patient shows an echogenic focus with acoustic shadowing, representing glass (*arrow*) in the soft tissues.

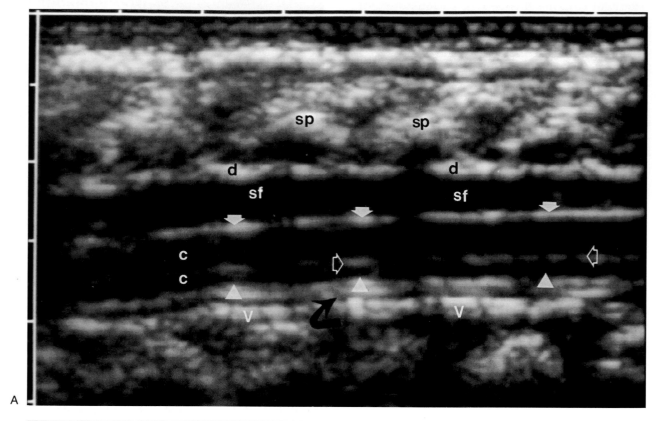

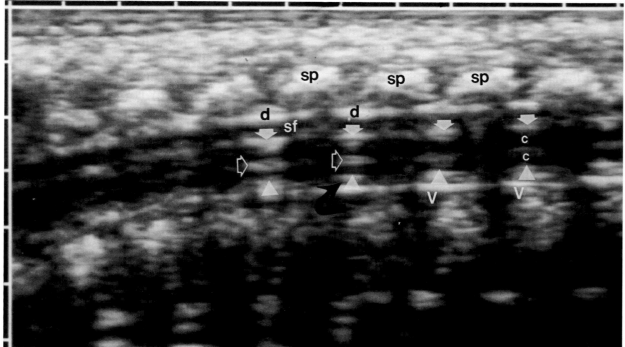

FIG. 30. Normal anatomy of spinal canal. **A,B:** Longitudinal scans of a neonate and 6-month-old infant, respectively, show the spinous processes (*sp*), posterior dura mater (*d*), posterior subarachnoid space with hypoechoic spinal fluid (*sf*), posterior wall of the spinal cord (*closed arrows*), hypoechoic cord (*c*), central echogenic complex of the anterior median fissure (*open arrow*), anterior wall of the cord (*triangles*), anterior subarachnoid space (*curved arrow*), and echogenic vertebral bodies (*V*).

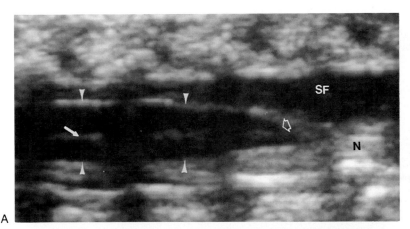

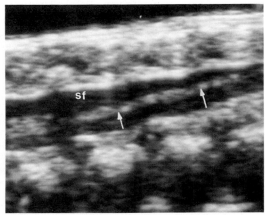

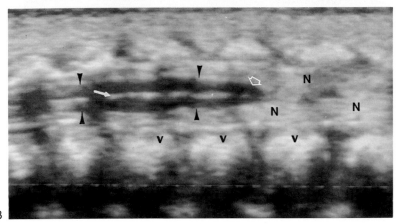

FIG. 31. Normal conus medullaris. **A,B:** Two longitudinal scans of the lumbar spine show the hypoechoic spinal cord (*arrowheads*), central echogenic complex (*closed arrow*), and the conus medullaris (*open arrow*) at the level of the second lumbar vertebral body. *SF,* spinal fluid. Echogenic nerve roots (*N*) are noted around the conus medullaris. *V,* vertebral bodies. **C:** Longitudinal scans of lower lumbar spine and sacrum below the level of the conus medullaris show a linear echogenic density (*arrows*) representing echogenic filum terminale surrounded by nerve roots. *sf,* spinal fluid.

Technique and Anatomy

Because the spinal cord is a superficial structure, high-frequency transducers are required for optimal scanning. Routinely, 5 or 10 MHz transducers are used and scans are obtained in both longitudinal and transverse planes with the patient prone and with a small pillow under the chest and abdomen to create a relatively kyphosis. This positioning produces splaying of the spinous processes, improving access to the spinal canal. In older children, angled, oblique, or parasagittal views may be helpful, especially in the thoracic spine. These approaches are useful to avoid the ossified spinous processes which interfere with transmission of the sound beam. Linear array transducers are preferred in infants and young children because they give a larger field of view. Sector scanners are useful in older children when the acoustic window is small (7).

On longitudinal scans, the posterior dura mater appears as an echogenic line paralleling the posterior subarachnoid space. The posterior subarachnoid space lies between the dura mater and the spinal cord and is anechoic. The spinal cord is visualized as a relatively hypoechoic tubular structure with echogenic anterior and posterior walls and a central echogenic complex

representing the anterior median fissure (Fig. 30) (56). It is surrounded anteriorly by the anechoic anterior subarachnoid space and echogenic vertebral bodies. The width of the spinal cord varies and is broadest in the cervical and lumbar regions. In the newborn, the sagittal diameters of the cervical, thoracic, and lumbar portions of the cord are 5.3, 4.4, and 5.8 mm, respectively (37). Enlargement of the cord in the cervical region corresponds to the origin of the nerves which supply the upper extremities, while the enlargement of the lumbar cord corresponds to the origin of the nerves which supply the lower extremities. At the level of the first or second lumbar vertebral bodies the cord tapers to form the conus medullaris. The conus medullaris is continuous with the filum terminale which extends into the sacral canal. On sonography, the filum terminale is an echogenic structure surrounded by nerve roots (Fig. 31).

On transverse images, the posterior dura mater appears as an echogenic band (Fig. 32). Beneath the dura mater is the anechoic posterior subarachnoid space. The spinal cord, beneath the posterior subarachnoid space, appears as an oval structure with a central echogenic complex. As it moves inferiorly, the spinal cord tapers, forming the conus medullaris. Paired echogenic anterior and posterior nerve roots border the conus in

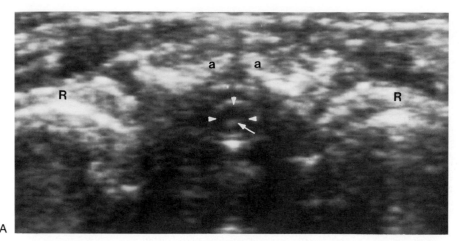

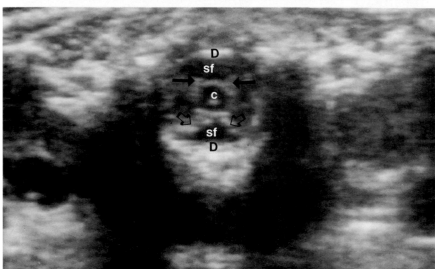

FIG. 32. Normal transverse scan of the spinal cord. **A:** Scan of lower thoracic spinal cord shows the neural arches (*a*), ribs (*R*), hypoechoic spinal cord (*arrowheads*), and central echo complex (*arrow*). **B:** Transverse scan of hypoechoic distal conus (*c*) shows paired echogenic anterior (*closed arrows*) and posterior (*open arrows*) nerve roots. The nerve roots are surrounded by anechoic cerebrospinal fluid (*sf*). *D*, dura.

the subarachnoid space. Transverse scans further caudally show the echogenic cauda equina or filum terminale surrounded by nerve roots. Anterior to the spinal cord are the anterior subarachnoid space and vertebral bodies. With real-time sonography, vascular pulsations within the cord and cauda equina can be demonstrated. In addition, anterior-posterior motion of the cord can be noted with episodes of crying, while longitudinal movement of the spinal cord can be observed with flexion-extension neck motion.

Identification of the conus medullaris, or termination of the spinal cord, is important in order to recognize patients with tethered cords. The level of termination of the conus medullaris can be determined sonographically by comparing its position with the position of two landmarks that can be palpated, namely, the tip of the last rib that usually lies at the L2 vertebral body and the top of the iliac crest that is about the level of the L4 vertebral body. Alternately, the position of the conus can be identified by identifying the rib sonographically and "counting" the vertebral bodies that lie caudad, or by identifying the sacral segments and "counting" vertebral bodies cranially. If

necessary, the vertebral level may be confirmed by obtaining a plain radiograph after a small radiopaque marker has been placed on the spine at the level in question. The normal conus medullaris lies at about the level of the L1-L2 vertebral bodies. Extension of the cord more caudally is an indication of a tethered cord.

Clinical Applications

Spinal Dysraphism

Spinal dysraphism refers to a group of disorders characterized by incomplete or absent fusion of midline structures. The disorders of spinal dysraphism include meningocele, diastematomyelia, and congenital dermal sinus. All of these can be associated with a tethered cord. Tethered cord may occur with minimal or no neurologic signs. It is important to identify patients with a tethered cord early so that surgical management can be undertaken to prevent neurologic dysfunction later in life. Sonography can be useful in newborns in screening evaluations of spinal dysraph-

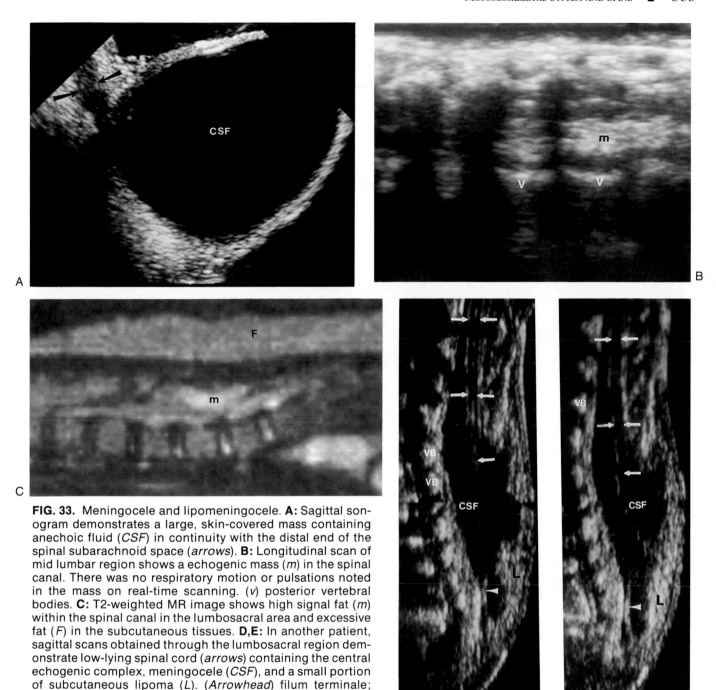

FIG. 33. Meningocele and lipomeningocele. **A:** Sagittal sonogram demonstrates a large, skin-covered mass containing anechoic fluid (*CSF*) in continuity with the distal end of the spinal subarachnoid space (*arrows*). **B:** Longitudinal scan of mid lumbar region shows a echogenic mass (*m*) in the spinal canal. There was no respiratory motion or pulsations noted in the mass on real-time scanning. (*v*) posterior vertebral bodies. **C:** T2-weighted MR image shows high signal fat (*m*) within the spinal canal in the lumbosacral area and excessive fat (*F*) in the subcutaneous tissues. **D,E:** In another patient, sagittal scans obtained through the lumbosacral region demonstrate low-lying spinal cord (*arrows*) containing the central echogenic complex, meningocele (*CSF*), and a small portion of subcutaneous lipoma (*L*). (*Arrowhead*) filum terminale; (*VB*) vertebral body. (Courtesy of T. Nadich, Miami, Florida)

ism, while in older children, CT myelography and MR imaging are necessary.

Meningoceles are congenital herniations of meninges through defects in the spinal column. When the contents of the herniated sac contain neural elements in addition to meninges and cerebral spinal fluid, the mass is termed a myelomeningocele. When fat and cerebral spinal fluid are present, the mass is referred to as a lipomeningocele. On sonography, the meningocele appears as a subcutaneous fluid-filled mass continuous with the spinal canal through open lamina. Often, the spinal cord is tethered and hydromelia may be present

(55). In these instances, the conus medullaris has an abnormally low position and abuts the posterior surface of the lumbosacral spine; the conus may or may not enter the meningocele sac. Absence of arterial pulsations within the nerve roots as well as decreased or absent motion of the distal cord suggest the presence of a tethered cord. When fat is present within the mass, the mass may be more echogenic than neural tissue (Fig. 33).

Congenital dermal sinuses are characterized by a small, fistulous tract extending from the skin into the spinal canal. Dermal sinuses are most common in the

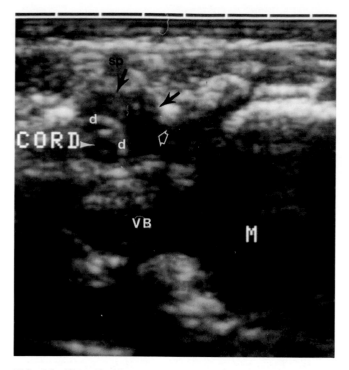

FIG. 34. Extradural tumor. Transverse scan through the posterior arches of upper thoracic spine shows a paraspinal mass (*M*) with an intraspinal component (*open arrow*) displacing the cord (*arrowhead*) and dura (*d*). *VB*, vertebral body; *sp*, spinous process (*arrows*). Intraspinal extension of neuroblastoma was shown at operation.

lumbosacral region, but may occur throughout the spinal canal. Because of the increased incidence of meningeal infection, early diagnosis is required. Physical exam reveals a small midline dimple with or without discharge. Sonography can be used to confirm or exclude a hypo- or hyperechoic tract extending from the dimple into the subcutaneous soft tissues, although the tract usually cannot be traced into the spinal canal (54). The presence of a low conus medullaris, suggesting a tethered cord, is indirect evidence of a fistulous tract between the skin and spinal canal. An intraspinal lipoma, which can accompany dermal sinuses, also may be noted.

In diastematomyelia, the spinal cord is divided into two separate components (63). In some cases a midline bony or fibrous spur arising from the back of a vertebral body may be found separating the cords. The cleft is most often in the lumbar region. If access to the spinal cord can be obtained through a parasagittal approach, sonography can demonstrate two cords and two central canals. The fibrous or bony spicules separating the cords and an associated hydromelia also may be imaged.

Tumors

Sonography can be used to diagnose primary neoplasms of the spinal canal as well as secondary neo-

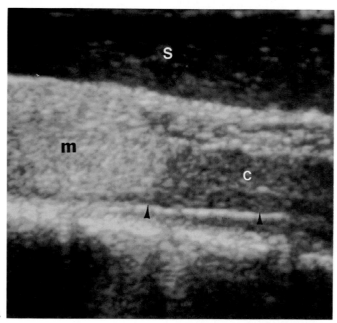

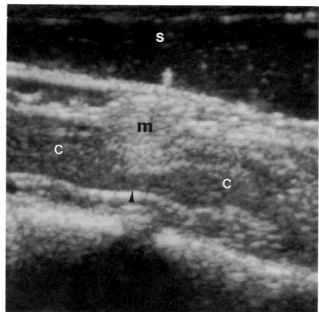

FIG. 35. Ependymoma. Intraoperative scanning. **A:** Longitudinal scan directly over the dura of the lower thoracic spinal cord (*c*) shows an echogenic intramedullary, intradural mass (*m*). *S*, saline bath; *arrowheads*, anterior margin of cord. **B:** Longitudinal scan over the dura of lumbar spine shows an extramedullary, intradural mass (*m*) displacing the spinal cord (*c*) anteriorly. The thoracic lesion was believed to be the primary tumor; the lumbar lesion presumably represented a drop metastasis.

plasms from contiguous spread of intrathoracic or intraabdominal tumors, such as neuroblastoma. Following laminectomy, sonography can be used to evaluate patients with symptoms of recurrent tumor. Tumors of the spinal cord may be intra- or extramedullary in origin. Intramedullary tumors may be solid or cystic and produce either focal or diffuse cord enlargement. The enlarged cord usually occupies the entire spinal canal, obliterating the subarachnoid space as well as the echogenic central canal. Motion of the affected segment of the cord is invariably diminished or absent. Extramedullary tumors appear as either echogenic or hypoechoic masses displacing the spinal cord to either side on transverse views, and either anteriorly or posteriorly on longitudinal scans (Fig. 34). Although the features of intramedullary and extramedullary tumors are different, in reality, sonography usually cannot identify the exact site of origin of the lesions. Separation of intraspinal tumors into intramedullary or extramedullary origin requires CT myelography or MR imaging.

Intraoperative Sonography

Intraoperative sonography is performed through a posterior laminectomy with the patient in a prone position. The laminectomy site is filled with sterile saline which acts as a coupling agents for the transducer. The most frequent use of intraoperative sonography is localization of spinal cord tumors (Fig. 35), arteriovenous malformations, cysts, areas of hydromelia, or the bony or cartilaginous septum in diastematomyelia. Such information is valuable in selecting the site of surgical resection. Intraoperative sonography also has been used to document the extent of residual gibbus deformity following straightening of spinal curvature (59–62,64–66).

REFERENCES

1. Aisen AM, McCune WJ, Macguire A, Carson PL, Silver TM, Jafri SZ, Martel W. Sonographic evaluation of the cartilage of the knee. *Radiology* 1984;153:781–784.
2. Bar-Ziv J, Barki Y, Maroko A, Mares AJ. Rib osteomyelitis in children. Early radiologic and ultrasonic findings. *Pediatr Radiol* 1985;15:315–318.
3. Berman L, Klenerman L. Ultrasound screening for hip abnormalities: Preliminary findings in 1001 neonates. *Br Med J* 1986; 293:719–722.
4. Boal DKB, Schwenkter EP. The infant hip: Assessment with real-time US. *Radiology* 1985;157:667–672.
5. Cardella JF, Young AT, Smith TP, Darcy MD, Hunter DW, Castaneda-Zuniga WR, Knighton D, Nelson D, Amplatz K. Lower-extremity venous thrombosis: Comparison of venography, impedance plethysmography, and intravenous manometry. *Radiology* 1988;168:109–112.
6. Clarke NMP, Clegg J, Al-Chalabi AN. Ultrasound screening of hips at risk for CDH. Failure to reduce the incidence of late cases. *J Bone Joint Surg* 1989;71-B:9–12.
7. Cramer BC, Jequier S, O'Gorman AM. Ultrasound of the neonatal craniocervical junction. *AJNR* 1986;7:449–455.
8. Cronan JJ, Dorfman GS, Grusmark J. Lower-extremity deep venous thrombosis: Further experience with and refinements of US assessment. *Radiology* 1988;168:101–107.
9. De Flaviis L, Nessi R, Scaglione P, Balconi G, Albisetti W, Derchi LE. Ultrasonic diagnosis of Osgood-Schlatter and Sinding-Larsen-Johansson diseases of the knee. *Skeletal Radiol* 1989;18:193–197.
10. Derchi LE, Balconi G, De Flaviis L, Oliva A, Rosso F. Sonographic appearances of hemangiomas of skeletal muscle. *J Ultrasound Med* 1989;8:263–267.
11. Dörr U, Zieger M, Hauke H. Ultrasonography of the painful hip. Prospective studies in 204 patients. *Pediatr Radiol* 1988; 19:36–40.
12. Falk RL, Smith DF. Thrombosis of upper extremity thoracic inlet veins: Diagnosis with Duplex Doppler sonography. *AJR* 1987;149:677–682.
13. Fornage BD. Soft-tissue changes in the hand in rheumatoid arthritis: Evaluation with US. *Radiology* 1989;173:735–737.
14. Fornage BD. Achilles tendon: US examination. *Radiology* 1986; 159:759–764.
15. Fornage BD. The hypoechoic normal tendon. A pitfall. *J Ultrasound Med* 1987;6:19–22.
16. Fornage BD, Eftekhari F. Sonographic diagnosis of myositis ossificans. *J Ultrasound Med* 1989;8:463–466.
17. Fornage BD, Schernberg FL. Sonographic diagnosis of foreign bodies of the distal extremities. *AJR* 1986;147:567–569.
18. Glasier CM, Seibert JJ, Williamson SL, Seibert RW, Corbitt SL, Rodgers AB, Lange TA. High resolution ultrasound characterization of soft tissue masses in children. *Pediatr Radiol* 1987; 17:233–237.
19. Gooding GAW. Tenosynovitis of the wrist. A sonographic demonstration. *J Ultrasound Med* 1988;7:225–226.
20. Gooding GAW, Hardiman T, Sumers M, Stress R, Graf P, Grunfeld C. Sonography of the hand and foot in foreign body detection. *J Ultrasound Med* 1987;6:441–447.
21. Graf R. Classification of hip dysplasia by means of sonography. *Arch Orthop Trauma Surg* 1984;102:248–255.
22. Graif M, Stahl-Kent V, Ben-Ami T, Strauss S, Amit Y, Itzchak Y. Sonographic detection of occult bone fractures. *Pediatr Radiol* 1988;18:382–385.
23. Gray DL, Crane JP, Rudloff MA. Prenatal diagnosis of neural tube defects: Origin of midtrimester vertebral ossification centers as determined by sonographic water-bath studies. *J Ultrasound Med* 1988;7:421–427.
24. Grissom LE, Harcke HT, Kumar SJ, Bassett GS, MacEwen GD. Ultrasound evaluation of hip position in the Pavlik harness. *J Ultrasound Med* 1988;7:1–6.
25. Gusnard DA, Naidich TP, Yousefzadeh DK, Haughton VM. Ultrasonic anatomy of the normal neonatal and infant spine: Correlation with cryomicrotome sections and CT. *Neuroradiology* 1986;28:493–511.
26. Harcke HT, Grissom LE. Sonographic evaluation of the infant hip. *Semin US, CT, MR* 1986;7:331–338.
27. Harcke HT, Lee MS, Sinning L, Clarke NMP, Borns PF, MacEwen GD. Ossification center of the infant hip: Sonographic and radiographic correlation. *AJR* 1986;147:317–321.
28. Harland U. Sonographic imaging of the shoulder and its pathological changes. *Electromedica* 1987;55:138–146.
29. Heaney RP, Avioli LV, Chesnut CH, Lappe J, Recker RR, Brandenburger GH. Osteoporotic bone fragility. Detection by ultrasound transmission velocity. *JAMA* 1989;261:2986–2990.
30. Heckmatt JZ, Pier N, Dubowitz V. Measurement of quadriceps muscle thickness and subcutaneous tissue thickness in normal children by real-time ultrasound imaging. *JCU* 1988;16:171–176.
31. Helvie MA, Rubin J. Evaluation of traumatic groin arteriovenous fistulas with Duplex Doppler sonography. *J Ultrasound Med* 1989;8:21–24.
32. Jeanty P, Kleinman G. Proximal femoral focal deficiency. *J Ultrasound Med* 1989;8:639–642.
33. Jones GT, Schoenecker PL, Dias LS. Pavlik harness pathology. Posterolateral acetabular deficiency after inappropriate use of the Pavlik harness *J Bone Joint Surg* 1990;in press.
34. Joseph B, Carver RA, Bell MJ, Sharrard WJW, Levick RK,

Aithal V, Chacko V, Murthy SV. Measurement of tibial torsion by ultrasound. *J Pediatr Orthop* 1987;7:317–323.

35. Kangarloo H, Gold RH, Diament MJ, Boechat MI, Barrett C. High-resolution spinal sonography in infants. *AJNR* 1984;5:191–195.

36. Katz R, Landman J, Dulitzky F, Bar-Ziv J. Fracture of the clavicle in the newborn. An ultrasound diagnosis. *J Ultrasound Med* 1988;7:21–23.

37. Kawahara H, Andou Y, Takashima S, Takeshita K, Maeda K. Normal development of the spinal cord in neonates and infants seen on ultrasonography. *Neuroradiology* 1987;29:50–52.

38. Keller MS, Chawla HS. Sonographic delineation of the neonatal acetabulum labrum. *J Ultrasound Med* 1985;4:501–502.

39. Keller MS, Weiss AA. Sonographic guidance for infant hip reduction under anesthesia. *Pediatr Radiol* 1988;18:174–175.

40. Keller MS, Weltin GG, Rattner Z, Taylor KJ, Rosenfield NS. Normal instability of the hip in the neonate: US standards. *Radiology* 1988;169:733–736.

41. Knudson GJ, Wiedmeyer DA, Erickson SJ. Color Doppler imaging in the assessment of upper-extremity deep venous thrombosis. *AJR* 1990;154:399–403.

42. Laasonen EM, Jokio P, Lindholm TS. Tibial torsion measured by computed tomography. *Acta Radiol Diag* 1984;25:325–329.

43. Laine HR, Harjula ALJ, Peltokallio P. Ultrasonography as a differential diagnostic aid in achillodynia. *J Ultrasound Med* 1987;6:351–362.

44. Laine HR, Harjula ALJ, Peltokallio P. Ultrasound in the evaluation of the knee and patellar regions. *J Ultrasound Med* 1987;6:33–36.

45. Lamminen A, Jaaskelainen J, Rapola J, Suramo I. High-frequency ultrasonography of skeletal muscle in children with neuromuscular disease. *J Ultrasound Med* 1988;7:505–509.

46. Langer R. Ultrasonic investigation of the hip in newborns in the diagnosis of congenital hip dislocation: Classification and results of a screening program. *Skeletal Radiol* 1987;16:275–279.

47. Lehto M, Alanen A. Healing of a muscle trauma. Correlation of sonographical and histological findings in an experimental study in rats. *J Ultrasound Med* 1987;6:425–429.

48. Lewis BD, James EM, Welch TJ. Current applications of duplex and color Doppler ultrasound imaging: Carotid and peripheral vascular system. *Mayo Clin Proc* 1989;64:1147–1157.

49. Marchal GJ, van Holsbeeck MT, Raes M, et al. Transient synovitis of the hip in children: Role of US. *Radiology* 1987;162:825–828.

50. Mayekawa DS, Ralls PW, Kerr RM, Lee KP, Boswell WD Jr, Halls JM. Sonographically guided arthrocentesis of the hip. *J Ultrasound Med* 1989;8:665–667.

51. Middleton WD, Edelstein G, Reinus WR, Melson GL, Totty WG, Murphy WA. Sonographic detection of rotator cuff tears. *AJR* 1985;144:349–353.

52. Miller CL, Karasick D, Kurtz AB, Fenlin JM Jr. Limited sensitivity of ultrasound for the detection of rotator cuff tears. *Skeletal Radiol* 1989;18:179–183.

53. Moulton A, Upadhyay SS. A direct method of measuring femoral anteversion using ultrasound. *J Bone Joint Surg [Br]* 1982;64:469–472.

54. Naidich TP, Fernbach SK, McLone DG, Scholnik A. Sonography of the caudal spine and back: Congenital anomalies in children. *AJNR* 1984;5:221–234.

55. Naidich TP, Radkowski MA, Britton J. Real-time sonographic display of caudal spinal anomalies. *Neuroradiology* 1986;28:512–527.

56. Nelson MD Jr, Sedler JA, Gilles FH. Spinal cord central echo complex: Histoanatomic correlation. *Radiology* 1989;170:479–481.

57. Novick G, Ghelman B, Schneider M. Sonography of the neonatal and infant hip. *AJR* 1983;141:639–645.

58. Novick GS. Sonography in pediatric hip disorders. *Radiol Clin North Am* 1988;26:29–53.

59. Pasto ME, Rifkin MD, Rubenstein JB, Northrup BE, Cotler JM, Goldberg BB. Real-time ultrasonography of the spinal cord: Intraoperative and postoperative imaging. *Neuroradiology* 1984;26:183–187.

60. Platt JF, Rubin JM, Chandler WF, Bowerman RA, DiPietro MA. Intraoperative spinal sonography in the evaluation of intramedullary tumors. *J Ultrasound Med* 1988;7:317–325.

61. Quencer RM, Montalvo BM, Eismont FJ, Green BA. Intraoperative spinal sonography in thoracic and lumbar fractures: Evaluation of Harrington rod instrumentation. *AJNR* 1985;6:353–359.

62. Quencer RM, Montalvo BM, Naidich TP, Post MJD, Green BA, Page LK. Intraoperative sonography in spinal dysraphism and syringohydromyelia. *AJNR* 1987;8:329–337.

63. Raghavendra BN, Epstein FJ, Pinto RS, Genieser NB, Horii SC. Sonographic diagnosis of diastematomyelia. *J Ultrasound Med* 1988;7:111–113.

64. Raghavendra BN, Epstein FJ, McCleary L. Intramedullary spinal cord tumors in children: Localization by intraoperative sonography. *AJNR* 1984;5:395–397.

65. Randel S, Gooding GAW, Dillon WP. Sonography of intraoperative spinal arteriovenous malformations. *J Ultrasound Med* 1987;6:539–544.

66. Rubin JM, DiPietro MA, Chandler WF, Venes JL. Spinal ultrasonography. Intraoperative and pediatric applications. *Radiol Clin North Am* 1988;26:1–27.

67. Sacks D, Robinson ML, Perlmutter GS. Femoral arterial injury following catheterization. Duplex evaluation. *J Ultrasound Med* 1989;8:241–246.

68. Scoles PV, Boyd A, Jones PK. Roentgenographic parameters of the normal infant hip. *J Pediatr Orthop* 1987;7:656–663.

69. van Holsbeeck M, van Holsbeeck K, Gevers G, et al. Staging and follow-up of rheumatoid arthritis of the knee. Comparison of sonography, thermography, and clinical assessment. *J Ultrasound Med* 1988;7:561–566.

70. Yousefzadeh DK, Ramilo JL. Normal hip in children: Correlation of US with anatomic and cryomicrotome sections. *Radiology* 1987;165:647–655.

71. Zieger M, Dorr U, Schulz RD. Sonography of slipped humeral epiphysis due to birth injury. *Pediatr Radiol* 1987;17:425–426.

72. Zeiger M, Dorr U, Schulz RD. Pediatric spinal sonography. Part II: Malformations and mass lesions. *Pediatr Radiol* 1988;18:105–111.

73. Zeiger M, Schulz RD. Ultrasonography of the infant hip. Part III. Clinical application. *Pediatr Radiol* 1987;17:226–232.

13

Interventional Sonography

Marshall E. Hicks, Marilyn J. Siegel, and Thomas E. Herman

Sonogram-guided percutaneous procedures in children have become increasingly popular over the past several years for diagnosis as well as treatment. Sonography has the advantage of being readily available and portable, and it offers three-dimensional localization of lesions for biopsy or drainage, permitting selection of the safest percutaneous access route. Sonography also allows precise depiction of the needle tip within a lesion, which increases the success rate of aspiration or drainage and decreases the risk of complications. Finally, biopsy or drainage can be performed with the patient in a variety of positions.

PATIENT PREPARATION

Sedation, Analgesia

A major problem in pediatric interventional radiology is the need for sedation and intravenous analgesia in infants and young children (4,15,30). Generally, patients under 12 or 13 years of age require either general anesthesia or intravenous sedation, usually with pentobarbital (Nembutal). Intravenous pentobarbital (5 mg/kg, to a maximum dose of 100 mg) is injected slowly in fractions of one-fourth to one-half the total dose and is titrated against the patient's response. The mean duration of drug activity from injection to the time it is safe to release the patient is 55 min (27). The relatively short duration of action is a major disadvantage if the interventional procedure is long, especially if catheter drainage is planned. Regardless of the regimen chosen, the use of parenteral sedation requires the facility and ability to resuscitate and maintain adequate cardiorespiratory support during and after the examination.

Local anesthesia usually is adequate for needle aspiration in older children. However, parenteral sedation may be required for catheter insertion. For painful procedures, the addition of a narcotic may be neces-

sary. Fentanyl (McNeil, Fort Washington, Pennsylvania) in an intravenous dose of 1 mcg/kg has been used safely.

To decrease the rate of complications, coagulation tests, prothrombin time, partial thromboplastin time, platelets, and hemoglobin should be performed prior to interventional procedures (15). Systemic antibiotics also are helpful to minimize the risk of septic shock following abscess drainage or decompression of an obstructed liver or kidney.

PERCUTANEOUS BIOPSY

Percutaneous biopsy is the most frequently performed sonogram-guided procedure. It is commonly used to diagnose complications of renal or hepatic transplantation. Less frequent indications include documentation of neoplastic or inflammatory disease. Its major advantage is that it may obviate surgery.

Transducers

Real-time scanners with needle-guiding mechanisms are preferred for interventional sonography. The main transducer types are: (a) linear array puncture transducer with a central canal through which the needle can be inserted perpendicular to the scan plane, and (b) linear array or sector scanner with an attachable needle guide that is clipped or screwed on to the end of the transducer. With the latter system, software modifications permit oblique angulation of the needle path.

Another method of biopsy is the free-hand puncture. This technique is performed by placing the needle and the transducer at a 90° angle from each other, jiggling the needle, and scanning the needle tip. The needle tip appears as a bright echo on the screen. In expert hands, this method is quick and capable of considerable accuracy, although small or deep lesions may not be amenable to this technique. Generally, sector scanners are preferred to linear transducers because their small head size allows angulation of the needle pathway and facilitates access to difficult-to-reach areas, such as the subcostal and intercostal spaces. These spaces are often used to gain access to the liver.

Needles

The character of the mass, its location, and the amount of tissue required for diagnosis are important factors in determining the choice of needle for biopsy. The more commonly used biopsy needles are depicted in Fig. 1.

Biopsy of a solid lesion to obtain a tissue core requires larger bore needles. These needles may be modified aspirating needles or cutting needles. Modified aspirating needles are available in 18, 20, and 22 gauge. Although there are a variety of these needles commercially available (including the Turner, Madayag, Greene, and Rotex needles), our choice is the Franseen needle (Cook, Bloomington, Indiana) because it is easy to manipulate and yields adequate tissue cores. Cutting needles, including Trucut, Lee, and Wescott needles, are available in sizes ranging from 14 to 20 gauge. These needles cut a large core of tissue and are

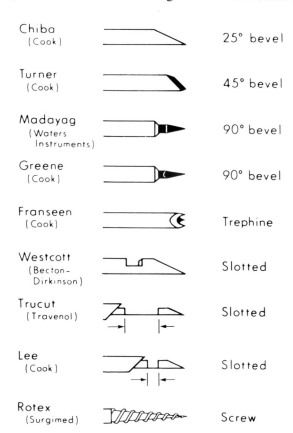

FIG. 1. Biopsy needles (From Picus et al., ref. 21, with permission.)

generally used for large lesions which are easily accessible and can be reached without traversing bowel or major vessels. Large bore or cutting needles are contraindicated if the lesion is hypervascular. Because of potential bleeding risks, we prefer to use a modified aspirating needle for obtaining tissue cores, reserving the cutting needle for repeat biopsies.

For aspiration biopsies, small gauge needles (20 or 22 gauge) are preferred. These are simple beveled needles that are used to obtain specimens for cytologic examination. The Chiba needle is one of the most frequently used. Small-gauge needles are useful when lesions are deep and bowel or vascular structures must be crossed to reach the lesion. The major disadvantage of the aspiration needle is its extreme flexibility, making it more difficult to direct. Multiple passes may be required.

Cytologic aspiration requires close cooperation with a pathologist. Optimally, the cytopathologist or a skilled technologist should be present in the radiology suite at the time of the procedure to determine the adequacy of the specimen and to provide a preliminary reading. This approach limits the number of passes required for positive diagnoses. If a pathologist is not immediately available, more than one sample should be obtained for cytology.

Besides the transducer and puncture needle, standard equipment necessary for a sonogram-guided aspiration biopsy consists of a sterile drape, syringes, sponges, local anesthesia, scalpel blades, and a sterile ruler. Most biopsies are now performed using equipment from prepackaged sterile trays.

Needle Placement

The initial step in a sonogram-guided biopsy is a review of the patient's previous diagnostic studies. After diagnostic imaging studies have been reviewed, optimal patient position (prone, oblique, or decubitus) for biopsy is chosen and the area of interest is localized. The phase of respiration that best allows access to the lesion is determined. Once the appropriate area is found, the site for needle entry is marked; the overlying skin is cleaned and draped; and in older patients, local anesthesia is administered subcutaneously. A sterile rubber sleeve or glove filled with a sterile coupling gel is placed over the transducer. Additional sterile gel is applied to the patient's skin directly over the biopsy area. The attachable guide is snapped onto the transducer over the rubber sleeve and the appropriate needle is inserted through the guide. The biopsy needle is then advanced to the correct depth. During passage of the needle, the patient is instructed to suspend respiration, if this is relevant. A shadowing artifact indicates that the tip of the needle is within the image plane.

Biopsy Techniques

Either a double-needle or tandem-needle approach may be used to obtain a tissue sample. The double-needle technique uses a large gauge needle (18 or 19 gauge) as a sleeve through which a smaller gauge (21 or 22 gauge) biopsy needle is placed to obtain the biopsy. The disadvantage of this method is that the larger gauge needle is inflexible and may cause damage to internal organs when there is respiratory motion.

The tandem-needle technique has largely replaced the double-needle technique. A thin needle is positioned in the center of the mass and left in place to act as a guide for placement of the biopsy needle. Subsequently, biopsy needles are placed around the guide needle to the same depth.

After the needle has been inserted in the proper location, a syringe is attached. Negative pressure is placed on the attached syringe while a twisting motion is applied to the barrel of the syringe. Once a biopsy attempt has been made, the suction is released before removing the needle from the body. This technique allows the specimen to remain in the needle, rather than being drawn into the syringe. The entire needle aspiration takes only a few seconds.

An alternative method for core biopsies in older children is the use of a spring loaded "biopsy gun" such as the Bard Biopty Gun (Bard Urologic Division, Convington, Georgia). The gun rapidly fires a modified cutting needle which extends approximately 2 cm into the tissue to acquire a specimen core. Advantages over conventional biopsy techniques include more uniform tissue sampling, reduced patient discomfort, and decreased procedure time (20). The gun technique has also shown promise in providing consistently high quality diagnostic samples using a relatively small needle (18 gauge) with fewer major complications (2,20).

Results and Complications

Sonogram-guided biopsies have a sensitivity of about 90% and a specificity close to 100%. False positive diagnoses are exceedingly rare. The sensitivity of this technique is directly correlated to the adequacy of the specimen.

Major complications are rare, occurring in about 1% of biopsies. These include bleeding, peritonitis, sepsis, pancreatitis, and pneumothorax (16,22). Minor complications include inadvertent puncture of the bowel, gallbladder, urinary bladder, and great vessels, and are almost always without sequelae.

Selected Biopsy Sites

Kidneys

The kidney is the most common site of sonogram-guided biopsy. Overall accuracy rates for percutaneous biopsy exceed 90%. The optimal biopsy site for biopsy of native kidneys is the lower pole, lateral to the collecting systems and below the ribs (Fig. 2) (37).

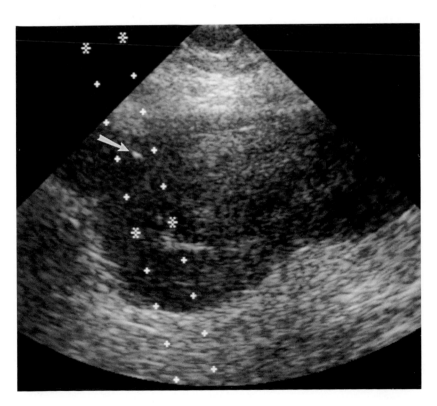

FIG. 2. Renal biopsy. A sector scan of a kidney during percutaneous biopsy. An attachable needle guide directs the biopsy needle between the dotted parallel lines and the needle tip is visible as a bright echo at the inferior pole of the kidney (*arrow*).

The needle should enter the renal cortex of the lower pole. Care must be taken to avoid the renal medulla, corticomedullary junction, and hilar vessels. Ideally, respiratory motion should be suspended at the time of biopsy. However, this procedure can be performed in sedated children who cannot hold their breath if respiratory excursion is reproducible and shallow. The incidence of postbiopsy hematuria or significant hemorrhage is low, possibly because of the high yield on the first attempt (37).

Biopsies of renal transplants with sonographic guidance are also frequently performed to diagnose the presence or absence of rejection. The ability of sonography to visualize directly the renal parenchyma and to avoid large vessels and the renal pelvis are advantages over blind biopsy. Respiratory motion is not as important in iliac fossa transplants as it is in biopsies of native kidneys. Sonography also is useful in the treatment of posttransplant fluid collections and hydronephrosis.

Muscle

Sonographic guidance can be used to confirm a site of abnormality for biopsy in a variety of myopathies. It is particularly helpful in cases of selective muscle involvement, such as congenital muscular dystrophy. Selective involvement of muscles is less common in Duchenne's muscular dystrophy.

In patients with congenital muscular dystrophy, the thigh initially is scanned anteriorly, and the echogenicity of the femoris muscle and vastus intermedius muscle are compared. Then the transducer is positioned laterally and the vastus intermedius and vastus lateralis muscles are imaged. In the upper arm, scans over the bicep muscle anteriorly and the deltoid muscle laterally should be performed (10). Scanning in multiple areas increases the likelihood of obtaining a diagnostic tissue sample. On sonography, an abnormal muscle group appears as an area of increased echogenicity, reflecting infiltration by adipose tissue and abnormal connective tissue. Once tissue sampling has been performed, staining is required for a specific diagnosis.

Thyroid

Fine-needle aspiration biopsy can facilitate selection of candidates for surgical removal of solitary thyroid nodules. This results in a major reduction in unnecessary surgical resections. The suspicious lesion is identified by sonography and then fixed between two fingers of one hand for immobilization. A fine needle (23 or 25 gauge) is used for aspiration. Rarely, a major neck vessel or the trachea is punctured, but this is usually without significant complications. Overall accuracy for thyroid biopsy is about 90%. False positive diagnoses suggesting cancer occur in about 5% of biopsies, usually in the presence of thyroiditis or colloid goiter (28). False-negative diagnoses are associated with large necrotic carcinomas.

Liver

Blind percutaneous biopsy is the procedure of choice to diagnose diffuse hepatic disease. However, sonogram-guided aspiration is a useful procedure to facilitate biopsy of small hepatic lesions. Overall sensitivity for this procedure is between 85% and 90% (1,19,24,38). It is particularly useful in children with unresectable lesions and those unable to undergo an operative procedure. Most lesions within the liver are well-visualized by sonography because the liver provides a good acoustic window. Either a thin needle (20 or 22 gauge) or an 18-gauge Franseen needle can be used for biopsy. The yield with 18-gauge needles is higher than with aspirating needles. A subcostal approach is preferred, avoiding the gallbladder and extrahepatic bile ducts and vessels. Infrequent complications include hemorrhage or passage of the needle through the gallbladder, interposed lung, or colon. Most complications can be avoided by meticulous attention to localization of the biopsy site.

PERCUTANEOUS FLUID DRAINAGE

Indications and Patient Selection

Sonography is a useful technique to guide drainage of a wide variety of fluid collections in the abdomen and pelvis. The subphrenic spaces, subhepatic space, and pelvis are well suited for sonographic drainage. Additionally, sonography can be useful for draining fluid collections in solid organs such as the liver, kidney, and spleen, and within the pleural space. The ability of sonography to follow the course of the needle into the fluid collection is particularly useful when performing drainage procedures.

There are limitations to this technology, especially in the mid abdomen where bowel gas can obscure detail. Open wounds, dressings, and surgical drains are also obstacles to scanning. In these patients computerized tomography (CT)-guided procedures are preferred.

Our current approach is to use sonographic guidance whenever the lesion can be easily imaged and when the access route is safe. Computerized tomography is indicated in the retroperitoneum, mediastinum, and for any lesion that is not easily shown by sonography.

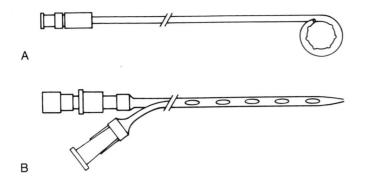

FIG. 3. Drainage catheters. Single lumen pigtail (**A**), and double lumen sump (**B**) catheters are shown diagrammatically. The cross-sectional view to the right of each catheter demonstrates the single lumen for the pigtail catheter and the double lumen of the sump catheter. The air-vent lumen of the sump catheter is indicated (*arrow*). (From Picus et al., ref. 21, with permission.)

Percutaneous drainage is most successful if the collection is well-defined and unilocular. However, it can be performed in multilocular lesions, especially if the patient is not a surgical candidate. Frequent catheter manipulation or multiple catheters may be necessary with loculated fluid collections.

Technique: Diagnostic Aspiration

The shortest and safest access route that avoids bowel loops, major vessels, and pleural space should be used for aspiration and drainage. Once the site for needle puncture is selected, the skin is prepped and draped in a sterile fashion. The depth and angulation of needle insertion is calculated from the sonogram images. A piece of sterile tape or a commercially available depth marker can be placed on the needle to indicate the measured distance from the skin surface to the lesion. The transducer selection and technique of needle placement is similar to that for percutaneous biopsy. When the needle is within the lesion, a diagnostic aspiration should be performed to determine whether the fluid is infected. Although sonography is sensitive for localizing a fluid collection, it cannot separate pus from blood, bile, lymph, or urine (18). Aspiration usually is performed with a 21- or 22-gauge needle. However, aspiration of viscid material may be difficult with a fine-gauge needle. If aspiration is unsuccessful and the needle tip is correctly positioned, a large gauge (18 gauge) needle may be helpful.

If purulent fluid is recovered, a drainage catheter can be placed immediately. If the fluid is not obviously infected, it should be sent for gram-stain, cultures, and chemical analysis. Catheter drainage may be delayed until the culture results are known. Alternatively, a catheter can be placed at the time of diagnostic aspiration, even if the collection is not clearly infected, and can be removed once infection or fistula has been ruled out. From a diagnostic standpoint, an erroneous diagnosis of abscess may be made if bowel contents are aspirated since the gram-stained specimen will contain bacteria.

Catheter Selection and Insertion

The selection of the drainage catheter depends on the size of the collection and nature of the fluid to be drained. Two catheter systems may be used: a single lumen catheter or sump catheter (Fig. 3) (8,18,31,33). Both systems are available with a straight or a curved distal tip. A curved or "pigtail" configuration of the distal tip of the catheter will help drainage to be maintained even as the cavity decompresses. Single lumen catheters are used primarily to drain collections of low viscosity, such as loculated ascites, seromas, and bilomas. The relatively small lumen, ranging in size from 8 to 12 French, and small side holes of most single lumen catheters limit their use in draining thick purulent collections. Larger single lumen catheters (12 or 14 French) are available for highly viscous fluid collections, but frequent irrigations with normal saline are required to maintain patency of the tube.

The system that is generally preferred for draining thick, viscous material is the vanSonnenberg sump catheter (Meditech, Inc., Watertown, MA) (33). This large caliber (12 to 14 French), double lumen tube with large side holes allows for simultaneous irrigation and drainage using low, intermittent suction. The air-vent lumen of the sump catheter allows air to enter the sump lumen, while suction is applied to the other lumen. This prevents the cavity wall from collapsing around the catheter and occluding the side holes, even when suction is applied to the wall. By contrast, the cavity walls often collapse and encroach on the side holes of the single lumen catheter when suction is applied to the catheter lumen.

Drainage catheters can be placed by either the Seldinger technique or the trocar technique. In the Seldinger technique, an 18-gauge needle is placed into the fluid collection. After diagnostic aspiration, a guide wire (0.035 inch or 0.038 inch) is passed through the needle or sheath into the fluid collection. Once the guide wire is in place, the remainder of the procedure can be performed with fluoroscopic guidance. The needle is then removed and a catheter is threaded over

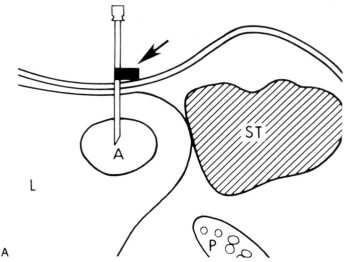

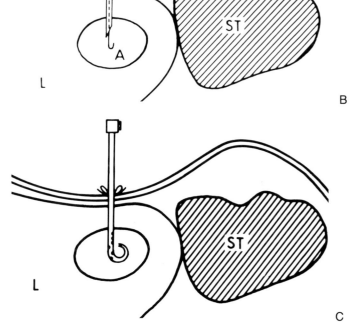

FIG. 4. Percutaneous abscess drainage using the Seldinger technique. **A:** Diagrammatic representation of a liver abscess. A needle is placed initially into the lesion for diagnostic aspiration. *Arrow* indicates a piece of sterile tape used as a depth marker. **B:** A guide wire is then passed through the needle into the collection. The needle is subsequently removed, leaving the guide wire in place. **C:** A catheter is threaded over the guide wire, and the guide wire is removed. The catheter is then sutured in place. *L*, liver; *A*, abscess; *ST*, stomach; *P*, pancreas; *Ao*, aorta. (From Picus et al., ref. 21, with permission.)

the guide wire into the lesion (Fig. 4). Adequate catheter placement can then be confirmed fluoroscopically by injection of contrast medium. If necessary, polyethylene dilators can be used to dilate the tract prior to catheter placement, particularly if the collections are deep or if scar tissue is traversed.

The trocar technique may be used when the fluid collection is large, superficial, and easily accessible. With the trocar technique the metal stylet and catheter function as a single unit. The entire unit is advanced through the front wall of the lesion into the fluid cavity. The catheter is advanced over the stylet into the lesion and the stylet is removed (Fig. 5). Because considerable force may be necessary to advance the catheter through the soft tissues of the abdominal wall, there is a risk of perforating the far wall of the abscess.

Management

After catheter placement, all purulent material is removed by syringe aspiration and the cavity is gently irrigated with saline until drainage is clear. Immediate irrigation is contraindicated if the patient is bacteremic or if there is ongoing sepsis. The catheter is then secured and left to dependent drainage or low suction.

Frequent irrigation may be necessary to keep the catheter patient. When catheter drainage stops, the cavity should be reimaged to document complete resolution before the catheter is withdrawn.

If output persists or increases, a fistulous communication may be present, or catheter position may be suboptimal. These complications can be confirmed with an injection of contrast medium into the catheter. Persistent elevation of the white blood cell count, fever, or an abnormal physical examination may indicate incomplete drainage, suboptimal catheter position, or loculated fluid. Repeat sonography or CT should be performed. If necessary, additional catheters can be placed into undrained locules or the existing catheter can be manipulated.

Results

Percutaneous drainage decreases hospital costs and avoids the risk of surgery and anesthesia. Success rates of approximately 80% to 90% have been reported and compare favorably with surgical management (3,8,14,18,32). Failure of complete resolution of the collections is usually due to loculations or septations, premature catheter removal, or a fistulous communi-

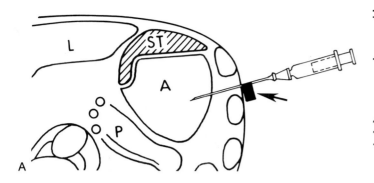

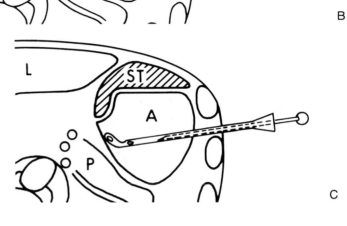

FIG. 5. Diagrammatic representation of a percutaneous abscess drainage using trocar technique. **A:** Aspiration of a retrogastric collection with a thin needle. The depth guide is indicated (*arrow*). **B:** The trocar unit is advanced to a previously determined distance with the depth marker in place to prevent puncture of the back wall of the abscess. **C:** With the stylet in place, the catheter is advanced until the drainage tube is well seated in the cavity. The trocar is removed and dependent drainage is begun. *L*, liver; *ST*, stomach; *A*, abscess; *P*, pancreas. (From Picus et al., ref. 21, with permission.)

cation with the bowel. Complications occur in 10% to 15% of patients. Major complications include significant hemorrhage and sepsis; minor complications include mild bleeding, transient bacteremia, bowel puncture, and superficial skin infection. Recurrence rates are approximately 5% (14,32).

Specific Sites

Right Upper Quadrant

The right subphrenic and subhepatic spaces are drained easily by percutaneous techniques. However, it is important to avoid entering the pleural space when draining the subphrenic area to prevent empyema formation.

Pelvis

The majority of pelvic abscesses in children are the result of intestinal perforation secondary to appendicitis or Crohn's disease, but they may follow pelvic surgery or trauma (Fig. 6). If there is a question of an infected pelvic fluid collection, percutaneous aspiration and drainage with sonogram guidance can easily be accomplished. An anterior approach is used most often for pelvic abscess drainage. Inadvertent punctures of the bowel or urinary bladder are occasional complications, although these are almost always without clinical sequelae.

Thorax

The most frequent indication for percutaneous intervention in the chest is pleural effusion. Sonographic guidance can be used to provide fluid for diagnosis. Percutaneous drainage can follow if indicated. Access to the pleural space may be obtained by scanning through subcostal or intercostal spaces or through the liver and spleen.

After the effusion has been recognized, the patient is placed in an upright position and the appropriate interspace for thoracentesis is marked. The patient may then return to the floor for thoracentesis, or the procedure may be performed in the radiology suite. If diagnostic thoracentesis is requested, a short 19- or 21-gauge needle is suitable for aspiration.

Thoracentesis is successful in 90% of patients (12). The most useful criteria for determining whether thoracentesis will be successful are: (a) presence of a change in shape of the fluid with inspiration and expiration, and (b) the absence of septations. Free-flowing fluid which changes shape with respiratory motion and nonseptated collections are more amenable to aspiration (17).

At times thoracentesis is unsuccessful even when the fluid is hypoechoic and the needle is in good position. Presumably the fluid in these cases is quite viscous or contains pus or clotted blood. In these instances, a larger gauge needle should be used for aspiration.

Empyema also can be drained percutaneously with

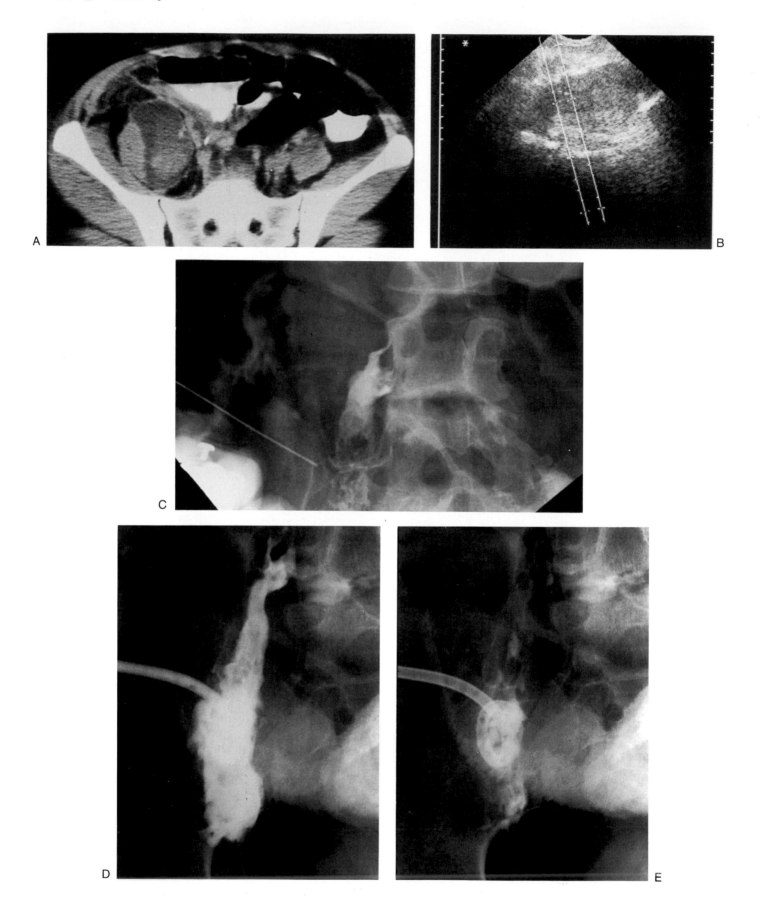

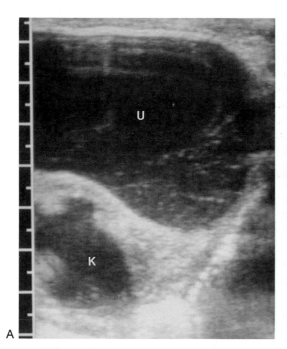

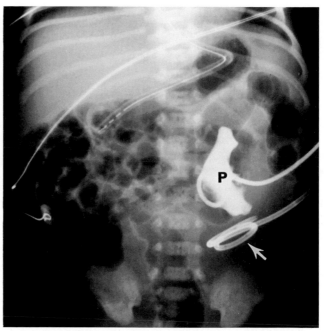

FIG. 7. Percutaneous nephrostomy and drainage of a urinoma. One-day-old male infant with abdominal distention and elevated serum creatinine. **A:** Sonogram demonstrates a large perirenal urinoma (*U*) and a hydronephrotic kidney (*K*). The urinoma was drained percutaneously prior to placement of the nephrostomy tube. **B:** A postprocedural nephrostogram documents the position of the drainage catheter in the urinoma (*arrow*) and the nephrostomy tube in the renal pelvis (*P*). The cause of the urinoma was a high-grade ureteropelvic junction obstruction.

sonographic guidance (13,34). For maximal drainage, the needle should be placed into the chest through a posterolateral approach. A large (12 or 14 French) sump catheter or single lumen, large hole catheter is necessary in order to drain thick viscid material. If a sump catheter is used, however, the sump portion should be clamped to avoid air leakage.

Miscellaneous Drainage Procedures

Adnexal Cyst Aspiration

Concern about the effect of operative procedures on future fertility has led to interest in sonogram-guided cyst aspiration in young women. Indications for cyst aspiration are the following: (a) patient age, 15 to 40 years; (b) mean cyst diameter greater than 30 mm; (c) cyst present for longer than 2 months; and (d) previous

laparoscopy for benign disease. The procedure often requires general anesthesia when done percutaneously. Cervical block anesthesia is used for endovaginal sonogram-guided puncture. The optimal lesion for aspiration is the unilocular cyst without internal echoes. Approximately 85% of cysts resolve completely after percutaneous drainage.

Nephrostomy Tube Placement

The development of sonogram-guided catheter placement techniques has made percutaneous nephrostomy and antegrade pyelography common procedures, even in children (26). Indications for percutaneous nephrostomy include evaluation of level of obstruction, short-term decompression, and treatment of infected collecting systems (Fig. 7). The technique requires a posterolateral approach below the twelfth

FIG. 6. Abscess drainage. Patient presenting with right lower quadrant mass, fever, and lethargy. **A:** CT reveals a complex, predominantly low attenuation mass in the right iliopsoas muscle, thought to represent an abscess. **B:** Sonographic guidance was then used for aspiration and drainage. On the sonogram the needle tip appears as an echogenic dot within the parallel guidelines. **C:** Contrast injection through the needle opacifies a fluid-filled cavity tracking within the iliopsoas muscle. **D:** A single lumen, self-retention, 14 French pigtail catheter was subsequently placed into the abscess cavity for drainage. **E:** Follow-up radiograph after aspiration demonstrates nearly complete resolution of the fluid-filled cavity.

rib. A transparenchymal approach is preferred over a transpelvic approach because the tube is less likely to kink when the patient changes position; there is less risk of renal vascular injury; and there is less extravasation of contrast medium.

After sonographic localization of the upper pole of the kidney, a 21- or 22-gauge needle is advanced into the collecting system. Generally, contrast medium is injected through the needle to delineate the collecting system and to identify a posterior calyx for nephrostomy tube placement. Alternatively, contrast and room air (or carbon dioxide) can be injected and with the patient in a prone position, the gas will fill the posterior calyces and the contrast will fill the dependent anterior calyces. An 18-gauge needle is then placed in the posterior calyx and a .038-inch, J-tipped guide wire is advanced through the needle into the renal pelvis. The needle is removed and polyethylene fascial dilators are inserted to enlarge the track. Finally, a self-retaining pigtail (single lumen) catheter is threaded over the wire and into the collecting system. When the tip of the pigtail is within the renal pelvis, the guide wire is removed and the tube is securely fastened to the skin. Dependent drainage is then begun.

An alternative method of percutaneous nephrostomy involves catheter introduction systems designed to convert a 21-gauge needle tract into a nephrostomy tube tract (5,23). This is particularly advantageous in neonates in whom 18-gauge needles are contraindicated. A 0.018-inch guide wire is passed through a 21-gauge needle into the collecting system. The needle is removed and a tapered catheter or a coaxial catheter system is passed over the wire, dilating the tract and allowing passage of a 0.038-inch guide wire. The procedure is then completed in the standard fashion described above, with fascial dilators and eventual placement of the nephrostomy tube. An advantage of this system is that it obviates the need for an additional puncture if the initial puncture to opacify the upper collecting system fortuitously enters the kidney in a satisfactory position for tube placement. Additionally, the conversion technique reduces the risks associated with larger needle (18 gauge) punctures especially in newborns (6).

Percutaneous nephrostomy also may be used to treat obstructive uropathy in patients with renal allografts (25). Sonographic guidance is helpful to avoid puncture of perinephric fluid collections and adjacent bowel

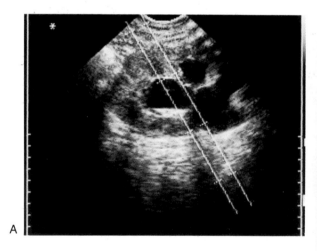

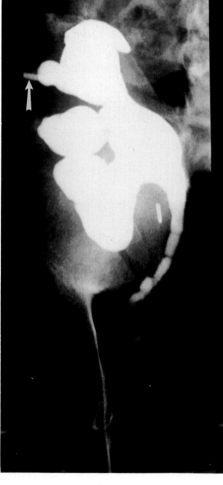

FIG. 8. Percutaneous nephrostomy and antegrade pyelography. Patient 3 months post-renal transplantation with a rising serum creatinine and hydronephrosis by diagnostic sonography. **A:** Sonography was used to guide nephrostomy tube placement into an anterior upper pole calyx. **B:** Contrast medium confirms positioning of an 8 French retention pigtail catheter (*arrow*) in an anterior calyx. Distal ureteral obstruction from a postoperative stricture was demonstrated to be the cause of the hydronephrosis.

loops (Fig. 8). In addition, sonography can help to identify an anterior calyx, which is the preferred location for nephrostomy placement in renal transplantation. This position minimizes damage to renal parenchyma and if percutaneous intervention is anticipated, it facilitates catheter manipulation within the ureter.

Percutaneous Gastrostomy

Percutaneous gastrostomy is a safe alternative to surgical gastrostomy and can be performed with local anesthesia. The most common indication in childhood is alimentation. Generally, percutaneous gastrostomy is performed best with fluoroscopic guidance. Fluoroscopy usually is sufficient to plan a safe access route for placement of a percutaneous gastrostomy or gastrojejunostomy tube (7,9,11,29,35,36). Sonographic guidance may be helpful in selected cases to avoid transhepatic catheter placement.

REFERENCES

1. Bernardino ME. Percutaneous biopsy. *AJR* 1984;142:41–45.
2. Bogan ML, Kopecky KK, Kraft JL, Holladay AO, Filo RS, Leapman SB, Thomalla JV. Needle biopsy of renal allografts: Comparison of two techniques. *Radiology* 1990;174:273–275.
3. Clark RA, Towbin R. Abscess drainage with CT and ultrasound guidance. *Radiol Clin North Am* 1983;21:445–459.
4. Committee on Drugs, Section on Anesthesiology, Guidelines for the elective use of conscious, deep sedation and general anesthesia in pediatric patients. *Pediatrics* 1985;76:317–321.
5. Cope C. Conversion from small (0.018 inch) to large (0.038 inch) guide wires in percutaneous drainage procedures. *AJR* 1982;138:170–171.
6. Cope C, Zeit RM. Pseudoaneurysms after nephrostomy. *AJR* 1982;139:255–261.
7. Cory DA, Fitzgerald JF, Cohen MD. Percutaneous nonendoscopic gastrostomy in children. *AJR* 1988;151:995–997.
8. Gerzof SG, Robbins AH, Johnson WC, Birkett DH, Nabseth DC. Percutaneous catheter drainage of abdominal abscesses. A five year experience. *N Engl J Med* 1981;305:653–657.
9. Halkier BK, Ho C-S, Yee ACN. Percutaneous feeding gastrostomy with the Seldinger technique: Review of 252 patients. *Radiology* 1989;171:359–362.
10. Heckmatt JZ, Dubowitz V. Ultrasound imaging and directed needle biopsy in the diagnosis of selective involvement in muscle disease. *J Child Neur* 1987;2:205–213.
11. Hicks ME, Surratt RS, Picus D, Marx MV, Lang EV. Fluoroscopically guided percutaneous gastrostomy and gastroenterostomy: Analysis of 158 consecutive cases *AJR* 1990;154:725–728.
12. Hirsch JH, Rogers JV, Mack LA. Real-time sonography of pleural opacities. *AJR* 1981;136:297–301.
13. Keller FS, Rosch J, Barker AF, Dotter CT. Percutaneous interventional catheter therapy for lesions of the chest and lungs. *Chest* 1982;81:407–412.
14. Lang EK, Springer RM, Glorioso LW, Cammarata CA. Abdominal abscess drainage under radiologic guidance: Causes of failure. *Radiology* 1986;159:329–336.
15. Liu P, Daneman A, Stringer DA, Ein SH. Percutaneous aspiration, drainage and biopsy in children. *J Ped Surg* 1989;24:865–866.
16. Livraghi T, Damascelli B, Lombardi C, Spagnoli I. Risk in fine-needle abdominal biopsy. *J Clin Ultrasound* 1983;11:77–81.
17. Marks WM, Filly RA, Callen PW. Real-time evaluation of pleural lesions: New observations regarding the probability of obtaining free fluid. *Radiology* 1982;142:163–164.
18. Mueller PR, vanSonnenberg E, Ferrucci JT. Percutaneous drainage of 250 abdominal abscesses and fluid collections. Part II: Current procedural concepts. *Radiology* 1984;151:343–347.
19. Pagani JJ. Biopsy of focal hepatic lesions. Comparison of 18 and 22 gauge needles. *Radiology* 1983;147:673–675.
20. Parker SH, Hopper KD, Yakes WF, Gibson MD, Owensbey JL, Carter TE. Image-directed percutaneous biopsies with a biopsy gun. *Radiology* 1989;171:663–669.
21. Picus D, Weyman PJ, Anderson DA. Interventional computed tomography. In: Lee JKT, ed. Computed Body Tomography with MR Correlation. New York: Raven Press, 1989;89–108.
22. Schnyder PA, Candardjis G, Anderegg A. Peritonitis after thin-needle aspiration biopsy of an abscess. *AJR* 1981;137:1271–1272.
23. Schwarz W. A new coaxial introducer system for percutaneous drainage. *AJR* 1985;144:1277–1278.
24. Schwerk WB, Schmitz-Moormann P. Ultrasonically guided fine-needle biopsies in neoplastic liver disease: Cytohistologic diagnoses and echo pattern of lesions. *Cancer* 1981;48:1469–1477.
25. Smith TP, Hunter DW, Letourneau JG, Cragg AH, Darcy MD, Castaneda-Zuniga WR, Amplatz K. Urinary obstruction in renal transplants: Diagnosis by antegrade pyelography and results of percutaneous treatment. *AJR* 1988;151:507–510.
26. Stanley P, Diament MJ. Pediatric percutaneous nephrostomy: Experience with 50 patients. *J Urol* 1986;135:1223–1226.
27. Strain JP, Harvey L, Foley C, Campbell JB. Intravenously administered pentobarbital sodium for sedation in pediatric CT. *Radiology* 1986;161:105–108.
28. Suen KC, Quenville NF. Fine needle aspiration biopsy of the thyroid gland: A study of 304 cases. *J Clin Pathol* 1983;36:1036–1045.
29. Towbin RB, Ball WS, Bissett GS. Percutaneous gastrostomy and percutaneous gastrojejunostomy in children: Antegrade approach. *Radiology* 1988;168:473–476.
30. Towbin RB, Strife JL. Percutaneous aspiration, drainage and biopsies in children. *Radiology* 1985;157:81–85.
31. vanSonnenberg E, Ferrucci JT, Mueller PR, Wittenberg J, Simeone JF. Percutaneous drainage of abscesses and fluid collections: Technique, results, and applications. *Radiology* 1982;142:1–10.
32. vanSonnenberg E, Mueller PR, Ferrucci JT. Percutaneous drainage of 250 abdominal abscesses and fluid collections. Part I: Results, failures, and complications. *Radiology* 1984;151:337–341.
33. vanSonnenberg E, Mueller PR, Ferrucci JT, Neff CC, Simeone JF, Wittenberg J. Sump catheter for percutaneous abscess and fluid drainage by trocar or Seldinger technique. *AJR* 1982;139:613–614.
34. vanSonnenberg E, Nakamoto SK, Mueller PR, Casola G, Neff CC, Friedman PJ, Ferrucci JT, Simeone JF. CT and ultrasound-guided catheter drainage of empyemas after chest-tube failure. *Radiology* 1984;151:349–353.
35. vanSonnenberg E, Wittich GR, Cabrera OA, Quinn SF, Casola G, Lee AA, Princenthal RA, Lyons JW. Percutaneous gastrostomy and gastroenterostomy: 2. Clinical experience. *AJR* 1986;146:581–586.
36. Wills JS, Oglesby JT. Percutaneous gastrostomy. *Radiology* 1988;167:41–43.
37. Yoshimoto M, Fujisawa S, Sudo M. Percutaneous renal biopsy well-visualized by orthogonal US application using linear scanning. *Clin Nephrol* 1988;30:106–110.
38. Zornoza J, Wallace S, Ordonez N, Lukeman J. Fine-needle aspiration biopsy of the liver. *AJR* 1980;134:331–334.

Subject Index